Clinical Neuroendocrinology

Contemporary Neurology Series:

Fred Plum, M.D. and Fletcher H. McDowell, M.D., *Editors-in-Chief*

Clinical Neuroendocrinology

JOSEPH B. MARTIN, M.D., Ph.D., F.R.C.P.(C.)

Professor of Neurology, Department of Neurology and Neurosurgery, McGill University; Neurologist-in-Chief, Montreal Neurological Institute and Royal Victoria Hospital; Senior Physician, Montreal General Hospital, Montreal

SEYMOUR REICHLIN, M.D., Ph.D.

Professor of Medicine, Tufts University School of Medicine; Chief, Endocrinology Division, New England Medical Center Hospital, Boston

GREGORY M. BROWN, M.D., Ph.D., F.R.C.P.(C.)

Professor, Department of Psychiatry, Faculty of Medicine, University of Toronto; Head, Neuroendocrinology Research Section, Clarke Institute of Psychiatry, Toronto

 F. A. DAVIS COMPANY, PHILADELPHIA

Library of Congress Cataloging in Publication Data

Martin, Joseph B.
    Clinical neuroendocrinology

    Includes bibliographies and index.
    1. Nervous system--Diseases. 2. Endocrine diseases. 3. Neuro-
endocrinology. I. Reichlin, Seymour, joint author. II. Brown,
Gregory C., joint author. III. Title.
RC361.M33   616.8   77-3601
ISBN 0-8036-5885-0

This book is dedicated to our wives.

Preface

The most conspicuous recent advances in neuroendocrinology have been the validation of the concept of neurosecretion and of the portal-vessel chemotransmitter hypothesis of anterior pituitary regulation, the demonstration of the role of biogenic amines as neurotransmitters in the control of the hypophysiotrophic neurons, and the chemical isolation and synthesis of three of the hypothalamic hormones. Neuroendocrinology has become an important and productive tool for the study and treatment of pituitary disease. New syndromes of isolated and combined hypophysiotrophic failure have been identified, and certain hypothalamic-pituitary diseases will likely be treated with synthetic hormones. One hypothalamic hormone, somatostatin, has been found outside the brain in gastric mucosa and pancreatic islet cells. Administration of somatostatin to man and animals inhibits secretion of gastrin, insulin, and glucagon, as well as growth hormone and TSH. This agent has already provided exciting new ideas about the pathogenesis and treatment of diabetes mellitus. The recent development of neuroendocrinology has paralleled the development of molecular biology and neuropharmacology so that many of the newer findings rest on a rigorous ultrastructural, biochemical, and neurophysiologic basis. A new and unanticipated dividend of current research is the observation that certain of the releasing hormones are distributed outside the hypothalamus and exert direct effects on brain function, thus raising the important possibility that they may be either true neurotransmitters, or that they modulate neurotransmitter actions. There is even some evidence for localized peptidergic neuron control systems unrelated to anterior pituitary function.

These advances have only partly made their way into the everyday analysis and management of a wide variety of clinical problems, some common, and some rare. Our purpose in writing this book is to summarize and integrate current knowledge of neuroendocrinology derived from laboratory and clinical investigation, and to apply it to the understanding of pathogenesis, diagnosis, and management of diseases of pituitary regulation and of the hypothalamus, and to disorders of brain function and behavior secondary to hormone disturbance.

JOSEPH B. MARTIN
SEYMOUR REICHLIN
GREGORY M. BROWN

Contents

PART I

BASIC NEUROENDOCRINOLOGY

CHAPTER 1

Neuroendocrine Transducers
and Neurosecretion

The central nervous system (CNS) controls the secretion of most glands, whether internal (endocrine) or external (exocrine). Exocrine glands (the secretory product of which leaves the gland by an external duct), for example, sweat, sebaceous, and salivary glands, are innervated by *secretomotor* postganglionic sympathetic or parasympathetic neurons. These end on the plasma membrane of the secretory cell, and the neurotransmitter substance, norepinephrine or acetylcholine, released at the neuroeffector synapse stimulates or inhibits secretion. Direct secretomotor control is far less important in the regulation of the glands of internal secretion, whose secretory products enter the blood stream and exert their effect at a more remote site. In fact, secretomotor control is of no importance for most endocrine glands (exceptions to this generalization occur and will be discussed later). Instead, neural control of the endocrine system is exerted through neurohumoral secretions arising either from specialized neurosecretory neurons or from secretory cells derived from nervous system elements. Once released, these secretions travel through the blood stream to act at a target site. The transformation of neural information to chemical control of secretion has been called *neuroendocrine transduction* by Axelrod[1] and by Wurtman and Anton-Tay.[19]

NEUROENDOCRINE TRANSDUCERS

Neuroendocrine transducers possess in common the capacity to change (transduce) neuronal (electric) signals into hormonally-mediated information (Table 1).[10, 11] Types of neuroendocrine transducer systems are shown in Figure 1. The adrenal medulla, the neurohypophysis, and the median eminence of the hypothalamus are three examples of neuroendocrine transducers.

The adrenal medulla, comprised of specialized chromaffin cells derived from the neural crest, is innervated by preganglionic sympathetic fibers which terminate directly on these specialized cells. Release of acetylcholine at the synapse causes the secretion of the catecholamines epinephrine and norepinephrine. This system illustrates the transducer concept: the input to the system is electric via transmitted action potentials in the axons of preganglionic sympathetic fibers; the outputs are blood-borne humoral agents which have widespread effects on specific receptor sites in various organs and tissues.

In the neurohypophysial system, supraoptic and paraventricular neurons give rise to axons which traverse the basal hypothalamus and pituitary stalk to end directly upon blood vessels in the neural lobe. Depolarization of these neurosecretory cells by acetyl-

Table 1. Neuroendocrine Transducer Systems

Neuroendocrine System	Hormones
1. Supraoptic-neurohypophysial Paraventricular-neurohypophysial	ADH Oxytocin
2. Tuberoinfundibular (tuberohypophysial)	Hypothalamic release and release-inhibiting hormones
3. Preganglionic cholinergic fibers— Adrenal medulla	Acetylcholine releases catecholamines
4. Postganglionic adrenergic fibers—Pineal gland	Norepinephrine releases melatonin
5. Postganglionic adrenergic fibers— Juxtaglomerular apparatus	Norepinephrine releases renin

choline released at synapses on the cell body leads to a propagated nerve action potential which ultimately causes release of stored hormones, antidiuretic hormone (ADH; vasopressin) and oxytocin.[7, 16, 17] These hormones rapidly diffuse into the blood and are transported to their appropriate target organs. In this instance the system's electric input via axonal impulses impinges on the neurohypophysial neurons, and the output is blood-borne hormones.

Hypothalamic regulation of the anterior pituitary is also achieved by a specialized transducer system.[17] Certain neurons of the medial basal hypothalamus are believed to synthesize and secrete specific hypothalamic *hypophysiotrophic* hormones (releasing factors) that stimulate (or inhibit) the secretion of anterior pituitary hormones. Axons of these hypothalamic hypophysiotrophic neurons terminate directly on the perivascular zone surrounding the capillaries of the median eminence, in a manner analogous to the interface between neurons and blood vessels in the posterior pituitary.[13] The hypophysiotrophic hormones enter the pituitary portal vessel system and are transported to the anterior pituitary trophic cells. Neural information is conveyed to the hypophysiotrophic cells by other cells in the CNS.

Several other examples of neuroendocrine transducers have recently been described. The pineal gland in the mammal, although attached by a stalk to the posterior-superior aspect of the diencephalon, contains no direct nerve fibers from the brain.[1, 19] Its innervation is derived circuitously from postganglionic adrenergic fibers which leave the superior cervical ganglia of the sympathetic chain, enter the cranium, and terminate with discrete synapse-like junctions upon parenchymal cells of the pineal gland (pinealocytes), which secrete melatonin (and perhaps other indoleamines) into the blood and/or cerebrospinal fluid. Release of norepinephrine from these neurons stimulates several of the enzymes involved in melatonin biosynthesis. Similarly, the juxtaglomerular apparatus of the kidney and the islets of Langerhans of the pancreas, both of which receive sympathetic innervation, can be considered as specialized types of neuroendocrine transducers.

NEUROSECRETION

Neurosecretory cells have a true dual function. They resemble typical neurons in their capability to be excited and to conduct action potentials; and on the other hand, they have the machinery to synthesize, transport, and release specific hormonal substances. In a sense, all neurons have a secretory function in that they release neuro-

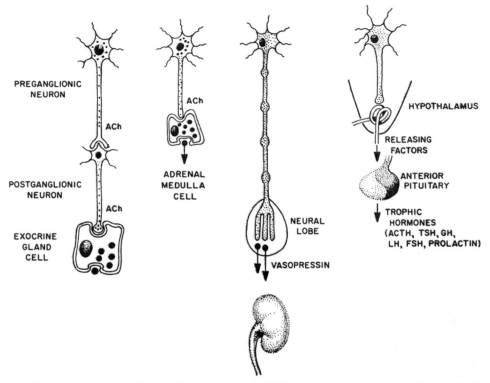

Figure 1. Types of neuroendocrine transducer systems. *Left,* Neurosecretomotor neurons. Postganglionic or preganglionic sympathetic fibers make direct synaptic contact with hormone-secreting cells. *Right,* Hypothalamic neurosecretory neurons. Neurosecretory neurons of the supraoptic system release ADH (vasopressin) into the systemic blood stream. Hypothalamic tuberoinfundibular neurons release hypophysiotrophic hormones (releasing factors) into the pituitary portal system to regulate secretion of hormones from the anterior pituitary. *Abbreviations:* ACh, acetylcholine; ACTH, adrenocorticotropin; TSH, thyroid-stimulating hormone (thyrotropin); GH, growth hormone (somatotropin); LH, luteinizing hormone; FSH, follicle-stimulating hormone.

transmitters into a synaptic cleft, but the neurosecretory cells differ in that their products have a true hormonal function: that is, they enter the circulation to affect remote structures.

The concept of a neuron serving as a specialized glandular secretory cell dates back to 1919 when Speidel,[18] working with the spinal cord of the fish, described giant neurons which had the appearance of secretory cells. Morphologically similar neurons were demonstrated in a variety of vertebrate and invertebrate species by Ernst and Berta Scharrer,[16, 17] who in 1940 showed that the axons of such cells as well as the perikarya (cell bodies) contain proteinaceous material with special staining characteristics. Subsequent research on the morphology and function of these systems has been vast.

Definition of Neurosecretion

The precise definition of neurosecretion has evolved through several stages over the years. In the mid-1950s, Knowles[11] introduced the term *neurohemal organ* to describe a neurosecretory cell system in which axons terminate directly upon blood vessels, distinguishing such cells from typical neurons that function to release chemical substances at localized synaptic regions. The cells formerly termed neurosecretory are truly *endo-*

5

crine, since their hormonal content is discharged directly into the blood — either into the general circulation, as in the neurohypophysis, or into a specialized local circulation, as in the case of the hypophysiotrophic neurons which release their hormones into the primary capillaries of the pituitary portal system.

Neurons that relay electric information from the nervous system to the endocrine system by synapse-like endings on a second cell were termed *neurosecretomotor* by Knowles and Bern.[11] Such synaptoid contacts occur in the corpora allata of insects, in the pars intermedia of vertebrates, and in the adrenal medullae and pineal glands. These neurosecretomotor cells resemble the postganglionic secretomotor cells that control certain exocrine structures such as the sweat glands. The postsynaptic cells that release the hormones are believed to be of CNS origin, being derived embryologically from the neural crest.

Neurosecretory neurons can thus be defined as specialized cells that provide an essential link between the nervous and endocrine systems. As such, they provide a final common pathway for endocrine regulation, and may be considered as analogous to the anterior horn cell which in the Sherringtonian view forms the final common pathway from the nervous system to the locomotor system. Electrophysiologic aspects of neurosecretory function have been extensively studied and are detailed in Chapters 2 and 4.

Synthesis and Transport of Neurosecretory Material

The cell bodies and axon processes of the supraoptic and paraventricular neurons stain intensely with specific stains that indicate the presence of a unique proteinaceous secretory product. Electron-microscopic studies have shown that the positive-staining material is membrane-bound in electron-dense granules with a diameter of 1,000 to 3,000 Å (Fig. 2).[2, 3, 13, 14] The active hormones have been localized within these neurosecretory granules by ultracentrifugation. The octapeptide hormones ADH and oxytocin are contained within the neurosecretory granules bound to a protein, neurophysin, that has a molecular weight of approximately 10,000 daltons.[7] The characteristic staining properties of this neurosecretory material are attributed to the high cysteine content of both the octapeptides and neurophysins.

The axons of the hypothalamic-neurohypophysial tract terminate in the posterior pituitary adjacent to capillaries, and are separated from them by a perivascular space and two basement membranes (see Fig. 2). Axonal swellings (Herring bodies, in the older literature),[4, 5] intra-axonal collections of packed neurosecretory granules, are found in the posterior pituitary and adjacent pituitary stalk. Interspersed between the axon terminals are specialized glial cells called pituicytes, the function of which is still unclear, although it has been postulated that they serve as scavengers in the degradation of products released from nerve endings.

The neurohormones are synthesized within the perikaryon of the neuron in the endoplasmic reticulum as part of a larger complex with neurophysin, and carried to the Golgi apparatus where they are packaged into granules.[9, 15] The evidence for transport of neurosecretory granules by axoplasmic flow down the axons to the neurohypophysis is convincing. Section of the hypothalamic-neurohypophysial tract results in distal depletion of stainable neurosecretory material with an accumulation proximal to the cut. Moreover, incorporation of labeled amino acids into ADH following administration of the label into the third ventricle occurs first in the hypothalamus and only later appears in the posterior pituitary;[15] section of the pituitary stalk prevents the appearance of labeled ADH in the neurohypophysis. In vitro incubation studies have shown that hypothalamic tissue can synthesize ADH de novo, whereas isolated neurohypo-

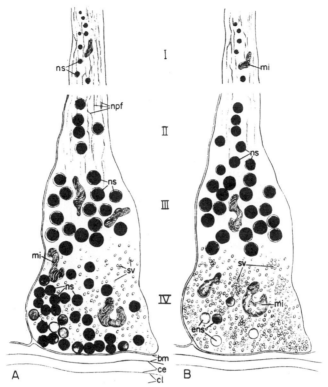

Figure 2. Diagram of electron photomicrograph of nerve terminals in neurohypophysis of the toad. *A*, Neurosecretory granules (ns) are shown as large electron-dense, membrane-bound structures. Small synaptic vesicles (sv) are also present. *B*, After dehydration and ADH release, there is depletion of neurosecretory granules and an increase in synaptic vesicles. The roman numerals refer to different portions of the axon from pituitary stalk to terminal in neurohypophysis. *Abbreviations:* bm, basement membrane; ce, capillary endothelium; cl, capillary lumen; mi, mitochondria; npf, neuroprotofibrils. (From Gerschenfeld H. M., et al.: *Ultrastructure and function in neurohypophysis of the toad.* Endocrinology 66:741, 1960, with permission.)

physial tissue cannot. Addition of protein-synthesis-inhibiting antibiotics, such as puromycin, prior to incubation prevents the incorporation of labeled amino acids into the polypeptide.

The discovery of an inherited form of diabetes insipidus in the Brattleboro strain of rats has provided a useful model for the study of hypothalamic production of polypeptide hormones. ADH is absent in the hypothalamus and neurohypophysis of such rats, while oxytocin can still be detected, indicating that the synthesis of the hormones is under separate genetic control. Such rats also have an abnormal neurophysin in hypothalamic-neurohypophysial tissue which suggests that the defect also includes a disturbance in synthesis of carrier protein.

Mechanisms of Hormonal Release from Neurosecretory Cells

Since the cells of the supraoptic and paraventricular nuclei are capable of generating and conducting axon potentials, it is reasonable to assume that depolarization of the axon terminals causes release of hormones.

Several questions arise concerning the sequence of events which lead to hormonal release. By what mechanism does depolarization of the axon terminal effect the rapid release of hormone from the cell into the perivascular space? Are the neurosecretory granules broken down within the cell and their products subsequently released from the cytoplasm, or are the granules released intact? Is the hormone present in a homogeneous pool within the terminals, or is there a free, readily releasable pool of hormone as well as a bound form?

Stimulus-Secretion-Coupling: The Calcium Hypothesis

In a series of elegant studies, Douglas and associates[6] clarified the sequence of events which transpire between depolarization and hormonal release. Using rat neurohypophyses, maintained in vitro, they were able to measure the rate of spontaneous hormonal release into the incubation media. Hormonal release increased following either electric stimulation or the addition of excess potassium ions into the media, both effects presumably resulting in depolarization of the terminals. (Actual measurement of transmembrane potential was not possible in this system, although the same workers did so in the chromaffin cells of the adrenal medulla.) Significantly, release of hormone occurred only in media containing calcium ions, and neither electric stimulation nor potassium addition increased hormonal release in the absence of calcium. Therefore, they postulated that the arrival of axon potentials at the axon terminals leads to depolarization. Increased membrane permeability during depolarization permits the influx of calcium ions into the cell and hormone release follows, a process that has been called stimulus-secretion-coupling by analogy with the stimulus-contraction-coupling mechanism of muscle. Measurements of ion flux with radioactive calcium 45 have confirmed that uptake of calcium does occur during depolarization of neural lobe terminals. The mechanism whereby calcium stimulates release is not known. The possibility has been suggested that calcium stimulates membrane phospholipases, with a resultant change in structure of the cell, or stimulates contraction of microtubules within the axon terminal (analogous to skeletal muscle) resulting in the approximation of the granule to the cell surface. The stabilization of the granule in contact with the cell surface is followed by a union of the opposing membranes and discharge of the granular contents.

This mechanism of release of cellular secretory products now appears to be fundamentally the same in all hormone-producing cells (Fig. 3). The final stage of hormonal release from intracellular granules appears to involve the union of granule membrane with the external cell membrane and the extrusion of the entire contents of the granule into the perivascular space. Recent electron-microscopic studies have been interpreted as showing morphologic evidence of such union of granule and cell membranes. If the contents of the granule were extruded as such, both neurophysin and the neural-lobe octapeptides would be discharged into the blood. After the recent development of radioimmunoassay methods, significant elevation of the carrier protein was detected in peripheral blood following either physiologic stimuli that are known to cause ADH release or electric stimulation of the supraoptic or paraventricular nuclei. The function, if any, of this release of neurophysin is unknown, since it does not appear to bind the octapeptides as a carrier protein in plasma.

Cholinergic Release

In addition to the neurosecretory granules found in the axon terminals of the neurohypophysis, small clear synaptic vesicles can also be identified by electron microscopy (see Fig. 2).[3, 14] Their appearance and size (300 to 500 Å) resemble vesicles which in other locations of the nervous system are known to contain acetylcholine. The posterior pituitary contains acetylcholine and true acetylcholinesterase is located in the

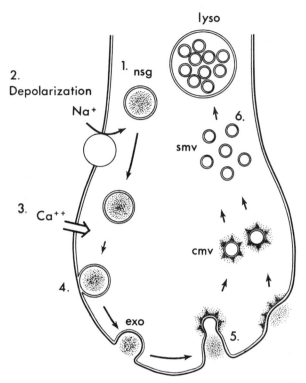

Figure 3. Diagram of neurohypophysial nerve terminal illustrating mechanisms of hormone secretion. The numbers show the sequential steps in transport and release of hormone and the recapture of granule membrane to form small synaptic vesicles. *1*, Neurosecretory granules, synthesized in the perikaryon of the cell are transported to the nerve terminal. *2*, Depolarization of the terminal is associated with Na^+ uptake. *3*, Depolarization triggers increased permeability to Ca^{++}. Uptake of Ca^{++} is essential to the secretory process. *4*, Membrane of neurosecretory granule fuses with external membrane of terminal. *5*, Entire contents of granule are extruded from the cell. *6*, The membrane of the empty vesicle is reincorporated into terminal to form synaptic vesicle. Lysosomes take up a portion of the empty vesicles and enzymatic degradation ensues. *Abbreviations:* nsg, neurosecretory granule; exo, exocytosis; cmv, coated microvesicles; smv, synaptic microvesicles; lyso, lysosomes. (Modified from Douglas, W. W.: *Mechanism of release of neurohypophisial hormone: stimulus-secretion coupling. In* Greep, R. O. and Astwood, E. B. (eds.): *Handbook of Physiology, Section 7: Endocrinology,* vol. 4, part 1. American Physiological Society. Williams & Wilkins, Baltimore, 1974, p. 211.)

neuronal cell bodies as well as throughout the entire axon of the hypothalamic-neurohypophysial tract. It has recently been demonstrated by combined biochemical and ultracentrifugation techniques that such small vesicles obtained from posterior pituitary actually do contain acetylcholine.[8]

The precise origin of the identified cholinergic vesicles is still in some doubt; some cholinergic neurons in the posterior pituitary may exist separate from those which contain ADH and oxytocin. Koelle[12] has made the interesting speculation that the arrival of the axon potential may first cause the terminal to release acetylcholine which then acts on its own cell membrane to cause release of peptide. Until recently, attempts to induce release of octapeptides by direct application of acetylcholine to the neurohypophysis in vivo were unsuccessful. Gosbee and Lederis[8] now indicate that acetylcholine is an effective stimulating substance.

An alternative explanation for the presence of the synaptic vesicles in neurosecretory axon terminals is that they represent fragmentation or breakdown components of neurosecretory granules, since they appear in increased numbers following physiologic stimuli associated with hormonal release.[6]

Releasable Pools of Hormone

Extensive studies by Sachs and associates[15] have shown that in the dog at least two storage pools of ADH can be identified, a readily releasable pool comprising 10 to 15 per cent of the total hormone content, and a more resistant pool comprising the remainder. Thus, an acute stimulus, such as hemorrhage, affects immediately only the first pool, allowing for more protracted hormonal secretion in situations that require it.

In summary, the supraoptic and paraventricular neurons serve as an excellent model in which to outline the concept of neuroendocrine transduction and neurosecretion. Although less well-documented experimentally, regulation of the anterior pituitary is believed to be similar, as will be described in Chapter 2.

REFERENCES

1. AXELROD, J.: *The pineal gland: a neurochemical transducer.* Science 184:1341, 1974.

2. BARER, R., HELLER, H. AND LEDERIS, K.: *The isolation, identification and properties of the hormonal granules of the neurohypophysis.* Proc. Roy. Soc. Lond., Ser. B 158:388, 1963.

3. BARER, R. AND LEDERIS, K.: *Ultrastructure of the rabbit neurohypophysis with special reference to the release of hormones.* Z. Zellforsch. Mikroskop. Anat. 75:201, 1966.

4. BODIAN, D.: *Herring bodies and neuro-apocrine secretion in the monkey. An electron microscopic study of the fate of the neurosecretory product.* Bull. Johns Hopkins Hosp. 118:282, 1966.

5. DELLMANN, H. D. AND RODRIGUEZ, E. M.: *Herring bodies; an electron microscopic study of local degeneration and regeneration of neurosecretory axons.* Z. Zellforsch. Mikroskop. Anat. 111:293, 1970.

6. DOUGLAS, W. W., NAGASAWA, J. AND SCHULTZ, R. A.: *Coated microvesicles in neurosecretory terminals of posterior pituitary glands shed their coats to become smooth "synaptic" vesicles.* Nature 232: 340, 1971.

7. DREIFUSS, J. J.: *A review on neurosecretory granules: their contents and mechanisms of release.* Ann. N.Y. Acad. Sci. 248:184, 1975.

8. GOSBEE, J. L. AND LEDERIS, K.: *In vivo release of antidiuretic hormone by direct application of acetylcholine or carbachol to the rat neurohypophysis.* Can. J. Physiol. Pharmacol. 50:618, 1972.

9. KNOWLES, F.: *Vesicle formation in the distal part of a neurosecretory system.* Proc. Roy. Soc. Lond., Ser. B 160:360, 1964.

10. KNOWLES, F.: *Neuronal properties of neurosecretory cells. In:* Stutinsky, F. (ed.): *Neurosecretion.* Springer-Verlag, Berlin, 1967, p. 8.

11. KNOWLES, F. AND BERN, H. A.: *The function of neurosecretion in endocrine regulation.* Nature 210: 271, 1966.

12. KOELLE, G. B.: *A proposed dual neurohumoral role of acetylcholine: its function at the pre- and post-synaptic sites.* Nature 190:208, 1961.

13. MONROE, B. G. AND SCOTT, D. E.: *Ultrastructural changes in the neural lobe of the hypophysis of the rat during lactation and suckling.* J. Ultrastruct. Res. 14:497, 1966.

14. RODRIGUEZ, E. M.: *Ulstrastructure of the neurohaemal region of the toad median eminence.* Z. Zellforsch. Mikroskop. Anat. 93:182, 1969.

15. SACHS, H., ET AL.: *Biosynthesis and release of vasopressin and neurophysin.* Recent Prog. Horm. Res. 25:447, 1969.

16. SCHARRER, B.: *The neurosecretory neuron in neuroendocrine regulatory mechanisms.* Am. Zoologist 7: 161, 1967.

17. SCHARRER, E.: *The final common path in neuroendocrine integration.* Arch. Anat. Microscop. Morphol. Exptl. 54:359, 1965.

18. SPEIDEL, C. C.: *Further comparative studies in other fishes of cells that are homologous to the large irregular glandular cells in the spinal cord of the skates.* J. Comp. Neurol. 34:303, 1922.

19. WURTMAN, R. J. AND ANTON-TAY, F.: *The mammalian pineal as a neuroendocrine transducer.* Recent Prog. Horm. Res. 25:493, 1969.

BIBLIOGRAPHY

BARGMANN, W.: *Neurosecretion.* Intern. Rev. Cytol. 19:183, 1966.

DOUGLAS, W. W.: *Mechanism of release of neurohypophysial hormones: stimulus-secretion coupling. In* Greep, R. O. and Astwood, E. B. (eds.): *Handbook of Physiology, Section 7: Endocrinology,* vol. 4, part 1. American Physiological Society. Williams & Wilkins, Baltimore, 1974, p. 191.

LEDERIS, K.: *Neurosecretion and the functional structure of the neurohypophysis. In* Greep, R. O. and Astwood. E. B. (eds.): *Handbook of Physiology, Section 7: Endocrinology,* vol. 4, part 1. American Physiological Society. Williams & Wilkins, Baltimore, 1974, p. 81.

SACHS, H.: *Neurosecretion. In* Lajtha, A. (ed.): *Handbook of Neurochemistry,* vol. 4. Plenum Press, New York, 1970, p. 373.

CHAPTER 2

Hypothalamic Control
of Anterior Pituitary Secretion

Early in the twentieth century, clinicians recognized that pituitary insufficiency could engender disease in the region of the hypothalamus, but were unable to resolve whether the effects were those of direct damage to the adjacent pituitary gland.[2, 12] On the basis of careful pathologic study, Erdheim[11] concluded that these changes could be caused by hypothalamic damage alone; and Aschner[3] in 1912 demonstrated that gonadal deficiency (now recognized as being due to gonadotropin failure) could be produced in dogs by hypothalamic lesions which spared the pituitary. Over the following four decades, many workers studied the effects of "denervation" of the pituitary by surgical section of the pituitary stalk, but the results were ambiguous and controversial. In a series of classic experiments, Harris and Jacobsohn[25] demonstrated the crucial role of the blood vessels of the stalk in this regulation. Stalk section in the rat caused loss of sexual function, which returned when the hypophysial-portal vessels regenerated. When a paper plate was inserted into the stalk section so as to prevent regeneration of the vessels, sexual function failed to return. In all animals, stalk section caused permanent destruction of neural connections. They also repeated and extended the earlier studies of Greep, who had shown that pituitaries transplanted to the pituitary fossa function normally, whereas pituitary transplants in other sites remained devoid of activity.[2] These observations showed that the pituitary fossa was a privileged site for the growth and function of the pituitary, and indicated that the crucial factor was the special blood supply from the hypothalamus. Some criticized the results of the Harris-Jacobsohn experiments as being due to damage to the pituitary caused by transplantation, but this reservation was resolved convincingly in the double-transplantation experiments of Nikitovitch-Winer and Everett,[38] who demonstrated in rats that the pituitary failure resulting from transplantation of the gland to the renal capsule was corrected by re-transplantation of the same pituitary to the region beneath the basal hypothalamus, if anatomic reconnection of the blood vessels occurred. Reconstitution of pituitary function did not occur in control experiments in which the pituitary was retransplanted to the temporal lobe (Fig. 1).

The local trophic function of the hypothalamus was also demonstrated in the early 1960s by transplantation of pituitary fragments directly into the hypothalamus. As reported independently by Halasz and coworkers[23] and by Knigge,[29] there is a region of the basal hypothalamus that contains trophic substances capable of maintaining the cellular structure and secretory function of the implants. The term *hypophysiotrophic area* was applied to this region (Fig. 2).

The hypophysial vessels themselves, now known to be the conduit of the hypotha-

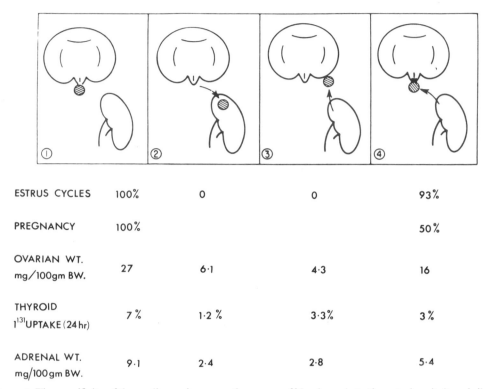

ESTRUS CYCLES	100%	0	0	93%
PREGNANCY	100%			50%
OVARIAN WT. mg/100gm BW.	27	6·1	4·3	16
THYROID I^{131}UPTAKE (24 hr)	7 %	1·2 %	3·3%	3 %
ADRENAL WT. mg/100gm BW.	9·1	2·4	2·8	5·4

Figure 1. The specificity of the median eminence as the source of blood supply to the anterior pituitary is illustrated in this diagrammatic representation of the work of Nikitovitch-Winer and Everett done in the rat. Pituitary tissue transplanted to the kidney and retransplanted to the median eminence, though twice insulted, could still restore toward normal the functions of gonads, thyroid, and adrenal glands. In other sites (kidney or temporal lobe of brain), transplants had virtually no function. (Modified from Bryson, M., and Reichlin, S.: *Neuroendocrine regulation of sexual function and growth.* Pediat. Clin. N. Amer. 13:423, 1966.)

lamic hypophysiotrophic hormones, were first described in 1930 by a Hungarian medical student, Popa,[39] following the lead given by his teacher, Ranier. The vessels were characterized by a peculiar group of coiled capillaries at the inferior extent of the hypothalamus that left the brain and joined to form long vessels that traversed the pituitary stalk. The blood in these vessels was incorrectly asserted by Popa, and his subsequent coworker Fielding,[39] to flow from the pituitary upwards to the base of the brain. In 1936, Wislocki and King[46] described similar vessels in the monkey and suggested on the basis of anatomic features that blood probably flowed from the hypothalamus to the pituitary. In 1947, Green and Harris[19, 20] confirmed this suggestion by direct observation in the rat that blood in the hypothalamic portal veins did indeed flow to the anterior pituitary, an observation which had been made previously in the toad by Houssay and coworkers.[27] Green and Harris proposed that the hypothalamus secretes into the portal capillaries of the median eminence specific pituitary-regulatory substances which are transported to the adenohypophysis by the portal vessels. This *portal vessel-chemotransmitter hypothesis* has continued to serve as the model for studies undertaken to clarify the details of this control.[24] A similar proposal was also made at about the same time by Friedgood[14] in a then unpublished lecture, and the earliest germs of this idea may be found in the writings of Hinsey and Marke a decade before.[2]

Vesalius, in *De Humani Corporis Fabrica* (1543) described the drainage of cerebro-

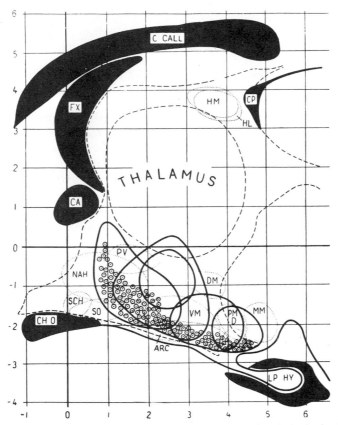

Figure 2. Diagram of hypophysiotrophic area of the hypothalamus. Anterior pituitaries implanted into various regions of the brain show morphologic differentiation and some trophic function. This observation indicates that there is a restricted area of the basal hypothalamus that functions to maintain pituitary cells. This area probably corresponds to the hypothalamic neurons that synthesize the hypothalamic hormones. ---------, Outline of third ventricle; ·········, hypothalamic nuclei; ———, borders of five midline pituitary grafts; ⊙, PAS-positive basophils; ARC, arcuate nucleus; CA, anterior commissure; C CALL, corpus callosum; CH O, optic chiasm, CP posterior commissure; DM, dorsomedial nucleus; FX, fornix; LP HY, posterior lobe of hypophysis, MM, medial mammillary nucleus; NAH, anterior hypophalamic nucleus; PM, pre-mammillary nucleus; PV, paraventricular nucleus; SCH, suprachiasmic nucleus; VM, ventromedial nucleus. (From Szentagothai, J., et al.: *Hypothalamic Control of the Anterior Pituitary.* Akademiai Kiado, Budapest, 1968, with permission.)

spinal fluid through the floor of the third ventricle (named *infundibulum* because of its resemblance to a funnel) into the pituitary and thence into the nose to form mucus *(pituita)* from which our modern term pituitary is derived. More recent studies indicating that certain hypophysiotrophic hormones may find their way to the anterior pituitary by way of the cerebrospinal fluid through the floor of the third ventricle and median eminence (see below) indicate how leisurely, at times, is the progress of scientific discovery.

Although the anterior pituitary gland lacks a direct nerve supply, the secretion of each of its hormones is under the control of the central nervous system. The pituitary and, in turn, its target glands respond to changes in the external and internal environments through specialized secretory neurons localized in the ventral hypothalamus. In addition, the neurohumoral connections of the anterior pituitary are important in the feedback regulations of a number of hormones, such as cortisol, the gonadal steroids, and thyroxine, and serve as part of the integrated mechanism by which behavior and metabolism are adapted to the external environment.

HYPOTHALAMIC NEUROSECRETION: HYPOPHYSIOTROPHIC NEURONS

Figure 3 shows the close anatomic relation of the pituitary gland to the hypothalamus. This relationship has both embryologic and functional significance. The anterior pituitary is derived from gut by an upward extension (Rathke's pouch) of the epithelium of the primitive mouth cavity (stomodeum). The neural or posterior lobe, however, develops as a downward evagination of the neural tube at the base of the hypothalamus, and, as such, represents a true extension of the brain. Neuroregulation of this structure is achieved by direct neuron connections.

Hormones of the Anterior Pituitary

The anterior lobe of the pituitary, or *adenohypophysis*, is divided into three parts: the *pars distalis* (the bulk of the gland, in man), the vestigial *pars intermedia,* and the *pars tuberalis* (Fig. 4). The last is an elongated collection of secretory cells that superficially envelop the pituitary stalk and extend upward as far as the basal hypothalmus.

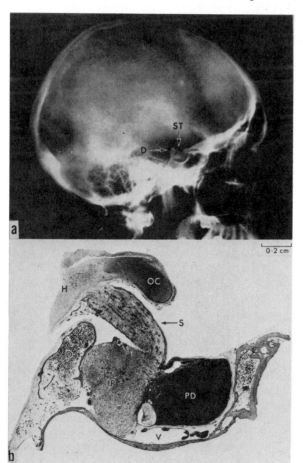

Figure 3. *a.* Lateral roentgenogram of the skull to show the sella turcica. ST, position of pituitary stalk; D, dorsum sella. *b,* Sagittal section of human pituitary and stalk (S) attached to hypothalamus (H). The pars intermedia is not shown. *Abbreviations:* OC, optic chiasm; IP, infundibular process or neurohypophysis; PD, pars distalis or adenohypophysis; D, dorsum sella. (From Daniel, P. M. and Pritchard, M. M. L.: *Studies of the hypothalamus and the pituitary gland.* Acta Endocrinol. Suppl. 201, 1975, with permission.)

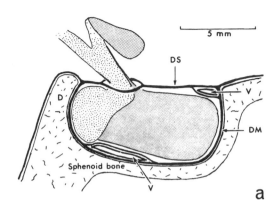

a

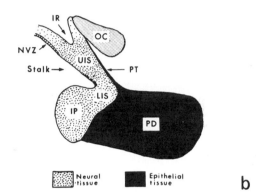

b

Figure 4. Diagram of human pituitary within sella turcica. The upper infundibular stalk (UIS), lower infundibular stalk (LIS) and infundibular process (IP) are all of neural origin. The pars distalis (PD) and pars tuberalis (PT) arise from epithelial tussue. *Abbreviations:* DS, diaphragma sella, V, veins; DM, dura mater lining sella turcica; IR, infundibular recess of third ventricle; NVZ, neurovascular zone of median eminence; OC, optic chiasm. (From Daniel, P. M. and Pritchard, M. M. L.: *Studies of the hypothalamus and the pituitary gland.* Acta Endocrinol. Suppl. 201, 1975, with permission.)

The pars distalis is a primary source of the six well-known pituitary hormones: thyrotropin (thyroid-stimulating hormone, TSH), adrenocorticotropin (ACTH), growth hormone (GH; somatotropin), luteinizing hormone (LH; interstitial-cell-stimulating hormone, ISCH), follicle-stimulating hormone (FSH), and prolactin (PRL; luteotropic hormone). In addition, melanocyte-stimulating hormone (MSH) appears to be produced in man primarily by cells of the pars distalis, rather than from the pars intermedia as in lower vertebrates. Several other active peptides have been extracted from anterior pituitary tissue whose physiologic functions have not been established. These include one or more lipolytic and lipotropic hormones and a factor that promotes cellular differentiation of fibroblasts. Since each cell type functions readily independent of the others, the adenohypophysis can be viewed as a complex of several glands, and it is not unlikely that the pituitary secretes other as yet unrecognized hormones.

With two known exceptions, morphologic and immunofluorescent evidence indicates that each adenohypophysial hormone is produced by a distinct and separate cell type. A proportion of gonadotrope cells secrete both LH and FSH, and most ACTH-secreting cells also secrete MSH or β-lipotropin. Simple staining methods such as hematoxylin and eosin or PAS-orange G are not adequate, however, to distinguish the specific secretory cell types. In the older literature, only three types of cells were described in the pars distalis, the acidophil (eosinophil), the basophil, and the chromophobe, named for their corresponding affinities to acidic, basic, or neutral dyes, respectively. More sophisticated staining methods reveal additional cell types.

The histochemical method developed by Ezrin and Murray has permitted identification of seven cell types in human pituitaries. Alpha cells (with staining affinity for orange G) correspond to the acidophil of the older classification, comprising approximately 50 per cent of

17

the cells within the gland, and secrete prolactin and GH. These cells tend to be regionalized to the posterolateral part of the gland. Five types of basophils (β_1, β_2, β_3 and δ_1, δ_2 cells) have been described. The β_1 and β_2 cells are associated with TSH and ACTH secretion, respectively. The δ_1 and δ_2 cells are thought to produce the gonadotropins LH and FSH. The β_3 cell has no known function, but may comprise part of the chromophobe cells, which according to this classification, are agranular cells with scanty cytoplasm that may represent a form of precursor or stem cell. A complete comparison of the various techniques for characterizing pituitary cell morphology is given by Baker.[4]

The use of peroxidase-labeled antibodies prepared against specific pituitary trophic hormones has further confirmed the separate identity of the different cell types of the adenohypophysis.[4] In addition, electron-microscopic studies have now clearly defined the structural characteristics of each cell type and its secretory granules. Such techniques have been widely used for the study of pituitary function in health and disease.

Functions of the Isolated Pituitary

As the hypothesis that the hypothalamus regulates the anterior pituitary was being developed, an important basis for it was the demonstration that separation of the pituitary from the hypothalamus resulted in significant morphologic and functional deterioration of the isolated pituitary. Structurally, interruption of the pituitary stalk is associated with degranulation of the anterior pituitary cells and loss of differential staining characteristics. The functional effects of stalk section vary with species, but as a general rule stalk section leads to hypopituitarism. This effect is not as severe as that following hypophysectomy; either some autonomous secretion of the pituitary remains in the absence of hypothalamic influence, or releasing hormones from the hypothalamus can reach the pituitary via the systemic circulation. The notable exception is prolactin secretion, which is enhanced after hypothalamus-pituitary disconnection. On the basis of modern hormone assay during disease in humans, it now appears that complete pituitary insufficiency can occur in hypothalamic failure; the so-called autonomous function of the isolated pituitary observed in experimental animals may be caused by blood-borne releasing factors (in the case of transplants and of stalk section), or may result from incomplete destruction (in the case of electrolytic lesions of the hypothalamus).

Pituitary infarction after stalk section or spontaneous disease of the stalk is a major component of the pituitary failure that follows gross stalk damage or postpartum pituitary necrosis. However, the finding that hypothalamic lesions can induce loss of specific pituitary functions in the complete absence of any vascular damage indicates that hypophysiotrophic hormone failure alone interferes with pituitary function, and that the vascular damage is but an additive and confounding factor.

Pituitary Hypophysial-Portal Blood Supply

The innervation of the anterior pituitary is remarkably sparse; the neurons present are probably exclusively of postganglionic sympathetic origin, and end predominantly on blood vessels. Hypothalamic control is obviously not simply neural. As outlined at the beginning of the chapter, the crucial regulating connection between the hypothalamus and anterior pituitary is by way of the hypophysial-portal vessels (Fig. 5).

The anatomy of the hypophysial system has been studied in detail in a number of species.[1, 9, 18, 40, 47] In man, the capillaries in the base of the hypothalamus are formed directly from branches of the superior hypophysial artery, which arises from the internal carotid prior to its entry into the subarachnoid space (see Fig. 5).[9] The blood supply

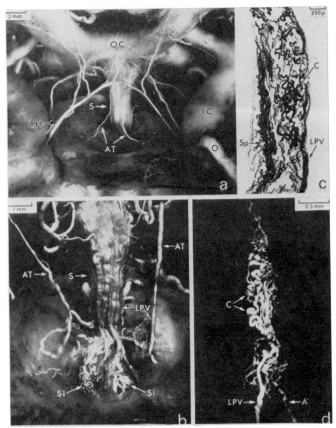

Figure 5. Pituitary portal vessels of human gland. *a,* View from above of superior hypophysial artery (SH), arising from internal carotid (IC). *Abbreviations:* OC, optic chiasm; S, stalk of pituitary; AT, artery of the trabecular; O, ophthalmic artery. *b,* Higher magnification of stalk vessels and long portal veins (LPV). *Abbreviation:* Si, sinusoidal capillaries in pituitary. *c,* Sagittal section of stalk-median eminence junction to show primary capillaries (C) and long portal veins (LPV). *Abbreviation:* Sp, short portal vessels. *d,* Cluster of capillaries and long portal vein. (From Daniel, P. M. and Pritchard, M. M. L.: *Studies of the hypothalamus and the pituitary gland.* Acta Endocrinol. Suppl. 201, 1975, with permission.)

to the posterior pituitary is largely separate, so that there is distinctly different regionalization of blood flow to the two portions of the gland. The average blood flow to the pars distalis, estimated to be 0.8 ml. per gram per minute, is the highest of any tissue identified in the mammal.

Blood flow to the pars distalis appears to be maintained at a relatively constant level under a variety of circumstances. Minimal changes in blood flow can be induced by pharmacologic doses of epinephrine, but it is unlikely that the sympathetic nervous system significantly affects the quantity of blood flow which reaches the pituitary. In the rat, for example, removal of both superior cervical ganglia does not affect pituitary blood flow.[18]

Hypophysiotrophic Hormones of the Hypothalamus

During the past thirty years an intense search has been carried out to identify the hormones of the hypothalamus that influence pituitary function.[6, 21, 44] Bioassays of various degrees of specificity and reliability have now demonstrated factors in hypothalamic extracts that stimulate the release of each of the known anterior pituitary hormones, and that inhibit the release of growth hormone, TSH, and prolactin. Thus, for the latter three hormones there may be a dual hypophysiotrophic control—both stimulatory and inhibitory. The hypophysiotrophic hormones have been named on the basis of their initially identified biologic activities (Table 1).

Three hypothalamic hormones have been identified structurally, their compositions proven by synthesis, and biologic effects in animals and man tested. The hormones were initially difficult to identify; they are present in extremely small concentration in animal tissue, early bioassays were relatively unreliable, and certain structural features are unique. Thyrotropin-releasing hormone (TRH), identified in 1969 by Schally[44] and by Guillemin[6, 21] and their respective collaborators, was the first of the hormones to be isolated. The second was luteinizing hormone-releasing hormone (LHRH), initially isolated in 1971 by Schally and collaborators,[44] and the third hormone to be chemically identified was somatostatin, reported in 1973 by Guillemin and collaborators. The chemical structures of these substances are shown in Figure 6, and their physiologic effects and other aspects are dealt with in subsequent sections. As far as is known, all of the hypothalamic hormones are small polypeptides, with the possible exception of PIF (prolactin release-inhibiting factor), which may be dopamine.

A tripeptide prolyl-leucyl-glycine amide which inhibits MSH secretion in the frog has been isolated from the hypothalamus and called MSH-inhibiting factor (MIF). This substance is identical to the terminal three amino acid residue of oxytocin and it

Table 1. Anterior Pituitary and Hypophysiotrophic Hormones

	Hypophysiotrophic Hormones	
Pituitary Hormone	*Name*	*Structure*
Thyrotropin (TSH)	Thyrotropin-releasing hormone (TRH)	Tripeptide
Adrenocorticotropin (ACTH)	Corticotropin-releasing factor (CRF)	Unknown
Luteinizing hormone (LH)	Luteinizing hormone-releasing hormone (LHRH) or	Decapeptide
Follicle stimulating hormone (FSH)	Gonadotropin-releasing hormone (GNRH)	
Growth hormone (GH)	Growth hormone-releasing factor (GRF)	Unknown
	Growth hormone release-inhibiting hormone* (somatostatin, GIH)	14 Amino acid peptide
Prolactin	Prolactin release-inhibiting factor (PIF)	Unknown
	Prolactin-releasing factor (PRF)†	Unknown
Melanocyte stimulating hormone (MSH)‡	MSH-inhibiting factor (MIF)	Tripeptide
	MSH-releasing factor (MRF)	Unknown

*Somatostatin also blocks TRH-stimulated TSH release.
†TRH stimulates prolactin release.
‡Recent work indicates that β-MSH may not exist as such in pituitary or blood but is in fact an artifactual breakdown product of the pituitary hormone β-lipotropin.

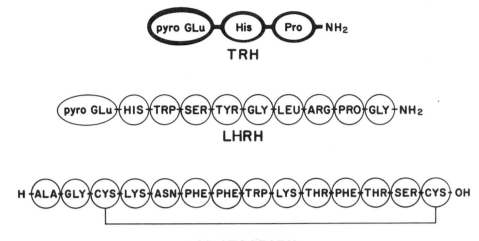

SOMATOSTATIN

Figure 6. Structures of the known hypothalamic hormones. *Top,* TRH (thyrotrophin releasing hormone). *Middle,* LHRH (luteinizing hormone-releasing hormone). *Bottom,* somatostatin (growth hormone release-inhibiting hormone).

has been proposed that the latter peptide may serve as a prohormone to MIF. The tripeptide has no effect on α- or β-MSH secretion in man, but a recent report has shown that large amounts of the substance are active in inhibition of GH secretion.

The availability of pure hypothalamic hormones has permitted the development of immunoassays and immunohistochemical studies, the demonstration of substantial amounts of releasing hormone in extrahypothalamic tissues, and extensive clinical trials. The use of synthetic hormones has clarified the question of specificity of the releasing factor. Certain of the factors may affect more than one pituitary function; for example, TRH causes release of both TSH and prolactin, somatostatin inhibits the secretion of GH and TSH, and LHRH releases both LH and FSH. In certain pathologic states, TRH can induce the secretion of GH and of ACTH.

On the basis of bioassays of crude extracts, there are potentially seven different releasing factors and three release-inhibiting factors, but the crossover effects noted above indicate that the number of hypothalamic hormones may be smaller, and that certain pituitary responses may be regulated by a specific secretory pattern of a more restricted number of hypothalamic hormones.

Tuberoinfundibular (Tuberohypophysial) System

Neurons of the medial basal hypothalamus which terminate directly on the capillaries of the portal vessels[5, 35] are called *tuberoinfundibular* or *tuberohypophysial*.* Because of their small size, they are often referred to as *parvicellular* neurons, to distinguish them from the large magnocellular neurons of the supraoptic and paraventricular system. The tuberohypophysial neurons are believed to synthesize, transport, and release the hypothalamic regulatory factors that control anterior pituitary hormone secretion. Hypothalamic-pituitary connections are shown in Figure 7.

---

*The terminology of the hypothalamic neurons that are believed to synthesize and secrete hormones for anterior pituitary regulation is confusing. In this text, the terms *tuberoinfundibular, tuberohypophysial* and *hypophysiotrophic* neurons are used interchangeably.

HYPOTHALAMIC-NEUROHYPOPHYSIAL
SYSTEM

HYPOTHALAMIC-ADENOHYPOPHYSIAL
SYSTEM

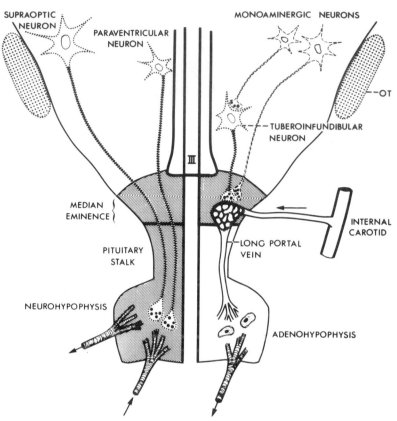

Figure 7. Diagram of the hypothalamic-pituitary axis in coronal section. *Left,* The hypothalamic-neurohypophysial system. Supraoptic and paraventricular axons terminate on blood vessels in the posterior pituitary (neurohypophysis). *Right,* The hypothalamic-adenohypophysial system. Tuberoinfundibular neurons, believed to be the source of the hypothalamic regulatory hormones, terminate on the capillary plexus in the median eminence. The pituitary portal system is derived from branches of the internal carotid which forms a primary capillary bed in the median eminence. The long portal veins drain the capillary plexus into the sinusoids of the anterior pituitary (adenohypophysis). Supraoptic, paraventricular, and tuberoinfundibular neurons are all classed as neurosecretory cells. The activity of tuberoinfundibular neurons is influenced by monoaminergic cells.

Structure of the Median Eminence

The anatomic arrangement of the basal hypothalamus is similar in members of the animal kingdom as remotely related as the frog and the primate. The term *median eminence* refers to a specialized area of the hypothalamus located beneath the inferior portion of the third ventricle. By gross inspection of the ventral surface, the median eminence is a small, highly vascular protrusion at the apex of the dome-shaped base of the hypothalamus, designated grossly as the tuber cinereum.[35, 45] The neural stalk of the neurohypophysis arises in the median eminence. The term *stalk-median eminence* (SME), widely used in neuroendocrinology, includes the median eminence and the upper part of the neural stalk; together these make up the contact zone between the endings of the hypophysiotrophic neurons and the capillaries of the hypophysial-portal

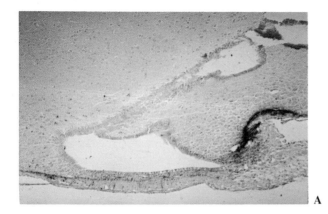

A

Figure 9. Distribution of LHRH and of somatostatin in the rodent hypothalamus as revealed by immunohistochemical methods.

A. Sagittal section of rat hypothalamus. LHRH demonstrated by the peroxidase technique of Sternberger. LHRH is found in cellular processes extending along the median eminence to terminate in the upper stalk. A large tract also enters the stalk from the mammillary region.

B. Frontal section at the level of median eminence in the rat. LHRH-containing cell processes are seen to sweep around the lateral walls to enter the contact zone of nerves and portal vessels in the median eminence.

C. Frontal section at level of the median eminence of the mouse. Higher power view shows LHRH-staining material in cellular processes oriented from ventricular lumen to external zone. The distribution at the light microscopic level does not distinguish between neuronal processes and tanycyte processes. However, electron microscopic work indicates that the bulk of the material is in nerve endings.

D. Beaded LHRH-containing nerve process in the anterior hypothalamus of the rat. It is believed that the localized swellings in the neuron are accumulations of secretory product. These are analogous to the Herring body of the supraoptic- and paraventricular-hypophysial pathway.

E. A somatostatin-containing cell body in the periventricular region of the anterior hypothalamus of the rat. Shown here are a large and a small cell containing material that reacts with antisomatostatin. These cells are believed to be the origin of the somatostatinergic pathway.

(Figure continues on next page.)

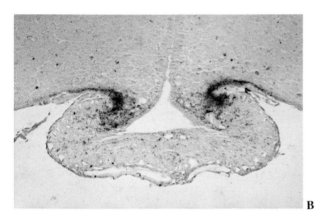

B

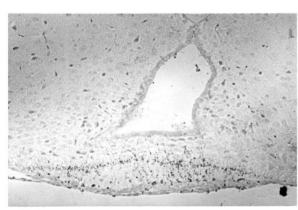

C

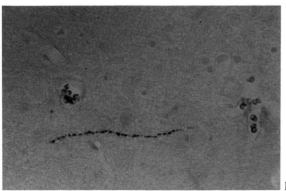

D

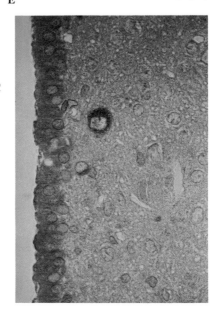

E

F

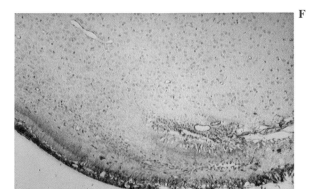

Figure 9. *Continued.*
F. Sagittal section showing distribution of somatostatin-containing neural processes. As shown here by the reddish stained material, somatostatin-containing processes are present in the base of the median eminence, somewhat deep to the superficial layer, but as the tract approaches the stalk itself, the neural processes descend ventrally to reach the region of the primary plexus of the hypophysial-portal vessels.

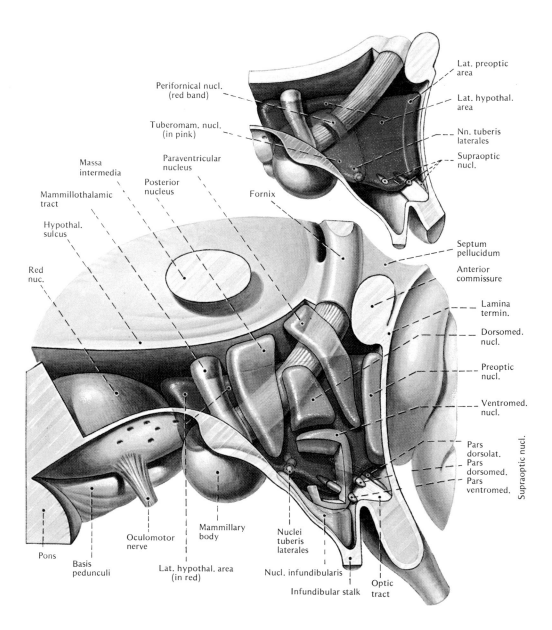

Perifornical nucl.
(red band)

Lat. preoptic
area

Lat. hypothal.
area

Tuberomam. nucl.
(in pink)

Nn. tuberis
laterales

Supraoptic
nucl.

Massa
intermedia

Paraventricular
nucleus

Posterior
nucleus

Fornix

Mammillothalamic
tract

Hypothal.
sulcus

Septum
pellucidum

Anterior
commissura

Red
nuc.

Lamina
termin.

Dorsomed.
nucl.

Preoptic
nucl.

Ventromed.
nucl.

Pars
dorsolat.
Pars
dorsomed.
Pars
ventromed.

Supraoptic nucl.

Pons

Basis
pedunculi

Oculomotor
nerve

Lat. hypothal. area
(in red)

Mammillary
body

Nuclei
tuberis
laterales

Nucl. infundibularis

Infundibular stalk

Optic
tract

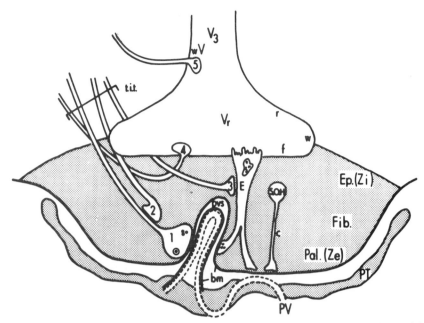

Figure 8. Schematic representation of basic structural arrangement and cellular composition of the median eminence. It is defined externally as that portion of the tuber cinereum in contact with the pars tuberalis (PT) of the anterior lobe and vascularized by the pituitary portal vessels (PV); internally it is demarcated by the wall (w) and floor (f) of the ventricular recess (V_r). The tissue between these two boundary planes constitutes the median eminence. No barrier exists between portal blood and the substance of the median eminence. It is generally organized into inner ependymal [Ep. (Zi)], middle fibrous (Fib.), and outer palisade [Pal. (Ze)] layers. The tuberoinfundibular tract (t.i.t.) constitutes the major afferent system; its terminals (1) abut in the palisade zone upon the perivascular space (pvs), may form axoaxonic contacts (2), make "synaptoid" contacts with ependymal cells (3), and also have terminals that protrude into the third ventricle (4). Ependyma (E) line the floor of the third ventricle and, in addition, extend processes that traverse the width of the median eminence to terminate on the portal perivascular space. The middle fibrous layer (Fib.) contains axons of the supraopticohypophysial tract (SOH) in transit to their termination of the neural lobe; some physiologic evidence, but no substantive morphologic data, suggests the possibility of collaterals (c) terminating in the palisade zone. (From Knigge, K. M.: *Anatomy of the endocrine hypothalamus. In* Greep, R. O. and Astwood, E. B. (eds.): *Handbook of Physiology, Section 7: Endocrinology,* vol. 4, part 1. American Physiological Society. Williams & Wilkins, Baltimore, 1974, p. 10, with permission.)

circulation. The median eminence and upper stalk have distinctive ependymal cells, capillary structures, and interstitial spaces, providing a functional definition in addition to the gross appearance (Fig. 8).

The blood supply to the median eminence has been calculated to be even greater than that of the pituitary. This region has a poorly developed blood-brain barrier.[31] Capillaries are fenestrated so that even relatively large molecules pass freely from blood into the perivascular spaces in the median eminence.[45]

The median eminence can be divided anatomically into three zones: 1) an inner

---

Figure 15. Diagram of dissected human brain, showing the major hypothalamic nuclei. Lateral to the fornix and the mammillothalamic tract is the lateral hypothalamic area *(in red),* in which the tuberomammillary nucleus *(in pink)* is situated. Situated rostrally in this area is the lateral preoptic nucleus. Surrounding the fornix is the perifornical nucleus *(represented as a red band),* which joins the lateral hypothalamic area with the posterior hypothalamic nucleus. The medially situated nuclei *(in yellow)* fill much of the region between the mammillothalamic tract and the lamina terminalis. The nuclei tuberis laterales *(in blue)* are situated at the base of the hypothalamus, mostly in the lateral hypothalamic area. The supraoptic nucleus *(in green)* consists of three parts. (From Haymaker, W., et al. (eds.): *The Hypothalamus.* Charles C Thomas, Springfield, 1969, with permission.)

ependymal zone, the lining of the inferior portion of the third ventricle; 2) an inner palisade layer that contains the hypothalamic-neurohypophysial neurons; and 3) an outer palisade layer, the zone of connection between the axons of the tuberohypophysial tract and the capillary loops of the portal plexus.[30] The capillary loops arise from the superior hypophysial arteries, which in turn originate from the internal carotids, and penetrate the surface of the median eminence to the region of the inner palisade layer. The outer zone of the median eminence is capped by a layer of anterior pituitary cells, the pars tuberalis. The function of these cells which lie in such close proximity to the median eminence is not known.

The axons which end on the portal capillaries appear to have their cells of origin largely along the outer inferior margin of the third ventricle. These groups of nuclei, which include the arcuate, anterior periventricular, and lateral tuberal groups, are composed of very small neurons, fusiform or triangular in shape.

The axons of these cells (forming the tuberohypophysial or tuberoinfundibular tract) can be traced inferiorly to the median eminence.[5, 9] As the axons descend through the median eminence, they criss-cross with the axons of the supraoptic and paraventricular-hypophysial tracts that are found in the deep portion of the median eminence clustered on either side of the midline.

The recent development of immunohistochemical techniques for the localization of hypothalamic hormones, utilizing antibodies developed against TRH, LHRH, and somatostatin, have confirmed and extended these observations. In several species of animals, TRH, LHRH, and somatostatin axons can be identified extending into the median eminence (Fig. 9, color plate, p. 23). It has now been demonstrated by the use of special methods, that LHRH-containing cell bodies are located as far anteriorly as the anterior septum of the hypothalamus and in the organum vasculosum of the lamina terminalis. A somewhat similar anterior hypothalamic somatostatinergic system has also been described.

ULTRASTRUCTURE OF THE MEDIAN EMINENCE. Electron-microscopic studies have contributed valuable information concerning the intimate relationships among various components of the median eminence. The outer palisade layer of the median eminence is composed of nerve endings and glial cells that are separated from the portal capillaries by a perivascular space. The structural arrangement closely parallels that in the neurohypophysis.[2, 9, 35] The fenestration of endothelial cells of the portal capillaries, unlike other brain capillaries, may partially explain the increased permeability of this region of the brain to substances like trypan blue. As in the neurohypophysis, the vessel lumen is separated from the perivascular space by a basement membrane, while a second basement membrane separates the axonal and glial endings from this space (Fig. 10).

On close examination of the axon terminals in the region of the portal vessels in mammals, both dense-core and synaptic types of granules can be identified.

The nature of the granular synaptic vesicles of the nerve terminals in the median eminence has not been fully resolved. Some contain catecholamines and others may contain releasing factors.[15, 16, 17] Certain of the intermediate size, dense-core vesicles resemble catecholamine-containing granules of the autonomic nervous system known to contain norepinephrine and dopamine. This is further indicated by the finding that nerve terminals stain intensely with formaldehyde vapor (Falck-Hillarp technique),[13] a method used to identify catecholamines and indolamines.[17] Many (perhaps 10 per cent) of the tuberohypophysial tract cell bodies, and a greater percentage of cell bodies of the arcuate nucleus, show catecholamine histofluorescence. With the possible exception of an effect on prolactin release, however, the biogenic amine nerve endings in the median eminence do not appear to alter anterior pituitary function directly, but rather regulate the release of the releasing factors. In the special case of prolactin secretion, dopamine, which has potent inhibitory effects on the pituitary, may act as a

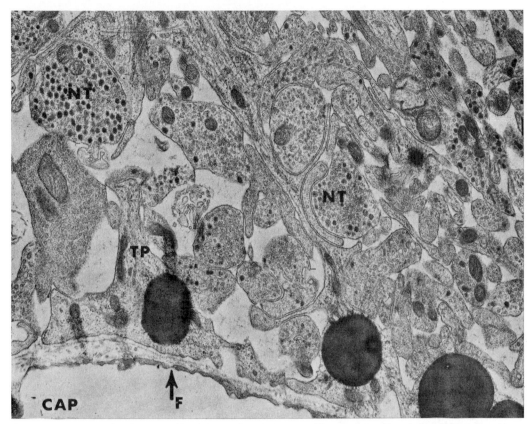

Figure 10. Electron photomicrograph of the median eminence of the rat. A capillary lumen (CAP) is evident in the lower left part of the figure. Fenestrations (F, arrow) of the capillary endothelium can be identified. The lipid droplets are contained in tanycyte processes (TP) which together with nerve terminals (NT) abut on the capillary. Dense core and "synaptic" vesicles are evident in the nerve terminals of neurosecretory neurons. These terminals are believed to contain the hypophysiotrophic hormones and the catecholamines norepinephrine and dopamine. (×18,000) (Courtesy of J. Brawer.)

prolactin release-inhibiting factor (PIF). There is evidence for a polypeptide PIF as well.

Other granules contain releasing factors. This has been shown for LHRH by differential centrifugation, and for LHRH and somatostatin by immunohistochemical study.

Conspicuously lacking from the outer zone of the median eminence are granules of the type associated with the supraoptic and paraventricular-hypophysial tracts, although these neurons pass through the inner zone. The neurohypophysis and median eminence, though occupying the same general anatomic area, may function independently, an interpretation supported by comparative anatomic studies of lower forms. Recently, however, immunohistochemical methods for study of neurophysin, a specific secretion of the neurohypophysis, have shown a striking distribution of neurons around the capillary loops of the primary portal plexus, indicating that neurons of the supraoptic and paraventricular-hypophysial tracts may also end in the median eminence. This finding, together with the demonstration of neurophysin and ADH in the portal vessels, has led to a reconsideration of the possible role of the neurohypophysial hormones in regulation of the anterior pituitary, and particularly of ACTH secretion.

The significance of the small vesicles of the median eminence is unknown; acetylcholine is present in significant amounts, but, as in the neurohypophysis, its function remains unclear.

Interspersed among the axons of the outer median eminence and also ending in intimate contact with the perivascular space are numerous glial and ependymal processes.[30, 45] The glial cells structurally resemble the pituicytes of the neurohypophysis. The ependymal processes are extensions that arise from ependymal cells lining the infundibular portion of the third ventricle (tanycytes).

The *inner palisade layer* of the median eminence is composed primarily of supraoptic and paraventricular neurons that traverse the zone anteroposteriorly to end in the infundibulum and neurohypophysis. These axons contain large (1500 Å) granules morphologically identical to those in the neurohypophysis.

The *inner ependymal zone* consists of the ependymal cells lining the third ventricle. The ependymal cells in this region of the ventricular system differ in several ways from typical ependymal cells (Fig. 11). The ventricular cell borders of these cells do not contain cilia, which is characteristic of ependyma elsewhere, but rather elongated pinocytotic apical processes that extend into the third ventricle lumen.[30, 31] Enlongated basal processes (hence the name *tanycytes*) extend throughout the entire thickness of the median eminence from the ventricle to the primary portal capillary plexus. These cells also contain vacuoles and vesicles.

Another unique anatomic finding of the ependymal cells of the third ventricle in the region of the median eminence is the presence of "tight" junctions between adjacent cells, which form a physical barrier to the movement of particles from the cerebrospinal fluid into the median eminence.[45] Since the tight junctions appear to prevent the passage of large molecules between cells (as shown by studies using horseradish peroxidase), the finding that hormones and ions placed into the third ventricle are transported to the

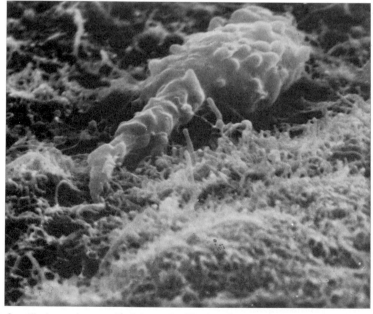

Figure 11. Scanning electron micrograph of the wall of the third ventricle in the region of the arcuate nucleus in the rat. This surface is comprised of tanycyte apices that exhibit profusions of microvilli and other surface irregularities. The large mace-shaped body lying on the tanycyte surface is a supraependymal cell characteristic of a variety commonly seen within the third ventricle. This micrograph is of tissue taken from a sexually mature, normally cycling female rat in proestrus. (×5,000) (Courtesy of J. Brawer.)

primary plexus has been interpreted to mean that transport has been via tanycyte cells. In fact, tanycytes have been shown to take up thyroxine in vitro against a concentration gradient by an energy-dependent concentrating mechanism. This property of the tanycyte has been invoked by Knigge and collaborators[31] (among others) as the basis of the transventricular transport of releasing factors for the control of pituitary function. Recently it has been reported that only some of the junctions between tanycytes are "tight," and that horseradish peroxidase can diffuse from the third ventricle through the median eminence.

Electrophysiologic Characteristics of the Tuberohypophysial System

By analogy to the supraoptic and paraventricular neurohypophysial system, it has been assumed that the smaller tuberohypophysial system also is neurosecretory, but because it is so much smaller, precise documentation of such function has been difficult. Recent electrophysiologic studies in the rat, combining antidromic stimulation (of the median eminence) with unit recording from the medial basal hypothalamus, indicate that tuberohypophysial neurons are located throughout the classic hypophysiotrophic area,[8, 10, 36, 42] including the periventricular region and the arcuate and ventromedial nuclei (Fig. 12).

These studies have localized tuberoinfundibular neurons that are thought to resemble those referred to in the anatomic and neuroendocrine literature as tuberoinfundibular or tuberohypophysial neurons. Electric stimulation of the median eminence produces antidromic invasion of tuberoinfundibular neurons; such stimulation also activates powerful recurrent inhibitory mechanisms which effectively silence spontaneously active tuberoinfundibular neurons for periods of 100–150 msec. The latency and duration of the inhibitory period are characteristic of a trans-synaptic response. Inhibition is also observed in tuberoinfundibular neurons whose excitability is enhanced postsynaptically by the microiontophoretic application of L-glutamate. The pathway(s) for postsynaptic recurrent inhibition may be either directly onto the cells of origin or through an inhibitory interneuron positioned in the recurrent pathway. According to Dale's principle, peptide released into the portal circulation should also be released at central connections of tuberoinfundibular neurons.

Electrophysiologic evidence from the studies of Renaud and Martin[42] suggests that other axon collaterals also exist in the tuberoinfundibular system. Terminal axonal branching of tuberoinfundibular neurons can be inferred from observations that some tuberoinfundibular neurons show antidromic invasion from more than one site within the hypothalamus (i.e., the anterior hypothalamic area and the paraventricular nucleus). Evidently, tuberoinfundib-

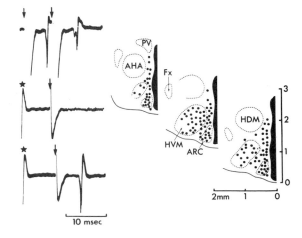

Figure 12. Distribution of cell bodies of antidromically-identified tuberoinfundibular cells. Neurons, shown by black dots, extend throughout the ventromedial (HVM) and arcuate (ARC) nuclei and the periventricular region. The third ventricle is shown in black. On the left, three oscilloscope sweeps illustrate the criteria for antidromic invasion utilized during this study. *Abbreviations:* AHA, anterior hypothalamic area; Fx, fornix; HDM, dorsomedial hypothalamic nucleus; PV, paraventricular nucleus. (From Renaud, L. P.: *Tuberoinfundibular neurons in the basomedial hypothalamus of the rat: Electrophysiological evidence for axon collaterals to hypothalamic and extrahypothalamic areas.* Brain Res. 105:59, 1976, with permission.)

ular cells establish connections at several local hypothalamic sites, in addition to terminations on the portal vessels.

Mechanism of Action of Hypophysiotrophic Hormones on the Anterior Pituitary

The hypothalamic regulatory factors appear to be authentic trophic hormones to the anterior pituitary. Not only do they stimulate almost-immediate release of preformed hormone, but they also stimulate the synthesis of new hormone and bring about the differentiation of specific pituitary cell types. Prolactin release-inhibiting factor (PIF) and somatostatin directly inhibit all functions of their target cells, acting on the pituitary in the same way that most peptide hormones act on their respective target tissues. The releasing factor is bound to specific receptor sites on the plasma membrane of the cell, which then activates membrane-bound adenyl cyclase, an enzyme which generates cyclic 3′,5′-adenosine monophosphate (cyclic AMP), the "second messenger of hormone action."[6, 44] Cyclic AMP in turn stimulates a cascade of cellular events which lead to activation of cellular enzymes, stimulation of the release process, and stimulation of new protein formation (Fig. 13). Crucial to the release process in the anterior pituitary (as in other endocrine organs) is the translocation of preformed product in secretory granules to the plasma membrane, fusion of the granular membrane with the plasma membrane, and the ejection of the product by reverse pinocytosis (emiocytosis, exocytosis) (Fig. 14). The active translocation process is believed to involve the contraction of cellular filamentous processes (microtubules) which, like actin in muscle cells, are contracted in the presence of adenosine triphosphate (ATP), one of the intracellular products of cyclic AMP, and by calcium ions.

A proposed alternative or additional mechanism of activation of secretion is by depolarization of the cell membrane, as has been observed in the adrenal medulla and posterior pituitary (stimulation-secretion-hypothesis). This view is given credence by the finding that potassium ions activate secretion, a response requiring calcium ions. How-

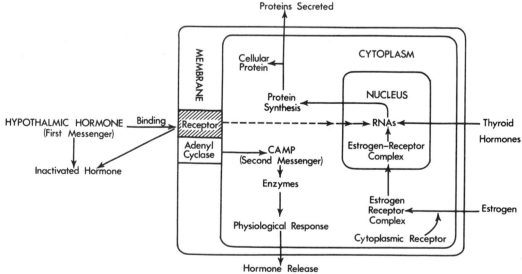

Figure 13. Diagrammatic representation of hypothalamic-hormone action. Binding to specific membrane receptors activates the enzyme adenyl cyclase which stimulates formation of cyclic AMP (CAMP). CAMP acts on intracellular enzymes to stimulate physiologic responses including hormone release. Peripheral hormones such as estrogen and thyroxine act on nuclear RNA to stimulate new protein synthesis. These feedback effects can alter subsequent responses of the cell to hypothalamic hormones.

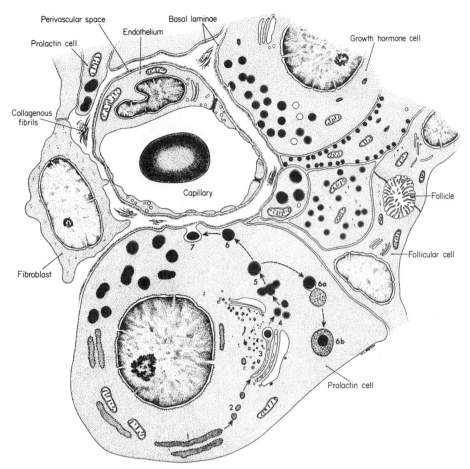

Figure 14. Diagram showing ultrastructural relationship of secretory cells to a capillary in rat anterior pituitary. Lower prolactin cell illustrates the steps in the secretory process. *1*, Synthesis of polypeptides in endoplasmic reticulum. *2*, Transport of polypeptide to Golgi system. *3*, Condensation into granules in Golgi apparatus. *4*, Liberation of membrane-enclosed granules from Golgi. *5*, Coalescence of granules. *6*, Movement of granules to peripheral plasmalemma. *7*, Extrusion of granule by exocytosis. Intracellular disposal of secretion in lysosomes is shown by *6a* and *6b*. (From Baker, B. L.: *Functional cytology of the hypophysial pars distalis and pars intermedia.* In Greep, R. O. and Astwood, E. B. (eds.): *Handbook of Physiology, Section 7: Endocrinology,* vol. 4, part 1. American Physiological Society. Williams & Wilkins, Baltimore, 1974, with permission.)

ever, direct proof that the releasing factors themselves act by depolarization has not been established. A number of ions such as zinc, nickel, and copper, as well as ammonium, can cause release of pituitary hormone in vitro. Although the metallic ions probably do not play a role in physiologic regulation, their presence in hypothalamic extracts is a potential artifact in the experimental study of pituitary control using incubation systems.

Although it was initially thought that the releasing factors were entirely specific, recent evidence indicates that there may be certain crossover effects with individual hypothalamic hormones. Systemic administration of TRH is not accompanied by any measurable release of GH, ACTH, FSH, or LH in normal individuals,[44] but TRH is a potent stimulus for prolactin release, and may also function physiologically as a prolactin-releasing factor. In addition, it has recently been reported that TRH releases GH in acromegalics and in isolated pituitary perfusion systems. Moreover, somatostatin, which inhibits GH release, has also been shown to inhibit TRH-stimulated TSH release without affecting TRH-induced prolactin release. Somatostatin also has been shown to have effects on other hormone-secreting tissues, such as the gut and pancreas. These observations, which indicate more widespread effects of the hypothalamic hormones, have increased the complexity of our understanding of hypothalamic-pituitary control functions.

HYPOTHALAMIC AND EXTRAHYPOTHALAMIC REGULATION OF THE HYPOTHALAMIC-ADENOHYPOPHYSIAL SYSTEM

Hypothalamus

In a true Sherringtonian sense, the neurosecretory neurons of the medial basal hypothalamus form a final common pathway for neuroendocrine regulation.[22] Inputs from other regions of the hypothalamus and ascending and descending tracts from other brain regions converge upon these neurons to subserve neuroendocrine reponses.[41] It has been suggested that certain neuroendocrine reflexes are mediated over quite specific and well-defined anatomic pathways. As an example, suckling stimulates breast receptors that signal via segmental nerves to the spinal cord, where impulses ascend to the midbrain and reach the hypothalamus via the medial forebrain bundle or the dorsal longitudinal bundle of Schütz where inputs to the paraventricular nuclei stimulate oxytocin release, and other connections to arcuate and/or anterior periventricular neurons effect prolactin release. This section reviews certain aspects of hypothalamic anatomy and the important afferent and efferent connections which probably comprise the connecting links for subserving various neuroendocrine responses.

Anatomy of the Hypothalamus

The hypothalamus can be divided both functionally and anatomically into *medial* and *lateral* portions, separated throughout a considerable portion of its length by the descending columns of the fornix (Fig. 15, color plate, p. 24). The medial hypothalamus contains the bulk of neuronal cell bodies controlling pituitary function, as well as important receptors of visceral functions; whereas the lateral hypothalamus is part of a multineuronal, multisynaptic system connecting the limbic forebrain with the mesencephalon. Anteriorly, the ill-defined anterior hypothalamic area blends without clear separation into the preoptic area. The latter is often considered not to be part of the hypothalamus, but its developmental origin and function are closely related to the hypothalamus, especially in regulation of body temperature, sex function, thyroid activity, and GH secretion. The posterior hypothalamic region joins directly with the reticular formation of the rostral midbrain. Dorsally, the hypothalamus merges with the thalamus, without clear demarcation except for the hypothalamic sulcus visible in the wall of the third ventricle. The major nuclei of the hypothalamus are listed in Table 2.

With the exception of the olfactory radiation to the hypothalamus by way of the medial forebrain bundle, the hypothalamus receives few if any direct connections from generally recognized sensory pathways. Its most massive associations are with the limbic forebrain structures and the paramedial region of the mesencephalon.[34] In addition to the pituitary-control system, the hypothalamus affects visceral motor function (i.e., parasympathetic and sympathetic outflow) by pathways through the reticular formation of the mesencephalon and lower brain stem.

In terms of neuroendocrine regulation these various anatomic pathways are impor-

Table 2. Major Hypothalamic Nuclei

Periventricular Zone	Medial Zone	Lateral Zone
Suprachiasmatic	Medial preoptic	Lateral preoptic
Paraventricular	Anterior hypothalamic	Supraoptic
Infundibular (arcuate)	Ventromedial	Lateral hypothalamic
	Dorsomedial	Mamillary
	Premammillary	
	Posterior hypothalamic	

tant for mediation of circadian rhythms in hormonal secretion and for integration of neuroendocrine and autonomic homeostatic responses. These structures also serve as the neural substrate for the perception and manifestation of drive states, and of emotion.

It has been far easier to determine how the hypothalamus regulates endocrine secretion than how it acts to integrate these complex regulatory and behavioral activities. Even in the sphere of endocrine control, certain anatomic peculiarities of the hypothalamus have made its study difficult, since functions are not readily assigned to circumscribed areas. The bulk of axons are unmyelinated and exceedingly small. They do not take classic stains well, and, as recently shown by Raisman and Field,[41] they appear to have unusual patterns of degeneration following section of tracts. With the exception of the paraventricular and supraoptic nuclei, characterized by large, easily-stained cells (magnocellular nuclei), the other nuclear groupings in the hypothalamus are much less distinct (parvicellular systems). Most of the hypothalamus is a matrix of interlaced neurons making up a true reticular formation, functionally, pharmacologically, and biochemically quite distinct, but anatomically largely coextensive.

Anatomic Localization of Releasing Hormones

Based on the pituitary microimplantation studies of Halasz and coworkers[23] and Knigge,[29] it appears that the cell bodies of origin of the releasing hormones and their axons lie in a crescentic zone on each size of the lower part of the ventricle (hypophysiotrophic area) and extend into the medial basal hypothalamus. This region is co-extensive with several of the named nuclei of the hypothalamus. Though difficult to demonstrate in some cases, certain general regions appear to form nuclei (see Table 2). The bulk of neurons which enter the tuberohypophysial tract (most are peptidergic and some dopaminergic) appear to arise in the arcuate nucleus, an elongated tract lying on either side of the lowermost portion of the lateral walls of the third ventricle. From this nucleus, the tuberohypophysial neurons sweep around the lower part of the third ventricle and enter the median eminence of the hypothalamus.

Electrophysiologic studies and microanatomic dissections of hypothalamic nuclei indicate that identified tuberoinfundibular neurons (see Fig. 12) are distributed throughout the entire medial basal hypothalamus.[43] Studies of the localization of the known hypothalamic regulatory hormones by microdissection and radioimmunoassay also have shown a widespread distribution (Fig. 16). These recent findings indicate that early functional descriptions of the hypophysiotrophic area were reliable indicators of the extent and distribution of the releasing hormones.

Other nuclear regions that probably also give rise to fibers ending in the median eminence include the suprachiasmatic nucleus, the preoptic area, and the dorsomedial nucleus.

It is inaccurate to ascribe specific functions to named nuclear groups of the hypothal-

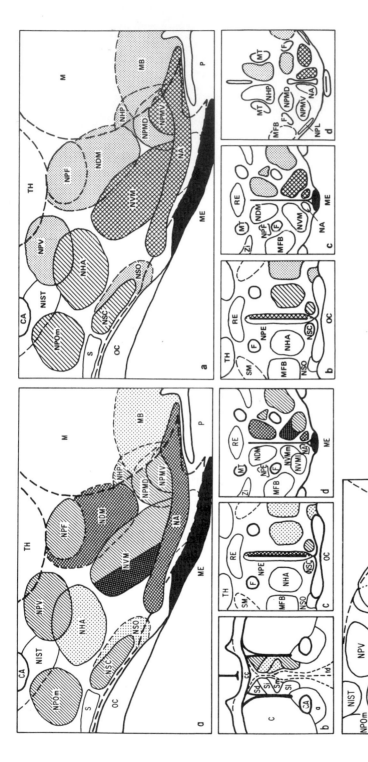

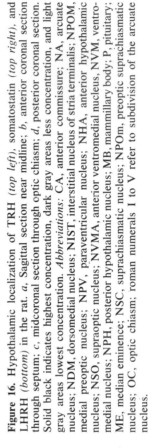

Figure 16. Hypothalamic localization of TRH *(top left)*, somatostatin *(top right)*, and LHRH *(bottom)* in the rat. *a*, Sagittal section near midline; *b*, anterior coronal section through septum; *c*, midcoronal section through optic chiasm; *d*, posterior coronal section. Solid black indicates highest concentration, dark gray areas less concentration, and light gray areas lowest concentration. *Abbreviations: CA*, anterior commissure; NA, arcuate nucleus; NDM, dorsomedial nucleus; NIST, interstitial nucleus of stria terminalis; NPOM, medial preoptic nucleus; NPV, paraventricular nucleus; NHA, anterior hypothalamic nucleus; NSO, supraoptic nucleus; NVMA, anterior ventromedial nucleus, NVM, ventromedial nucleus; NPH, posterior hypothalamic nucleus; MB, mammillary body; P, pituitary; ME, median eminence; NSC, suprachiasmatic nucleus; NPOm, preoptic suprachiasmatic nucleus; OC, optic chiasm; roman numerals I to V refer to subdivision of the arcuate nucleus.

(Top left figure from Brownstein, M., et al.: Thyrotropin-releasing hormone in specific nuclei of rat brain. Science 185:267, 1974, with permission. Top right figure from Brownstein, M., et al.: The regional distribution of somatostatin in rat brain. Endocrinology 96:1460, 1975, with permission. Bottom figure from Palkovits, M., et al.: Luteinizing hormone-releasing hormone (LH-RH) content of the hypothalamic nuclei in the rat. Endocrinology 95:557, 1974, with permission.)

amus; functions of a given region often extend beyond the anatomic margins of the nucleus. For example, the ventromedial nuclei in the mid-hypothalamus, on either side of the median eminence, dorsolateral to the arcuate, appear to be a major area of control of GH and insulin secretion, and in addition have a glucoreceptor function which is involved in the regulation of food intake. Because of its crucial role in determining the intake of nutrients and hormonal control of metabolism, the ventromedial nucleus has been regarded as important in integrating metabolic homeostatis. However, recent studies have suggested that glucoreceptors also exist in the lateral hypothalamus, and clear separation of ventromedial function from lateral hypothalamic function is not always possible.

The other named nuclei of the medial hypothalamus, i.e., dorsomedial and anterior, have no clearly-defined, specific function. The mammillary nuclei, properly part of the hypothalamus, although they have major anatomic connections with the "visceral brain,"[32] are, surprisingly, without known influence on endocrine function. Both anterior-posterior and lateral intrahypothalamic neural connections have been described which appear to link certain regions of the hypothalamus. These have not been completely defined in any species, and have been difficult to study because extensive descending and ascending pathways enter the hypothalamus from other parts of the brain. Connections of the hypothalamus with extrahypothalamic structures, however, have received intensive study.

Monoaminergic Regulation of Hypophysiotrophic Neurons

Certain biogenic amines (in particular, norepinepherine, dopamine, and serotonin) appear to play a crucial role in modulating the secretion of anterior pituitary trophic hormones, although they generally do not act directly on the pituitary itself.[17, 33] The monoamines appear to function in anterior pituitary control by their action at a hypothalamic level on the hypophysiotrophic neurons to modulate the release of releasing hormone. This view has taken some time to reach its present form, depending as it did on the development of histochemical methods for demonstration of monoamines by Falck and associates,[13] and of modern neuropharmacologic techniques for measuring biogenic-amine synthesis and degradation.

The majority of monoaminergic neural cell bodies which synthesize the biogenic amines are located in the mesencephalon and lower brain stem[17] (Fig. 17). Their axons ascend in the medial forebrain bundle to terminate in various forebrain structures including the hypothalamus, striatum, hippocampus, amygdala, and cortex. Dopaminergic inputs to the prosencephalon arise primarily from cell bodies in the substantia nigra, and serotonergic fibers arise from cells in the mesencephalic and pontine raphe nuclei. Central noradrenergic neurons arise principally in the locus ceruleus. The concentration of the monoamines in the axon terminals of these fiber systems accounts for the high concentrations of these substances in certain specific brain regions. Within the hypothalamus, the highest concentrations of norepinephrine, for example, are found in the region of the supraoptic and paraventricular nuclei, the periventricular nucleus (which is immediately adjacent to the third ventricle), the retrochiasmatic nucleus, and the dorsomedial nucleus. Terminations also are present in the middle and external zone of the median eminence. A few terminations have been identified in the ventromedial and anterior hypothalamic nuclei. The importance of this noradrenergic-input pathway has been demonstrated by the fact that lesions in the posterior part of the medial forebrain bundle result in a decrease in fluorescence of forebrain structures and a marked reduction in their norepinephrine content.

The processes of the dopaminergic system also ascend in the medial forebrain bundle and a major component reaches structures of the striatum (putamen and caudate nucle-

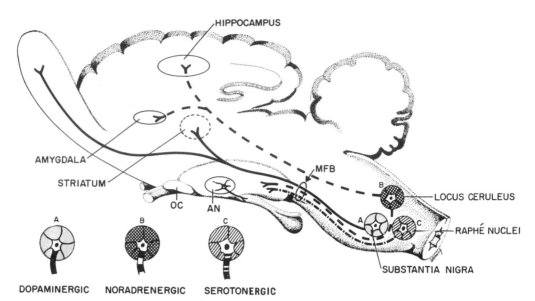

Figure 17. Monoaminergic pathways in mammalian brain. The principal localization of the neurons containing norepinephrine, dopamine, and serotonin is in the mesencephalon and pons. Axons of these cells are distributed to widespread areas of cortex, limbic system, and striatum. The dopaminergic system of the arcuate is an exception to this general scheme of distribution. *Abbreviations:* MFB, medial forebrain bundle; AN, arcuate nucleus; OC, optic chiasm.

us). A few dopaminergic-system axons are believed to end in the medial hypothalamic nuclei. A second prominent dopaminergic system arises and ends entirely within the medial basal hypothalamus.[15, 16, 26] The neuronal cell bodies of this system, as described above, are located in the arcuate and anterior periventricular nuclei, and their processes end directly in the perivascular space surrounding the capillaries of the median eminence. An estimated 10 to 15 per cent of the neurons of these nuclei are dopaminergic, and as many as one third of the terminal axonal boutons which abut on the neurovascular zone of the median eminence are monoaminergic. This is in striking contrast to other dopaminergic regions of the brain such as the striatum where it is estimated that only 4 per cent of the terminals are dopaminergic. In addition to the profuse dopaminergic endings in the external zone of the median eminence there are other terminals, identified as noradrenergic endings, the precise cellular origin of which have not been determined.

The apposition of axon terminals containing dopamine to other neuronal processes in the median eminence has afforded a morphologic basis for the hypothesis that dopaminergic terminals may stimulate releasing-factor release from hypophysiotrophic neurons through axo-axonic connections (Fig. 18). Such connections may function by facilitating depolarization of releasing-factor neuron terminals, with subsequent release of the releasing factor to diffuse into the portal capillary system for eventual transport to the anterior pituitary. Serotonergic cell systems have also been linked to neuroendocrine regulation. Some of the neurons ascending from the mesencephalic and pontine raphe nuclei terminate in the hypothalamus (particularly in the suprachiasmatic region); others continue to other regions of the forebrain, including the limbic system and cortex.

Evidently, the complex system of innervation of the hypothalamus by these monoaminergic systems provides important inputs from midbrain reticular systems which may be involved in mediation of neuroendocrine reflexes. Neuropharmacologic studies in

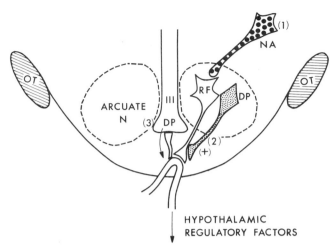

Figure 18. Axoaxonic connections in the median eminence. *Abbreviations:* DP, dopamine neuron; NA, noradrenergic neuron; OT, optic tract; RF, releasing factor neuron. The numbers indicate possible mechanisms by which catecholamines might influence releasing factor release: 1) NA stimulation of RF neurons, 2) Axoaxonic stimulation of RF by DP, and 3) transependymal transport of DP by tanycytes. (From Martin, J. B.: *Neural regulation of growth hormone secretion.* N. Engl. J. Med. 288:1384, 1973, with permission.)

experimental animals provide the most impressive support for the hypothesis that biogenic amines may play a fundamental role in neuroendocrine regulation. Agents known to deplete central catecholamines significantly alter neuroendocrine function in the rat. Reserpine, a drug which interferes with re-uptake of catecholamines and serotonin into storage granules of axon terminals, blocks ovulatory LH release, causes an increase in corticosterone levels, inhibits thyroid function, and increases prolactin secretion. Similar effects are elicited by inhibition of catecholamine synthesis by α-methyl-p-tyrosine, a substance which inhibits tyrosine hydroxylase, the first enzyme in the synthesis pathway of dopamine and norepinephrine. That these monoamines function at a hypothalamic level and not at a pituitary level is suggested by several lines of evidence. For example, infusion of catecholamines into the pituitary portal vessels does not cause secretion of any pituitary trophic hormone, whereas the administration of the appropriate releasing factor is effective. Pituitary fragments incubated in vitro do not release hormones following addition of small amounts of dopamine or norepinephrine, nor do the catecholamines potentiate the effect of the releasing factor at the pituitary level. An exception to these general principles is the observation that dopamine acts directly on the pituitary to inhibit prolactin secretion.

On the other hand, injection of dopamine into the hypothalamus or ventricular system is effective in altering anterior pituitary hormone release.[28, 33] In the rat, intraventricular dopamine has been shown to stimulate LH and FSH release and to inhibit the release of prolactin and GH. By contrast, norepinephrine has little if any effect in this species. In the baboon, however, intrahypothalamic injection of norepinephrine elicits GH release. It has also been shown that dopamine can release the releasing factor from nerve terminals in vitro.

In man also, catecholaminergic systems are important in neuroendocrine regulation. The oral administration of L-dopa, the precursor of both dopamine and norepinephrine, causes a prompt increase in plasma GH levels and inhibition of prolactin. These effects are so striking that they have been used as a secretory reserve test for pituitary failure. The response is specific for these hormones, since the secretion of the other trophic hormones in unaltered. In the case of GH, the presence of a dopaminergic receptor

37

appears important for activation of GH release, since administration of apomorphine, a specific agonist of dopamine receptors in brain, causes prompt release of GH. Apomorphine, like L-dopa, also causes inhibition of prolactin. Administration of clonidine, a noradrenergic-receptor-stimulating agent, is also effective in releasing GH in both man and higher primates.

It appears that serotonergic systems also are important for neuroendocrine regulation, although these have not been as fully clarified. In the rat, serotonin administered intraventricularly causes inhibition of LH and FSH release and stimulation of prolactin and GH secretion. In higher primates including man, the intravenous administration of tryptophan or 5-hydroxytryptophan (precursor of serotonin) is effective in causing both prolactin and GH secretion. It has been postulated that certain types of GH release, such as that which accompanies slow-wave sleep, may be induced by serotonergic mechanisms. More detailed consideration of certain of these effects is given in Chapter 3 and in various sections devoted to the regulation of individual hormones.

Extrahypothalamic Regulation of Hypophysiotrophic Function

The functions of the hypothalamus in visceral and endocrine regulation, and in behavior, drive, affect, and consciousness arise in part from within the hypothalamus itself but to a greater extent from the interactions between the hypothalamus and the limbic lobe or limbic system. The limbic lobe as first described by Broca[7] consisted of several brain regions distributed largely as a fringe (limbus) around the diencephalon, including cingulate and hippocampal gyri, amygdala, and adjacent cerebral cortex. Because of prominent anatomic relationships of these structures with the olfactory system and their large size in lower forms in which smell is important, it was believed for a long time that the limbic lobe (also called rhinencephalon) was primarily concerned with smell afferents and smell-related behavior. This restricted view of the limbic lobe was modified in the first few decades of the twentieth century as a result of increased anatomic knowledge and clinical observations of behavioral effects of lesions in these structures. In 1937, Papez proposed the existence of a "hypothalamic-anterior-thalamic-cingulate cortex-hippocampal-fornix-hypothalamic circuit" that subserved certain aspects of emotion.[32] Deliberate production of lesions in the amygdaloid nuclei of the monkey were shown in the same year by Klüver and Bucy to produce changes in visual and food discrimination and in sexuality, thus confirming the relationship of this structure to non-olfactory behavior.[32] MacLean in 1949 expanded the concept of the "limbic system" to that of the "visceral brain" as the integrator of emotional and vegetative information concerned with internal events of the organism.[32] The limbic system was now defined anatomically in a much broader sense to include the interconnections of the limbic lobe with thalamic, hypothalamic, and midbrain regions.

The precise way in which these regions are integrated, the full extent of anatomic connections within and without the limbic system, and its neurophysiologic and neuropharmacologic control have not been resolved adequately. Nevertheless, on the basis of the effects of lesions of the limbic system, of electric stimulation, and of neuropharmacologic manipulations, one can gain some insight into the mechanism by which brain structures modulate hypothalamic activity.

Anatomy of the Limbic System

The limbic system as now defined anatomically includes the medial part of the mesencephalic reticular formation (the so-called midbrain limbic system), hypothalamus, hippocampus, septum, amygdala, and cingulate, orbitofrontal, and pyriform cortex areas (Fig. 19). The main pathway that connects these areas is the medial forebrain

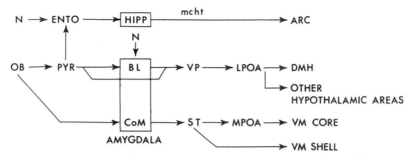

Figure 19. A schematic representation of some of the principal connections of the limbic system, indicating the main neocortical and olfactory afferents and the major pathways from the hippocampus and the amygdala to the hypothalamus. *Abbreviations:* ARC, arcuate nucleus; BL, basolateral nucleus; CoM, corticomedial nucleus; DMH, dorsomedial hypothalamic nucleus; ENTO, entorhinal area; HIPP, hippocampus; LPOA, lateral preoptic area; mcht, medial corticohypothalamic tract; MPOA, medial preoptic area; N, neocortex; OB, olfactory bulb; PYR, pyriform cortex; ST, stria terminalis; VM, ventromedial nucleus; VP, ventral amygdalofugal pathway. (From Raisman G. and Field, P. M.: *Anatomical considerations relevant to the interpretation of neuroendocrine experiments. In* Martini, L. and Ganong, W. F. (eds.): *Frontiers in Neuroendocrinology, 1971.* Oxford University Press, New York, 1971, with permission.)

bundle, which is characterized by an admixture of cells and nerve fibers in a multineuronal, multisynaptic system.[34, 41] Frequent collateral branchings from the medial forebrain bundle reach adjacent structures. Particularly important with respect to neuroendocrine regulation are relays to the medial hypothalamus, which serve to connect the medial "endocrine" hypothalamus with the limbic system.

The hypothalamic and extrahypothalamic components of the limbic system lack direct input from primary sensory systems. It is probable that neuroendocrine effects derived from olfactory, somatosensory, visual, or auditory stimuli are relayed through the reticular formation of the brain stem and thalamus (or in the case of olfaction, through the pyriform cortex of the temporal lobe). A possible exception to this generalization is the direct retinohypothalamic connection to the suprachiasmatic nucleus of the hypothalamus. This input may have a role in determining diurnal rhythmicity in hypothalamic function, particularly with respect to pineal and pituitary-adrenal activity.

Specific functions in the limbic system cannot be readily assigned to specific anatomic structures, because, as pointed out by Isaacson, "many if not all effects produced by stimulation or lesions of the extrahypothalamic limbic structures can be replicated by stimulation or lesions of the hypothalamus."[48] This is particularly true when one attempts to define the anatomic basis of emotionality, of feeling state, of drives (such as thirst and hunger), and of visceral integration. The major divisions of the limbic system and their connections are described in the remainder of this chapter.

Hippocampus

Isaacson[48] argues persuasively for a role of the hippocampus in learning and discriminatory behavior. Animals with hippocampal destruction or with septal lesions (the two structures are intimately related anatomically) tend to initiate responses more rapidly and more frequently than intact animals. Learning is impaired and can be ascribed to a defect in transference from one learning experience to another. The prior learning appears to interfere with subsequent attentiveness to another aspect of the same problem. Correspondingly, bilateral hippocampal lesions in man are associated with the amnestic syndrome (Korsakoff's psychosis). Such patients are unable to learn new information; registration is intact but the memory is not imprinted and is rapidly lost. In the rat and monkey, stimulation of the hippocampus results in GH release.

The principal efferent system of the hippocampus is the fornix which, in addition to its major distribution to the mammillary bodies also has direct (monosynaptic) inputs to the arcuate and ventromedial hypothalamic nuclei. Electrophysiologic studies have shown that some of these inputs terminate directly on tuberoinfundibular neurons. Raisman and Field[41] have described one component of the fornix in the rat that originates in the prosubiculum of the hippocampus and deviates medially at the level of the anterior commissure to form the medial corticohypothalamic tract. This group of fibers terminates in the anterior pole of the arcuate nucleus. The remainder of the fornix distributes to other hypothalamic and adjacent structures including the septum, the anterior thalamic nuclei, preoptic area, and periventricular zone of the hypothalamus, as well as the mammillary bodies. The exact distribution from the fornix to these nuclear groups varies considerably with different species.

Afferent connections to the hippocampus arise predominantly in the entorhinal cortex of the temporal lobe. This region in turn receives afferents from the olfactory system and the pyriform cortex. In addition, virtually every structure that receives inputs from the hippocampus also sends fibers reciprocally to it. Particularly important in this regard is the septum, but fibers arising from the midbrain and hypothalamus also reach the hippocampus.

Amygdala

The amygdala functions to determine emotionality by supplying affect to perceptual responses. Animals with lesions of the amygdala show reduced reactivity to environmental changes and may consequently show a defect in acquisition of information. The extremes of emotion are lost. A wild animal shows increased tameness, even lethargy. Bilateral lesions of the amygdala also affect appetitive behavior, although the results are not consistent. Aphagia and adipsia, or excessive food intake have been reported to follow amygdaloid lesions in experimental animals. In the Klüver-Bucy syndrome abnormalities of appetitive behavior occur characterized by loss of discrimination. Inedible objects are mouthed and sexual hyperactivity may be evident, copulation occurring inappropriately (e.g., with inanimate objects). The lesions in these animals were extensive and included destruction of the amygdala and the adjacent medial temporal lobe. Similar clinical disturbances have been described in humans with bilateral temporal lobe lesions.

The amygdaloid complex is comprised of a number of subdivisions. According to the classification of Johnston, the amygdala can be divided into basolateral and corticomedial nuclear groups. The basis of this division is both anatomic and phylogenetic. In terms of comparative neuroanatomy, the corticomedial subdivisions are the most primitive, the basolateral groups appearing later in evolutionary development.

Anatomic studies suggest a functional distinction between these groups. The corticomedial nuclei send fibers through the stria terminalis to the septum, preoptic area, and the external border of the hypothalamic ventromedial nuclei. This efferent system is partly crossed so that bilateral inputs from each amygdala reach the hypothalamus. The primary efferents of the basolateral amygdala reach the lateral hypothalamus via a ventral amygdalofugal pathway. The precise anatomic termination of this pathway is in some doubt. Direct connections are described to the lateral and anterior hypothalamus. Presumably information from the basolateral amygdala is relayed to the medial hypothalamus via synaptic connections in the medial forebrain bundle or the anterior hypothalamus.

Electrophysiologic studies support a distinction between these two efferent amygdaloid pathways. Murphy and Renaud[37] reported that neurons of the ventromedial nucleus are affected differently by stimuli applied to the stria terminalis or to the basolateral amygdala. Stimulation of the basolateral amygdala caused excitation of ventromedial hypothalamic neurons, whereas stimulation of the stria terminalis was inhibitory. Electric stimulation studies in the rat also have confirmed a difference of function of these areas with respect to GH control. Thus, the basolateral amygdala is excitatory and the corticomedial amygdala inhibitory to GH release in this species.

The amygdala also receives afferent connections from the hypothalamus. The possibility should be considered that these recurrent connections function in a feedback modulation of neuroendocrine responses. Connections between the amygdala and ventromedial nucleus, for instance, may partake in the control of GH secretion. Both regions are reported to contain significant concentrations of somatostatin.

Septum

Rodents with lesions in the septal area exhibit rage reactions and hyperemotionality. This effect is particularly prominent in rats and mice, but is less evident in cats and difficult to produce in monkeys. Animals with septal lesions show increased reactivity both emotionally and hormonally, as shown by the studies of Seggie and Brown (see Chapter 8). The septal area is also concerned with regulation of water intake. In higher animals, the septal area is smaller than other components of the limbic system. In man, the septum is small and limited to a few cells in the septum pellucidum and the medial cortex beneath the genu of the corpus callosum. Lesions in this area, such as may be produced by subarachnoid hemorrhage after rupture of an anterior communicating aneurysm, may produce remarkable disturbances in personality. Such patients frequently are belligerent, uncooperative, and emotionally unstable.

Corticohypothalamic Inputs

The existence and potential significance of cortical inputs to the hypothalamus have long been debated. Several recent neuroanatomic and neurophysiologic studies indicate that direct connections do exist. Use of the horseradish peroxidase technique to trace neuronal connections has convincingly shown that direct hypothalamic cortical projections also exist in the monkey. This is important since it contributes further evidence that the hypothalamus has extraordinarily widespread connections with other brain regions.

Limbic Midbrain Connections

In addition to descending connections to the hypothalamus, there are important ascending inputs from the midbrain reticular formation and from midbrain nuclear groups that contain the cells of origin of the monoaminergic fiber system. Most of these diffuse and monosynaptic inputs are relayed to the hypothalamus through the mammillary peduncle or the medial forebrain bundle. A midline periventricular system also ascends from the periaqueductal gray substance of the midbrain, to become continuous with the periventricular gray of the third ventricle. This system is co-extensive with the dorsal longitudinal fasciculus of Schütz, which carries fibers to and from the hypothalamus and brain stem.

Summary

In terms of neuroendocrine regulation, the various hypothalamic and extrahypothalamic pathways described above are assumed to mediate 1) circadian rhythms in hormonal secretion; 2) stress-induced alterations in hormone secretion; 3) integration of neuroendocrine activity with autonomic nervous system responses; 4) neuroendocrine effects triggered by olfactory and peripheral sensory responses; and 5) elaboration of neurosecretomotor activation for regulation of organs such as the pancreas, pineal gland, and the renal juxtaglomerular apparatus. These aspects of neuroendocrine regulation are discussed further in relation to control of individual trophic hormones.

REFERENCES

1. ADAMS, J. H., DANIEL, P. M. AND PRICHARD, M. M. L.: *Distribution of hypophysial portal blood in the anterior lobe of the pituitary gland.* Endocrinology 75:120, 1964.

2. ANDERSON, E. AND HAYMAKER, W.: *Breakthroughs in hypothalamic and pituitary research. In:* Swaab, D. F. and Schade, J. P. (eds.): *Progress in Brain Research,* vol. 41. Elsevier, New York, 1974, p. 1.

3. ASCHNER, B.: *Ueber die Fuktion der Hypophyse.* Pfluegers Arch. Ges. Physiol. 146:1, 1912.

4. BAKER, B. L.: *In* Greep, R. O. and Astwood, E. B. (eds.): *Handbook of Physiology, Section 7: Endocrinology,* vol. 4, part 1. American Physiological Society. Williams & Wilkins, Baltimore, 1974, p. 45.

5. BJORKLUND, A., ET AL.: *Identification and terminal distribution of the tuberohypophysial monoamine fibre systems in the rat by means of stereotaxic and microspectrofluorimetric techniques.* Brain Res. 17: 1, 1970.

6. BLACKWELL, R. E. AND GUILLEMIN, R.: *Hypothalamic control of adenohypophysial secretions.* Annu. Rev. Physiol. 35:357, 1973.

7. BROCA, P.: *Anatomie comparee des circonvolutions cerebrales. Le grand lobe limbique et la scissurs limbique dans la serie des mammiferes.* Rev. Anthrop. Ser. 2 1:385, 1878.

8. CROSS, B. A. AND SILVER, I. A.: *Electrophysiological studies on the hypothalamus.* Br. Med. Bull. 22: 254, 1966.

9. DEROOIJ, J. A. M. AND HOMMES, O. R.: *The tuberoinfundibular region in man: Structure-monoamines-karyometrics. In* Swaab, D. F. and Schade, J. P. (eds.): *Progress in Brain Research,* vol. 41. Elsevier, New York, 1974, p. 79.

10. DYER, R. G.: *The electrophysiology of the hypothalamus and its endocrinological implications. In* Swaab, D. F. and Schade, J. P. (eds.): *Progress in Brain Research,* vol. 41. Elsevier, New York, 1974, p. 133.

11. ERDHEIM, J. AND STUMME, E.: *Ueber die Schwangerschaftsveranderung der Hypophyse.* Beitr. Pathol. Anat. Allgem. Pathol. 46:1, 1909.

12. EVANS, H. M.: *Clinical manifestations of dysfunction of the anterior pituitary.* In: *Glandular Physiology and Therapy.* American Medical Association, Chicago, 1935, p. 7.

13. FALCK, B., ET AL.: *Fluorescence of catecholamines and related compound condensed with formaldehyde.* J. Histochem. Cytochem. 10:348, 1962.

14. FRIEDGOOD, H. B.: *The nervous control of the anterior hypophysis* (originally presented at the Harvard Tercentenary Celebrations, Sept. 15, 1936). J. Reprod. Fertil. [Suppl.] 10:3, 1970.

15. FUXE, K.: *Cellular localization of monoamines in the median eminence and in the fundibular stem of some mammals.* Acta Physiol. Scand. 58:383, 1963.

16. FUXE, K. AND HOKFELT, T.: *Further evidence for the existence of tubero-infundibular dopamine neurons.* Acta Physiol. Scand. 66:245, 1966.

17. FUXE, K. AND HOKFELT, T.: *Catecholamines in the hypothalamus and the pituitary gland. In:* Ganong, W. F. and Martini, L. (eds.): *Frontiers in Neuroendocrinology, 1969.* Oxford University Press, New York, 1969, p. 47.

18. GOLDMAN, H. AND SAPIRSTEIN, L. A.: *Determination of blood flow to the rat pituitary gland.* Am. J. Physiol. 194:433, 1958.

19. GREEN, J. D.: *Comparative anatomy of hypophysis, with special reference to its blood supply and innervation.* Am. J. Anat. 88:225, 1951.

20. GREEN, J. D. AND HARRIS, G. W.: *Neurovascular link between neurohypophysis and adenohypophysis.* J. Endocrinol. 5:136, 1947.

21. GUILLEMIN, R., BURGUS, R. AND VALE, W.: *The hypothalamic hypophysiotropic thyrotropin releasing factor.* Vitam. Horm. 29:1, 1971.

22. HALASZ, B.: *The endocrine effects of isolation of the hypothalamus from the rest of the brain. In* Ganong, W. F. and Martini, L. (eds.): *Frontiers in Neuroendocrinology, 1969.* Oxford University Press, New York, 1969, p. 307.

23. HALASZ, B., PUPP, L. AND UHLARIK, S.: *Hypophysiotrophic area in the hypothalamus.* J. Endocrinol. 25:147, 1962.

24. HARRIS, G. W.: *Electrical stimulation of hypothalamus and mechanism of neural control of adenohypophysis.* J. Physiol. (Lond.) 107:418, 1948.

25. HARRIS, G. W. AND JACOBSOHN, D.: *Functional grafts of anterior pituitary gland.* Proc. Roy Soc. Ser. B 139:263, 1952.

26. HOKFELT, T. AND FUXE, K.: *On the morphology and the neuroendocrine role of the hypothalamic cate-cholamine neurons. In* Knigge, K. M., Scott, D. E. and Weindl, W. (eds.): *Brain-Endocrine Interaction: Median Eminence: Structure and Function.* Karger, Basel, 1972, p. 181.

27. HOUSSAY, B. A., BIASOTTI, A. AND SAMMARTINO: *Modifications functionelles de l'hypophyse apres les lesions infundibulotuberiennes chez le crapaud.* C. R. Soc. Biol. (Paris) 120:725, 1935.

28. KAMBERI, I. A., MICAL, R. S. AND PORTER, J. C.: *Luteinizing hormone-releasing activity in hypophysial stalk blood and elevation by dopamine.* Science 166:388, 1969.

29. KNIGGE, K. M.: *Gonadotropic activity of neonatal pituitary glands implanted in the rat brain.* Am. J. Physiol. 202:387, 1962.

30. KNIGGE, K. M. AND SCOTT, D. E.: *Structure and function of the median eminence.* Am. J. Anat. 129: 223, 1970.

31. KNIGGE, K. M. AND SILVERMAN, A. J.: *Transport capacity of the median eminence. In* Knigge, K. M., Scott, D. E. and Weindl, A. (eds.): *Brain-Endocrine Interaction: Median Eminence: Structure and Function.* Karger, Basel, 1972, p. 350.

32. MACLEAN, P. D.: *Influence of limbic cortex on hypothalmus. In* Lederis, K. and Cooper, K. E. (eds.): *Recent Studies of Hypothalamic Function.* Basel, Karger, 1974, p. 216.

33. MCCANN, S. M., ET AL.: *The role of monoamines in the control of gonadotropin and prolactin secretion. In* Knigge, K. M., Scott, D. E. and Weindl, A. (eds.): *Brain-Endocrine Interaction: Median Eminence: Structure and Function.* Karger, Basel, 1972, p. 224.

34. MILLHOUSE, O. E.: *A Golgi study of the descending medial forebrain bundle.* Brain Res. 15:341, 1969.

35. MONROE, B. G.: *A comparative study of the ultrastructure of the median eminence, infundibular stem and neural lobe of the hypophysis of the rat.* Z. Zellforsch. 76:405, 1967.

36. MOSS, R. M.: *Unit responses of arcuate and other hypothalamic neurons. In:* Martini, L. and Ganong, W. F. (eds.): *Frontiers in Neuroendocrinology,* vol. 4. Raven Press, 1975, p. 95.

37. MURPHY, J. T. AND RENAUD, L. P.: *Mechanisms of inhibition in the ventromedial nucleus of the hypothalamus.* J. Neurophysiol. 32:85, 1969.

38. NIKITOVITCH-WINER, M. AND EVERETT, J. W.: *Functional restitution of pituitary grafts re-transplanted from kidney to median eminence.* Endocrinology 63:916, 1958.

39. POPA, G. AND FIELDING, U.: *A portal circulation from the pituitary to the hypothalamic region.* J. Anat. 65:88, 1930.

40. PORTER, J. C., ONDO, J. G. AND CRAMER, O. M.: *Nervous and vascular supply of the pituitary gland. In* Greep, R. O. and Astwood, E. B. (eds.): *Handbook of Physiology, Section 7: Endocrinology,* vol. 4, part 1. American Physiological Society. Williams & Wilkins, Baltimore, 1974, p. 33.

41. RAISMAN, G. AND FIELD, P. M.: *Anatomical considerations relevant to the interpretation of neuroendocrine experiments. In* Martini, L. and Ganong, W. F. (eds.): *Frontiers in Neuroendocrinology, 1971.* Oxford University Press, New York, 1971, p. 3.

42. RENAUD, L. P. AND MARTIN, J. B.: *Electrophysiological studies of connections of hypothalamic ventromedial nucleus neurons in the rat: Evidence for a role in neuroendocrine regulation.* Brain Res. 93:145, 1975.

43. RENAUD, L. P.: *Tuberoinfundibular neurons in the basomedial hypothalamus of the rat: Electrophysiological evidence for axon collaterals to hypothalamic and extrahypothalamic areas.* Brain Res. 105: 59, 1976.

44. SCHALLY, A. V., ARIMURA, A. AND KASTIN, A. J.: *Hypothalamic regulatory hormones.* Science 179: 341, 1973.

45. WEINDL, A. AND JOYNT, R. J.: *The median eminence as a circumventricular organ. In:* Knigge, K. M., Scott, D. E. and Weindl, A. (eds.): *Brain-Endocrine Interaction: Median Eminence: Structure and Function.* Karger, Basel, 1972, p. 280.

46. WISLOCKI, G. B. AND KING, L. S.: *Permeability of the hypophysis and hypothalamus to vital dyes, with study of hypophyseal supply.* Am. J. Anat. 58:421, 1936.

47. XUEREB, G. P., PRICHARD, M. M. L. AND DANIEL, P. M.: *Arterial supply and venous drainage of human hypophysis cerebri.* Q. J. Exp. Physiol. 39:199, 1954.

48. ISAACSON, R. L.: *The Limbic System.* Plenum Press, New York, 1974.

BIBLIOGRAPHY

DANIEL, P. M. AND PRICHARD, M. M. L.: *Studies of the hypothalamus and the pituitary gland. With special reference to the effects of transection of the pituitary stalk.* Acta Endocrinol. [Suppl.] 80:201, 1975.

GREEP, R. O. AND ASTWOOD, E. B. (EDS.): *Handbook of Physiology, Section 7: Endocrinology,* vol. 4, parts 1 and 2. American Physiological Society. Williams & Wilkins, Baltimore, 1974.

HARRIS, G. W. AND DONOVAN, B. (EDS.): *The Pituitary Gland,* vols. 1–3. University of California Press, Berkely, 1966.

HAYMAKER, W., ANDERSON, E. AND NAUTA, W. J. H. (EDS.): *The Hypothalamus.* Charles C Thomas, Springfield, 1969.

LEDERIS, K. AND COOPER, K. E.: *Recent Studies of Hypothalamic Function.* Karger, Basel, 1974.

LOCKE, W. AND SCHALLY, A. V.: *The Hypothalamus and Pituitary in Health and Disease.* Charles C Thomas, Springfield, 1972.

MARTINI, L. AND GANONG, W. F. (EDS.): *Frontiers in Neuroendocrinology,* vol. 4. Raven Press, New York, 1975.

MEITES, J.: *Hypophysiotrophic Hormones of the Hypothalamus.* Williams & Wilkins, Baltimore, 1970.

MOGENSON, G. J. AND CALARESU, F. R. (EDS.): *Neural Integration of Physiological Mechanisms and Behaviour.* University of Toronto Press, Toronto, 1975.

SZENTAGOTHAI, J., *Hypothalamic Control of the Anterior Pituitary,* ed. 3. Akademiai Kiado, Budapest, 1968.

TIXIER-VIDAL, A. AND FARQUHAR, M. G. (EDS.): *The Anterior Pituitary.* Academic Press, New York, 1975.

CHAPTER 3

Neuropharmacology of Anterior Pituitary Control

Since studies of sex function provided the first unequivocal evidence of neural control of the anterior pituitary, it is not surprising that the earliest attempts to identify chemical factors in the brain capable of affecting pituitary function also used endpoints of reproductive physiology. The first efforts to determine the effect of catecholamines on anterior pituitary function were those of Sawyer, Markee, and Townsend,[36] who in 1949 observed that ovulation followed infusion of epinephrine into the anterior pituitary of the rabbit under stereotaxic control. In 1956, Donovan and Harris[13] attempted to repeat this work, taking pains to use minimal amounts of epinephrine over prolonged periods of time so as to avoid the backtracking of injected material along the needle to the hypothalamus. When these precautions were taken, gonadotropins were not released by direct intrapituitary injections of epinephrine. It seemed likely, therefore, that the earlier experiments of Sawyer and colleagues had been due to hypothalamic stimulation. At about the same time, Vogt[44] showed by bioassay methods that the hypothalamus contained large amounts of norepinephrine, and soon thereafter Carlsson and coworkers[5] demonstrated substantial concentrations of dopamine in the brain. These observations clearly indicated that the hypothalamus was rich in catecholamines, which might participate in regulation of the pituitary through effects mediated at the hypothalamic level.[22, 30, 31, 37, 43]

As outlined in the preceding chapter, subsequent advances were made by the anatomic mapping of catecholaminergic and serotonergic pathways within the brain using the fluorescence microscopic techniques of Falck and associates,[14] by administration of neuropharmacologic agents that interfered with various aspects of neurotransmitter action in the brain,[27] and by the study of enzymes involved in the biosynthesis of the biogenic amines norepinephrine, dopamine, and serotonin. From these studies, it now appears that biogenic aminergic neurons constitute a major intermediate route for neural influence on the function of hypophysiotrophic neurons in the hypothalamus.[12, 18, 47, 48]

In this chapter, the basic and clinical neuropharmacology of central aminergic neurons is reviewed. Specific effects of various manipulations of central neurotransmitters on pituitary function will be discussed in subsequent chapters dealing with regulation of individual hormones.

HYPOTHALAMIC BIOGENIC AMINES

The principal biogenic monoamines considered to be central nervous system neurotransmitters regulating hypophysiotrophic function are dopamine, norepinephrine, and serotonin (Fig. 1).[3, 36, 47] Acetylcholine also is important in regulation of hypophysiotrophic neurons, although the evidence is less complete.[28, 36] These substances satisfy classic criteria as neurotransmitters: they are localized in nerve terminals, they are released after depolarization, and enzymatic mechanisms exist in the central nervous system for both their synthesis and metabolism. When delivered to single neurons by microiontophoresis they cause excitation or inhibition of cellular electric activity.[3] Histamine[5, 39] and epinephrine[21] have also been detected in the hypothalamus, but little is known of their possible physiologic importance in hypophysiotrophic hormone regulation. The demonstration by Saavedra and collaborators[35] that the enzyme phenylethanolamine N-methyltransferase (PNMT), which converts norepinephrine to epinephrine, is distributed throughout noradrenergic pathways raises the possibility that epinephrine is more important than previously thought. The metabolic pathways for synthesis of dopamine, norepinephrine, and epinephrine are shown in Figure 2.

Monaminergic neurons in the hypothalamus terminate on tuberoinfundibular neurons, either by synaptic connections on the dendrites of such cells, or via axo-axonic connections in the median eminence.[18] As outlined in Chapter 2, noradrenergic and serotonergic nerve cell perikarya are almost entirely, if not exclusively, situated in brain stem nuclear groups, the locus ceruleus and raphe nuclei, respectively.[10, 19] That most hypothalamic norepinephrine and serotonin arise from extrahypothalamic sites is indicated by the work of Wiener[46] who found that deafferented hypothalamic "islands" contain less than 10 per cent of the normal concentration of norepinephrine and less than 30 per cent of serotonin. In contrast, the content of dopamine is normal in hypothalamic islands. This evidence provides strong support for the contention that hypothalamic dopaminergic neurons that regulate the anterior pituitary are located principally within the medial basal hypothalamus. This conclusion is further supported by the anatomic finding that a significant proportion of tuberoinfundibular neurons, in particular those located within the confines of the arcuate nucleus, are dopaminergic.[18, 46]

The median eminence itself contains large concentrations of serotonin, norepinephrine, and dopamine.[32, 34] Dopamine is located almost exclusively in the external zone of the median eminence, in nerve terminals adjacent to other fibers thought to contain the releasing factors (Fig. 3a). This juxtaposition led Fuxe and Hökfelt[18, 19] to postulate that dopamine may act on axon terminals of releasing-factor neurons through axo-axonic connections, to facilitate or inhibit the release of releasing factors. Electron-micro-

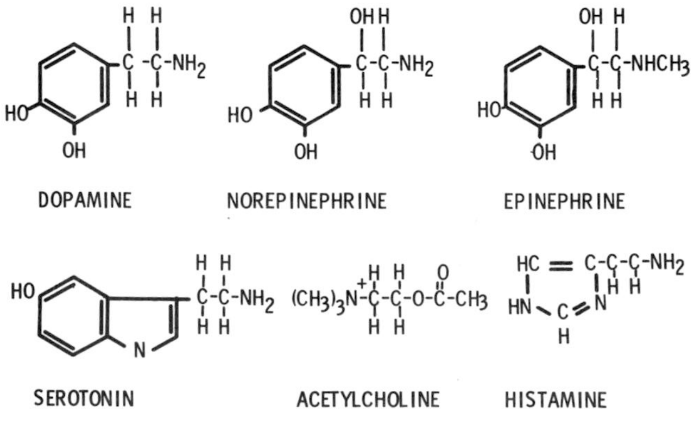

Figure 1. Structures of neurotransmitters which may be involved in hypophysiotropic hormone control.

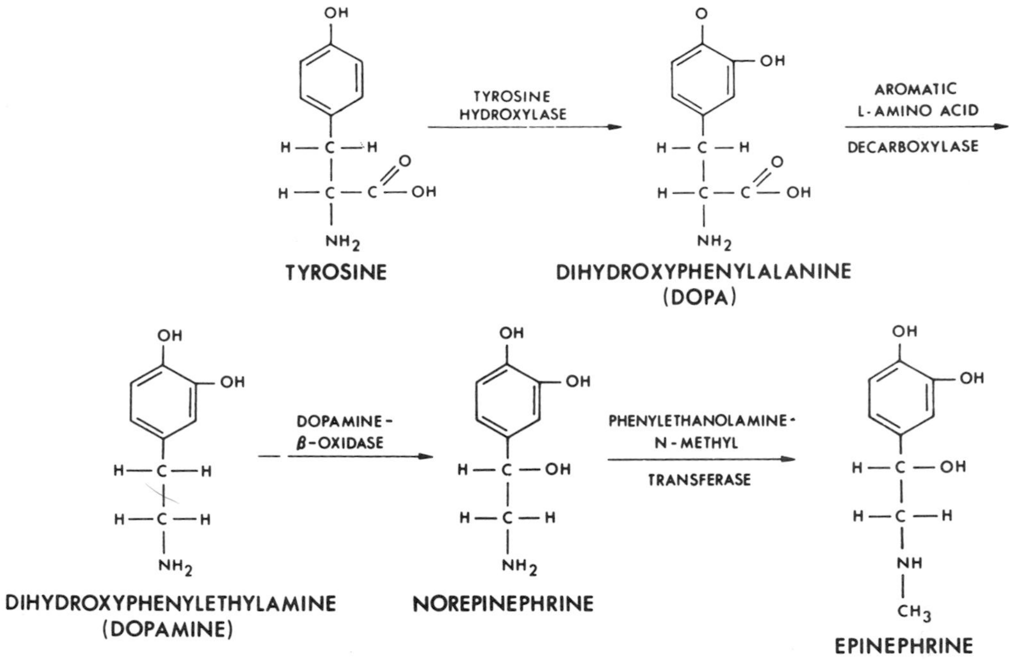

Figure 2. Metabolic pathway for synthesis of dopamine, norepinephrine and epinephrine.

scopic studies have not confirmed more than a rare synapse-like connection between such nerve terminals, however, and no other evidence is available either to support or refute this interesting suggestion.

Norepinephrine is located in both the external and internal palisade layers of the median eminence (Fig. 3b).[18, 32] Serotonin is diffusely distributed throughout the median eminence (Fig. 3c).[34] The precise origin of the cells that contribute terminals to these layers has not been identified.

Electrophysiologic studies have shown that each of the three monoamines, when applied by microiontophoresis,[3] affects single neurons in the hypothalamus. The effects vary from cell to cell and may be either depressant or stimulatory. Until the exact cell under study can be further identified and correlated with pituitary function, such studies will probably not provide much information of precise effect-mechanisms in terms of anterior pituitary control.

Significant amounts of dopamine and serotonin are present in the anterior pituitary itself.[35] The origin of the amines has not been clarified. They are not present in nerve terminals and it is possible that they may be produced by specialized mast cells. The serotonin found in the pituitary may originate in the hypothalamus, since lesions of the raphe nuclei reduce serotonin content in the anterior pituitary. The fact that dopamine is present in the anterior pituitary further supports the possibility of a direct pituitary function for biogenic amines, particularly in prolactin control.

It should be readily apparent that systemic or intraventricular administration of various pharmacologic agents provides little evidence as to precise sites of action.[47] A noradrenergic agent, for example, might affect a noradrenergic cell body in the brain stem, act on connections to a second neuron that could in turn affect hypothalamic cells, act directly on noradrenergic synapses on tuberoinfundibular cells, influence axon terminals in the median eminence, or directly stimulate or inhibit pituitary secretion.

47

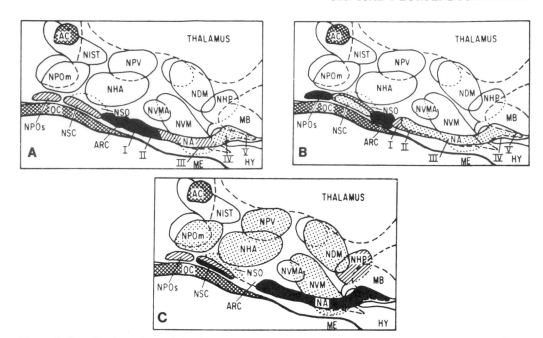

Figure 3. Localization of *(A)* dopamine, *(B)* norepinephrine, and *(C)* serotonin in sections of rat hypothalamus. Darkness corresponds to degree of concentration. *Abbreviations:* AC, anterior commissure; ARC and NA, arcuate nucleus; NDM, dorsomedial nucleus; NIST, interstitial nucleus of stria terminalis; NPOm, medial preoptic nucleus; NPV, paraventricular nucleus; NHA, anterior hypothalamic nucleus; NSO, supraoptic nucleus; NVMA, anterior ventromedial nucleus; NVM, ventromedial nucleus; NPH, posterior hypothalamic nucleus; MB, mammillary body; HY, pituitary; ME, median eminence, NSC, suprachiasmatic nucleus; NPOs, Preoptic suprachiasmatic nucleus; Roman numerals I to V refer to subdivision of the arcuate nucleus. (*A* and *B* from Palkovits, M., et al.: *Norepinephrine and dopamine content of hypothalamic nuclei of the rat.* Brain Res. 77:137, 1974, with permission. *C* from Saavedra, J. M., et al.: *Serotonin distribution in the nuclei of the rat hypothalamus and preoptic region.* Brain Res. 77:157, 1974, with permission.)

FUNCTION OF BIOGENIC AMINERGIC NEURONS

Some understanding of aminergic-neuron function has been derived from the study of both central and peripheral autonomic structures. Based on these studies, a model for the function of aminergic neurons has been developed that probably also applies to the function of the aminergic neurons that regulate hypophysiotrophic function. Cooper, Bloom, and Roth[8] have outlined this model and identified the steps in the synthesis and secretory process. The following description is modified from their monograph.

Central Catecholaminergic Neurons

Step 1: Uptake of Amino Acids into Aminergic Neurons

Although tyrosine, an essential amino acid and precursor of dopamine, norepinephrine, and epinephrine, is transported actively into brain, no known agent selectively blocks its uptake into cells. Other large neutral amino acids compete with tyrosine for uptake into brain, but it is not known whether this is true for specific catecholaminergic neurons in brain. Wurtman and Fernstrom[15, 49] reviewed in detail the possible role of tyrosine availability as a regulator of catecholamine synthesis, suggesting that variations in dietary intake may significantly alter central neurotransmitter function. The amino acid L-dopa is also taken up actively by catecholaminergic neurons, and by virtue of its activity as a substrate, increases synthesis and content of brain dopamine and norepinephrine.[7] This is the basis of its therapeutic action in Parkinson's disease (Fig. 4).

Step 2: Enzymatic Synthesis

After its entry into cells, tyrosine is hydroxylated in a rate-limiting step by the synaptosomal enzyme tyrosine hydroxylase to form L-dihydroxyphenylalanine (L-dopa).[45] Tyrosine hydroxylase has been purified and its cofactors and kinetic properties have been carefully studied. The drug α-methyltyrosine, an inhibitor of tyrosine hydroxylase, blocks L-dopa formation. L-dopa is decarboxylated by a nonspecific enzyme, L-aminodecarboxylase, to dopamine (DA) which is in turn hydroxylated by the enzyme dopamine β-hydroxylase to norepinephrine (NE). Norepinephrine can be methylated to form epinephrine by phenylethanolamine N-methyltransferase (PNMT), an enzyme present in adrenal medulla, and as mentioned above, also in certain areas of the brain.

Step 3: Storage Phase

After their synthesis, NE and DA are stored in specific granules within nerve terminals, probably bound to ATP and other carrier substances. They are protected within the granules from degradation. In peripheral sympathetic nerves, but not in brain, these storage-receptor sites are also accessible to NE and DA when the latter is introduced into the systemic circulation. These substances do not, however, readily cross the blood-brain barrier, and therefore do not reach central monoaminergic neurons. Interference (as by reserpine) with the capacity to store amines in the granules of nerve endings leads to depletion of aminergic stores, both centrally and peripherally. The administration of reserpine leads to a prompt liberation of catecholamines from the storage phase in autonomic tissues generally, and the effect is long-lasting, probably because the granules are damaged irreversibly.

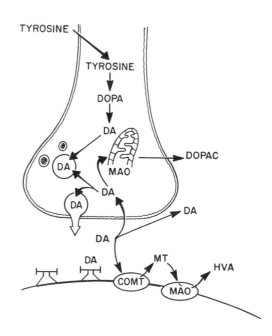

Figure 4. Schematic representation of a central dopaminergic synapse. See text for abbreviations. (Modified from Cooper, J. C., Bloom, F. E. and Roth, R. H.: *The Biochemical Basis of Neuropharmacology.* Oxford University Press, New York, 1974.)

Step 4: Release of Preformed Granules

In response to neuronal depolarization, granules are extruded from the nerve endings. This comes about through the effects of a propagated action potential and, by analogy with the adrenal medulla, probably is preceded by an influx of Ca^{++}. Amphetamines act, at least in part, by stimulating the release of preformed NE and possibly DA.

Step 5: Interaction of Catecholamines with Receptors Located on the Postsynaptic Neuron

Specific binding sites for NE and DA are present on the postsynaptic cell body in catecholamine-responsive tissue such as fat cells and cardiac muscle. It is assumed that similar receptors are present on hypophysiotrophic neurons. By analogy with peripheral autonomic pharmacology and the study of central nervous system control, it may be assumed that there are two classes of norepinephrine receptors on hypophysiotrophic neurons, one corresponding to α-receptors, and the other corresponding to β-receptors. This has not, however, been shown conclusively to be true in brain. Dopamine receptors are probably also present in certain hypophysiotrophic neurons.[24, 25, 38] From an analysis of pituitary control, it appears likely that some hypophysiotrophic neurons may have more than one type of receptor. Agents that duplicate the effects of the biogenic amines are called *agonists,* and agents that block agonist effects are called receptor-blockers or *antagonists.* Central β-adrenergic agonist effects are produced by the drug isoproterenol, and α-adrenergic agonist effects are duplicated by the drug clonidine. Dopamine receptors are stimulated by apomorphine, lergotrile mesylate, and bromergocryptine. Alpha-receptor blocking drugs in common use are phentolamine and phenoxybenzamine; a commonly used β-blocker is propranolol. Because these classes of agents have important potential therapeutic applications, an enormous amount of development work is under way and a number of new blockers have been synthesized and tested.[42]

The nature of the dopamine receptor and aberrations in dopamine metabolism have become increasingly important areas of investigation in both basic research and clinical medicine. As is well known, Parkinson's disease results from a deficiency in dopamine agonist effects in the caudate and putamen, and dopamine agonists such as L-dopa and bromergocryptine can ameliorate many of the manifestations of this disorder. Dopamine agonists are also potent inhibitors of prolactin secretion and stimulators of GH release.[26, 29] Dopamine receptors are widely distributed throughout the body, including parenchymal organs, heart, brain, and spinal cord. On the basis of the findings that all drugs that relieve schizophrenia are dopamine-receptor blockers and that dopamine agonists provoke psychotic behavior in animals, the theory has evolved that excessive dopamine-receptor stimulation may be responsible for certain human psychoses. Important drugs of this type are chlorpromazine, perphenazine, haloperidol, and pimozide (Fig. 5).

Step 6: Re-Uptake Process

Following the release of preformed hormone, free neurotransmitter in the synaptic cleft that has not reacted with receptor is taken up into the presynaptic nerve ending where it is either destroyed (see below) or incorporated again into a storage granule. The re-uptake process is the principal mechanism responsible for terminating the effects of postsynaptic nerve cell stimulation. A number of drugs cause increased noradrenergic effects by blocking the re-uptake process, thus making more norepinephrine

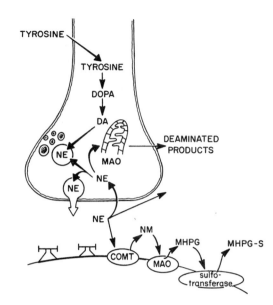

Figure 5. Schematic representation of a central noradrenergic synapse. See text for abbreviations. Modified from Cooper, J. C., Bloom, F. E. and Roth, R. H.: *The Biochemical Basis of Neuropharmacology.* Oxford University Press, New York, 1974.)

available at the postsynaptic receptor site. These include cocaine and the tricyclic antidepressants desipramine, chlorimipramine, and amitryptyline. Amphetamine may also act in part by this mechanism. It is likely that DA release and re-uptake is also regulated in this manner.

Step 7: Degradation of Neurotransmitter

Norepinephrine bound to postsynaptic membranes, or free (nongranule-bound) in the presynaptic nerve ending is vulnerable to destruction by the enzyme monoamine oxidase (MAO) that converts NE to its aldehyde, 3,4-dihydroxymandelic acid (see Fig. 5). This enzyme is also active against DA, converting it to homovanillic acid and dihydroxyphenylacetic acid. Increased noradrenergic activity results from administration of drugs that block monoamine oxidase activity such as pargyline, isocarboxazid, and tranylcypromine. By inhibition of the degradating enzyme, more neurotransmitter becomes available to the postsynaptic cell.

A second enzyme responsible for inactivating NE and DA is catechol-O-methyltransferase (COMT). The precise site at which this reaction takes place is unknown, but in brain, the metabolic products of the reaction find their way into the cerebrospinal fluid where they may serve as an index of turnover. The principal products of DA are 3-methoxytyramine and homovanillic acid, and those of NE are normetanephrine (NM), 3-methyoxy-4-hydroxyphenylglycol (MHPG), and its sulfate, MHPG-sulfate. The drug tropolone is believed to act as an inhibitor of COMT. Turnover of catecholamines in brain is influenced by various endocrine states.[1, 2, 12]

Axonal Transport of Catecholamines

Labeling and ligature experiments indicate that the protein-binding matrix of catecholaminergic storage granules is synthesized in the cell body and transported down the nerve by axoplasmic flow to its site in the nerve ending. The principal site of synthesis of the catecholamines, however, is in the terminal itself.

Mechanism of Action of Catecholamines on Hypophysiotrophic Neurons

The precise mechanism of action of catecholamines on hypophysiotrophic neurons has not been identified. Nevertheless, on the basis of studies of DA effects in sympathetic ganglia and caudate nucleus, of NE effects on the Purkinje cell, and of extensive work on catecholamine effects in parenchymal tissues and fat, it is reasonable to assume that hypophysiotrophic neurons are influenced by catecholamines through the second messenger, cyclic AMP.

According to the second-messenger hypothesis, catecholamines react with specific receptors on cell membranes to activate an enzyme, adenyl cyclase, that catalyses the conversion of ATP to cyclic AMP. Cyclic AMP initiates a cascade of intermediary chemical events such as new protein formation, increased metabolic activity, and cellular secretion. All of the characteristic enzymes and intermediary products of this reaction are found in brain. In fact, the brain is the richest source of the enzyme adenyl cyclase. The finding of Grimm and Reichlin[20] that the cyclic AMP analogue, dibutyryl cyclic AMP, causes the release of TRH in vitro from mouse hypothalami suggests that the hypophysiotrophic neuron is similarly affected by catecholamines.

Serotonergic Neurons

Serotonin (5-hydroxytryptamine) is widespread throughout the body. About 90 per cent is in enterochromaffin cells of the intestinal tract, and only 1 to 2 per cent is present in the central nervous system and pineal gland. This indolalkylamine is formed from the precursor essential amino acid tryptophan. The concentration of plasma tryptophan, as shown by Wurtman and Fernstrom[49] determines the rate of synthesis of serotonin, and this plasma level varies markedly with diet. In the neuron, tryptophan is converted by the enzyme tryptophan hydroxylase to 5-hydroxytryptophan, and thence to serotonin by the enzyme amino acid decarboxylase. As noted in Chapter 2, the serotonergic pathway arises in the raphe nuclei of the lower pons and upper brain stem and is distributed to the forebrain and to the hypothalamus. The function of serotonin as a putative neurotransmitter, and its neuropharmacology, have not been as well characterized as have the catecholaminergic neuronal functions, but a hypothetical model of control can be constructed that explains most of the available information. The function of these neurons can be described in a manner paralleling that of dopamine and norepinephrine neurons (Fig. 6).

Step 1: Uptake of Tryptophan

Tryptophan, like other large neutral amino acids is taken up actively by brain cells. Cellular concentration of the amino acids depends upon dietary intake, and varies rapidly within a few minutes to hours with changes in circulating levels in the blood. Uptake into brain is suppressed by excess amounts of other amino acids of the same class.

Step 2: Enzymatic Synthesis

Tryptophan is converted to 5-hydroxytryptophan by the enzyme tryptophan hydroxylase. The subsequent conversion to serotonin is accomplished by the enzyme L-aminodecarboxylase, which appears to be identical to that responsible for the synthesis of norepinephrine.[49] The conversion of tryptophan to 5-hydroxytryptophan can be blocked by p-chlorophenylalanine, and the conversion to serotonin can be blocked by disulfiram. In tissues, such as the pineal gland and the retina, serotonin is converted to

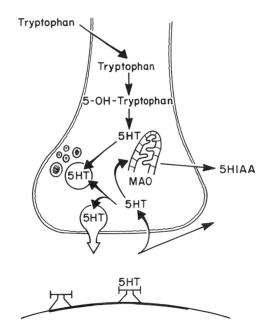

Figure 6. Schematic representation of a central serotonergic synapse. See text for abbreviations. (Modified from Cooper, J. C., Bloom, F. E. and Roth, R. H.: *The Biochemical Basis of Neuropharmacology.* Oxford University Press, New York, 1974.)

melatonin, an indoleamine that is also present in the brain and which may function as a neurotransmitter, although the evidence is not compelling at this time.[40] Evidence is also accumulating that serotonin can be converted to N-acetylserotonin in cerebellum and brain stem; the function of this substance is unknown.

Step 3: Storage Phase

Serotonin, like NE and DA, is stored in granules in nerve endings, complexed with a protein carrier and ATP. The storage mechanism for serotonin is also analogous to that of the catecholamines, since it is abolished by the same drugs, reserpine and tetrabenazine, which cause a depletion of serotonin.

Step 4: Release Phase

The control of the release process has not been completely established. It is likely that release of storage granules at nerve terminals occurs in response to a propagated action potential.

Step 5: Interaction of Serotonin with Receptors Located on the Postsynaptic Membrane

Serotonin probably intereacts with specific receptors on the postsynaptic membrane. A number of serotonin analogues may mimic serotonin-agonist functions, including quipazine and the hallucinogenic drug LSD which may act in some way to increase effective serotonin levels at the receptor site. Important serotonin antagonists that have been widely used for study of hypophysiotrophic neuropharmacology are methysergide and cyproheptadine.[29, 33] The specificity of these antagonists has not been established with complete certainty, particularly in the central nervous system.

Table 1. Actions of Pharmacologic Agents and Effects on Anterior Pituitary Secretion

Drug	Trade Name	Mechanisms of Action	Effect on Monoamines
Precursors			
L-dopa	Larodopa	Increases substrate for DA and NE formation	Increases DA and NE levels in brain
Tryptophan and 5-OH-tryptophan		Increases substrate for serotonin formation	Increases serotonin level in brain
Receptor Agonists (Stimulators)			
Apomorphine Bromergocryptine	CB-154	Stimulate dopamine receptors	Mimics dopamine effects
Clonidine	Catapres	Stimulates α-adrenergic receptors	Mimics α-receptor effects
Isoproterenol	Isuprel	Stimulates β-adrenergic receptors	Mimics β-receptor effects
Quipazine LSD		Stimulates serotonin receptors	Mimics serotonin effects
Receptor Blockers			
Pimozide Haloperidol Chlorpromazine	Haldol Largactil Thorazine	Blocks dopamine receptors (and NE receptors in large doses)	Prevents dopamine effects
Phentolamine Phenoxybenazmine	Rogitine Dibenzylene	α-adrenergic blocker	Blocks peripheral and central α-receptors
Propranolol	Inderal	β-adrenergic blocker	Blocks peripheral and central β-receptors
Cyproheptadine Methysergide	Periactin Sansert	Serotonin receptor blocker	Blocks peripheral and central serotonin receptors
Enzyme Inhibitors			
α-methyl-p-tyrosine		Inhibits tyrosine hydroxylase	Blocks formation of DA and NE
Disulfram fusaric acid	Antabuse	Blocks dopamine-β-oxidase	Blocks formation of norepinephrine
p-chlorophenylalanine		Blocks tryptophan hydroxylase	Blocks formation of serotonin
Precursor Analogues			
α-methyldopa	Aldomet	Converted into methylated monoamine	Acts as a false transmitter
Presynaptic Storage Blockers			
Reserpine	Serpasil	Inhibits storage and reuptake of biogenic amines by granules	Depletion of DA, NE and serotonin in terminals
Tricyclic antidepressants	Imipramine, Chlorimipramine, etc.	Blocks reuptake by nerve terminals	Depletes terminals of catecholamines and serotonin
Mixed Function			
Amphetamines		Releases biogenic amines, blocks reuptake	Increases NE turnover, increases availability of NE
Catecholaminergic Nerve Ending Poisons			
6-hydroxydopamine		Localizes to catecholamine nerve endings	Destroys dopaminergic and noradrenergic terminals

Key: ↑ increases; ↓ decreases; → no effect; ? not tested

Data are based chiefly on work in rats, monkey and man. Since there are species differences in effects of these agents, and all agents have not been tested in all three species, this table is incomplete and possibly inaccurate in some details.
*Data are conflicting; partially blocks insulin-induced GH release, but increases sleep release.

54

Effect on Anterior Pituitary Secretion				
Growth Hormone	Prolactin	Gonadotropin	TSH	ACTH
↑	↓	→	blocks response to TRH	→
↑	↑	→	↓	↑
↑	↓	→	→	→
↑	→	→	→	→
↓	→	?	?	?
?	?	?	?	?
↓	↑	↓ blocks ovulation	→	→
↓ GH responses	→	→	→	↓ response to insulin
↑ GH responses	→	→	→	↑ response to insulin
↓↑ GH responses* sleep release	↓ stress and sleep release	→	→	↓ response to insulin hypoglycemia
↓↑	↑ suckling response	blocks ovulation ?	?	↑ ?
↓	↓	?	?	?
?	↑	?	?	?
↓ GH sleep release	↑	blocks ovulation →	→	↑ →
↑	↑	?	?	↑
?	↑	?	?	?

Step 6: Re-Uptake Process

As with catecholamines, the action of the neurotransmitter is terminated by re-uptake from the synaptic cleft into the presynaptic nerve ending. Drugs such as the tricyclic antidepressants imipramine and amitryptyline potentiate serotonin effects by inhibiting the re-uptake process.

Step 7: Enzymatic Degradation

As with catecholamines, the enzyme monoamine oxidase (MAO) degrades free serotonin in the nerve ending. The product of this metabolism is 5-hydroxyindoleacetic acid (5-HIAA). Agents such as pargyline that interfere with MAO also potentiate serotonin effects.

Effects of Serotonin on Hypophysiotrophic Neurons

Understanding the role of serotonergic neurons in anterior pituitary regulation is based largely on pharmacologic manipulations, all of which have inherent limitations. 5-Hydroxytryptophan administration, known to increase serotonin formation, is followed by the release of prolactin,[23] suggesting that there is an excitatory serotonergic pathway. This hypothesis is confirmed by the finding that stress-induced prolactin release is blocked by methysergide, a serotonin antagonist. Suckling-induced prolactin release in the rat is also reported to be blocked by administration of parachlorophenylalanine, an inhibitor of serotonin synthesis. Electric stimulation of the raphe nucleus in the rat results in growth-hormone release.

It is reasonable to postulate that serotonin receptors on certain classes of hypophysiotrophic neurons activate the cyclic AMP mechanism, leading to biosynthesis of releasing factors and possibly to release mechanisms analogous to those postulated for the catecholamine-dependent neurons.

A summary of drugs used clinically and in the experimental elucidation of neurotransmitter control of hypophysiotrophic function is presented in Table 1.[9, 11, 12, 16, 17]

Central Histaminergic Pathways

Histamine is a normal brain constituent; approximately 50 per cent is present in perivascular mast cells, and the remainder is postulated to be in neurons. Histamine is localized in both the hypothalamus and anterior and posterior pituitary; in the hypothalamus, highest concentrations are found in the median eminence.[5, 39, 41] A specific enzyme, histidine decarboxylase, is present in selective regions of the brain including the hypothalamus, and acts on the precursor amino acid histidine to form histamine. Selective unilateral lesions in the lateral hypothalamus that interrupt the medial forebrain bundle cause depletion of histamine in the cortex, hippocampus, and hypothalamus of the same side. Histamine is also present in synaptosome preparations of cortex, and microintophoresis onto single nerve cells causes excitation or, more rarely, depression of cellular activity. On the basis of these observations, Schwartz[39] has postulated that a histaminergic system exists in the brain analogous to the catecholaminergic and serotonergic systems and that histamine may act as a neurotransmitter.

Relatively little is known of the functional significance of histamine in neuroendocrine control. Hypothalamic lesions cause depletion of histamine in the posterior pituitary. Histamine is reported to release GH in man but the effects may be nonspecific via a stress mechanism.

Cholinergic Pathways in Neuroendocrine Regulation

The detailed knowledge now available about central biogenic amine pathways summarized above is a reflection of the intensity of research into neuroleptic drugs and biogenic amine localization in the brain, including the hypothalamus. However, there is evidence that cholinergic pathways are also involved in pituitary regulation.[28, 36] The classic example of this is the neurohypophysial neuron which is activated functionally and electrically by cholinergic drugs, contains membrane-bound acetylcholinesterase and is blocked by anticholinergic agents (see Chapter 4). In the rabbit, reflex ovulation is blocked by large doses of atropine, and pharamacologic studies by Krieger[28] suggest that ACTH is stimulated by a cholinergic system. Unfortunately, surprisingly little is known about the function of cholinergic structures in the brain. The enzyme choline acetyltransferase functions in brain to induce acetylcholine formation. Both muscarinic and nicotinic receptors are present in brain; their role in neurohypophysial control is outlined in Chapter 4. Acetylcholinesterase, a membrane-bound enzyme that inactivates acetylcholine has widespread distribution in the brain.

Most drugs that block cholinergic systems do not penetrate the blood-brain barrier. The few that do (atropine, scopolamine, and diisopropyl phosphorofluoridate) produce marked behavioral effects including nightmares, confusion, hallucinations, agitation, and slowing of intellectual and motor processes; the specific neuroanatomic sites of action are unknown. Among the unsolved problems preventing delineation of central cholinergic mechanisms in pituitary regulation are those summarized by Baldessarini and Karobath:

> The general unavailability of potent and specific inhibitors of choline acetyltransferase and the toxicity of the potent acetylcholinesterase inhibitors have limited attempts to study the physiological role of ACH in the CNS by altering its metabolism. Another difficulty is the lack of methods to delineate precisely central cholinergic pathways. Histochemical methods for acetylcholinesterase demonstrate its rather diffuse distribution throughout the CNS. Furthermore there are no specific and sufficiently sensitive histochemical reactions for ACH which are suitable for use in mammalian brain tissue. Newer histochemical methods for choline acetyltransferase may provide a more specific means of localizing cholinergic cells.[4]

These uncertainties suggest that the study of cholinergic control of pituitary function, particularly of the neurohypophysis, may be a potent tool for the elucidation of the role of acetylcholine in central synapses.

REFERENCES

1. ANTON-TAY, F., PELHAM, R. W., WURTMAN, R. J.: *Increased turnover of ³H-norepinephrine in rat brain following castration or treatment with ovine follicle stimulating hormone.* Endocrinology 84: 1489, 1969.

2. ANTON-TAY, F. AND WURTMAN, R. J.: *Norepinephrine: turnover in rat brains after gonadectomy.* Science 159:1245, 1968.

3. AXELROD, J.: *Neurotransmitters.* Sci. Am. 230(6):59, 1974.

4. BALDESSARINI, R. J. AND KOROBATH, M.: *Biochemical physiology of central synapses.* Ann. Rev. Physiol. 35:273, 1973.

5. BROWNSTEIN, M. J., ET AL.: *Histamine content of hypothalamic nuclei of the rat.* Brain Res. 77:151, 1974.

6. CARLSSON, A., FALCK, B. AND HILLARP, N. A.: *Cellular localization of brain monoamines.* Acta Physiol. Scand. [Suppl.] 196:1, 1962.

7. CHALMERS, J. P., BALDESSARINI, R. J. AND WURTMAN, R. J.: *Effects of L-dopa on norepinephrine metabolism in the brain.* Proc. Natl. Acad. Sci. USA 68:662, 1971.

8. COOPER, J. R., BLOOM, F. E. AND ROTH, R. H.: *The Biochemical Basis of Neuropharmacology.* Oxford University Press, New York.

9. CORRODI, H., ET AL.: *Effect of ergot drugs on central catecholamine neurons: Evidence for a stimulation of central dopamine neurons.* J. Pharm. Pharmacol. 25:409, 1973.

10. DAHLSTROM, A. AND FUXE, K.: *Evidence for the existence of monoamine neurons in the central nervous system. II. Experimentally induced changes in the intraneuronal amine levels of bulbospinal neuron system.* Acta Physiol. Scand. [Suppl.] 247:1, 1965.

11. DEWIED, D. AND DE JONG, W.: *Drug effects and hypothalamic anterior pituitary function.* Ann. Rev. Pharmacol. 14:389, 1974.

12. DONOSO, A. O., ET AL.: *Effects of drugs that modify brain monoamine concentrations of plasma gonadotropin and prolactin levels in the rat.* Endocrinology 89:774, 1971.

13. DONOVAN, B. T. AND HARRIS, G. W.: *Adrenergic agents and the release of gonadotrophic hormone in the rabbit.* J. Physiol. (London) 132:577, 1956.

14. FALCK, B., HILLARP, N. A. AND TORP, A.: *Fluorescence of catecholamines and related compounds condensed with formaldehyde.* J. Histochem. Cytochem. 10:348, 1962.

15. FERNSTROM, J. D. AND WURTMAN, R. J.: *Brain serotonin content: physiological dependence on plasma tryptophan levels.* Science 173:149, 1971.

16. FROHMAN, L. A.: *Clinical neuropharmacology of hypothalamic releasing factors.* N. Engl. J. Med. 286: 1391, 1972.

17. FROHMAN, L. A. AND STACHURA, M. E.: *Neuropharmacologic control of neuroendocrine function in man.* Metabolism 24:211, 1975.

18. FUXE, K. AND HOKFELT, T.: *Catecholamines in the hypothalamus and the pituitary gland. In:* Ganong, W. F. and Martini, L. (eds.): *Frontiers in Neuroendocrinology, 1969.* Oxford University Press, New York, 1969, p. 47.

19. FUXE, K.: *Evidence for the existence of monoamine neurons in the central nervous system. IV. Distribution of monoamine nerve terminals in the central nervous system.* Acta Physiol. Scand. [Suppl] 247:39, 1965.

20. GRIMM, Y. AND REICHLIN, S.: *Thyrotropin releasing hormone (TPH): neurotransmitter regulation of secretion by mouse hypothalamic tissue in vitro.* Endocrinology 93:626, 1973.

21. HOKFELT, T., ET AL.: *Immunohistochemical evidence for the existence of adrenaline neurons in the rat brain.* Brain Res. 66:235, 1974.

22. IMURA, H., NAKAI, Y. AND YOSHIMA, T.: *Effect of 5-hydroxytryptophan on growth hormone and ACTH release in man.* J. Clin. Endocrinol. Metab. 35:204, 1973.

23. KATO, Y., ET AL.: *Effect of 5-hydroxytroptophan (5-HTP) on plasma prolactin levels in man.* J. Clin. Endocrinol. Metab. 38:695, 1974.

24. KAMBERI, I. A., SCHNEIDER, H. P. G. AND McCANN, S. M.: *Action of dopamine to induce release of FSH-releasing factor (FRF) from hypothalamic tissue in vitro.* Endocrinology 86:278, 1970.

25. KAMBERI, I. A., MICAL, R. S. AND PORTER, J. C.: *Luteinizing hormone-releasing activity in hypophysial stalk blood and elevation by dopamine.* Science 166:388, 1969.

26. KLEINBERG, D. L., NOEL, G. L. AND FRANTZ, A. G.: *Chlorpromazine stimulation and L-dopa suppression of plasma prolactin in man.* J. Clin. Endocrinol. Metab. 33:873, 1971.

27. KOPIN, I. J.: *False adrenergic transmitters.* Annu. Rev. Pharmacol. 8:377, 1968.

28. KRIEGER, D. T.: *Neurotransmitter regulation of ACTH release.* Mt. Sinai J. Med. NY, 40:302, 1973.

29. LAL, S., ET AL.: *Effect of apomorphine on growth hormone, prolactin, luteinizing hormone and follicle stimulating hormone levels in human serum.* J. Clin. Endocrinol. Metab. 37:719, 1973.

30. LICHTENSTEIGER, W.: *Cyclic variations of catecholamine content in hypothalamic nerve cells during the estrous cycle of the rat, with a concomitant study of the substantia nigra.* J. Pharmacol. Exp. Ther. 165: 204, 1969.

31. NAKAI, Y., ET AL.: *Effect of cyproheptadine on human growth hormone secretion.* J. Clin. Endocrinol. Metab. 38:446, 1974.

32. PALKOVITS, M., ET AL.: *Norepinephrine and dopamine content of hypothalamic nuclei of the rat.* Brain Res. 77:137, 1974.

33. PLONK, J. W., BIVENS, C. H. AND FELDMAN, J. M.: *Inhibition of hypoglycemia-induced cortisol secretion by the serotonin antagonist cyproheptadine.* J. Clin. Endocrinol. Metab. 38:836, 1974.

34. SAAVEDRA, J. M., ET AL.: *Serotonin distribution in the nuclei of the rat hypothalamus and preoptic region.* Brain Res. 77:157, 1974.

35. SAAVEDRA, J. M., ET AL.: *Distribution of biogenic amines and related enzymes in the rat pituitary gland.* J. Neurochem. 25:257, 1975.

36. SAWYER, C. H., MARKEE, J.E. AND TOWNSEND, B. F.: *Cholinergic and adrenergic components in neurohumoral control of release of LH in rabbits.* Endocrinology 44:18, 1949.

37. SAWYER, C. H.: *First Geoffrey Harris Memorial Lecture—Some recent developments in brain-pituitary ovarian physiology.* Neuroendocrinology 17:97, 1974.

38. SCHNEIDER, H. P. G. AND McCANN, S. M.: *Release of LH-releasing factor (LRF) into the peripheral circulation of hypophysectomized rats by dopamine and its blockage by estradiol.* Endocrinology 87: 249, 1970b.

39. SCHWARTZ, J. C.: *Histamine as a transmitter in brain.* Life Sci. 17:503, 1975.

40. SMYTHE, G. A. AND LAZARUS, L.: *Growth hormone regulation by melatonin and serotonin.* Nature 244: 230, 1973.

41. SNYDER, S. H. AND TAYLOR, K. M.: *Histamine in the brain: a neurotransmitter? In* Snyder, S. (ed.): *Perspectives in Neuropharmacology.* Oxford University Press, New York, p. 43, 1972.

42. SULSER, F. AND SANDERS-BUSH, E.: *Effect of drugs on amines in the CNS.* Annu. Rev. Pharmacol. 11: 209, 1971.

43. VANLOON, G. R., ET AL.: *Effect of intraventricular administration of adrenergic drugs on the adrenal venous 17-hydroxycorticosteroid response to surgical stress in the dog.* Neuroendocrinology 8:257, 1971.

44. VOGT, M.: *Concentration of sympathin in different parts of central nervous system under normal conditions and after administration of drugs.* J. Physiol. (Lond.) 123:451, 1954.

45. WEINER, N.: *Regulation of norepinephrine biosynthesis.* Annu. Rev. Pharmacol. 10:273, 1970.

46. WEINER, R. I.: *Hypothalamic monoamine levels and gonadotrophin secretion following differentiation of the medial basal hypothalamus.* Progr. Brain Res. 39:165, 1973.

47. WURTMAN, R. J.: *Brain catecholamines and the control of secretion from the anterior pituitary gland. In* Meites, J. (ed.): *Hypophysiotropic Hormones of the Hypothalamus: Assay and Chemistry.* Williams & Wilkins, Baltimore, 1970, p. 184.

48. WURTMAN, R. J.: *Brain monoamines and endocrine function.* Neurosci. Res. Program Bull. 9:172, 1971.

49. WURTMAN, R. J. AND FERNSTOM, J. D.: *L-tryptophan, L-tyrosine, and the control of brain monoamine biosynthesis. In* Snyder, S. H.(ed.): *Perspectives in Neuropharmacology.* Oxford University Press, New York, 1972, p. 143.

BIBLIOGRAPHY

COOPER, J. R., BLOOM, F. E. AND ROTH, R. H.: *The Biochemical Basis of Neuropharmacology.* Oxford University Press, New York, 1974.

FUXE, K. AND HOKFELT, T.: *Catecholamines in the hypothalamus and the pituitary gland. In* Ganong, W. F. and Martini, L. (eds.): *Frontiers In Neuroendocrinology, 1969.* Oxford University Press, New York, 1969.

IVERSEN, L. L.: *How do antipsychotic drugs work? The F. O. Schmitt Lecture in Neuroscience, 1974.* Neurosci. Res. Program Bull. 13 [Suppl]: 29, 1975.

KOPIN, I. J. (ED.): *Neurotransmitters.* Williams & Wilkins, Baltimore, 1972.

SAWYER, C. H.: *First Geoffrey Harris Memorial Lecture—Some recent developments in brain-pituitary ovarian physiology.* Neuroendocrinology 17:97, 1974.

SNYDER, S. H. (ED.): *Perspectives in Neuropharmacology.* Oxford University Press, New York, 1971.

WURTMAN, R. J.: *Catecholamines.* Little, Brown and Co., Boston, 1966.

WURTMAN, R. J.: *Brain catecholamines and the control of secretion from the anterior pituitary gland. In* Meites, J. (ed.): *Hypophysiotrophic Hormones of the Hypothalamus: Assay and Chemistry.* Williams & Wilkins, Baltimore, 1970, p. 184.

PART II

CLINICAL NEUROENDOCRINOLOGY

Neural Regulation of Water and Salt Metabolism: Physiologic Function and Disease

Plasma osmolarity and effective circulating blood volume are among the most jealously guarded features of the internal milieu. Homeostatic mechanisms maintain their constancy by regulating the excretion and intake of water and salt, physiologic processes both of which depend heavily on central nervous system integrating mechanisms. These include:

1. Regulation of the secretion of antidiuretic hormone (ADH, vasopressin) which controls free-water clearance of the kidney through its actions on tubular reabsorption of water.
2. Regulation of the thirst mechanism by peripheral blood volume receptors, by central neural receptors of blood osmolarity, and possibly by circulating angiotensin.
3. Regulation of renin secretion, which in turn determines the activity of the angiotensin-aldosterone system, the principal salt-regulating hormonal system.

Neural factors have also been implicated in the regulation of sodium ion excretion by kidney tubules, through control of intrarenal circulatory dynamics or through a postulated hormonal "third factor" believed to be secreted by the hypothalamus. In this chapter, the elements of these mechanisms will be discussed and related to clinical disorders of salt and water metabolism.

THE NEUROHYPOPHYSIS

The neural lobe develops embryologically as a downgrowth from the ventral diencephalon and retains its neural connections and neural character in adult life. The dominating features of the neurohypophysis are the supraoptic-hypophysial and paraventricular-hypophysial nerve tracts.[9, 37] These unmyelinated nerve tracts arise from the supraoptic and paraventricular nuclei within the hypothalamus, and descend through the infundibulum and neural stalk to terminate in the neural lobe (posterior pituitary) (Fig. 1).[14, 43]

Neurohypophysial Hormones

The function of the posterior pituitary was a mystery as late as the end of the nineteenth century. Oliver and Schafer[49] in 1895 injected extracts of bovine posterior lobe and demonstrated increases in blood pressure. These pressor effects, seen only with large doses of extract, are now regarded as being physiologically unimportant for blood

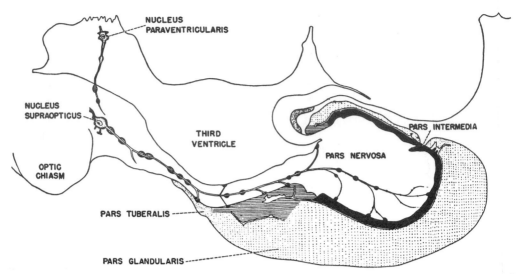

Figure 1. Diagram of hypothalamic-neurohypophysial system in the dog. Axons of neurons in the supraoptic and paraventricular nuclei traverse the pituitary stalk to end in the posterior pituitary (pars nervosa). The dilated areas on the axon represent neurosecretory material (NSM). Electron microscopy indicates that the NSM is within the unmyelinated axons. (From Bargmann, W. and Scharrer, E.: *The site of origin of hormones of the posterior pituitary. Am. Scient. 39:225, 1951, with permission.)*

pressure regulation; but over the succeeding twenty years, additional biologic effects of neurohypophysial extracts were defined, including antidiuretic, oxytocic (uterine-contraction stimulating), and milk-ejecting effects, the latter mediated by contraction of periacinar myoepithelial cells in the breast. Not until 1949, however, was the chemical nature of these substances identified by DuVigneaud and associates, who isolated oxytocin and determined its structure.[17] Subsequently, between 1951 and 1953, these workers elucidated the structure of ADH. Their landmark work established that the neurohypophysial hormones were small polypeptides, composed of eight amino acids, and paved the way for the structural elucidation of larger, more complex polypeptide hormones of the pituitary, and of other glands. DuVigneaud's studies have been the model for the attack on the structure of the hypophysiotrophic hormones of the hypothalamus, and the practical and theoretic benefits that have arisen from the ability to synthesize these hormones have provided a continuing stimulus to workers in this field. The structures of ADH and oxytocin in the human are remarkably similar, differing by only two amino acids. Each octapeptide contains a disulfide link and a terminal amide group (Fig. 2). The chemistry and phylogenetic implications of neurohypophysial hormone structure have been studied in detail by Sawyer.[59] These hormones have also been the subject of intense study of structure-activity relationships, molecular configuration, and molecular-receptor binding. To a very real degree, development of understanding of hypothalamic-hypophysiotrophic function at the molecular level has followed understanding of the more readily-approached neurohypophysial system.

Regulation of ADH Secretion

The classic experiments which led to an identification of the mechanisms regulating ADH secretion were those of Verney[66] who demonstrated in dogs the effects of increased plasma osmolarity, exercise, and emotional stress. In 1947 he showed that systemically ineffective amounts of hypertonic sodium chloride are highly effective as an antidiuretic agent when injected directly into the carotid arteries. Sucrose, but not glu-

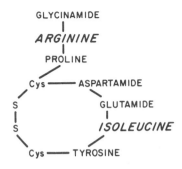

ARGININE VASOTOCIN

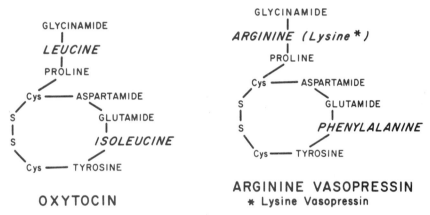

OXYTOCIN

ARGININE VASOPRESSIN
* Lysine Vasopressin

Figure 2. Structures of oxytocin, arginine vasopressin, and arginine vasotocin. The latter is present in the human pineal gland. Lysine vasopressin is present in the pig.

cose or urea, produced a similar effect. From these observations, he concluded that the brain was sensitive to alterations in osmolarity when the osmotic stimulus was produced by substances that were largely excluded from cells. The necessary role of the neurohypophysis in the antidiuretic effect was shown by appropriate ablation experiments. A decade later, he localized the region of the brain which is critical for this antidiuretic effect to the anterior hypothalamus, in the region of the supraoptic and paraventricular nuclei. As a consequence of Verney's work, the term *osmoreceptor* was applied to cells within the brain which monitor extracellular osmolality. Characteristically, such cells show alterations in electrical firing rates in association with osmotic stimuli. Verney pioneered in his delineation of neural control of osmotic balance, but his work was also important in the development of a strategy in neuroendocrine investigations. He showed that emotional factors were important in ADH regulation, thus pointing out, for the first time, the role of such stress in neuroendocrine regulation. He also adapted the classic Sherringtonian approach of the neurologist to identify a neuroendocrine reflex analogous to a spinal reflex. This involves the identification of a receptor for afferent stimuli, and a motor component effecting hormone secretion. Like Sherrington, Verney emphasized the use of selective neurologic ablations to identify neural pathways of neuroendocrine control. This approach, now taken for granted, has been widely used for studies of anterior as well as posterior pituitary secretion.

65

Specificity of Control of ADH and Oxytocin Secretion

The concept of a distinct neuronal control mechanism for the two neurohypophysial hormones is supported by the fact that each of the hormones can be discharged in response to appropriate stimuli, with little or no release of the other hormone. For example, suckling causes prompt release of oxytocin without significant effects on diuresis; and conversely, osmotic stimuli have little effect on oxytocin release. While there is some overlap in the secretion of these hormones, earlier ablative and electric stimulation studies suggested that ADH was synthesized mainly by cells of the supraoptic nuclei, whereas oxytocin arises from paraventricular cells. Bilateral lesions in the paraventricular nuclei cause depletion of oxytocin in the neural lobe without detectable change in the ADH content, and oxytocin and ADH can be released relatively independently by selective hypothalamic electrical stimulation of the appropriate nuclear group.

The problem of specificity of localization and function has recently been approached by Zimmerman and colleagues[71] with the aid of immunohistochemical techniques utilizing antisera reacting either with ADH or oxytocin. In man (and rat) ADH is found in virtually all cells of the supraoptic nuclei and in many but not all of the cells of the paraventricular nucleus as well. Oxytocin-containing cells were also found in both neurohypophysial nuclei. Both oxytocin and ADH were present in many of the same cells. The characteristic neurophysins which bind ADH or oxytocin were found in cells containing the appropriate neurohypophysial hormone (Fig. 3).

Neurohypophysial Hormone Synthesis

The neurohypophysial hormones are synthesized as part of a prohormone in the perikaryon (cell body) by classic protein-synthetic pathways[31] which include formation on ribosomes, condensation in the Golgi apparatus, and storage in granules.[58] The hormones appear to be formed in association with, or as part of, a larger molecule, neurophysin, which has the role of a carrier substance in the granule.[12, 13, 67] There are two major classes of neurophysin, one that binds oxytocin, and another that binds ADH. The characteristic staining of neurosecretory granules in the supraoptic and paraventricular pathways (the Gomorri staining of neurosecretions of Scharrer[60] and Bargmann[6]) is due to the high cysteine content of both neurophysin and the octapeptides. From the cell body, the neurosecretory vesicles pass into nerve endings by axonal streaming. The rate of transport is estimated to be several hundred mm. per day, which is considerably faster than the overall rate of axoplasmic flow (as estimated from regeneration of nerves) and is the same order of magnitude as the rate of flow of neuronal catecholaminergic secretory granules.[25] These findings suggest that there is a form of saltatory progression, possibly mediated by contractile neurotubular elements in the neurons.

Electrophysiology of Neurohypophysial Control

Current evidence supports the hypothesis that release of ADH and oxytocin from the neurohypophysis is initiated by the summated depolarization of the axon terminals of the neurosecretory neurons that comprise the hypothalamic-neurohypophysial system.[4, 5] An increased rate of neuronal firing results in increased hormone release, whereas diminished cellular activity causes decreased hormone secretion. Although not strictly proven, this concept has been widely used as the basis for experimental analysis of the factors which influence the secretion of the octapeptides.

The spontaneous discharge rate of hypothalamic neurosecretory cells is slow, usually

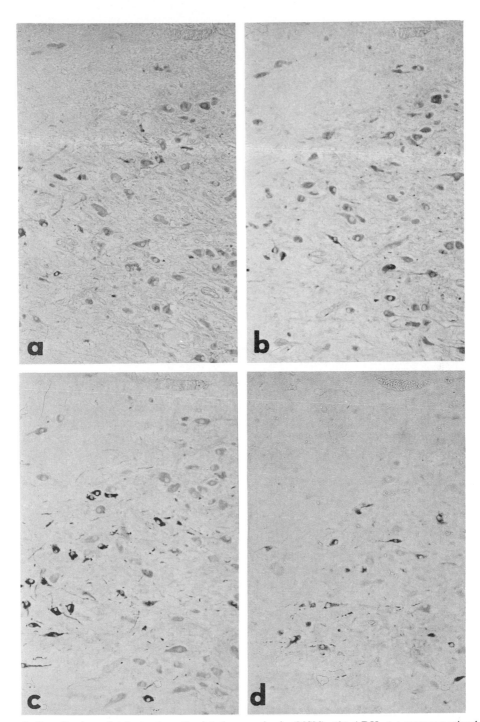

Figure 3. Localization of *(a)* nicotine-stimulated neurophysin (NSN), *(b)* ADH, *(c)* estrogen-stimulated neurophysin (ESN), and *(d)* oxytocin, in serial sections of human supraoptic nucleus by immunoperoxidase method. NSN and ADH appear to be contained in virtually all perikarya, while ESN and oxytocin are found together in a smaller population of cells. (×100) *(a, b* and *c* from Zimmerman, E. A., et al.: *The distribution of neurophysin-secreting pathways in mammalian brain: Light microscopic studies using the immunoperoxidase technique.* Ann. N. Y. Acad. Sci. 248:92, 1975; *d* from Zimmerman, E. A.: *Localization of hypothalamic hormones by immunocytochemical techniques.* In Martini, L. and Ganong, W. F. (eds.): *Frontiers in Neuroendocrinology,* vol. 4, Raven Press, New York, 1976, with permission.)

less than one discharge per second.[4, 19, 34-36] A number of investigators (using extracellular electrodes) have reported changes in cellular firing rates in the supraoptic nucleus following administration of hypertonic saline.[4, 26, 33] More recently, intracellular recordings have been successfully made in supraoptic neurons in the dog and cat.[42] The cells possess resting transmembrane potentials of -50 to -80 mV. and both excitatory and inhibitory postsynaptic potentials have been identified in these cells. By a combination of single-unit recording and antidromic stimulation, Koizumi and Yamashita[42] found that not all osmoreceptive cells are antidromically excitable. These findings suggest that at least some cells sensitive to osmotic changes are separate from the large neurosecretory cells, and perhaps function as interneurons. Conversely, not all antidromically excitable cells were influenced by osmotic changes. Although osmoreceptor cells have also been identified in other regions of the brain and spinal cord, it has been repeatedly shown that animals with hypothalamic islands are capable of maintaining normal water balance, indicating that the necessary components for basal fluid regulation reside within this region of the brain. The mechanisms by which cells in the brain (neuronal or otherwise) monitor osmotic changes are unknown. It has been proposed that such cells are responsive to altered size as mechanoreceptors, or that the membrane is specifically altered by minor changes in hydration.[37]

Hayward and Jennings,[34-36] in a series of neurophysiologic experiments, have further characterized neurosecretory cells in the unanesthetized monkey. Using antidromic stimulation, several types of cells were identified. The majority of cells were characterized by a steady but irregular firing pattern. Presumably these cells are tonically active and release steady-state quantities of the neurohypophysial hormones. A smaller number of cells (21 per cent) were found to be activated in a regular, repetitive, periodic-burst pattern which was immediately influenced by osmotic stimuli but not by other stimuli such as stress, sensory inputs, or changes in the waking state. These findings suggest that stimulus-specific populations of cells exist within the supraoptic nucleus. Although cell bodies of the supraoptic nucleus are large, the axons are small (0.1 to 0.3 μ in diameter), unmyelinated, and their conduction velocity (0.4 to 0.9 m./sec.) estimated by antidromic stimulation is similar to that of unmyelinated peripheral nerve fibers of comparable size.

Recurrent Collateral Inhibition

Neuroendocrine cells in the supraoptic nucleus of the monkey show excitatory-inhibitory sequences following activation. A recurrent collateral inhibitory mechanism analogous to the Renshaw cell in the spinal cord is suggested by these findings.[19, 35, 36, 47] It may be postulated that this mechanism functions to prevent excessive discharges from such cells. Disorders of the inhibitory impulse could conceivably account for the inappropriate antidiuretic hormone secretion which occurs in certain brain diseases.

The fact that direct electric stimulation of the neurohypophysis discharges supraoptic neurons antidromically has been useful in clarifying the mechanism of responses in these cells. Such experiments have suggested that supraoptic neurons receive recurrent collateral inhibition. This inhibition is accompanied by hyperpolarization of the transmembrane potential within supraoptic cells, indicating the presence of true inhibitory postsynaptic potentials (IPSP) and giving support to the hypothesis that neurosecretory neurons are capable of forming synapses on other neurons. It has been proposed that either the neurosecretory product itself (ADH or oxytocin) or some other transmitter substance formed in the neuron might be implicated in recurrent inhibition. The microiontophoretic studies of Nicoll and Barker[47] suggest that either a muscarinic cholinergic receptor or a norepinephrine receptor, or both, can induce this inhibition. Norepinephrine was considered an unlikely possibility because treatment of animals with 6-hydroxydopamine (with attendant destruction of catecholaminergic neurons in the brain) did not prevent the recurrent inhibitory response. Significant inhibition after antidromic activation occurred in many cells after the application of ADH to the supraoptic nucleus, raising the interesting possibility that release of ADH at recurrent synapses might function in a negative feedback fashion to regulate its own secretion.

Volume Receptor Control

In addition to local osmoreceptor responses, afferent inputs from volume receptors outside the brain to the supraoptic neurons also influence ADH secretion.[3] Changes in "effective" blood volume after depletion in total blood volume, or following fluid shifts within the cardiovascular system, stimulate the afferent limb of the ADH reflex arc which is located in aortic baroreceptors and in cardiac stretch receptors within the subendocardial portion of the left atrium.[26, 62] Mechanical stretch of the atrium leads to a rapid and effective diuretic response (presumably through inhibition of ADH secretion) which can be blocked by cooling or sectioning of the vagus nerve.[62] The central pathways by which these responses are relayed to the neurosecretory neurons of the hypothalamus have not been entirely elucidated. However, direct stimulations of both the vagus and carotid sinus nerves have been shown to produce increased firing rates in supraoptic neurons. Transverse sections through the midbrain abolish the reflex, whereas section at the cervical-medullary level does not.

ADH Secretion in Man

The recent development of radioimmunoassay for plasma ADH in man has confirmed the extensive earlier studies of osmotic control of ADH secretion, based on physiologic studies of renal free-water clearance.[8, 38, 56, 63] Recumbent normal subjects studied by Robertson and coworkers[53] had a plasma osmolality of 287 ± 2.1 mOsm./ml. and a plasma ADH level of 2.7 ± 1.4 pg./ml. After 16 to 20 hours of fluid deprivation which resulted in a significant rise in plasma osmolality to 292 mOsm./ml., plasma ADH rose to 5.4 ± 3.4 pg./ml. Conversely, administration of a water load resulted in a reduction in ADH levels to 1.4 ± 0.8 pg./ml. These are surprisingly small changes in plasma hormone levels when compared with anterior pituitary hormone fluctuations in plasma. Responses to stressful stimuli and to hemorrhage are much greater than to osmotic perturbations.

The importance of the baroreceptor regulation of ADH release has also been demonstrated in man. Assumption of the upright position is accompanied by a significant, abrupt increase in plasma ADH levels. Acute stresses also increase the secretion of ADH in man as well as animals. This response accounts for the well-established antidiuretic effects of pain or anxiety.

ADH circulates unbound in the plasma, where its half-life is about 15 to 25 minutes. It is removed from the circulation predominantly by renal and hepatic routes. Factors that influence ADH secretion in man are summarized in Figure 4 and Table 1.

Neurotransmitter Regulation

In addition to the direct osmotic control of ADH by osmoreceptors, there is evidence that cholinergic and adrenergic inputs to the magnocellular neurons influence cellular activity and mediate reflex control of secretion.[5, 19, 46, 68] An excitatory role for acetylcholine in ADH release was proposed as early as 1939, when Pickford[51] reported that intravenous administration of acetylcholine caused inhibition of water diuresis in dogs, a response dependent on an intact neurohypophysis. She later reported that direct

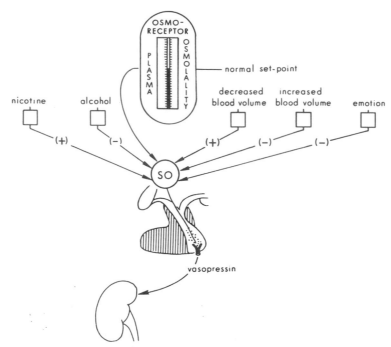

Figure 4. Control of ADH (vasopressin) release. The normal stimulus for ADH release is plasma osmolality higher than the normal setpoint, which is usually constant but may be altered in disease. ADH release can also be increased by severe decrease in blood volume or by administration of nicotine (or its absorption in tobacco smoking). ADH release can be decreased by reduction in plasma osmolality, increase in blood volume, or administration of alcohol. Generally, emotional stress results in decreased ADH release and hence produces polyuria. (From Ezrin, C., et al.: *Systematic Endocrinology*. Harper and Row, New York, 1973, p. 19, with permission.)

injection of acetylcholine into the supraoptic region of anesthetized dogs also caused antidiuresis. Intracarotid or intraventricular injection of acetylcholine or its analogues, carbachol and methylcholine, caused an increased firing rate of the supraoptic neurons which was accompanied by release of ADH.

In contrast to the excitatory effects of cholinergic agents, adrenergic drugs such as norepinephrine inhibit the release of ADH.[5, 46] Systemic administration of epinephrine or norepinephrine effectively causes inhibition of ADH release, predominantly by effects mediated through peripheral baroreceptor mechanisms, but central adrenergic mechanisms are also important since norepinephrine administered into the third ventricle also will inhibit ADH release.

Anatomic studies using the Falck fluorescence method show that noradrenergic fibers terminate directly on neurons of the supraoptic and paraventricular nuclei. Since similar terminals are not found in the neurohypophysis, it is likely that the effects of noradrenergic agents are mediated by direct effects on the perikarya of neurosecretory cells.

> Studies using direct iontophoresis of these putative neurotransmitters upon the cells of the supraoptic nuclei have provided additional evidence for their role in synaptic regulation of ADH secretion. Barker and coworkers,[5] using antidromically identified neurosecretory cells in the cat, found that the monoamines dopamine, norepinephrine, and serotonin uniformly reduced the activity of these cells. The inhibition of activity was blocked by β-adrenergic blocking agents. Acetylcholine, on the other hand, produced a dual effect consisting of a de-

Table 1. Factors That Influence ADH Secretion in Man

Physiologic (Appropriate)	Pathologic	Pharmacologic or Hormonal
Increase in ADH		
1. Upright position	1. Inappropriate ADH syndrome	1. Morphine
2. Decrease in blood pressure	a. Hypothalamic disease	2. Barbiturates
3. Hyperosmolality	b. Cerebral disease	3. Carbamazepine
4. Hypovolemia	c. Chest disease	4. Nicotine
5. Myocardial failure, edematous states with hyponatremia	d. Tumors	5. Cholinergic drugs (carbachol, methacholine)
6. Emotional stress	e. Drugs (chlorpropamide)	6. ? Beta-adrenergic agents
7. Elevated central temperature	f. Vincristine[52]	7. Angiotensin II
	g. Hypothyroidism	8. Clofibrate[44]
Decrease in ADH		
1. Recumbent position	1. Diabetes insipidus	1. Alcohol
2. Increase in blood pressure		2. Phenytoin
3. Hypo-osmolality		3. ? Adrenergic agents
4. Increase in blood volume		4. Anticholinergic drugs
5. Decrease in central temperature		

Drugs That Facilitate ADH Action
1. Chlorpropamide[45]
2. Chlorthiazides
3. Adrenal cortical steroids

crease in activity which was found to be mimicked by nicotine. This is of interest because smoking, presumably by a nicotine effect, results in a *several hundredfold* rise in plasma ADH levels in man (as measured by radioimmunoassay). The acetylcholinesterase inhibitor physostigmine potentiated the action of acetylcholine. These workers postulated that supraoptic neurons may have both excitatory (nicotinic) and inhibitory (muscarinic) cholinergic receptors.

Other drugs exert important effects on ADH secretion. Alcohol strongly inhibits ADH release, both decreasing basal levels and preventing normal ADH responses to stimuli such as reduced blood volume. Phenytoin also inhibits ADH release transiently. On the other hand, ADH release is stimulated by morphine, barbiturates, and other hypnotics, and these agents can cause significant antidiuresis. From a practical point of view, drug-induced ADH release leads to impaired water excretion and may be responsible in part for water intoxication in hospitalized patients given intravenous fluids. Pain and stress, which also stimulate ADH secretion, can intensify the defect in water clearance.

Neurophysin

Release of ADH from the axonal granules of the neural lobe is achieved by fusion of the secretory granule membrane with the external limiting membrane of the axon terminal. The entire content of the secretory granule is then discharged into the perivascular space of the posterior pituitary.[9, 12] It is not surprising, therefore, that the carrier protein, neurophysin, which is synthesized within the cell body and transported down the axon bound to ADH, is also released into the blood (Fig. 5).[12, 13] The neurophysins are a group of similar proteins of at least three different types, with a molecular weight of approximately 10,000 daltons.[67] Neurophysins probably are combined with ADH and oxytocin as a prohormone (Fig. 6).

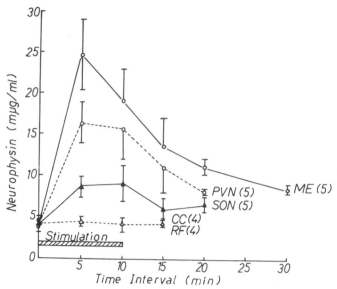

Figure 5. Release of neurophysin after electrical stimulation of several regions in the hypothalamus of the rat. Stimulation of median eminence (ME), supraoptic nuclei (SON), and paraventricular nuclei (PVN) causes neurophysin release. Stimulation of brain stem reticular formation (RF) or cerebral cortex (CC) had no effect. (From Cheng, K. W., Martin, J. B. and Friesen, H. G.: *Studies of neurophysin release.* Endocrinology 91:177, 1972, with permission.)

The development of radioimmunoassays for neurophysin in the rat, pig, and man have confirmed that neurophysin is released concurrently with ADH in a variety of experimental situations.[12, 55] In studies in the rat, it has been shown that neurophysin is released following stimuli which are known to release ADH, including dehydration, ingestion of hypertonic saline, and intravenous infusion of hypertonic solution. Neuro-

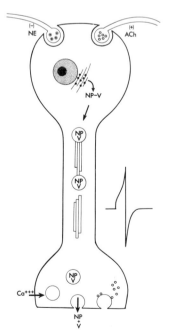

Figure 6. Schematic of vasopressin (ADH) secreting neuron to show synthesis, transport, and release of vasopressin and neurophysin. Neurophysin and vasopressin are synthesized in Golgi system and packaged into granules to be transported by axoplasmic flow to the nerve terminal. Axon terminal depolarization is followed by calcium uptake, union of granule membrane with cell membrane, and release of both neurophysin and vasopressin. The vasopressin neuron receives both noradrenergic (inhibitory) and cholinergic (excitatory) inputs. *Abbreviations:* NE, norepinephrine; ACh, acetylcholine; NP-V, neurophysin-vasopressin; Ca^{+++}, calcium ions.

physin and ADH are released concurrently after hemorrhage in the dog.[58] The serum concentration of neurophysin under basal conditions in the adult human was found to be 2.0 ± 1.0 ng./ml. Plasma neurophysin is elevated in man in many situations in which ADH secretion is enhanced, such as dehydration, and in some cases of the syndrome of inappropriate secretion of ADH.[56]

Release of neurophysin can be demonstrated in patients given nicotine, a potent stimulator of ADH release, and after suckling, a potent stimulator of oxytocin release.[55] Neurophysin levels rise in the last two trimesters of pregnancy and remain elevated during the immediate postpartum period. Elevated levels of neurophysin have also been observed in patients with acromegaly and galactorrhea.

The recent work of Robinson[55] has shown selective mechanisms of neurophysin release. Using assays directed against different neurophysins, he has found one neurophysin which is apparently increased by stimuli commonly associated with ADH release, and another which is influenced by estrogen administration. The estrogen-stimulated neurophysin is probably responsible for the pregnancy-related changes, and recently has been shown to be related to oxytocin release. Oxytocin-containing cells contain estrogen-induced neurophysin, whereas nicotine-induced neurophysin is associated with ADH-containing cells (Fig. 7).

Elevated neurophysin levels are occasionally seen in patients with diabetes insipidus. As in the hereditary diabetes insipidus strain of rats (Brattleboro), such individuals appear to have a defect in synthesis of ADH (but not of neurophysin) and manifest compensatory hyperfunction of the supraoptic-hypophysial system.[20]

By means of immunohistochemical methods, neurophysin has been demonstrated surrounding the primary plexus of the portal capillaries, and by immunoassay to be present in the portal vessel blood.[50, 70] Neurophysin is also found in the pineal gland, without ADH, although vasotocin, a closely related peptide, is present there, Its function in this tissue is unknown. Neurophysin together with ADH, but not with oxytocin, is found in certain ADH-secreting nonendocrine tumors such as the oat cell tumor of

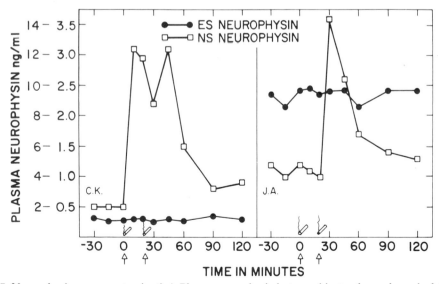

Figure 7. Neurophysin response to nicotine. Plasma neurophysin in two subjects who each smoked two cigarettes as indicated. The subject on the right was taking oral contraceptives containing estrogen, resulting in elevated estrogen-stimulated neurophysin release. (From Robinson, A. G.: *Radioimmunoassy of neurophysin proteins: Utilization of specific neurophysin assays to demonstrate independent secretion of different neurophysins in vivo.* Ann. N. Y. Acad. Sc. 248:246, 1975, with permission.)

73

the lung.[29] Secretion of ADH from these tumors is responsible in some cases for the syndrome of inappropriate ADH secretion (dilutional hyponatremia due to excess water retention), one of the several causes of this syndrome, and an example of an ectopic paraendocrine disorder. The abnormal secretion from the tumor, commonly considered to be due to dedifferentiation of cells, indicates that genetic control of ADH and neurophysin synthesis are closely linked. Elevated levels of neurophysin are frequently present during renal failure.

The functional significance of plasma neurophysin has been reviewed by Cheng and Friesen.[12] It appears that neurophysin does not function significantly as a carrier of ADH in the blood, since the affinity for the octapeptide is too low to provide significant binding at the low concentrations of the substances in the blood. On the other hand, in view of its high concentration in portal-vessel blood, it may exert an effect on anterior pituitary secretion.

A few preliminary studies have suggested a peripheral function for neurophysin. Neurophysin is reported to increase the contractility of the heart, a reaction that would serve the teleologically valuable purpose of providing a compensatory mechanism for maintenance of blood pressure. Neurophysin has also been reported to promote sodium excretion by the kidney (i.e., act as a potential natriuretic factor). How this effect is integrated into a total system for electrolyte regulation is not known.[41]

Since the immunoassay for neurophysin is technically simpler than that for ADH and oxytocin and concentrations in the peripheral blood are much higher, and measurements of neurophysin may prove to have practical value in the clinical delineation of hyponatremic syndromes.[50]

Suprahypothalamic Regulation of ADH Secretion

In addition to the effects of osmotic and other reflex stimuli for ADH secretion, a number of other mechanisms appear to be involved in ADH regulation, certain of which probably arise from higher brain centers.[32, 69] It is well known that pain and emotional stress bring about a rapid release of ADH accompanied by antidiuresis. This effect is mimicked by a number of drugs such as meperidine, barbiturates, and morphine, although some of these effects may be mediated through baroreceptor mechanisms rather than by a direct pharmacologic effect on the neurohypophysial system. A diurnal pattern of ADH release has been identified. In the normal individual, assumption of the recumbent posture is associated with a decrease in ADH secretion, which would be expected to result in an enhanced urinary output. However, such a diuresis providently does not occur during the night; sleep is accompanied by a period of antidiuresis, presumably mediated by release of ADH. Although this has not been conclusively proven, this nocturnal antidiuresis apparently overrides the inhibitory stimulus of the reclining posture.

A number of limbic system structures influence ADH secretion.

Electric stimulation of either the medial or basolateral nuclei of the amygdala causes ADH release in the rhesus monkey, as indicated by an abrupt decrease in water secretion. Similarly, stimulation of limbic midbrain areas including the ventral tegmental area of Tsai, the periaqueductal gray matter, and the midbrain reticular formation are effective in inducing antidiuretic responses in unanesthetized monkeys.[32] Responses to stimulation of the thalamus, tectum, and pyramidal tract are negative. Many of these same limbic-hypothalamic-midbrain areas also mediate drinking responses following osmotic, electric, or cholinergic stimuli.

Neurosecretory cells in both the supraoptic and paraventricular nuclei can be excited by single-pulse stimulations of widespread areas of the brain including the septum, the midbrain reticular formation and central gray matter, the anterior commissure, and the hippocampus.[69]

Such excitations are frequently followed by a prolonged inhibitory period, lasting as long as 500 msec. after application of a single pulse. These effects are of more than passing interest in view of the frequent clinical findings of excessive ADH secretion in association with a variety of intracranial disease processes, many of which are not restricted to hypothalamic centers.

Taken together, these findings indicate that neural inputs impinging upon the supraoptic and paraventricular nuclei vary greatly and are integrated for the regulation of ADH output. Some of these inputs are probably cholinergic, others, in particular those from the brain stem, are noradrenergic. Such inputs not only mediate reflex release via ascending vagal and sympathetic nervous system impulses, but also probably regulate the complex neuroendocrine responses by which ADH secretion is integrated with other homeostatic mechanisms such as temperature regulation, drinking, and eating.

MECHANISMS OF THIRST REGULATION

Hypothalamic Mechanisms

The control of drinking behavior is integrated with ADH release in the homeostatic control of water content of the body. It has long been recognized that either a decrease in blood volume or an increase in plasma osmolarity arouses the sensation of thirst.[24] This response is mediated by both central and peripheral receptors. Hypothalamic receptors for thirst sensation have been localized by studying the effects of lesions and of electrical, hyperosmotic, and pharmacologic stimulations. Investigations by Stevenson and colleagues[65] in 1949 showed that rats with lesions in the hypothalamic ventromedial nuclei increased their food intake and drank less.[62] In these animals a combination of diabetes insipidus and decreased thirst led to a chronic state of dehydration manifested by hypernatremia. Subsequently, Andersson and McCann[1] showed that in the dog, lesions restricted to the anterior hypothalamus (sparing the supraoptic nuclei and tracts) caused adipsia without either diabetes insipidus or disturbance in food intake. Results of more restricted lesions in the rat have indicated that a region exists in the lateral hypothalamus (within the medial forebrain bundle), destruction of which induces severe adipsia without aphagia. It is likely that lesions in the lateral hypothalmus cause adipsia because of interruption of pathways related to limbic system structures.

Several extrahypothalamic regions of the brain also have been shown to be important in the modulation of drinking. Septal lesions in the rat cause increased water intake.[24] Regions of the hippocampal complex and of the amygdala also have been implicated in control of water intake; an excitatory "center" for drinking appears to exist in the anteroventral portion of the amygdala in some species. In the rat, bilateral lesions in this region cause a combination of aphagia and adipsia. Lesions of the amygdala in the dog are also reported to produce an adipsia-aphagia syndrome. The failure of complete circumsection of the hypothalamus in the cat to result in adipsia indicates the importance of extrahypothalamic mechanisms in normal thirst-drinking responses.

Drinking can be induced by intrahypothalamic microinjections of hypertonic saline, by electric stimulation, or by artificial elevation of hypothalamic temperature. In the goat, Andersson and coworkers showed that intraventricular or intrahypothalamic infusions of a small volume (3 to 10 μl.) of hypertonic saline (2 to 3 per cent) elicited drinking.[24] The region from which such responses were most consistently obtained was the perifornical area of the anterior hypothalamus. Similar results can be obtained with electric stimulation (see Fig. 6). Effective stimulation sites include the region between the anterior column of the fornix and the mammillothalamic tracts, extending from dorsal to ventral hypothalamus. In the monkey, stimulation of extrahypothalamic sites, in particular the anterior cingulate gyrus and the substantia nigra, also have been effective in eliciting drinking. Studies have shown that effective sites for stimulation of drinking are similar to those which are effective for self-stimulation; concurrent drinking and self-stimulation could be induced by stimulation of a number of sites in the lateral hypothalamus. Sites which induced eating have been clearly separate from those which cause drinking in several studies.

Local warming of the preoptic region of the hypothalamus also induces drinking, even in the water-replete animal. Local cooling has the opposite effect, in some instances causing instead an increase in food intake. Thus, increased environmental temperature may cause an increase in water intake by activation of both peripheral and central receptors, as well as by the osmotic effects of sensible and insensible water loss.

It has been proposed by Grossman[28] and Fitzsimmons[24] that the system for control of drinking has a specific neuropharmacologic basis. It was shown that the direct instillation of cholinergic substances into the hypothalamus of the rat led to increased drinking, and adrenergic substances elicited feeding behavior. Although carbachol-induced polydipsia is blocked by atropine, thirst secondary to hypovolemia or dehydration is not. A number of other noncholinergic pharmacologic agents, such as barbiturates, chlordiazepoxide, and levorphanol, also may increase thirst, and thirst is inhibited by alcohol. These findings make it unlikely (as pointed out by Fitzsimmons) that there is precise neuropharmacologic coding for drinking behavior.

Renal Mechanisms

Recently, a renal hormonal component of thirst regulation has been disclosed by the experiments of Andersson[2] and of Fitzsimmons.[24] The kidney was implicated in CNS control of drinking when it was shown that decreased renal blood flow caused by loss in effective blood volume (ligation of the inferior vena cava, hemorrhage) led to increased fluid intake, and that this response was blocked by removal of both kidneys.

> The renin-angiotensin system has been implicated in this effect by a number of experimental findings. Reduced renal perfusion is known to stimulate the secretion of the enzyme renin from the renal juxtaglomerular apparatus, both directly and through sympathetic secretomotor control. Renin catalyzes the conversion of circulating angiotensinogen to angiotensin I, which is altered to angiotensin II by a converting enzyme localized in the lung. The active peptide, angiotensin II, causes both constriction of blood vessels and release of aldosterone. Angiotensin II also has been shown to stimulate drinking behavior in experimental animals, whether administered systemically or by direct intrahypothalamic injection. The effects are not mediated through aldosterone release, since aldosterone does not stimulate drinking, and the peptide is active even in adrenalectomized animals. Effects of angiotensin II in the hypothalamus synergize with local osmolarity. The effects of angiotensin are blocked by haloperidol, implicating a catecholaminergic mechanism in thirst as well as feeding.

The theoretic importance of this hypothesis is that a hormonal signal, generated in the kidney in response to a volume stimulus, may be integrated with other neural and osmotic stimuli in the regulation of water intake through a hypothalamic mechanism. Parallel studies have also been carried out on the effects of angiotensin II on ADH release, but findings are still controversial. This peptide stimulates unit activity of supraoptic neurons exposed to iontophoretically applied hormone.[48] A formulation of the proposed role of angiotensin in thirst mechanisms is shown in Figure 8.

The effects of angiotensin II on drinking appear to explain the syndrome of malignant thirst occasionally seen in patients with renal failure. Several cases have been reported of severe thirst present in renal failure despite restitution of normal blood electrolytes and normal blood volume by hemodialysis. Nephrectomy was followed by a return to

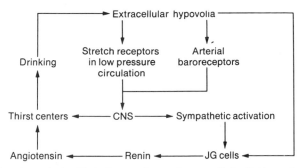

Figure 8. Function of angiotensin in thirst. Low volume of extracellular fluid results in CNS activation of thirst centers and via the juxtaglomerular (JG) cells stimulates renin release. Renin induces formation of angiotensin, which may act centrally to stimulate thirst centers (From Fitzsimons, J. T.: *The renin-angiotensin system in the control of drinking. In* Martini, L., et al. (eds.): *The Hypothalamus.* Academic Press, New York, 1970, p. 210, with permission.)

the normal drinking pattern. The angiotensin hypothesis may also explain the severe thirst of patients with hypovolemic shock, a situation in which the renin-angiotensin system is strongly activated (see Fig. 8).

NEUROENDOCRINE REGULATION OF SODIUM METABOLISM

Sodium chloride has long been of great value to man. Salt craving develops in individuals on a low-salt diet, or salt-depleted by diuretics or adrenal failure.[62] But salt appetite is only one of the mechanisms by which sodium homeostasis is achieved. Renal control is more important and can compensate for sodium inputs over an extraordinary range. Renal control is mediated by two major factors: the rate of glomerular blood flow (a function of blood volume and of cardiac output), and the active reabsorption of sodium from the renal tubular fluid under the action of aldosterone. Many nephrologists believe that there is a third factor in renal-tubule control of sodium excretion.[62] They believe this because under certain experimental conditions it can be shown that a salt load can be excreted appropriately even when aldosterone secretion is maintained constant and when there has been no detectable change in renal plasma flow. As in salt appetite, neurogenic factors are involved in aldosterone regulation and may also be responsible for "third factor" effects.

Central Sodium Appetite

In his admirable review of the neural control of salt and water balance, Fitzsimmons[24] points out that the evolutionary development of a specific appetite for sodium probably determined the success of the migratory steps of organisms from the sea to fresh water and ultimately to dry land. Organisms which do not make wise evolutionary choices do not survive, and the intake of sodium in proper amounts is wise. Sodium governs the volumes of plasma and extracellular fluid and exerts ionic effects on cell membranes generally. In line with this importance, specific taste receptors for sodium are distributed widely in terrestrial vertebrates and some lower forms. Sodium receptors are also important in the behavioral responses to salt deficiency. In the rat, salt restriction or adrenalectomy (which causes sodium depletion) leads to an increased intake of salt. Rats, given their choice, take high-sodium in preference to low-sodium diets.

The mechanism by which sodium balance determines sodium intake is not fully understood. The most important factor appears to be blood volume and not blood osmolarity, since any means used to lower effective circulating blood volume increases salt intake even in the presence of normal sodium concentration. Volume receptors may serve as the afferent arm of a reflex sodium intake control system, or a more remote, hormonal control system (like the angiotensin system) may be involved. It should be emphasized that salt appetite is not merely a homeostatic response; both rats and man prefer salty foods far in excess of homeostatic needs.

Neuroendocrine Regulation of Aldosterone Secretion

Aldosterone, the principal mineralocorticoid hormone of the adrenal cortex, regulates the proximal-tubule resorption of sodium ion by an active, energy-requiring process in exchange for potassium. In the absence of aldosterone (e.g., in adrenal insufficiency) or when aldosterone blockers such as spironolactone are administered, this exchange does not take place, so that sodium is lost in excess and potassium is retained.[62] The secretion of aldosterone, like that of the other adrenal hormones, is under the control of adrenocorticotropic hormone (ACTH) from the anterior pituitary. ACTH injection stimulates the release of aldosterone, and anterior-pituitary deficiency brings about a reduction in aldosterone secretion. But ACTH is not the main regulator of aldosterone secretion. A more important control system is linked to the renal-angiotensin system described above in relation to control of fluid intake.

> The renal component of the system is localized to a peculiar glandular structure which lies on the afferent blood vessels at their point of entry into the glomerulus. This juxtaglomerular apparatus is an endocrine gland as revealed by special stains and by electron microscopy, the product of which is an enzyme, renin, which is secreted into the blood. Since the concentrations of angiotensinogen and of angiotensin I are great, the rate-limiting step for the formation of angiotensin II is renin concentration so that the secretion of the kidney is the major determinant of the rate of formation of angiotensin II. This substance, a powerful pressor agent, also directly stimulates the adrenal cortex to form and release aldosterone. Through this circuitous route, the secretion of specialized glandular cells within the kidney normally regulates renal tubular function.

The mechanism(s) by which juxtaglomerular-apparatus secretion is regulated has received much study. At first it was shown that the secretion of renin was regulated by renal blood flow; when perfusion was low, renin was released in increased amounts. More recently it has been shown that the juxtaglomerular apparatus receives a significant direct postganglionic noradrenergic innervation. A number of stimuli which are known to cause activation of the sympathetic nervous system (such as hypoglycemia, hemorrhage, and assumption of the upright position) are associated with an increase in renin secretion, and these reactions are prevented by drugs which block β-adrenergic receptors. Thus the secretion of aldosterone is controlled in part by the central nervous system.

Feedback effects of angiotensin II on central nervous control of water balance introduce an additional neuroendocrine loop into this system. As described above, angiotensin appears to stimulate drinking behavior and to stimulate the release of ADH, both effects being mediated through direct actions on the hypothalamus. It has been proposed that the homeostatic defense against decreased blood volume includes a major neuroendocrine control system, the primary link of which is the juxtaglomerular apparatus (Fig. 9).

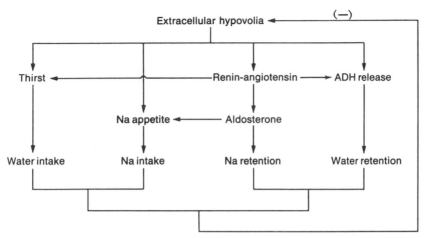

Figure 9. Function of renal mechanisms and aldosterone in regulation of salt and water. Low volume extracellular fluid stimulates renin-angiotensin system; aldosterone may act directly in CNS to stimulate sodium appetite, in addition to stimulating sodium retention in the kidney. (From Fitzsimons, J. T.: *The hormonal control of water and sodium intake. In* Martini, L. and Ganong, W. F. (eds.): *Frontiers in Neuroendocrinology.* Oxford University Press, London, 1971, p. 103, with permission.)

Natriuretic ("Third") Factor

Although the renin-angiotensin system plays a major role in renal electrolyte control, other important mechanisms are independent of the adrenal gland. In an adrenalectomized animal maintained on constant doses of aldosterone, the infusion of hypertonic saline solution is followed by an appropriate saline diuresis. The simplest explanation of this phenomenon, held by many nephrologists, is that the saline load increases the circulating blood volume and, secondarily, the cardiac output and the renal plasma flow. Since an increase in renal plasma flow increases the salt load presented to the kidney, it is reasonable to suppose that at a constant level of aldosterone effect, more salt will be lost to the urine. However, in many studies of this question, it has not been easy to demonstrate increased renal plasma flow. This failure has led to speculation about the existence of an unknown hormonal factor, released during sodium loading, which acts on renal tubules to promote saline diuresis.

Bricker and colleagues[11, 72] have found a substance in the urine of animals undergoing salt loading which stimulated sodium excretion. But other studies designed to test the existence of this factor have been extremely controversial, and at this time, the hypothesis still has not been proven. Candidates for this hormonal function have been ADH, oxytocin, MSH, and most recently, neurophysin. The most conservative view is that third-factor effects are best explained on the basis of hemodynamic changes within the kidney as the result of increased renal plasma flow, and that it is not necessary to postulate additional hormonal control.

SUMMARY OF MECHANISMS

The mechanisms which regulate water and sodium excretion are extremely complex. In addition to simple reflex osmoreceptor release of ADH from the neurohypophysis and the secretion of renin from the kidney, the secretions of the end-organ hormones act on neural structures in a feedback regulatory fashion. Thus renin and angiotensin appear to be involved in the regulation of thirst, and aldosterone in the regulation of sodium appetite. The threshold level of sensitivity remains to be determined for each of these pathways in terms of homeostatic mechanisms, and we have yet to define the place of each in the hierarchy of controls that maintain water and salt balance.

NEUROLOGIC DISORDERS OF WATER AND SALT REGULATION

In this section we consider disorders of water and salt regulation caused by disturbances of CNS regulatory mechanisms. Many disorders which resemble those of neurologic origin may be due to remote systemic disease or to intrinsic renal abnormalities; they are not considered in detail here. The major neurologic disorders of water and salt balance are diabetes insipidus (ADH deficiency), compulsive water drinking, hypodipsia, essential hypernatremia, and inappropriate ADH secretion.

Diabetes Insipidus

Diabetes insipidus is a disorder of excessive renal water loss due to deficiency in the secretion of ADH.[41] The condition may be congenital, or may be due to acquired disturbance of the hypothalamic-neurohypophysial axis. A superficially similar clinical picture may be produced by hereditary nephrogenic diabetes insipidus in which the renal tubules are insensitive to ADH, or to acquired disease of the renal tubules.

A reduction in ADH secretion sufficient to interfere with normal renal water-conservation mechanisms is normally accompanied by appropriate increased H_2O intake (polydipsia), unless central thirst mechanisms are also disordered. In the latter case, impaired perception of hypovolemia or hyperosmolality may result in further dehydration and in severe cases, death. Thus, it is generally agreed that the polydipsia of diabetes insipidus is appropriate, i.e., a corrective mechanism to maintain water balance. Because functions for ADH release and thirst overlap, diabetes insipidus patients rarely present abnormal stimulation of central thirst mechanisms early in the course of the disorder. In one case studied by the authors, repeated admissions for compulsive water drinking occurred before a hypothalamic teratoma was diagnosed; this subsequently progressed to cause diabetes insipidus. Compulsive water drinking is ordinarily a psychologic disturbance (see below).

Causes

The main causes of diabetes insipidus are summarized in Table 2.

Familial or congenital diabetes insipidus is an exceedingly rare disorder that occurs in infancy or childhood and affects either sex. A few cases have been autopsied and these show failure of development of the supraoptic neurons; the paraventricular neurons may also be involved, and the posterior pituitary is reduced in size.[27] Congenital diabetes insipidus must be distinguished from the superficially similar congenital nephrogenic diabetes insipidus, due to an inherited defect in renal tubule responsiveness to ADH. The latter condition is largely a disease of young men or boys.

Idiopathic diabetes insipidus is a far more common cause of ADH deficiency, comprising approximately half of the cases of acquired disease. As well shown in the classic series accumulated by Blotner,[10] the "spontaneous disease" may occur at any age in either sex. Absence of other clinical signs of hypothalamic destruction or of disturbance in other pituitary functions, and failure to develop other hypothalamic abnormalities over prolonged periods of time indicate that the disease is restricted to the hypothalamic-neurohypophysial axis.

Post-traumatic diabetes insipidus is brought about by damage to the upper stalk and infundibulum in head injury: in acute deceleration, the stalk may be compressed on the sharp edge of the diaphragma sellae. This form of the disease may be temporary

Table 2. Principal Causes of Diabetes Insipidus

1. Familial or congenital
2. Idiopathic
3. Post-traumatic—basal skull fractures
4. Neoplastic—primary or secondary, including leukemia and lymphoma
5. Histiocytosis X
6. Granulomatous disease (sarcoidosis, tuberculosis, meningovascular syphilis)
7. Vascular lesions
8. Infections—pyogenic meningitis
9. Neurosurgery

or permanent. Some patients follow a water-balance pattern like that seen in cats following the classic stalk-section studies of Ranson and in a proportion of humans subjected to high surgical stalk section. This three-stage response begins with severe diabetes insipidus due to damage to the neural mechanism controlling ADH release. As the neurohypophysis degenerates and releases its product into the blood, the diabetes insipidus pattern abates, occasionally giving rise to excessive ADH release; the third stage, permanent diabetes insipidus, follows. Other patients show only a relatively delayed permanent diabetes insipidus, and in still others, the somewhat delayed diabetes insipidus is followed after a long period by resumption of normal water balance. For this reason, in post-traumatic cases it is important to re-evaluate the status of diabetes insipidus periodically for as long as two years.

Neoplastic and granulomatous infiltration may also cause diabetes insipidus. Destruction of the posterior pituitary is rarely the cause, because diabetes insipidus does not usually occur in pituitary disease unless the basal hypothalamus or upper stalk is damaged. This feature is due to the anatomic fact that some axons of the supraoptic-hypophysial tract terminate on blood vessels high in the stalk or in the median eminence. Moreover, fibers of the neurohypophysial system show some capacity for regeneration; following hypophysectomy in the sheep, rat, or goat, a vestigial but nevertheless functional neural lobe regenerates as a stump and re-establishes a neurovascular anastomosis. When neoplastic or inflammatory conditions cause diabetes insipidus, they usually do so by destruction in the upper stalk and in the median eminence, where the neurohypophysial neurons streaming into the neural lobe converge in a relatively superficial position. At this point they are extremely vulnerable to destruction by relatively circumscribed lesions which may not be apparent by conventional neuroradiologic methods. Tumor infiltration and granulomatous basilar meningitides invade the hypothalamus via the vascular mantle of the infundibulum. The diabetes insipidus of suprasellar tumors also comes about mainly through damage in the infundibular region and upper stalk. Inflammatory conditions of the infundibulum causing diabetes insipidus, such as sarcoidosis, may show spinal-fluid abnormalities. Sarcoidosis is the most common of the granulomatous causes of diabetes insipidus, but tuberculosis, syphilis, and cryptococcosis have also been observed. Almost any tumor metastatic to the brain may lodge in the infundibulum or upper stalk and cause diabetes insipidus; carcinoma of the lung is notorious in this regard.

Vascular lesions may cause diabetes insipidus in several ways. Aneurysm of the circle of Willis, most commonly of the anterior communicating artery, may cause infundibular damage as well as anterior pituitary deficiency. Postpartum pituitary necrosis (Sheehan's syndrome) occasionally causes diabetes insipidus in addition to anterior lobe deficiency, presumably through vascular damage to the upper stalk. Rupture of aneurysms of the anterior circle of Willis may damage the supraoptic nuclei or the infundibulum as an acute event.

Neurosurgical intervention is one of the commoner causes of diabetes insipidus. This may come about inadvertently or by necessity in the removal of tumors of the hypothalamus or pituitary. Surgical stalk section also has been used as an alternative to the more difficult hypophysectomy in the treatment of carcinoma of the breast and other endocrine-dependent tumors, and for the management of rapidly progressive diabetic retinopathy. The occurrence of diabetes insipidus depends on the stalk-section level for reasons listed above; high section causes ADH deficiency and low section generally does not. The general consequences of surgical stalk section in man have been discussed in Chapter 2.

Diagnosis

The diagnosis of diabetes insipidus must be considered in patients who pass large amounts of low-osmolality urine. Nocturia and increased thirst at night are almost always present; these features may help to distinguish true polydipsia due to excessive water loss from psychogenic polydipsia. If thirst mechanisms are intact, neither dehydration nor hypovolemia will develop, although most patients usually fall slightly behind in fluid replacement, as shown by a modest (not diagnostically useful) elevation in plasma osmolality.

On the other hand, the results may be catastrophic if diabetes insipidus is accompanied by a defect in thirst sensation. The accompanying hypovolemia, hyperosmolality, and dehydration may lead to fever, hyperpnea, stupor, coma, and death, often *without* seizures. Dehydration may not be clinically striking, and normal skin turgor is often preserved even in severe water depletion.

The diagnosis of diabetes insipidus requires two elements: proof that the kidney is capable of responding to ADH and proof that stimuli to water conservation are ineffective in bringing about decreased urine volume and increased urine concentration. Since the diagnosis of diabetes insipidus usually means that the patient will be treated for life with replacement medications, it is essential that there be no question about the diagnosis. Normally, plasma osmolarity ranges from 285 to 290 mOsm./l. Many patients with diabetes insipidus have slightly elevated plasma osmolarity when given free access to drinking water, while patients with compulsive water drinking tend to have low normal plasma osmolarity. Proof that the kidney can respond to exogenous hormone is demonstrated by the subcutaneous injection of ADH (5 pressor units) which should bring about a marked decrease in urine volume and an increase in urinary osmolarity to at least 300 to 350 mOsm./l. (specific gravity greater than 1.011). The preparation is usually well tolerated, but it does have pressor and coronary vasoconstrictor properties and should not be administered in full dosage to patients with known heart disease or hypertension. Smaller doses should be given to such individuals, under careful supervision. The second precaution about the use of ADH as a diagnostic aid is that patients with long-standing compulsive water drinking may show only modest responses to the hormone. They may in fact mimic patients with intrinsic renal disease. It may therefore be necessary to reduce excess water intake for several days in order to clarify the diagnosis. If the patient then fails to respond to exogenous ADH, intrinsic renal disease of some type is probably present. Kleeman and Vorherr[41] give an excellent discussion of the nephrogenic diabetes insipidus syndromes.

The simplest way to determine the ability to conserve water is a 6- to 8-hour dehydration test. The patient must be observed very closely and not permitted to lose more than 3 per cent of body weight, because water deficiency can lead to severe mental disturbance, fever, and profound prostration. In normal individuals, 6 to 8 hours without water will produce an increase in urine osmolarity to that of plasma or as much as twice that value (urine specific gravity greater than 1.015) with no change in plasma osmolarity. In severe diabetes insipidus, urine volume remains high and concentration low.

However, in severe dehydration, even diabetes insipidus patients may show a modest increase in urine concentration, and a decline in urinary volume due to severe blood volume contraction with decreased renal plasma flow. The compulsive water drinker poses a major diagnostic problem, and it may be necessary to extend the dehydration period for as long as 18 hours, by which time compulsive water drinkers are always able to concentrate their urine.

Radioimmunoassays for ADH are available only as research tools but will likely prove to be of value in diagnosis. Husain and collaborators[38] reported that ADH could not be detected in plasma of patients with diabetes insipidus, and Robertson and coworkers[53] found reduced levels of ADH (0.8 ± 0.3 compared with 2.7 ± 1.4 pg./ml. in normals). These patients did not show normal secretory response to fluid restriction.

A number of other tests for diabetes insipidus have been reported in the literature. These include the hypertonic saline infusion test (Hickey-Hare or Carter-Robbins), a procedure that increases blood solute concentration, and the nicotine test which stimulates acetylcholine receptors on the supraoptic neurons. The former test is not superior to the dehydration procedure and, although it is quicker, requires more effort on the part of patient and doctor. Nicotine (which can be supplied by smoking one or two cigarettes quickly) stimulates ADH release in normal persons, but not in diabetes insipidus patients. Unfortunately, chronic smokers lose their sensitivity to nicotine, and even in normal persons, results are somewhat variable. It has been proposed by Dingman[16] that the use of dehydration and nicotine tests permits the delineation of a syndrome of loss of osmoreceptor function, with retained neuronal responsiveness to direct pharmacologic stimulation. However, this distinction may be quantitative rather than qualitative.

Management

CHRONIC MILD DIABETES INSIPIDUS. In patients with partial or incomplete diabetes insipidus who are capable of normal regulation of water intake, an effort should be made to control polyuria by means of either chlorpropamide 100 to 200 mg. per day or hydrochlorthiazide 50 to 100 mg. per day. These agents synergize with residual endogenous ADH at the renal tubule and may provide a useful amount of control using relatively simple oral medications. These agents may, rarely, cause severe water retention and hyponatremia even in partial diabetes insipidus, and chlorpropamide can cause hypoglycemia. If the oral agents are not effective, one of the forms of ADH therapy is indicated.

SEVERE DIABETES INSIPIDUS. Several forms of ADH therapy are available: aqueous vasopressin, vasopressin tannate in oil, synthetic lysine vasopressin nasal spray, vasopressin snuff, and DDAVP (D_1D_1 arginine vasopressin). The last-named compound, a synthetic long-acting analogue of arginine vasopressin, may well be the best form of therapy, but at this writing, it has not been released for use in the United States, although it has been used extensively in England and Europe for the past five years.

Aqueous vasopressin (20 U./ml.) is a partially-purified extract of neurohypophyses, standardized by bioassay. Because its effect after subcutaneous injection is short-lived (two hours or less), it is used mainly as a diagnostic aid in differentiating central from renal polyuria, and as treatment for the acute diabetes insipidus that develops after brain surgery or head trauma. In the latter cases, the neurosurgeon may be reluctant to use longer-acting vasopressin tannate in oil for fear of inducing cerebral edema.

Vasopressin tannate in oil (5 U./ml.) is a tannic acid salt of partially-purified vasopressin suspended in oil. Antidiuretic action is observed for 6 to 72 hours after administration of 0.1 to 1.0 ml. intramuscularly. In starting therapy it is advisable to begin with lower doses (0.3 ml. or less) and adjust the amount and the timing of subsequent doses according to the response. For most patients this is the best therapy now available but several important practical precautions must be observed.

1. The ampoules containing vasopressin tannate must be shaken thoroughly to ensure complete suspension. Failure to respond is almost always due to faulty mixing or injection techniques. Suspension is easier if the ampoule is first warmed. The ampoules should not be stored upside down, because the active compound will then settle in the tip and may be discarded inadvertently when the ampoule is opened.

2. If the patient does not require the full 1.0 ml. dose, the remaining amount can be stored safely in a disposable plastic syringe until the next injection.

3. Successive doses of vasopressin tannate in oil are usually give before the previous dose has worn off completely. Consequently, unless care is taken, patients may show excessive water retention and the syndrome of inappropriate ADH secretion. Plasma sodium or osmolarity should be monitored from time to time. An easy way to detect excessive water retention is by daily standardized weighings. Weight gain of 2 to 4 pounds in a day may indicate excessive ADH action. In patients with long-standing ADH deficiency, the renal tubule may become relatively insensitive to exogenous hormone and initially may require larger doses than will be needed later.

Allergic reactions to vasopressin may occur because it is derived from animal sources and is contaminated with trace amounts of bovine tissue proteins, neurophysins, and anterior pituitary hormones. In addition to hives, and even anaphylactic reactions, antibodies to GH, ACTH and prolactin may be detected in patients under treatment. This immune response does not have important physiologic effects but may cause spurious radioimmunoassay values.

Lysine 8-vasopressin, available in a nasal spray form containing 50 U./ml., provides good control of diabetes insipidus in most patients, but must be taken every 3 to 4 hours. It does not control symptoms in all patients with severe diabetes insipidus, but is useful in conjunction with other treatment even in cases in which it is not the sole therapy. Some patients show nasal irritation, most do not. Nasal spray has supplanted the use of *vasopressin snuff* which has the same limitations of duration of action, but in addition, as a crude compound, is more likely to cause local sensitization.

DDAVP is a synthetic analogue of arginine vasopressin which can be taken by nasal insufflation and gives great promise for the treatment of diabetes insipidus.[21, 54] The analogue is relatively resistent to degradation in plasma and therefore has prolonged action, most patients being controlled with two insufflations a day. The proper dose is determined by a series of preliminary test doses. We believe that DDAVP will prove to be the best treatment for patients with diabetes insipidus who cannot be controlled on chlorpropamide or chlorthiazide.

Central "Essential" Hypernatremia

In some cases of partial diabetes insipidus a compensatory intermediate homeostatic state develops, characterized by chronic hypernatremia, mild dehydration, and hypovolemia in which net water balance is adequate because ADH secretion is driven by the hypovolemic state.[18, 29, 64] In isolated descriptions of such cases, the diagnosis had been "essential hypernatremia." In some instances, hypernatremia and hyperosmolarity persist chronically for may months or years. The possibility exists that in such cases, the regulatory osmoreceptor center(s) in the hypothalamus operate at a new "setpoint." Serum sodium levels as high as 170 to 190 mEq./l. may occur without significant symptoms.

In addition to neurologic causes, hyperosmolarity may also occur in diabetic patients with or without acidosis. The hyperosmotic coma syndrome without acidosis is caused by partial insulin deficiency which has led to hyperglycemia and marked urinary fluid loss. Hyperosmolar coma may also be induced by peritoneal dialysis (if hypertonic glucose is used) and therapeutically by attempts at osmotic diuresis using mannitol or urea.

It should not be assumed that the brain disturbance in dehydration is fully reversible, since permanent brain damage can occur following hyperosmotic coma in diabetes.

Inappropriate Secretion of ADH (Schwartz-Bartter Syndrome)

Dilutional hyponatremia due to excessive water retention is a relatively common disorder seen in many different clinical states. Because the syndrome closely resembles that produced experimentally by prolonged administration of ADH, it was named the syndrome of inappropriate ADH secretion by Schwartz and Bartter.[61] Recent studies have confirmed that plasma ADH is inappropriately high for the degree of plasma hyposmolarity present.[7] In cases of idiopathic or central abnormalities, the ADH levels are usually only slightly elevated above normal, but there is a failure to suppress further secretion in the face of the hypo-osmolar state. This implies a functional derangement of osmoreceptor-ADH control. In patients with ADH-secreting neoplasm, plasma levels of ADH are commonly very high, reaching 10 to 100 times those in normal subjects. In one patient with vincristine neurotoxicity, the ADH levels were also markedly elevated.[52] These observations support the original hypotheses of Schwartz and Bartter that the syndrome is caused by increased ADH secretion.

Although the drinking mechanism is regulated in part by plasma osmolarity, most individuals continue to ingest water even in the face of low serum osmolarity and increased effective blood volume. Persistent water intake together with excessive ADH leads to the critical disturbance in this syndrome: excessive body water.

Etiology

The main causes of inappropriate secretion of ADH are summarized in Table 3. The syndrome may be caused by:
1. Excessive activity of the neurohypophysial system, secondary to suprahypothalamic brain disease.
2. Hypothalamic disturbances due to local processes which lead to damage and "leakage" of ADH from the supraoptic neurons.
3. Abnormal reflex ADH release due to persistent drive from baroreceptors or volume receptors, secondary to diseases in the chest or heart or to prolonged recumbent posture.
4. Exogenous or ectopic production of ADH by inflammatory or neoplastic tissue.
5. Drug administration.

The first and fourth are the most common causes of the syndrome.

SUPRAHYPOTHALAMIC BRAIN DISEASE. Acute subarachnoid hemorrhage, concussion, transfrontal lobotomy, craniotomy, subdural hematoma, and brain tumors are among the common central causes of inappropriate ADH secretion. The localization of the disturbance is not specific. Also seen as causes of the syndrome are cerebral infarction, brain abscess, and meningitis.[23] Rarely, the disorder occurs in diffuse brain disease due to encephalitis, metabolic encephalopathy, and disseminated microvascular disease. The enormous variety and lack of anatomic specificity of lesions capable of causing excessive ADH secretion have not been explained. An earlier view that the suprahypothalamic brain exerts a predominantly inhibitory effect on basal ADH secretion, and that hypersecretion in this syndrome is due to "denervation" hyperactivity, has not been supported by experimental studies. Animal preparations with "hypothalamic islands" in which the supraoptic nuclei or the medial basal hypothalamus has been

Table 3. Causes of Inappropriate ADH Secretion

I. Central hypersecretion of ADH
   A. Hypothalamic disorders
      1. Trauma
      2. Surgery
      3. Metabolic encephalapathy
      4. Acute intermittent porphyria
      5. Myxedema
      6. Subarachnoid hemorrhage
      7. Vascular lesions
   B. Suprahypothalamic disorders
      1. Cerebral infarcts
      2. Subdural hematoma
      3. Infections, meningitis (tuberculosis)
II. Peripheral hypersecretion
   A. Excessive stimulation in recumbent posture (coma)
III. Excessive production from nonhypothalamic sites (ectopic ADH)
   A. Pulmonary infections—TB
   B. Tumors—lung, etc.
IV. Drugs
      1. Vincristine
      2. Chlorpropamide
      3. Chlorthiazide
      4. Cyclophosphamide
      5. Carbamazepine
      6. Clofibrate
      7. Chlorpromazine

separated from the overlying brain, maintain water balance in response to osmotic stimuli much as intact animals do. In one report, two patients with central pontine myelinolysis developed features of the disorder.[23] Selective inhibitory pathways from the limbic system cortex or brain stem may be responsible for some cases of inappropriate ADH secretion, but there is no evidence to support or disprove this possibility.

One potential pathogenetic feature common to many cases of inappropriate ADH secretion is coma. It has been proposed that in patients with a variety of brain disturbances, a prolonged stay in the supine position may lead to ADH hypersecretion through stimulation of peripheral baroreceptors.[3]

ECTOPIC HUMORAL SYNDROMES. The other major cause of inappropriate ADH secretion is the ectopic production of the hormone by certain types of malignant tumor. The most common variety causing the syndrome is the oat cell tumor of lung, which may present clinically with little or no evidence of thoracic disease. In a few cases, ADH has been isolated from the tumor itself, together with the carrier protein neurophysin.[29] Electron micrographs of the tumor cells show secretory granules resembling those found in neural lobe axon terminals.

DRUGS. Patients experiencing severe stress, particularly in the immediate postoperative period, or treated with a variety of pain-relieving or tranquilizing drugs (see Table 3) may also show inappropriate ADH secretion.[40] This possibility should be borne in mind in patients with unexplained hyponatremia.

Recently, attention has been drawn to a peculiar form of the syndrome of inappropriate ADH secretion caused by drugs such as chlorpropamide, an oral hypoglycemic agent, and chlorthiazide, a diuretic which potentiates the action of ADH at the level of the renal tubule.[40, 41] These agents were accidently discovered to have therapeutic benefit in diabetes insipidus through their facilitating effects at the renal level in patients with minimal ADH secretion. They also may cause hyponatremia in both normal individuals and in patients with diabetes insipidus.

Vincristine, by an unknown mechanism, may also cause the disorder,[52] as may clofibrate.[44]

Manifestations

Neurologic manifestations of inappropriate ADH secretion are identical to those of water intoxication, and correlate to some extent with the degree of hyponatremia. Associated brain disturbance, for example cerebral arteriosclerosis, hypoxemia, or anemia, may interact with hyposmolarity to modify the neurologic picture. Symptoms do not usually occur until serum sodium levels fall below 120 to 125 mEq./l. Early symptoms are anorexia, nausea, vomiting, lethargy, and irritability. Subtle personality changes, inattentiveness, and forgetfulness may progress to paranoia and delusions. With a further fall in serum sodium to 100 to 110 mEq./l. the neurologic disturbance becomes even more severe and includes stupor, coma, and intractable generalized seizures which are usually refractory to treatment with anticonvulsants.

Attempts have been made to define experimentally the neurologic disturbance in the syndrome of inappropriate ADH secretion, but the results are somewhat conflicting.[57] Severe hyponatremia (and water intoxication) is not associated with significant increase in intracranial pressure, i.e., cerebral edema is not present. CSF pressure is normal on lumbar puncture. Dila and Pappius[15] found in rats in which water intoxication was induced by exogenous ADH administration that loss of potassium occurred from cerebral tissues (and from muscle), and postulated that this loss may contribute to the symptoms. In contrast, the sodium content was less markedly decreased. Rymer and Fishman[59] confirmed these findings in the rat but found that these metabolic derangements persisted for a time after neurologic recovery. They speculated that the potassium defect in brain is in fact protective, minimizing brain swelling. They concluded that the critical factor in the level of consciousness was the level of brain water, not sodium or potassium levels. Although these observations received different interpretations by the two teams of investigators, they both show that cerebral swelling is not a significant factor in the disorder. Administration of corticosteroids has no effect in the condition, either beneficially or adversely.[22]

Diagnosis and Management

Since hyponatremia may be a sign of sodium depletion (such as that seen after prolonged vomiting or in adrenal insufficiency) the clinician is commonly faced with the differential diagnosis of disorders which require distinctly different treatments. In inappropriate ADH secretion, salt administration does not raise plasma sodium levels (except transiently), and adrenal corticoids are without effect. In this syndrome blood volume is normal, signs of peripheral circulation are normal (normal pulse and blood pressure), renal clearance is normal, and plasma BUN and creatinine as a consequence are also normal, or even lower than normal. In sharp contrast, hyponatremia due to sodium depletion is accompanied by contraction of blood volume (low blood pressure, tachycardia), decreased renal blood flow, and renal retention of BUN and creatinine (prerenal azotemia). Occasionally mixed types of the disease are observed.

In the syndrome of inappropriate ADH secretion, the treatment is strict water restriction (400 to 600 ml. per day). This regimen, both therapeutic and diagnostic, is all that is needed in mild or non-urgent cases. If serious brain disturbance demands urgent treatment, administration of hypertonic sodium chloride (3 to 5 per cent) is indicated. Unless water intake is simultaneously restricted, the salt load will be quickly excreted (see below under pathogenesis). The treatment for sodium depletion is the administration of isotonic or slightly hypertonic salt, and if adrenal cortical deficiency is present, glucocorticoids and mineralocorticoids. When the diagnosis is in doubt, the patient should be given slightly hypertonic sodium chloride intravenously, with or without cortisol, because this treatment is lifesaving in depleted patients and will usually have no detrimental (or beneficial) effect on patients with inappropriate ADH.

Several investigators have advocated the use of furosemide for rapid correction of hyponatremia.[30] This may be important in congestive heart failure due to the fluid overload. Furosemide usually causes a diuresis sufficient to reduce cardiac overload. When furosemide is given, careful attention must be paid to correction of potassium and other electrolyte losses induced by the drug. Once the hyponatremia has been corrected, careful adherence to a regimen of fluid restriction is important to prevent recurrence of water intoxication. Treatment should then be directed at the underlying problem.

Pathogenesis

The combination of excess water retention and water intake leads to expansion of the extracellular fluid volume and increases in renal plasma flow, glomerular filtration rate, and sodium load in the glomerular filtrate. Thus the apparently paradoxic situation arises in which urine sodium excretion is high in the face of low plasma sodium concentration, and patients excrete as much sodium as they are given. Because renal clearance is not low, nitrogeous waste products are adequately cleared from the blood, and blood urea and creatinine remain normal.

Another aspect of the clinical picture presented by these patients is the excretion of hyperosmolar urine with sodium concentration higher than that of plasma. No intrinsic disease of the adrenal or the kidney is present. Water administration does not cause water diuresis, but salt diuresis occurs after salt loading. The syndrome reverses relatively rapidly after water restriction, which may have to be extreme. Most patients continue to drink water (may complain of severe thirst) and will often steal water even in the presence of severe hyponatremia.

REGULATION AND FUNCTION OF OXYTOCIN IN THE HUMAN

Although oxytocin has been shown to be released in response to suckling in women, its physiologic role in milk letdown, so thoroughly studied in experimental animals, has not been clearly defined in the human. Milk letdown does occur in women; it may be inhibited by emotional stress, and initiated by such conditioned stimuli as the cry of a hungry baby. The release mechanisms for ADH and oxytocin seem to be separate. Nicotine and hypertonic saline induce release of ADH with minimal effects on oxytocin; suckling has the reverse effect.[56]

In man, the functions of oxytocin and ADH overlap somewhat, but ADH is 100 times as potent as oxytocin in its antidiuretic effects, and oxytocin is 100 times as potent as ADH in inducing milk ejection. Species differ considerably in the relative effects of the two hormones.

In spite of extensive investigation of the physiologic actions of oxytocin and the common use of the drug to induce uterine contraction, there is no convincing evidence that the hormone's function in parturition or lactation in humans is critical. Women with diabetes insipidus have delivered babies normally and nursed them. Plasma oxytocin has not been measured directly in the plasma of such patients, however, to establish that no oxytocin is released. Oxytocin has no known physiologic effect in the male.

During orgasm in women oxytocin is released, as shown by milk letdown in lactating women; increased uterine contractions also accompany sexual excitement in the human and the cow. In the latter species, responses are due to oxytocin release. Analogous studies have not been done in man. Increased uterine motility is said to be one of the mechanisms for enhancing sperm transport, but in the human, the progressive action of the uterus is from the fundus down, and hence this cannot be a significant mechanism.

REFERENCES

1. ANDERSSON, B. AND MCCANN, S. M.: *Drinking, antidiuresis and milk ejection from electrical stimulation within the hypothalamus of the goat.* Acta Physiol. Scand. 35:191, 1955.
2. ANDERSSON, B. AND WESTBYE, O.: *Synergistic action of sodium and angiotensin on brain mechanisms controlling water and salt balance.* Nature 228:75, 1970.
3. AUGER, R. G., ET AL.: *Position effect on antidiuretic hormone: Blood levels in bedfast patients.* Arch. Neurol. 23:513, 1970.
4. BARKER, J. L., CRAYTON, J. W. AND NICOLL, R. A.: *Antidromic and orthodromic responses of paraventricular and supraoptic neurosecretory cells.* Brain Res. 33:353, 1971.
5. BARKER, J. L., CRAYTON, J. W. AND NICOLL, R. A.: *Noradrenaline and acetylcholine responses of supraoptic neurosecretory cells.* J. Physiol. (Lond.) 218:19, 1971.
6. BARGMANN, W. AND SCHARRER, E.: *The site of origin of the hormones of the posterior pituitary.* Am. Sci. 39:255, 1951
7. BAUMANN, G., LOPEZ-AMOR, E. AND DINGMAN, J. F.: *Plasma arginine vasopressin in the syndrome of inappropriate antidiuretic hormone secretion.* Am. J. Med. 52:19, 1972.
8. BEARDWELL, C. G.: *Radioimmunoassay of arginine vasopressin in human plasma.* J. Clin. Endocrinol. Metab. 33:254, 1971.
9. BISSET, G. W., CLARK, B. J. AND ERRINGTON, M. L.: *The hypothalamic neurosecretory pathways for the release of oxytocin and vasopressin in the cat.* J. Physiol. (Lond.) 217:111–131, 1971.
10. BLOTNER, H.: *The inheritance of diabetes insipidus.* Am. J. Med. Sci. 204:261, 1942.
11. BRICKER, N. S., ET AL.: *In vitro assay for a humoral substance present during volume expansion and uremia.* Nature 219:1058, 1968.
12. CHENG, K. W. AND FRIESEN, H. G.: *Physiological factors regulating secretion of neurophysin.* Metabolism 19:876, 1970.
13. CHENG, K. W., FRIESEN, H. G. AND MARTIN, J. B.: *Neurophysin in rats with hereditary hypothalamic diabetes insipidus (Brattleboro strain).* Endocrinology 90:1055, 1972.
14. DANIEL, P. M. AND PRICHARD, M. M. L.: *The human hypothalamus and pituitary stalk after hypophysectomy or pituitary stalk section.* Brain 95:813, 1972.
15. DILA, C. J. AND PAPPIUS, H. M.: *Cerebral water and electrolytes.* Arch. Neurol. 26:85, 1972.
16. DINGMAN, J.: Personal communication.
17. DU VIGNEAUD, V.: *Hormones of the posterior pituitary gland: oxytocin and vasopressin.* Harvey Lectures Sec. 50:1, 1954–1955.
18. DERUBERTIS, F. R., ET AL.: *"Essential" hypernatremia due to ineffective osmotic and intact volume regulation of vasopressin secretion.* J. Clin. Invest. 50:97, 1971.
19. DREIFUSS, J. J. AND KELLY, J. S.: *The activity of identified supraoptic neurones and their response to acetylocholine applied by iontophoresis.* J. Physiol. 220:105, 1972.
20. DYBALL, R. E. J.: *Single unit activity in the hypothalamo-neurohypophysial system of Brattleboro rats.* J. Endocrinol. 60:135, 1974.
21. EDWARDS, C. R. W., ET AL.: *Vasopressin analogue DDAVP in diabetes insipidous: Clinical and laboratory studies.* Br. Med. J. 3:375, 1973.
22. FICHMAN, M. P. AND BETHUNE, J. E.: *The role of adrenocorticoids in the inappropriate antidiuretic hormone syndrome.* Ann. Int. Med. 68:806, 1968.
23. FINLAYSON, M. H., ET AL.: *Cerebral and pontine myelinolysis: Two cases with fluid and electrolyte imbalance and hypotension.* J. Neurol. Sci. 18: 399, 1973.
24. FITZSIMMONS, J. T.: *Thirst.* Physiol. Rev. 52:468, 1972.
25. FLAMENT-DURAND, J. AND DISTIN, P.: *Studies on the transport of secretory granules in the magnocellu-*

lar hypothalamic neurones. I. Action of colchicine on axonal flow and neurotubules in the paraventricular nuclei. Z. Zellforsch. Mikrosk. Anat. 130:440, 1972.

26. GAUER, O. H., HENRY, J. P. AND BEHN, C.: *The regulation of extracellular fluid volume.* Annu. Rev. Physiol. 32:547, 1970.

27. GREEN, J. R., ET AL.: *Hereditary and idiopathic types of diabetes insipidus.* Brain 90:707, 1967.

28. GROSSMAN, S. P.: *Eating or drinking elicited by direct adrenergic or cholinergic stimulation of hypothalamus.* Science 132:301, 1960.

29. HAMILTON, B. P. M., UPTON, G. V. AND AMATRUDA, T. T., JR.: *Evidence for the presence of neurophysin in tumors producing the syndrome of inappropriate antidiuresis.* J. Clin. Endocrinol. Metab. 35: 764, 1972.

30. HANTMAN, D., ET AL.: *Rapid correction of hyponatremia in the syndrome of inappropriate secretion of antidiuretic hormone. An alternative treatment to hypertonic saline.* Ann. Int. Med. 78:870, 1973.

31. HATTON, G. I. AND WALTER, J. K.: *Induced multiple nucleoli, nucleolar margination, and cell size changes in supraoptic neurons during dehydration and rehydration in the rat.* Brain Res. 59:137, 1973.

32. HAYWARD, J. N.: *The amygdaloid nuclear complex and mechanisms of release of vasopressin from the neurohypophysis. In* Eleftheriou, B. E. (ed.): *Neurobiology of the Amygdala.* Plenum Press, New York, 1972, p. 685.

33. HAYWARD, J. N.: *Physiological and morphological identification of hypothalmic magnocellular neuroendocrine cells in goldfish preoptic nucleus.* J. Physiol. 239:103, 1974.

34. HAYWARD, J. N. AND JENNINGS, D. P.: *Influence of sleep waking and nociceptor-induced behavior on the activity of supraoptic neurons in the hypothalamus of the monkey.* Brain Res. 57:461, 1973.

35. HAYWARD, J. N. AND JENNINGS, D. P.: *Activity of magnocellular neuroendocrine cells in the hypothalamus of unanaesthetized monkeys. I. Functional cell types and their anatomical distribution in the supraoptic nucleus and the internuclear zone.* J. Physiol. 232:515, 1973.

36. HAYWARD, J. N. AND JENNINGS, D. P.: *Activity of magnocellular neuroendocrine cells in the hypothalamus of unanaesthetized monkeys. II. Osmosensitivity of functional cell types in the supraoptic nucleus and the internuclear zone.* J. Physiol. 232:545, 1973.

37. HAYWARD, J. N.: *Neural control of the posterior pituitary.* Annu. Rev. Physiol. 37:191, 1975.

38. HUSAIN, M. K., ET AL.: *Radioimmunoassay of arginine vasopressin in human plasma.* J. Clin. Endocrinol. Metab. 37:616, 1973.

39. KASTIN, A. J., ET AL.: *Asymptomatic hypernatremia.* Am. J. Med. 38:306, 1965.

40. KIMURA, T., ET AL.: *Mechanism of carbamazepine (Tegretol)-induced antidiuresis: evidence for release of antidiuretic hormone and impaired excretion of a water load.* J. Clin. Endorcrinol. Metab. 38:356, 1974.

41. KLEEMAN, C. R. AND VORHERR, H.: *Water metabolism and the neurohypophysial hormones. In:* Bondy, P. K. and Rosenberg, L. E. (eds.): *Duncan's Diseases of Metabolism.* W. B. Saunders, Philadelphia, 1974, p. 1459.

42. KOIZUMI, K. AND YAMASHITA, H.: *Studies of antidromically identified neurosecretory cells of the hypothalamus by intracellular and extracellular recordings.* J. Physiol. 221:683, 1972.

43. MARTINI, L.: *Neurohypophysis and anterior pituitary activity. In* Harris, G. W. and Donovan, B. T. (eds.): *The Pituitary Gland,* vol. 3. University of California Press, Berkeley, 1966, p. 535.

44. MOSES, A. M., ET AL.: *Clofibrate-induced antidiuresis.* J. Clin. Invest. 52:535, 1973.

45. MOSES, A. M., NUMANN, P. AND MILLER, M.: *Mechanism of chlorpropamide-induced antidiuresis in man: evidence for release of ADH and enhancement of peripheral action.* Metabolism 22:59, 1973.

46. MOSS, R. L., DYBALL, R. E. J. AND CROSS, B. A.: *Responses of antidromically identified supraoptic and paraventricular units to acetylcholine, noradrenaline and glutamate applied iontophoretically.* Brain Res. 35:573, 1971.

47. NICOLL, R. A. AND BARKER, J. L.: *The pharmacology of recurrent inhibition in the supraoptic neurosecretory system.* Brain Res. 35:501, 1971.

48. NICOLL, R. A. AND BARKER, J. L.: *Excitation of supraoptic neurosecretory cells by angiotensin II.* Nature [New Biol.] 233:172, 1971.

49. OLIVER, G. AND SCHAFER, E. A.: *On the physiological action of extracts of pituitary body and certain other glandular organs.* J. Physiol. (Lond.) 18:277, 1895.

50. PARRY, H. B. AND LIVETT, B. G.: *A new hypothalamic pathway to the median eminence containing neurophysin and its hypertrophy in sheep with natural scrapie.* Nature 242:63, 1973.

51. PICKFORD, M.: *Inhibitory effect of acetylcholine on water diuresis in dog, and its pituitary transmission.* J. Physiol. (Lond.) 95:226, 1939.

52. ROBERTSON, G. L., BHOOPALAM, N. AND ZELKOWITZ, L. J.: *Vincristine neurotoxicity and abnormal secretion of antidiuretic hormone.* Arch. Int. Med. 132:717, 1973

53. ROBERTSON, G. L., ET AL.: *Development and clinical application of a new method for the radioimmunoassay of arginine vasopressin in human plasma.* J. Clin. Invest. 52:2340, 1973.

54. ROBINSON, A. G.: *DDAVP in the treatment of central diabetes insipidus.* N. Engl. J. Med. 294:507, 1976.

55. ROBINSON, A. G., ARCHER, D. F. AND TOLSTOI, L. F.: *Neurophysin in women during oxytocin-related events.* J. Clin. Endocrinol. Metab. 37:645, 1973.

56. ROBINSON, A. G. AND FRANTZ, A. G.: *Radioimmunoassay of posterior pituitary peptides: a review.* Metabolism 22:1047, 1973.

57. RYMER, M. M. AND FISHMAN, R. A.: *Protective adaptation of brain to water intoxication.* Arch. Neurol. 28:49, 1973.

58. SACHS, H., ET AL.: *Supraoptic neurosecretary neurons of the guinea pig in organ culture. Biosynthesis of vasopressin and neurophysin.* Proc. Natl. Acad. Sci. 68:2781, 1971.

59. SAWYER, W. H.: *The mammalian antidiuretic response. In* Greep, R. O. and Astwood, E. B. (eds.): *Handbook of Physiology, Section 7: Endocrinology,* vol. 4, part 1. American Physiological Society. Williams & Wilkins, Baltimore, 1974, p. 443.

60. SCHARRER, E.: *Principles of neuroendocrine integration.* Res. Publ. Assoc. Res. Nerv. Ment. Dis. 43:1, 1966.

61. SCHWARTZ, W. B. AND BARTTER, F. C.: *The syndrome of inappropriate secretion of antidiuretic hormone.* Am. J. Med. 42:790, 1967.

62. SHARE, L. AND CLAYBAUGH, J. R.: *Regulation of body fluids.* Ann. Rev. Physiol. 34:235, 1972.

63. SKOWSKY, W. R., ROSENBLOOM, A. A. AND FISHER, D. A.: *Radioimmunoassay measurement of arginine vasopressin in serum: development and application.* J. Clin. Endocrinol. Metab. 38:278, 1974.

64. SRIDHAR, C. B., CALVERT, G. D. AND IBBERTSON, H. K.: *Syndrome of hypernatremia, hypodipsia and partial diabetes insipidus: a new interpretation.* J. Clin. Endocrinol. Metab. 38:890, 1974.

65. STEVENSON, J. A. F.: *Effects of hypothalamic lesions on water and energy metabolisms in the rat.* Recent Prog. Horm. Res. 4:363, 1949.

66. VERNEY, E. B.: *The antidiuretic hormone and the factors which determine its release.* Proc. Roy. Soc. (Ser.) B 135:25, 1947.

67. WATKINS, W. B.: *The tentative identification of three neurophysins from the rat posterior pituitary gland.* J. Endocrinol. 55:577, 1972.

68. WHITAKER, S. AND LABELLA, F. S.: *Cholinesterase in the posterior and intermediate lobes of the pituitary. Species differences as determined by light and electron microscopic histochemistry.* Z. Zellforsch. Mikrosk. Anat. 142:69, 1973.

69. WOODS, W. H., HOLLAND, R. C. AND POWELL, E. W.: *Connections of cerebral structures functioning in neurohypophysial hormone release.* Brain Res. 12:26, 1969.

70. ZIMMERMAN, E. A., ET AL.: *Vasopressin and neurophysin: High concentrations in monkey hypophyseal portal blood.* Science 182:925, 1973.

71. ZIMMERMAN, E. A., ET AL.: *Studies of neurophysin secreting neurons with immunoperoxidase techniques employing antibody to bovine neurophysin. I. Light microscopic findings in monkey and bovine tissues.* Endocrinology 92:931, 1973.

72. WEBER, H., BOURGOIGNIE, J. J. AND BRICKER, N. S.: *Effects of the natriuretic serum fraction on proximal tubular sodium reabsorption.* Am. J. Physiol. 226:419, 1974.

BIBLIOGRAPHY

FITZSIMMONS, J. T.: *Endocrine mechanisms in the control of water intake. In* Mogenson, G. J. and Calaresu, F. R. (eds.): *Neural Integration of Physiological Mechanisms and Behavior.* University of Toronto Press, Toronto, 1975, p. 226.

HALL, E.: *Anatomy of the limbic system. In* Morgenson, G. J. and Calaresu, F. R. (eds.): *Neural Integration of Physiological Mechanisms and Behavior.* University of Toronto Press, Toronto, 1975, p. 68.

HAYWARD, J. N.: *Neurohumoral regulation of neuroendocrine cells in the hypothalamus. In* Lederis, K. and Cooper, K. E. (eds.): *Recent Studies of Hypothalamic Function.* Karger, Basel, 1974, p. 166.

KLEEMAN, C. R. AND VORHERR, H.: *Water metabolism and the neurohypophysial hormones. In* Bondy, P. K. and Rosenberg, L. E. (eds.): *Duncan's Diseases of Metabolism.* W. B. Saunders, Philadelphia, 1974, p. 1459.

SACHS, H., ET AL.: *Biosynthesis and release of vasopressin and neurophysin.* Recent Prog. Horm. Res. 25:447, 1969.

SAWYER, W. H.: *The mammalian antidiuretic response. In* Greep, R. O. and Astwood, E. B. (eds.): *Handbook of Physiology, Section 7: Endocrinology,* vol. 4, part 1. American Physiological Society. Williams & Wilkins, Baltimore, 1974, p. 443.

CHAPTER 5

Neuroendocrinology of Reproduction

To ensure the perpetuation of the species, mating behavior must be correlated with gametogenesis in ovary and testis. Complex neuroendocrine mechanisms involving the brain, the pituitary, and the sex steroid hormones integrate these functions. Neural factors also determine the onset of puberty and the initiation and maintenance of lactation. That neural control is involved in human pituitary-gonad function is clear from the clinical effects of disease of the hypothalamus, emotional stress, psychopharmacologic drugs and electroshock therapy. In intense research over the past three decades, the chemical nature of the hormones involved has been elucidated and much insight gained into the underlying neural mechanisms.

HORMONES INVOLVED IN PITUITARY-GONAD REGULATION

Pituitary Hormones

The two hormones of the pituitary responsible for regulation of the gonads are follicle-stimulating hormone (FSH) and luteinizing hormone (LH).[1, 6, 21, 45, 53, 62, 63, 72, 73] Together they are termed *gonadotropins*. The luteinizing hormone has also been called interstitial cell stimulating hormone (ICSH) because in the male it stimulates the secretion of interstitial cells (Leydig cells) of the testes, the cellular source of the secretion of testosterone. No chemical difference between LH and ICSH is known. The use of the term ICSH is rather old fashioned and confusing to new generations of endocrinologists. Luteinizing hormone is not to be confused with luteotropic hormone (LTH), also known as prolactin because it stimulates the production of milk. The earlier designation was derived from an action of prolactin in rats to maintain the life and secretory activity of the corpus luteum after ovulation has taken place. To avoid confusion this hormone should be called prolactin.

Both FSH and LH are glycoproteins,[63] that is, they contain an appreciable amount of carbohydrate, a component which is responsible for the characteristic basophilic staining of the anterior pituitary gonadotrope cells. They also stain with the periodic acid-Schiff reagent. The two pituitary gonadotropins are chemically related to a third, placental gonadotropin. This substance, human chorionic gonadotropin (HCG), appears as early as the ninth day of pregnancy and is detected by the common pregnancy tests. In its biologic actions HCG closely resembles LH, and in fact is used in women to induce ovulation. HCG is important in clinical medicine also because of the occasional abnormal (ectopic) secretion of HCG by hydatidiform mole and choriocarcinoma, both derived from placenta. Tumors of the testes and teratomas of the lung, the medial basal hypothalamus, and the pineal gland may also secrete HCG.[16] Recent work indicates that traces of HCG occur in normal testes. In some nonendocrine tumor conditions the abnormal secretion may serve as a marker of cancer.

Human menopausal gonadotropin (HMG), a slightly altered mixture of pituitary gonadotropins (mainly FSH-like), is excreted in large amounts by menopausal and castrated women. HMG is used together with HCG to induce ovulation in women.

The various gonadotropic hormones are standardized by bioassay and different units are used. The advent of immunoassay has rendered obsolete the bioassay measurement of urinary gonadotropin excretion as an index of pituitary secretion. The older bioassay is expensive, time consuming, only semiquantitative, and does not distinguish adequately between LH and FSH. Instead, highly reliable measurements of both LH and FSH can be made routinely by radioimmunoassay of plasma.[1, 6] The main problems with radioimmunoassay at the present time are the confusion over unitage of standards, the claim by some workers that the immunassayable form of the hormone may not correspond to the biologically active form, and the fact that values may vary markedly from minute to minute, particularly in patients with high levels, thus reflecting the pulsitile release of gonadotropins.[60] By agreement, most workers relate the potency of LH and FSH to an international reference preparation (IRP) of partially purified urinary menopausal gonadotropin, maintained in the biologic standards laboratory of the National Research Council in Mill Hill, England. The National Pituitary Agency of the National Institutes of Health has provided an immunoassay reference preparation from human pituitary extract which has been standardized by bioassay, using the IRP as reference. Values for immunoassayable LH and FSH now appearing in current literature are usually related to equivalents of the IRP and are given as international units (IU). Some workers give values in relationship to actual weights of hormones measured, but since preparations vary in purity, these measurements vary. Normal values for LH and FSH are shown in Table 1.

All the gonadotropic hormones (both pituitary and placental) and thyrotropin (thyroid-stimulating hormone, TSH) are composed of two chains, termed α and β, which are dissociable under relatively mild conditions. The α chains of all five hor-

Table 1. Serum Gonadotropins in Children and Adults: Radioimmunoassay

Sexual Stage and Age (yr)	FSH*	LH*	Sexual Stage and Age (yr)	FSH*	LH*
Prepubertal (5–11)	4.5 ± 0.2	3.9 ± 0.2	Prepubertal (2–12)	4.2 ± 0.2	2.9 ± 0.4
Adult	7.4 ± 0.7	10.9 ± 1.4	Adult†	8.3 ± 0.3	12.8 ± 1.0
Prepubertal (>5)	2.4 ± 0.1	9.6 ± 0.2	Prepubertal (>5)	3.0 ± 0.1	8.8 ± 0.4
Adult	9.6 ± 0.2	12.2 ± 0.4	Adult†	7.1 ± 0.8	11.8 ± 0.7
Prepubertal (8)	3.2 ± 0.2	1.1 ± 0.3	Prepubertal (8)	4.4 ± 0.3	1.9 ± 0.1
Adult (age 15)	9.1 ± 0.5	4.0 ± 0.5	Adult†	12.5 ± 0.6	13.6 ± 1.1
Prepubertal (1–10)	4.6 ± 0.2	2.8 ± 0.2	Prepubertal (1–10)	5.4 ± 0.3	2.7 ± 0.2
Adult	11.0 ± 0.3	11.1 ± 0.3		12.3 ± 0.3	9.2 ± 0.3
Prepubertal (0.2–12)	4.9 ± 0.2	7.7 ± 0.5			
Adult	8.3 ± 0.3	18.0 ± 0.9			

*X ± SE in mIU/ml 2nd IRP/HMG, immunoassay.
†Follicular phase of cycle.
(Adapted from Kulin, H. E. and Reiter, E. O.: *Gonadotropins during childhood and adolescence: A review.* Pediatrics 51:260, 1973.)

mones are virtually identical in chemical behavior and amino acid sequence. Specificity is a function of the β chain which is different for each hormone. Immunoassays can now use this property to measure the characteristic β chain of each hormone and thus provide specific measurements.

Gonadal Hormones

In addition to the two pituitary gonadotropins, the secretions of the gonads are involved in pituitary-gonad control as well as in the determination of secondary sex characteristics. There are three main classes of sex steroids: estrogens, progestins, and androgens (Fig. 1). The names of these hormones are derived from Greek and Latin words which provide an excellent clue to their key actions. *Estrogens* (*oistros*, mad desire + *gennan*, to produce) are substances which bring about estrus i.e., sexual receptivity in the female. The term has been extended now to mean a hormone which brings about characteristic changes such as growth of the uterus and breasts, female type of skeletal structure, and female pattern of fat distribution on buttocks, thighs, and abdomen. *Progestins* (*pro*, before + *gestare*, to bear) prepare the uterus for implantation of a zygote and maintain gestation. Hormones of this type are also involved in the differentiation of the breast. *Androgens* (*andros*, man + *gennan*, to produce) stimulate the development of characteristic male features such as hair on face and chest, growth of the accessory sex organs (penis, prostate, seminal vesicles, etc.), skeleton and muscle development, deepening of the voice (growth of the larynx), and regression of scalp hair in genetically susceptible individuals.

All three classes of steroid hormones are synthesized from acetate through cholesterol by a series of enzymatic transformations in both the cytosol and the mitochondria of hormone-producing cells in the gonads. Analogous syntheses take place in the adrenal cortex: hence the occasional abnormal estrogen or androgen production by adrenal tumors, and the abnormal production of estrogens by testicular tumors, or the secretion of testosterone by the ovary. The precise chemical details of the synthesis are beyond the scope of this text, but a schematic outline is shown in Figure 2. It is important to recognize that particular steps in hormone biosynthesis can be blocked in certain genetic diseases of the adrenal, or by certain drugs.

Of the hormones secreted by the ovary, 17β-estradiol is the most important of the estrogens, and progesterone is the most important of the progestins. The principal androgen secreted by the testis is testosterone, but in certain target glands such as male

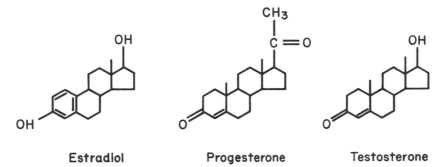

| Estradiol | Progesterone | Testosterone |

Figure 1. Structural formulae of principal sex steroids. The three classes of steroids involved in sexual function are estrogens, progestogens (gestagens), and androgens. 17β-Estradiol, progesterone, and testosterone are the most important steroids of these classes. The ovary secretes other related estrogens and progestins as well as testosterone. The testis secretes testosterone and small amounts of 17β-estradiol. Some conversion of testosterone to estrogenic hormones can take place in peripheral tissues, including fat and brain.

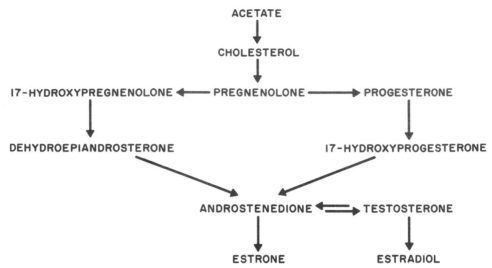

Figure 2. Pathways of enzymatic synthesis of gonadal steroids. The biosynthetic pathways of sex steroids in both ovary and testis are outlined. Many intermediate steps up to pregnenolone are omitted. From acetate as precursor the steroid nucleus is synthesized by way of cholesterol. In both ovary and testis, testosterone is a precursor of estradiol. Thus, in tumors or synthetic defects of the ovary, excessive testosterone may be synthesized to cause virilization, and tumors of the testis may produce estradiol. The weakly androgenic steroid compounds dehydroepiandrosterone and androstenedione may also be secreted in primary disease of the ovary or testis (or adrenal cortex).

accessory structures, testosterone is converted to dihydrotestosterone, the tissue-active form of the hormone. The adrenal glands of both males and females secrete androgenic hormones which are less potent than testosterone, but if secreted in increased amounts may bring about mild or even severe masculinization.[43] The adrenal androgens are necessary for maintaining libido in women.

Hypothalamic Hypophysiotrophic Hormones

The third hormonal link in pituitary-gonad regulation is the hypothalamic *luteinizing hormone-releasing hormone* (LHRH).[82, 83, 97] This substance, originally isolated from the porcine hypothalamus by Schally and collaborators,[84] is a linear decapeptide (Fig. 3) which has all the hormonal properties of the native hormone isolated from both porcine and ovine hypothalamic tissue. Immunoassays indicate that a similar or identical compound is found in the hypothalamus, blood, and cerebrospinal fluid of man. A breakdown product of LHRH is found in urine. The injection of the LHRH decapeptide brings about the release of both of the gonadotropic hormones, LH and FSH (Fig. 4), and for this reason, most workers now believe that this material is the only hypophysiotrophic factor regulating gonadotropin release.[8, 27, 38, 57] Some call this hormone gonadotropin-releasing hormone (GnRH). It has been proposed that there is a second FSH-releasing factor distinct from LHRH, but the chemical evidence on which this claim is based is not extensive,[83, 98] and gonadotropic hormone-releasing effects of hy-

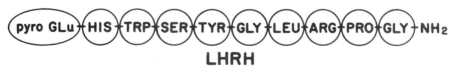

LHRH

Figure 3. The amino-acid sequence in luteinizing-hormone-releasing hormone (LHRH).

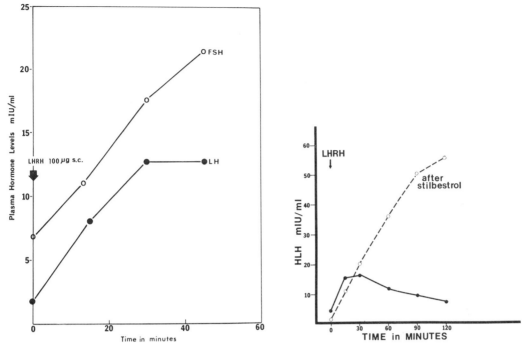

Figure 4. *Left,* effect of intravenous injection of LHRH on plasma LH and FSH levels in a patient with galac-torrhea-amenorrhea due to pituitary adenoma. The stimulating effects of LHRH on plasma FSH and LH are illustrated. The FSH secretory response to LHRH is more marked than is the LH response, and the time of onset of response is earlier. *Right,* following treatment with an estrogenic hormone for several days, the re-sponse of LH to LHRH is enhanced, illustrating that one effect of estrogens in females is to sensitize the pituitary to the hypothalamic hormone. If given for short periods of time, estradiol inhibits the response to LHRH (see Fig. 14). (Left figure from Reichlin, S.: *The control of anterior pituitary secretion. In* Beeson, P. B. and McDermott, W. (eds.): *Textbook of Medicine.* W. B. Saunders, Philadelphia, 1975, p. 1671, with permission.)

pothalamic extracts are blocked by antibody to the LHRH decapeptide. All the known effects of the hypothalamus on both FSH and LH release can be explained by varia-tions in dose, time course, and steroid hormone interaction at the pituitary level with a single GnRH. The pituitary-stimulating effects of LHRH are specifically restricted to changes in gonadotropic hormone secretion, none of the other anterior pituitary hormones being released in response to injection of this hypothalamic hormone. The one exception to this generalization is the finding that LHRH releases GH in some pa-tients with acromegaly.[23]

LEVELS OF HYPOTHALAMIC FUNCTION IN PITUITARY-GONAD CONTROL

Secretion of LHRH by LHRH-peptidergic neurons constitutes the final common pathway of gonadotropin control.[73] The function of these neurons is, in turn, involved in many aspects of gonadotropin regulation (Fig. 5). These aspects include the mainte-nance of "basal" levels of secretion, generation of the phasic release of gonadotropins responsible for ovulation, determination of the time of onset of puberty, and integration of mating behavior with gonadal readiness. Although much information has been gained about each of these functional "levels," the precise mechanisms involved are still poor-ly understood.

97

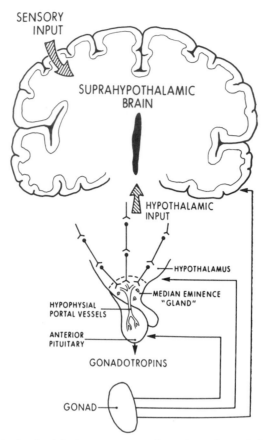

Figure 5. The various anatomic-physiologic components of gonadotropic regulation. The neural component can be visualized as operating at several levels. LHRH, the secretion of the tuberohyophysial neurons ("median-eminence" gland) enters the hypophysial-portal vessels and then stimulates the synthesis and release of the gonadotropic hormones. This system of neurons and blood vessels constitutes the "final common pathway" of neuroendocrine control. The secretion of LHRH neurons is responsible for maintenance of the tonic secretion of LH and FSH, and is also responsible for phasic influences which bring about the surge of LH at midcycle. The tonic type of secretion is commonly referred to as the "male pattern," and the phasic type as the "female pattern." The time of onset of puberty is determined by neural signals. Determination of puberty, of gondal maturation, and ripeness of the gamete is integrated with sexual behavior so as to permit mating to occur when appropriate. (From Reichlin, S.: *Summation. In* Mack, H. C. and Sherman, A. I. (eds.): *Neuroendocrinology of Human Reproduction.* Charles C Thomas, Springfield, Ill., 1971, p. 198, with permission.)

Under basal conditions in both men and women, pituitary secretion of LH and FSH is episodic, one secretory burst occurring approximately each hour (Fig. 6).[14, 15, 19] The amplitude of the bursts is greater in castrated or hypogonadal individuals. Based on pharmacologic studies in monkeys, who manifest similar secretory bursts, it seems likely that the spiking of secretion is due to changes in hypothalamic secretion of LHRH. This interpretation is further supported in man by the finding of rapidly changing peripheral levels of LHRH. In sexually mature women, the "ovulatory surge" of gonadotropin secretion is imposed upon the basal secretion pattern. The occurrence of an ovulatory surge is widely considered to be characteristic of the "female" pattern of gonadotropin secretion,[19, 69] whereas the tonic phase (with minor spiking) is considered typical of the "male" gonadotropin pattern. Most workers believe that the ability to re-

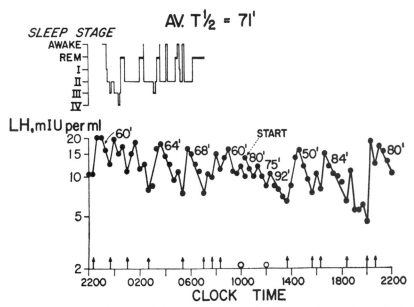

Figure 6. Plasma LH concentration sampled every 20 minutes for 24 hours in an adult male. In the mature subject, cyclic changes in plasma gonadotrophic hormones occur throughout the day and night, and are unrelated to cyclic brain activity. (From Boyar, R., et al.: *Twenty-four hour pattern of luteinizing hormone secretion in normal men with sleep stage recording.* J. Clin. Endocrinol. Metab. 35:73, 1972, with permission.)

lease gonadotropins in an ovulatory surge pattern means that the hypothalamic-pituitary axis has a positive-feedback capacity, but the exact site of the positive-feedback receptor(s) is still under study (see below). The rise in LH that preceeds ovulation is composed of a series of progressively larger surges.[59]

The hypothalamus is also involved in determining the time of onset of puberty. Destruction of anterior hypothalamic structures in the rat, or spontaneous lesions of various poorly-defined hypothalamic areas in man, can lead to precocious puberty.[34, 37, 72, 94, 96] This effect should be regarded as a *deficit* phenomenon due to an age-related loss of tonic inhibitory hypothalamic influence on LHRH secretion. The physiologic trigger which initiates puberty in man is poorly understood. It has been generally considered that the loss of inhibition is due to an intrinsic pattern of brain development analogous to other genetically-determined brain functions, such as walking, talking, and sphincter control. More recently, however, it appears that this genetic program may be modified by critical changes in body weight or body composition. As emphasized by Frisch and Revelle,[25, 26] puberty in women begins when a critical weight has been reached which is virtually the same for all Caucasian groups. This observation has been interpreted teleologically to mean that reproductive behavior cannot begin until the female is big enough and has enough storage calories to sustain pregnancy and lactation. The precise pathway by which fat stores may signal hypothalamic function is unknown, but the mechanism is important even after puberty in such disorders as anorexia nervosa (see below).

As emphasized by Boyar and associates,[12, 14, 15] the earliest endocrinologic sign of puberty is the episodic release of LH during sleep (Fig. 7). Studies in monkeys have indicated that LHRH is secreted episodically into the portal blood during ovulation.

Finally, the hypothalamus, at a fourth level of function, is responsible for integrating sexual behavior with the function of the gonads. Patterned sexual behavior, so read-

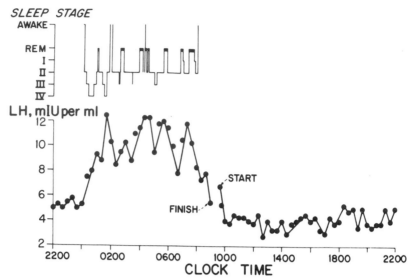

Figure 7. Plasma LH concentration sampled every 20 minutes for 24 hours in a boy in early puberty. Unlike the man (shown in Fig. 6), the boy shows a striking increase in LH secretion during the night. In this study all pubertal patients had significantly higher LH levels at night, and the number of LH secretory episodes corresponded to the number of sleep cycles of rapid (REM) and nonrapid eye movements. Boyar and colleagues[14] regard the sleep-associated increase in LH secretory activity as a "biologic index for the identification of puberty." (From Boyar, R., et al.: *Synchronization of augmented luteinizing hormone secretion with sleep during puberty.* N. Engl. J. Med. 387:582, 1972, with permission.)

ily induced in lower forms by sex hormones, facilitates mating so that insemination can occur when the egg is ripe. The far more complex nature of the hormonal control of human sexual behavior will be discussed in Chapter 12.

NEURAL PATHWAYS OF CONTROL OF GONADOTROPIN SECRETION

Maintenance of basal levels of gonadotropin secretion appears to depend on tonic hypothalamic influences arising from the medial tuberohypophysial system. The neural triggering mechanisms responsible for mediating ovulation appear to have a more extensive anatomic distribution.[19, 53] In the rat, the species in which most experimental work has been done, several workers have proposed on the basis of lesion and electric stimulation studies that the medial preoptic region is the site of origin of neurons responsible for the midcycle ovulatory surge.[17, 19] In such studies, for example, electric stimulation of the preoptic area was shown to bring about the release of LH (Fig. 8). Other electrically excitable areas include a region of the brain beginning in the medial septum, extending through the preoptic and anterior hypothalamic areas, and terminating in the median eminence-arcuate nucleus complex (Fig. 9a). Negative results from stimulation were obtained from the olfactory tubercle, dorsal hippocampus, and lateral amygdala. In another study, the hippocampus was shown to exert an inhibitory effect on gonadotropin secretion.[39] FSH-secretion responses accompany LH-secretion responses in only 80 per cent of stimulations, and FSH response lags appreciably behind the LH response. Dissociation of responses of the two gonadotropins could be taken as evidence that they are regulated independently. It is more likely, however, that these differences are due to the intrinsically greater responsiveness of the pituitary to LHRH.

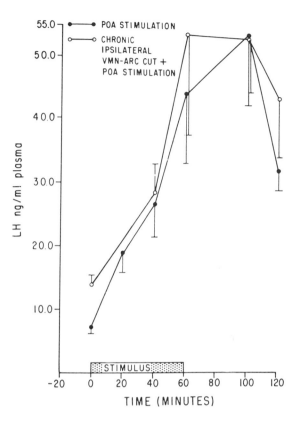

Figure 8. Effect of electrical stimulation of the preoptic area (POA) of the hypothalamus on plasma LH in the rat. This experiment illustrates the presence of electrically excitable neurons in the POA that regulate secretion of LHRH. Hemisections in the region of the ventromedial nucleus (VMN-arc) failed to interfere with ipsilateral preoptic stimulations; evidently fibers from the POA to the median eminence do not cross anterior to this region. On the other hand, there is evidence from other transection studies for crossover between the VMN-arcuate complex and the median eminence itself. (From Cramer, O. M. and Barraclough, C. A.: *Effects of preoptic electrical stimulation on pituitary LH release following interruption of components of the preoptico-tuberal pathway in rats.* Endocrinology 93:369, 1973, with permission.)

It has been shown that injection of LHRH leads to a more brisk and earlier release of LH than of FSH.[8, 57]

Recent studies using specific immunohistochemical methods have confirmed that these electrically excitable regions correspond to the site of origin of LHRH-containing peptidergic neurones (Fig. 9b). These are summarized by Barry and Dubois,[7] based on their anatomic studies in the dog, as follows: precommissural, preoptic, tuberal, premammillary. A few are found in the ventromedial and dorsomedial regions and the rostral mesencephalon. The distribution conforms generally to that in other species, including localization in the region of the "organum vasculosum of the lamina terminalis."

Impinging on the LHRH peptidergic system are neurons arising elsewhere in the brain. The most important group is believed to be noradrenergic fibers arising from the locus ceruleus of the midbrain, a region known to have connections with the limbic system. Impulses arising in the limbic system may thus alter LHRH and, thereby, gonadotropin secretion.[53]

Little is known about the pathways in man. In the rhesus monkey, both the tonic and the episodic secretory mechanisms appear to be localized within the medial basal hypothalamus, as shown by Knobil.[45] Perhaps in the primate all LHRH pathways have been condensed into the basal hypothalamus. Primates and rats also differ in the development of the cyclic LH release mechanism in that androgen treatment early in life supresses this response in the rat, but not in the monkey. It is not known where these differences in morphology and susceptibility to androgens occur. In the human, both the tonic and episodic releases of LH are impaired by destruction of the hypothalamus.

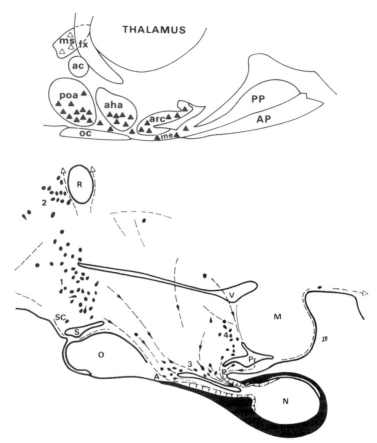

Figure 9. *Top,* localization of sites in the rat hypothalamus electrically excitable for LH secretion, and *bottom,* of neuron cell bodies staining for LHRH by immunofluorescent methods in the dog. These sites generally outline the distribution of the LHRH peptidergic pathway from preoptic hypothalamus to median eminence (see also Chapter 2). (Top figure from Clemens, J. A., et al.: *Areas of the brain stimulatory to LH and FSH secretion.* Endocrinology 88:180, 1971; bottom figure from Barry, J. and Dubois, M. P.: *Immunofluorescent study of LRF-producing neurones in the cat and the dog.* Neuroendocrinology 18:290, 1975, with permission.)

BIOGENIC AMINES AND GONADOTROPIN REGULATION

There is considerable evidence in experimental animals that the hypophysiotrophic neurons that release LHRH are in turn regulated by biogenic amines.[53] Dopamine and norepinephrine content in the median eminence changes with different stages of the estrus cycle in the rat. Dopamine can stimulate LHRH release when incubated with hypothalamic fragments in vitro, but fails to elicit LH and FSH when added directly to pituitary incubates.[85] Intraventricular injections of dopamine cause LH and FSH release, but similar doses have no effect when placed into the portal vessels.

Despite these observations in the rat, little evidence is available to indicate a role for biogenic amines in LH or FSH control in man. Acute administration of L-dopa, apomorphine, or clonidine has no effect on either hormone. A recent report indicated that pimozide, a dopamine receptor-blocking agent, administered for several days caused a slight reduction in serum LH and testosterone levels in men; perhaps a facilitatory dopaminergic mechanism exists. Adrenergic blockade with phenoxybenzamine abolishes pulsatile LH secretion in the ovariectomized monkey.

FEEDBACK CONTROL OF GONADOTROPIC HORMONE SECRETION

Deficiency of gonad secretion, whether occurring "spontaneously" as in menopausal women, after castration in males and females, or developmentally as in certain chromosomal disorders, leads to increased secretion of both LH and FSH. Long-term administration of estrogens or androgens leads to a fall in plasma gonadotropin levels (Fig. 10). These observations indicate that sex steroids regulate gonadotropic hormones through a negative-feedback mechanism (Figs. 11 and 12). The bulk of evidence suggests that long-term estrogen administration in women and testosterone administration in men inhibits gonadotropin secretion at the hypothalamic level.[40, 42, 89] In men, estrogen is a potent direct inhibitor of pituitary secretion.[90]

Although this negative-feedback mechanism is readily demonstrated in man and experimental animals, much current evidence indicates that the phasic gonadotropin secretion responsible for ovulation is brought about through a positive-feedback control system which also involves the hypothalamus and pituitary. The detailed workings of these interacting negative and positive control loops have not been fully clarified, but are important to the understanding of normal and abnormal menstrual function.

REGULATION OF THE MENSTRUAL CYCLE

Under usual circumstances, women menstruate regularly at approximately 28-day intervals and ovulate on the fourteenth day of the cycle[1, 11, 21, 62, 108] (by convention, the

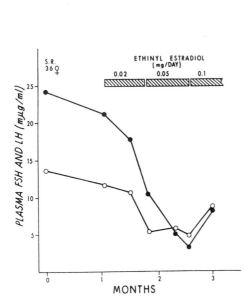
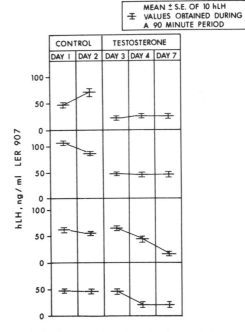

Figure 10. Inhibitory effects of sex steroids on LH secretion. *Left,* the administration of estrogen to hypogonadal (menopausal) women or *right,* of testosterone to men results in a fall in plasma LH, demonstrating the negative-feedback control (Left figure from Schalch, D. S.: *Gonadotropin secretion in the human. In* Mack, H. C. and Sherman, A. E. (eds.): *Neuroendocrinology of Human Reproduction.* Charles C Thomas, Springfield, Ill., 1971, with permission.)

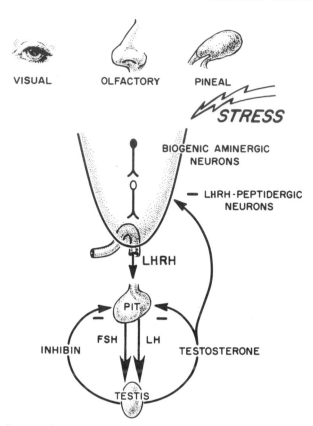

Figure 11. Schematic diagram of gonadotropin control system in men, showing the interactions of neural and hormonal feedback controls. Pituitary and testis are connected by a negative feedback link. Secretion of testosterone by the testis is stimulated by LH; maturation and growth of the tubule cells by FSH. The secretion of testosterone in turn inhibits the secretion of LH. It is likely that the major target of negative feedback is the hypothalamus; long-term testosterone administration in man does not interfere with the effectiveness of LHRH (pituitary sensitivity is relatively unaltered). A newly discovered peptide secretion of the testis, "inhibin," is believed to be secreted by tubular epithelium and to exert a direct inhibitory effect on FSH secretion. It is not known whether inhibin affects the hypothalamus directly. The LHRH-peptidergic neurons are in turn regulated by a biogenic amine neural system that links gonadotropin regulation to the remainder of the brain. Through this system a wide variety of impulses can be brought to bear on reproductive function. Stimuli affecting male gonadotropic function have been well demonstrated in experimental animals, though they are not as well worked out in the human. Visual influences include light-induced changes in seasonal breeders such as domestic cattle, deer, and birds. Olfactory signals in male rats influence gonadal function. The pineal gland in many species of animals inhibits gonadotropin secretion by a direct effect of a pineal secretion either on the hypothalamus or on the pituitary.

first day of bleeding is day 1). The menses represent withdrawal bleeding due to the loss of the endometrium-stimulating effects of estrogens and progesterone, the plasma levels of which drop dramatically toward the end of the cycle.[82]

    If one uses modern methods to follow plasma levels of the pituitary and gonad secretions through a normal cycle, a characteristic pattern emerges (Fig. 13). During the menses, plasma levels of progesterone and 17β-estradiol are at the lowest levels of the cycle. During the first half of the cycle the follicle grows and matures under the influence of FSH and LH. Early in this follicular phase, the hormonal secretion of the ovary is quite modest, but toward the middle of the cycle a burst of estrogen secretion occurs, accompanied by a modest increase in 20α-progesterone, a progesterone analogue. This hormonal secretion comes from the follicle itself and appears to be due to a

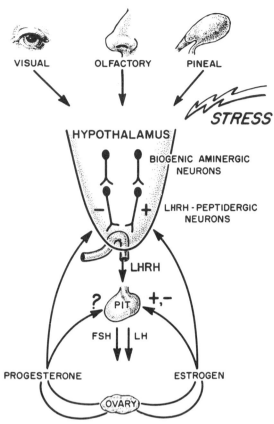

Figure 12. Schematic diagram of gonadotropin control systems in women, showing the interactions of neural and hormonal feedback controls. The development of the ovarian follicle is largely under control of the follicle-stimulating hormone (FSH). Secretion of estrogens by the developing follicle is both FSH- and LH-dependent. Ovulation is brought about by the luteinizing hormone (LH), which stimulates the secretion of progesterone in addition to estrogenic hormones. Estrogenic hormones have complex effects on the feedback control mechanism of LH and FSH secretion. Depending upon dose, time course, and prior hormonal status, estrogens can either inhibit or stimulate the secretion of LH through effects at both hypothalamic and pituitary levels. Thus, there is evidence for both negative and positive feedback control. Progesterone also can either stimulate or inhibit LHRH secretion, depending upon the setting in which it is given, but its effects at the pituitary level are relatively insignificant. Secretions of the LHRH peptidergic neurons are in turn regulated by the biogenic-aminergic system through which a variety of nonhormonal signals can influence reproductive function. Visual stimuli in many lower animals can influence onset of sexual function (as in seasonal breeders). Olfactory signals through "pheromones" influence estrus cycles in many rodents, and may do so in women. Pineal factors in lower animals delay onset of puberty.

continuing secretion of FSH and an increasingly responsive follicular cell. This time-course of sensitization is programmed genetically, and is not due to increasing stimulation by FSH. The spurt of estrogen appears to be crucial in triggering the neuroendocrine mechanisms which bring about ovulation.[11, 99] The importance of estrogen in this response is shown by studies in which anti-estrogen antibodies are found to block ovulation in the rat when given at a critical time, and by the duplication of this response in man by appropriate estrogen administration. Chronic estrogen exposure appears to sensitize the pituitary to, and probably increases the secretion of, LHRH (Fig. 14).[42] A third mechanism of the ovulatory surge appears to be sensitization of the pituitary LH-releasing mechanism to LHRH by exposure to LHRH.[2] Recent evidence indicates that LHRH injections increase the response of the pituitary to a subsequent LHRH injec-

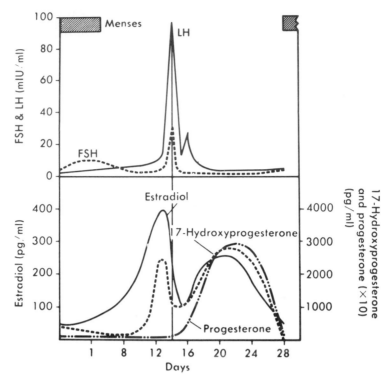

Figure 13. Pattern of secretion of sex steroids and gonadotropins during the reproductive cycle in women. The complex hormonal events leading to ovulation involve interaction among two classes of ovarian hormones, two pituitary hormones, and a hypothalamic hormone (LHRH). Early development of the follicle during the first half (follicular stage) of the menstrual cycle is stimulated by the secretion of FSH. At midcycle there is surge of secretion of LH which is responsible for ovulation. The accompanying less marked surge of FSH secretion does not have a clearly defined function. The follicular phase is associated with developing ovarian function. Immediately preceding the ovulatory surge, there is a rise in plasma estradiol and 17-hydroxyprogesterone. The preovulatory estradiol secretion is mainly responsible for triggering the release of LH, but progesterone may be needed for this response to occur. Following ovulation the luteinized follicle secretes progesterone (luteal phase of the cycle). The crucial event for neuroendocrine control of ovulation is believed to be the trigger to hypothalamus and pituitary from the rising estrogen level. (From Odell, W. D. and Moyer, D. L.: *Physiology of Reproduction.* C. V. Mosby, St. Louis, 1971, p. 66, with permission.)

tion,[2] and that this response is most readily observed in the presence of estrogen (Fig. 15).[108] According to this view, the timing of regular cycles is attributable to the programmed cycle of intrinsic ovarian function ("the clock is in the pelvis," as Knobil[45] puts it), but alterations in brain function which prevent normal LHRH responses at appropriate times can cause menstrual disturbance by interfering with LHRH secretion. Thus, in the normal cycle, the ovary signals its readiness to ovulate by secreting preovulatory estrogen. In the abnormal cycle due to brain disease, the ovary signals but the hypothalamus does not respond.

To explain how both negative- and positive-feedback elements may be present in hypothalamic-pituitary control, we have postulated (Fig. 12) that there are two sets of neurons, one activated by estrogen deficiency (negative-feedback loop) and the other by estrogen excess (positive loop).[73] Probably the cycles' levels of sensitivity and time courses of response and refractoriness are different, thus accounting for the time characteristics of onset and cessation of gonadotropin secretion.

Following the release of LH at midcycle (accompanied by FSH release), the developed egg leaves the ovary, and the remaining follicular cells in the ovary, under the

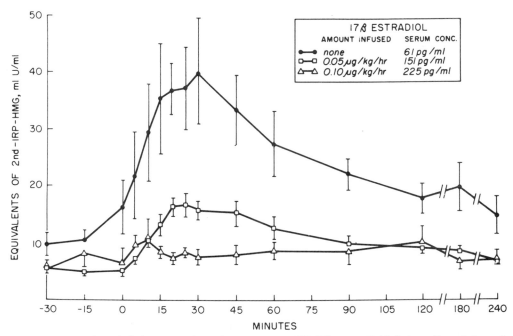

Figure 14. Modulation of pituitary gonadotropin response to LHRH by estradiol infusions. Estradiol was infused intravenously so as to maintain levels of hormone within the physiologic range. Increasing levels of estradiol were found to inhibit pituitary responses to LHRH. This illustrates the negative-feedback component of estrogen effect on the pituitary. If given for longer periods of time, estradiol sensitizes the pituitary to exogenous LHRH (see Figure 4). (From Keye, W. R., Jr., and Jaffe, R. B.: *Modulation of pituitary gonadotropin response to gonadotropin-releasing hormone by estradiol.* J. Clin. Endocrinol. Metab. 38:805, 1974, with permission.)

influence of LH, undergo luteinization, the conversion to a progesterone-secreting structure, the corpus luteum. The life history of the corpus luteum is largely determined genetically, and it involutes after about 12 days of secretion. The consequent fall in plasma estrogens and progesterone leads to withdrawal uterine bleeding, and the cycle begins again. In the rat, the life of the corpus luteum is regulated by still another pituitary hormone, prolactin, which in this species has a luteotropic function. Under experimental conditions, the rat corpus luteum, which ordinarily involutes in 48 hours, may persist for up to 16 days in a condition called pseudopregnancy. Some of the stimuli which can cause this reaction are mating (with a sterile male), severe stress, and mechanical or electric direct stimulation of the cervix of the uterus. Pseudopregnancy is believed to be due to increased prolactin secretion.[53]

It has long been suspected that an analogous reaction might be responsible for certain cases of false pregnancy (pseudocyesis), but evidence that prolactin is luteotropic in man or in primates has been lacking. Recently it has been shown that prolactin is luteotropic in rhesus monkeys, and women with pseudocyesis may have high prolactin levels (see below).

REGULATION OF GONADOTROPIN SECRETION IN THE MALE

Unlike the phasic pattern of gonadotropin secretion in the female which is enforced by the intrinsic ovarian cyclic rhythm, the function of the testes develops under the tonic influence of LH and FSH secretion. The maturation of spermatozoa requires sustained gonadotropin stimulation over a 70-day period.[62] Spermatozoa form from primi-

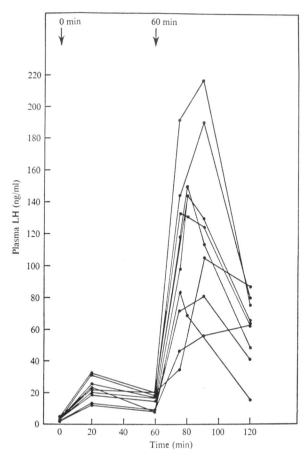

Figure 15. The "priming" effect of LHRH on subsequent response to LHRH in the rat. Female rats were injected with two equal doses of LHRH at one hour intervals. Note that the response to the second injection is much greater than to the first. It has been proposed that due to the continuing secretion of modestly increased LHRH at the time of the midcycle surge, there is an accelerating secretory responsiveness contributing to the ovulatory increase in LH secretion characteristic of midcycle. Similar experiments in humans indicate that estrogens must be present to produce this effect. (From Aiyer, M.S., Chiappa, S. A. and Fink, G.: *A priming effect of luteinizing hormone releasing factor on the anterior pituitary gland in the female rat.* J. Endocrinol. 62:573, 1974, with permission.)

tive spermatogonia in the testicular tubules which divide all through reproductive life. This is in contrast to the eggs of the ovary which are all formed by the time of birth (primordial follicles), and remain dormant until stimulated by the pituitary.

Testosterone, an androgenic hormone, is secreted by the interstitial cells of the testis (Leydig cells) under the influence of LH. The maturation of the spermatozoa requires stimulation by both FSH and LH. Androgenic hormones play a role in sperm maturation as well, and under certain well-defined experimental conditions, androgen administration can maintain spermatogenesis even after hypophysectomy. It has been proposed that even the effects of LH and FSH on spermatogenesis are mediated through changes in testicular androgen economy. LH stimulates the secretion of androgen by Leydig cells and FSH stimulates the secretion of an androgen-binding protein by one of the components of the testicular tubule, the Sertoli cell, which has a sustaining function in the maintenance of the maturing sperm cell. The androgen-binding protein, it is believed, brings about extremely high local concentrations of testosterone in the immediate vicinity of the sperm, stimulating their development.

Although castration leads to elevation of both FSH and LH, and testosterone administration leads to a depression of both LH and FSH, there is evidence that the negative-feedback control of gonadotropins by the testes is not mediated solely by an androgenic hormone. It has been shown that selective destruction of the tubules (for example, by the antitumor agent cyclophosphamide) leads to selective increase in FSH secretion. Occasionally, a similar syndrome develops in patients with isolated testicular tubular disease. The nature of the tubular component responsible for feedback regulation of FSH was unknown for many years, although the biologic activity had been suspected, and it had been given the name "inhibin." Recently a number of laboratories have found that inhibin is a polypeptide, a nonsteroid substance, and efforts have been made to isolate this material and determine its amino acid sequence. Through its selective suppression of FSH, inhibin can inhibit maturation of the germinal element of the testes without affecting the secretory function.

Studies of response to LHRH injection suggest that inhibin inhibits FSH secretion through action at the level of the pituitary gland. Inhibin-like activity has been identified in ovarian cyst fluid.

NEUROENDOCRINE CONTROL OF LACTATION

Almost all of the hormones of the pituitary and its target glands are involved in one way or another in the development of the breast, the control of milk production, and the delivery of milk at the nipple. This richness of endocrine control may reflect the evolutionary fact that the differentiation of sebaceous glands into an apocrine milk-producing gland is characteristic only of mammals. Early breast development requires normal amounts of glucocorticoids and growth hormone, and the added effects of estrogen (from the adolescent ovaries). These three hormones are essential for the growth of the breast bud, characteristic of early puberty, due largely to the formation of ducts and stroma. The lobular alveoli of the breast develop under the influence of progesterone and prolactin. During pregnancy, the increased secretion of both steroid hormones as well as increased secretion of the prolactin-like hormone of the placenta (human placental lactogen, HPL), lead to the characteristic breast growth. Lactation is initiated at the time of delivery by the sudden decline in plasma levels of placental estrogens, which during pregnancy have suppressed milk production by direct action on breast acinar membranes. The continued manufacture of milk requires the repetitive suckling stimulus, which initiates a neuroendocrine reflex leading to release of prolactin (see Chapter 6). The afferent arc of this reflex is carried to the upper thoracic segment of the spinal cord through the midbrain to hypothalamus. It is likely that this stimulus leads to the release of prolactin-releasing factor (PRF) which in turn stimulates release of prolactin. It is also possible (and represents a more conventional hypothesis) that suckling causes the inhibition of secretion of prolactin-inhibiting factor (PIF). Some evidence indicates that this activating component of prolactin release may be mediated by a serotonergic hypothalamic link, but critical studies of this problem have not been carried out in man.

The neural pathways involved in prolactin release are vulnerable to neurologic disorder. As will be discussed in the section on galactorrhea (Chapter 6), the tonic inhibitory component of prolactin regulation may be disrupted by stalk section or other disease of the hypothalamic-stalk region. This situation appears to be due to the deficiency of PIF secretion, the hormone which is believed to inhibit prolactin secretion under normal conditions. Irritative lesions of the upper thoracic wall (such as herpes zoster, or postthoracotomy inflammation), or lesions of the upper cord (such as extrinsic tumors or ependymomas).have all at times been reported to be associated with inappropriate lactation. Frequent nipple stimulation also can cause milk production, a reflex which has been exploited by foster mothers so that they can nurse their adopted child. Prolactin release also follows stimulation of the breast in men but requires a particular psychologic "set." For example, self-stimulation fails to release prolactin, but stimulation of the subject by his wife is effective. This observation suggests a "gating" phenomenon permitting the nipple stimulation reflex to occur.

Nipple stimulation also is involved in the milk "let-down" reflex. If one observes the nursing process closely in humans or in animals, it is apparent that the initial sucking of the infant is not followed immediately by the appearance of milk at the nipple. There is a delay of twenty or thirty seconds before quantities of milk can be removed from the nipple. This response is due to the contraction of specialized myoepithelial cells which surround the terminal acinar lobules of the breast and expel contained milk through the lobular ducts. The let-down is attributable to the release of oxytocin through a reflex arc involving the hypothalamus and the neurohypophysis. If blocked (e.g., by lesions of the hypothalamus), the nursling may be unable to get milk from the breast. In the rat, this leads to death of the litter. Let-down can be duplicated by oxytocin injection which has been used in women who are having difficulty in providing milk to their infants.

Oxytocin release is probably mediated by cholinergic pathways, impinging on a population of neurons in both the supraoptic-hypophysial and the paraventricular-hypophysial pathways. Emotional stress can block this response, as can the administration of epinephrine. In part this is due to the inhibitory effect of catecholamines on the myoepithelial cells of the breast, and in part to central inhibitory adrenergic effects at the hypothalamic level.

An important accompaniment of nursing is anovulation lasting for up to eight or more months after delivery. From a teleologic point of view, this protects the mother from another pregnancy while the child is still an infant, and has a biologic effect on populations in that it spaces pregnancies, and is a natural form of birth control. Of course, the birth control offered is only relative, since prevention of conception is not complete and the recovery of ovulatory cycles is variable. The suppression of ovulation by suckling has been attributed to neurogenic inhibition of release of the gonadotropin-releasing hormone. On the basis of the recent finding that high plasma prolactin levels suppress gonadotropin secretion through an action at the hypothalamic level, it appears more likely that hyperprolactinemia caused by suckling is the mediating factor in this reaction. The intensity of suckling-induced prolactin release gradually declines in the months after delivery, roughly paralleling the return of menses, but the correlation has not been established fully.

The act of breast feeding has for most women a strong psychologic effect associated with enhanced maternal feelings and tranquility. This phenomenon is striking in some individuals, and is emphasized by such groups as the La Leche League (a voluntary association of women interested in furthering breast feeding) as one of the personal rewards of nursing. The nature of this response is not fully understood. That there is a strong associative component cannot be denied, and nipple stimulation in the nursing setting may also have a central tranquilizing effect through the release of central biogenic amines. On the other hand, it is possible that the prolactin released during suckling has a direct effect on the affective state, by mechanisms analogous to its short-loop-feedback hypothalamic effect on prolactin and gonadotropin release. From animal studies it might be anticipated that prolactin would have behavioral effects. In lower forms, prolactin induces maternal behavior, for example, broodiness in hens, nest building and pup recovery in rats, and egg-guarding behavior in fish. Unfortunately, this question has not been subjected to critical inquiry. Primate prolactin (the only form available which would have biologic action in man) is unavailable for clinical testing. As an alternative, TRH, which can induce prolactin release, may have direct effects of its own on the brain (see Chapter 9). The possible central effect of prolactin and peptides is a promising area for psychosomatic research.[65]

DISEASES OF GONADOTROPIN REGULATION

Hypogonadism

From an historic point of view, the 1901 description by Frölich (see Chapter 11) of adiposogenital dystrophy in a young boy with pituitary tumor must be looked upon as a landmark in the recognition of the role of the pituitary in the control of human sex function. In 1904, Erdheim determined by careful pathologic study of a suprasellar cyst that hypogonadism could result from damage to the regions of the hypothalamus controlling gonadotropin secretion.[3] Today this all seems very simple, but for a long time the claim that hypogonadism could be produced by selective hypothalamic damage was controversial. The clinical endocrinologist recognizes two general types of hypogonadism: one, caused by local damage to the gonad, termed primary hypogonadism, and the other which is secondary to disease of the hypothalamus or pituitary. Intrinsic gonad disease with consequent failure of steroid secretion leads to secondary activation of pituitary gonadotropin secretion through the operation of the negative-feedback control system (see above). This group is sometimes termed *hyper*gonadotropic hypogonadism. Secondary hypogonadism is recognized when gonadotropic secretion is inappropriately low in the face of gonadal steroid deficiency (*hypo*gonadotropic hypogonadism). Hypogonadotropic hypogonadism due to hypothalamic disorder is also termed hypophysiotropic hypogonadism. Primary and secondary hypogonadism are readily differentiated by measurement of plasma gonadotropins (see Chapter 16). On the other hand, in the absence of clear-cut evidence of local pituitary or hypothalamic disease, the differential diagnosis of pituitary and hypothalamic failure is not always easy. The pituitary in many cases of undoubted hypothalamic failure fails to respond to a single injection of LHRH, responding only after a series of injections.[58, 61] LHRH deficiency probably leads to loss of pituitary sensitivity to LHRH, so that in cases of hypothalamic failure, the pituitary becomes abnormal. Only the hypogonadotropic disorder is discussed here, since intrinsic gonad disease properly relates to endocrine rather than neuroendocrine disease. See Table 1 for normal values of gonadotropic hormones.

Hypogonadotropic Hypogonadism in Women

Of all pituitary functions, gonadotropin secretion is second only to growth hormone secretion in its vulnerability to lesions of the hypothalamic-pituitary unit.[109] Preservation of normal menstrual cycles or male gonadal function, therefore, usually indicates normal pituitary function, although there may be occasional exceptions. All the known causes of disease in this region (see Chapter 11) cause amenorrhea and hypogonadism. Of greater numeric importance are the far more common instances of nonstructural abnormalities in ovulatory control.

It must be emphasized that intrinsic pituitary disease may rarely cause relatively isolated deficiency of gonadotropin secretion. Recently, isolated FSH deficiency has been described, thought to be due to congenital absence or deficiency of this group of cells.[68]

SECONDARY AMENORRHEA. Secondary amenorrhea (defined as amenorrhea occurring after normal menstrual cycles have been established) is by far the most common symptom attributable to disordered pituitary function.[70] In the great majority of cases, the amenorrhea is unaccompanied by evident deficiency of other pituitary hormones, and careful study will not show structural abnormality of ovary, pituitary, or hypothalamus. The possibility of pregnancy must be considered. The amenorrhea usually is temporary, and its spontaneous regression indicates that significant structural disease was not the cause of the illness. Amenorrhea of this type is commonly termed "functional," "psychogenic," or "hypothalamic."[78] Psychogenic amenorrhea occurs in several clearly-defined clinical settings as the sole manifestation of pituitary insufficiency. If the pituitary disorder begins before menarche, delayed puberty may result.[66] It commonly occurs in young women undergoing minor stresses such as going away to school. Isolated deficiency of the gonadotropins due to intrinsic pituitary disease has been described.[51, 68]

Many psychotropic drugs, including reserpine and the phenothiazines (see Chapter 6), can cause amenorrhea. In general, any agent which interferes with central catecholamine function can have this effect. These drugs probably act on the biogenic amine control of LHRH and prolactin secretion. Drug-induced amenorrhea is almost always accompanied by elevated levels of prolactin, and sometimes by galactorrhea. Amenorrhea can be a sign of severe depressive illness, and can also be precipitated by a course of electroshock therapy for psychosis.

PSEUDOCYESIS. Pseudocyesis is one of the forms of "grand hysteria," recognized since the time of Hippocrates, but is now uncommon, as are other manifestations of gross conversion states. In its full-blown form, the affected woman complains of amenorrhea and numerous sensations commonly associated with pregnancy, and believes herself to be pregnant. The patients commonly desire strongly to be pregnant, or conversely fear being pregnant. Some of the manifestations include enlargement and bloating of the abdomen, sensation of fetal movements, engorgement and tenderness of the breasts (sometimes with galactorrhea), nausea, morning sickness, and even labor pains. Although an apparent misnomer, pseudocyesis has been reported to occur even with normal periods. In the earlier literature, pseudocyesis was apparently not uncommon, and one series reported as many as one in 250 maternity clinic admissions, many of which had misled one or more unwary obstetricians. The precise pathogenesis of pseudocyesis is unknown, though it is clearly psychogenic. By analogy with the syndrome of pseudopregnancy in the rat which is brought on by stress or cervical stimulation, it has been proposed that the crucial feature of the condition is persistence of the corpus luteum secondary to inappropriate prolactin secretion. In fact, a persistent corpus luteum has been observed in few human cases at laparotomy and recently several cases with elevated plasma levels of prolactin have been reported.

Endocrinologically there is no difference between pseudocyesis and the galactorrhea-amenorrhea syndrome (see Chapter 6). Indeed, some cases of pseudocyesis may represent examples of the galactorrhea-amenorrhea syndrome, perhaps brought on by psychic stress and interpreted by suggestable, hysterical, or unsophisticated women as being due to pregnancy because of their need or fear of pregnancy. The psychiatric treatment of pseudocyesis, like that of hysteria is relatively unsuccessful. In one series of patients, 27 individuals were informed that they were not pregnant. More than half refused to accept the diagnosis. Even those who did usually developed pseudocyesis again in a few months. There is no generally applicable way of handling these cases. The approach to psychotherapy is related to the formulation of the individual patient's psychic state, but it is usually recommended that a menstrual period be induced by exogenous hormone to demonstrate the normal function of the uterus. The subject of pseudocyesis has received remarkably little recent study with the aid of new endocrinologic and psychologic approaches.

ANOREXIA NERVOSA. Amenorrhea is almost always found in active anorexia nervosa, but does not dominate the clinical picture as does the marked wasting and disturbed feeding behavior.[13, 92]

There is no generally satisfactory definition of anorexia nervosa. Some psychiatrists define it as the condition of any patient who has lost 25 pounds or more for psychologic reasons. In many patients, anorexia nervosa can be looked on as a symptom clearly related to definable psychiatric illness such as depression, schizophrenia, or anxiety. But most patients with anorexia nervosa, though disturbed psychologically, have no other clearly-defined psychiatric disease, and the disturbance in eating dominates the clinical picture. A relatively high proportion give a history of excessive weight, and the anorectic state results from a dieting excess "which never stopped." There is no explanation for the high frequency in young women, the rarity in males, and the high incidences in the middle and the upper income groups. Many patients with anorexia nervosa deny that they have an eating problem, and may hide their abnormality by inducing vomiting after eating a full meal, or by surreptitious disposal of food. Characteristic of most patients is a disturbed body image of size. They regard themselves as being fat, bloated, or ugly at commonly accepted normal weight levels and may promote a slender appearance by secret abuse of laxatives. The combination of restricted food, vomiting, and laxative abuse can lead to profound disturbance in electrolyte balance, notably sodium depletion, potassium depletion, alkalosis, secondary hyperaldosteronism, and hypotension. For this reason (and because patients commonly conceal their disturbance), unexplained electrolyte depletion must always suggest to the physician the existence of anorexia nervosa.

It is traditional to interpret many of the feeding problems of these patients in terms of serious psychosexual conflict, such as "fear of impregnation," and it is true that many are extremely immature sexually and may show a curious manipulative form of seductive behavior. On the other hand, many patients appear to be completely within normal limits in their sexual activity and are capable of normal marital life. Even though one can interpret the amenorrhea in this condition to mean symbolically that the patient does not wish to become pregnant, it has been reported in one study that two of three anorexia nervosa patients in whom ovulation was induced by hormone injections resumed normal cycling after pregnancy.

With respect to the menstrual disturbance, some patients stop menstruating within a month of onset of anorexia, thus indicating that both are manifestations of a common disorder. On the other hand, amenorrhea may not develop until substantial weight has been lost. In all cases, normal periods will not return until weight has risen to a critical level. In this regard, the loss and resumption of menses is analogous to the normal appearance of menstruation at puberty, a point emphasized by the work of Frisch and Revelle.[25, 26] Further insight into the nature of the gonadotropin regulatory defect in anorexia nervosa has come from the work of Boyar and colleagues.[13] Using a technique which permits the sampling of blood gonadotropin levels at short intervals over 24 hours, they found that some patients showed a very flat curve and barely detectable levels of LH, whereas others showed the spiking LH pattern which is characteristic of an earlier stage of maturity. It is evident, therefore, that in the majority of cases both psychogenic and nutritional factors determine the menstrual state.

Other evidence of hypothalamic disorder has been demonstrated in anorexia nervosa, such as disturbances of thermal and vasomotor homeostasis. There is increased growth of lanugo-type body hair.

Anorexia nervosa is not benign; 20 per cent of earlier series of patients have died, although the figure is closer to 5 to 10 per cent today. There is a critical weight for each patient beyond which weight loss may be fatal. Early hospitalization is recommended in borderline cases.

In addition to hypogonadism, a number of other endocrine manifestations of anorexia nervosa, all attributable to malnutrition, are observed. These include borderline low-normal plasma thyroxine levels, often with extremely low levels of plasma triiodothyronine and elevated plasma levels of growth hormone, with normal plasma cortisol.[54] An important feature differentiating the condition from hypopituitarism is retention of pituitary-adrenal responsiveness. The normal adrenal cortical function of the patient with anorexia nervosa permits retention of normal pubic and axillary hair, a helpful clinical clue. Since the amenorrhea in this disorder is neurogenic, it would appear reasonable to suppose that such patients have a normal pituitary response to injections of LHRH. This assumption is correct in only a proportion of cases. About half show no response to a single injection of LHRH, attributable to long-standing LHRH deficiency and not to intrinsic pituitary disease. Responsiveness returns when weight is regained.[90]

PSYCHOGENIC AMENORRHEA. Anorexia nervosa and pseudocyesis are the clearest examples of neurogenic (psychogenic) amenorrhea. But these make up the minority of cases of functional amenorrhea or oligomenorrhea. Amenorrhea may occur as a response to relatively trivial events (even ones with generally pleasant associations) such as going away to college or to summer camp, and is also seen after profoundly disturbing stress such as an automobile accident, rape, or incarceration in a concentration camp. In the famous series of cases observed during the London Blitz, each of four women who stopped cycling in response to a bombing attack was shown by endometrial biopsy to be arrested at the age of the cycle present at the time of the emotional stress.

Unfortunately for the diagnostician, many cases of hypothalamic amenorrhea do not fit the categories of psychic disorder mentioned above. These women are not apparently different psychologically from comparable groups of normal women, and the diagnosis is usually made by exclusion, and by prolonged follow-up. We have had the experience in about one fifth of these women of observing resumption of normal periods after careful medical evaluation.

The clinician is commonly called on to decide how extensively to pursue neurologic diagnostic procedures in patients with unexplained hypothalamic-pituitary hypogonadism. The rare occurrence of isolated FSH deficiency should be kept in mind.[68] The question of invasive diagnostic procedures such as pneumoencephalography is often raised. It is our practice to obtain roentgenograms of the pituitary fossa, and to evaluate the other endocrine functions of the pituitary, particularly pituitary-thyroid, pituitary-adrenal, growth hormone secretory reserve, and plasma prolactin. The LHRH secretory reserve test is being introduced into clinical medicine, but in most cases a single injection is not a powerful discriminatory tool.[58, 77, 109] The administration of clomiphene will bring about an ovulatory LH surge with or without subsequent menses in about 50 per cent of cases of functional amenorrhea, and is a useful diagnostic aid, for it will only be effective in the presence of an intact hypothalamic-pituitary-gonad axis. Even if clomiphene is ineffective, if other pituitary functions (including prolactin) and conventional roentgenograms are normal, it is our recommendation to do no further diagnostic procedures, but to observe the patient for prolonged periods of time. It is important to reassure the patient that in great likelihood this is a self-limited condition, and that the use of drugs such as clomiphene or gonadotropins will permit the induction of ovulation (with subsequent pregnancy) in up to 80 per cent of cases when pregnancy is desired. The plan of treatment depends on the patient's needs. If she is severely hypogonadal (secondary to gonadotropin deficiency), substitution therapy is indicated, as is also the case if the patient wants to have regular menses. Drugs to induce ovulation are indicated if the patient wishes to become pregnant. The decision as to psychotherapy is determined by psychologic evaluation and criteria. Psychologic distress and malfunction are the indications for therapy, and not anovulation per se, because the latter is not closely correlated with the severity of psychic disturbance.

Hypogonadotropic Hypogonadism in Males

Deficiency of LHRH secretion in males, as in females, results in hypogonadism. Acquired structural disease of the hypothalamus and stalk can be the cause of LHRH deficiency, and there appears to be at least one type of isolated congenital hypophysi-otropic-hormone failure.[4, 50] Specific causes of acquired disease include craniopharyngioma, internal hydrocephalus (of any cause), neoplasms of many types including leukemia, granuloma (eosinophilic granuloma, histiocytosis X, sarcoidosis, tuberculosis), encephalitis, microcephaly, Freidreich's ataxia, and demyelinating disorders. Although any of these conditions can cause isolated gonadotropin failure, usually other pituitary deficiencies are present or develop in time. On the other hand, the congenital form of hypogonadism appears to be a developmental problem and remains fixed throughout the individual's life.

With the benefit of modern knowledge, one can review early case reports of neurologic developmental abnormalities accompanied by hypogonadism such as those quoted in *Psychopathia Sexualis* by Krafft-Ebbing:

> A case mentioned by *Heschl* ("Wiener Zeitschrift f. pract. Heilkunde," 22d March, 1861) is remarkable, where the absence of both olfactory lobes was accompanied by imperfectly developed genitals. It was the case of a man aged forty-five, in all respects well developed, with the exception of the testicles, which were not larger than beans and contained no seminal canals, and the larynx, which seemed to be of feminine dimensions. Every trace of olfactory nerves was wanting, and the *trigona olfactoria* and the furrow on the under surface of the anterior lobes were absent. The perforations of the ethmoid plate were sparingly present, and occupied by nerveless processes of the dura instead of by nerves. In the mucous membrane of the nose there was also an absence of nerves.[46]

Cases of this type are probably due to maldevelopment of the olfactory brain with associated abnormalities of gonadotropin-regulating areas. A key manifestation in some, but not all, individuals is hyposmia.[4, 50] The full-blown syndrome (Kallmann's syndrome) is also known as olfactory-genital dysplasia and is often associated with other neurologic defects such as color blindness and nerve deafness. Kallmann's syndrome is a genetic disorder, probably inherited as an X-linked dominant gene with incomplete penetrance. Variations may occur, including males with hyposmia but with normal sex function. Females may also have hyposmia but almost always have normal sex function. Sporadic cases of this syndrome also occur, and many cases have been reported of isolated gonadotropin deficiency with normal olfaction. Whether the latter type of case is related to Kallmann's syndrome is not known. The hyposmia is a convenient diagnostic clue to the diagnosis because in the usual type of hypopituitarism, olfactory thresholds are lowered with the result that olfactory sensation is enhanced.

In the differential diagnosis of isolated hypogonadotropic hypogonadism, LHRH administration is being used with increasing frequency. As noted above, a single injection of LHRH may have little or no effect.[35, 51] Repeated subcutaneous injections, however, gradually restore gonadotropin secretory responsiveness, and in fact can bring about maturation of normal spermatozoal function. In one reported case, repeated LHRH injections led to antibody formation and subsequent loss of effectiveness.[101] Insemination has been successful in a few cases after this treatment. The testis in isolated hypogonadotropic hypogonadism is also somewhat unresponsive to stimulation by its tropic hormone, in this case LH, and this responsivity is gradually restored by successive injections. Such studies indicate that both ends of the pituitary-gonad axis are abnormal.

A well-established cause of neurogenic hypogonadism in males is inflammatory or traumatic spinal cord lesions. The testosterone deficiency is sometimes accompanied by gynecomastia. It is tempting to speculate that genital sensations normally exert a regulatory influence on gonadotropic secretion, but convincing evidence of this in humans has been difficult to obtain. Sexual excitement and orgasm in men or women does not lead (on a short-term basis at any rate) to alterations in plasma gonadotropin level. This is in contrast to the situation in many animals in which stimulation of the cervix leads to an acute release of LH capable of triggering ovulation. The regulatory effects of neural afferents from the human genitalia on gonadotropin secretion remain to be studied.

There is suggestive evidence that a form of neurogenic hypogonadism in men is analogous to the more readily detectable amenorrhea of women. In the studies of Kreus and coworkers,[47] plasma testosterone was observed in detail during military training of officers. During the period recognized by the subjects as being extremely stressful, plasma testosterone levels reached their nadir (Fig. 16). In a particularly convincing experiment carried out in a rhesus monkey colony, loss of status in the dominance hierarchy brought about by introduction of a more aggressive male led to a marked decline in plasma testosterone levels.

The various forms of hypogonadotropic hypogonadism are generally considered in the differential diagnosis of boys who fail to mature sexually at the usual age (10 to 16).[48] However, most cases of delayed puberty are not caused by structural disease of the hypothalamus or pituitary, but appear related to inborn patterns of development. Delayed puberty commonly, but not always, runs in families, is often accompanied by delay in psychosexual maturation as well, and is frequently accompanied by obesity. So common, in fact, is the association of obesity and delayed puberty that it has been considered that hypogonadism may be caused by the obesity, or that both are manifesta-

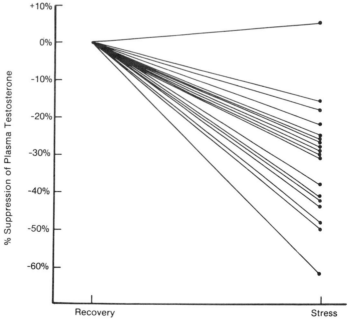

Figure 16. Changes in plasma testosterone level in male subjects undergoing the stress of officer candidate school. Each individual serves as his own control, a value being obtained during the most stressful period (third week) and again during the last phase of the training period, perceived by the students as being much less stressful. Only one individual showed no significant difference in values between the two periods. (From Kreuz, L. E., Rose, R. M. and Jennings, J. R.: *Suppression of plasma testosterone levels and psychological stress.* Arch. Gen. Psychiatry 26:479, 1972, with permission.)

tions of the same functional hypothalamic disorder.[52, 64, 86, 93] The endocrinologist should always determine whether the apparent small size of the penis is due to a large pubic fat pad. A very small penis is suggestive evidence of extremely marked hypogonadism of long standing, and suggests that the disorder is true gonadotropin deficiency, and not delayed puberty.

Because delayed puberty must be differentiated from the more serious causes of hypogonadism, and because of the severe psychologic consequences of prolonged infantilism in adolescent-age boys, efforts should be made before age 15 to establish the diagnosis with certainty and initiate some form of treatment.[22] It is important to treat testosterone deficiency at an early age, because normal psychosocial development in the male requires testosterone at a critical period. Late replacement (e.g., after the age of 20) is generally unsatisfactory in restoring normal sexual vigor and a normal male aggressive personality.[97]

The differential diagnosis of delayed puberty in boys is difficult.[41] If routine roentgenograms show that the pituitary fossa is normal, visual fields are normal, and other tests of pituitary function (particularly growth hormone reserve) are normal, most causes of pituitary failure are excluded, but isolated hypogonadotropic hypogonadism cannot be excluded. Injection of LHRH elicits only modest or no response in the prepubertal child and is not helpful in differential diagnosis,[77] nor do children with delayed puberty respond to clomiphene, a widely used test of pituitary-gonad reserve. Normal sense of smell does not exclude the diagnosis of isolated hypogonadotropic failure. Given a child with completely normal neurologic examination, normal pituitary fossa, and normal anterior pituitary function (except for gonadotropins), most clinical endocrinologists will not recommend further neuroradiologic measures but will observe the case over a period of time. For psychologic reasons it is recommended that replacement androgenic hormones be given by age 15. Some believe that this treatment may trigger the onset of normal sexual maturation by stimulating maturation of the hypothalamus, but in any case, it does not prevent the normal process if it is to occur. Testes development is clear evidence of onset of gonadotropic function, but in any case, treatment is stopped for a month every year up to the age of 20 to determine whether normal sexual function has begun. Of course, neurologic status and other pituitary functions should also be evaluated. It is generally assumed that if sexual maturity does not occur by age 20 to 22, normal spontaneous gonadotropic functions will never develop.

Delayed Puberty In Women

Many of the considerations discussed above for boys also govern the diagnosis and management of girls with delayed onset of sexual development. Age 16 is commonly taken as the criterion of delay, even though the normal age range for this development is from 11 to 13 in healthy Caucasian girls. Nutrition plays an even greater role in the female than the male, either obesity or extreme inanition delaying the onset of menses. In both girls and boys, gonadal failure and hypothalamic-pituitary failure can readily be differentiated because at the normal time of puberty, children with gonadal failure show an increased secretion of gonadotropic hormones.

Precocious Puberty

The term *precocious puberty* is used when otherwise normal pituitary-gonad function appears at an abnormally early age.[9, 30, 37, 49, 55] In boys this means onset of androgen secretion and spermatogenesis, and in girls onset of estrogen secretion and cyclic ovarian activity. In *primary* disease of testis or ovary, causing early hypersecretion of androgens and estrogens (in boys and girls respectively), physical sex characteristics

117

develop prematurely, but in contrast to the situation in true precocious puberty, gametogenesis does not develop similarly. Examples are the adrenogenital syndrome due to enzymatic defects of the adrenal cortex, or tumors of ovary or testis. These disorders are classified as *pseudoprecocious puberty*.

True precocious puberty always arises from disturbed neural function, which may or may not have an identifiable structural basis. Only this form of neurogenic disorder is considered in this text; pseudoprecocious puberty is classified here as a primary endocrine problem.

Normal Age of Onset of Puberty

For the past century and a half, the average age at menarche in Western European countries has decreased by about 3 to 4 months per decade. Thus, from 1840 to 1973, in representative Scandinavian populations, the decrease has been from age 17.2 to 12.7. This *secular* trend appears to be leveling off in developed countries, and it seems that the major factor now determining pubertal onset is genetic, if environmental factors such as food and infection are generally adequate. The work of Frisch and Revelle[25, 26] suggests strongly that the critical factor for initiation of puberty is the achievement of a certain body weight, about 48 kg. for average Caucasian populations. Due to improved nutrition and decreased infection, this weight is achieved sooner now than in earlier times, thus accounting for the secular change. The fact that critical weight is associated with a certain amount of stored calories as fat, has led to the teleologic interpretation that puberty begins when there are sufficient calories in storage form to sustain a woman through pregnancy and lactation. The mechanism by which a critical mass of fat stores can trigger the neural events underlying puberty is unknown.

Owing to the fact that there is no event in males that so dramatically signals onset of sexual development as does menarche in females, analogous data have not been compiled for boys.

The mean age at menarche in the United States was estimated recently as 12.6 ± 1.1 years (S.D.). In the studies of Tanner,[96] the mean onset of the growth spurt in girls was 10.7 years, of breast development 10.8 years, of the appearance of pubic hair 11.3 years, and of menarche 10.5 to 15.5 years (Tables 2 and 3). The diagnosis of precocity is usually made if the age at menarche is under 8 years. Partial puberty is not uncommon in girls. *Precocious thelarche* refers to premature development of breasts unaccompanied by other signs of puberty, and *precocious pubarche* (adrenarche) refers to

Table 2. Sequence of Appearance of Sexual Characteristics in Normal Puberty

Onset	Mean (Years)	Range (Years)
Male		
Testes growth	11.5	9.5 – 13.5
Pubic hair	12.0	10.5 – 14.5
Penis growth	12.5	10.5 – 14.5
Growth spurt	12.7	10.5 – 16.0
Female		
Growth spurt	10.7	
Breast development	10.8	8.0 – 13.0
Pubic hair	11.3	
Menarche	12.7	10.5 – 15.5

(Adapted from Tanner, J. M.: *Growth and Endocrinology of the Adolescent. In* Gardner, L. I. (ed.): *Endocrine and Genetic Diseases of Childhood and Adolescence,* ed. 2. W. B. Saunders, Philadelphia, 1975.)

Table 3. Representative Ages at Menarche in Various Groups

Country	Year	Age at Menarche
England	1965	13.0 ± 0.2 (S.E.M.)
United States	1968	
Whites		12.8 ± 0.04
Blacks		12.5 ± 0.11
Istanbul	1965	
Rich		12.3 ± 0.15
Average		12.8 ± 0.11
Poor		13.2 ± 0.10
Hong Kong (Chinese)	1962	
Rich		12.5 ± 0.18
Average		12.8 ± 0.20
Poor		13.3 ± 0.19

(Adapted from Tanner, J. M.: *Growth and Endocrinology of the Adolescent. In* Gardner, L. I. (ed.): *Endocrine and Genetic Diseases of Childhood and Adolescence,* ed. 2. W. B. Saunders, Philadelphia, 1975.)

premature development of pubic hair. The mechanisms underlying these partial forms of puberty have not been elucidated. They do not have the same clinical significance as does precocious menstruation.

In boys, testes growth begins at a mean age of 11.8 ± 1 years (S.D.). In Tanner's series, the age of normal onset of testes growth was as low as 9.5 years, of penis growth 10.5 to 14.5 years, and of the growth spurt 10.5 to 16 years (see Table 2). It is common to use the term precocious puberty if spermatogenesis is present before the age of 10 years, but it is obvious that in the age range 9 to 10 the diagnosis of precocity may be ambiguous.

Incidence and Causes of Precocious Puberty

True precocious puberty is at least twice as common in girls as in boys.[100] In girls this diagnosis is less serious than in boys because less than 10 per cent of the cases have organic structural intracranial lesions, whereas 20 to 40 per cent of cases in boys have significant intracranial lesions.

IDIOPATHIC SEXUAL PRECOCITY. This is the largest category of true precocity.[9, 30] There is an hereditary form, largely confined to males, but familial occurrence is uncommon. In the studies of Liu and coworkers,[49] girls with true precocity were found to have a high incidence of abnormal electroencephalograms and behavioral disturbance, suggesting the presence of an underlying brain disturbance. Beirich[9] disputes this contention and claims that precocious puberty is unaccompanied by even occult brain damage. The pathogenesis of this disorder therefore remains a matter of controversy.

NEUROGENIC PRECOCIOUS PUBERTY. The site of hypothalamic lesions that influence the timing of puberty are not well localized in the human, since most cases coming to autopsy have relatively widespread disease. In the classic compilation of Weinberger and Grant,[103] approximately two thirds of the cases in which anatomic correlations could be made had destruction of the posterior hypothalamus. This is in contrast to the situation in the rat, in which localized lesions in the preoptic hypothalamus induce precocious puberty. Invasive lesions that have been recognized to cause precocity[10] include craniopharyngioma (although delayed puberty is more common), hamartoma,[74] astrocytoma,[103] pineal lesion (see below), encephalitis, miliary tuberculosis, tuberous sclerosis, Sturge-Weber syndrome, porencephaly, craniostenosis, microcephaly, hydrocephalus, and Tay-Sachs disease.[70]

One category of neoplasms of the hypothalamus that merits special mention is the hamartoma.[74] This lesion is a possible exception to the generalization that tumors of the brain cause precocious puberty by destructive effects on the regions that normally suppress gonadotropin secretion. A *hamartoma* may be defined neuropathologically as a tumor-like collection of normal nerve tissue lodged in an abnormal location. One type of hypothalamic hamartoma consists of a sharply encapsulated nodule of nerve tissue attached to the posterior hypothalamus at a point between the anterior portion of the mammillary body and the posterior region of the tuber cinereum. These differ from glial tumors that may occupy the same region, but are invasive.

The hypothalamic hamartoma grows into the cisternal space between the cerebral peduncles, often adapting itself to the pyramidal shape of the cisternal space, and may produce signs of early puberty before other neural effects occur. Tumors of this type are rare, fewer than 50 having been reported up to 1972, but miniature "hamartomatous" nodular formations of the tuber cinereum are commonly seen in normal brains. Many hypothalamic hamartomas are asymptomatic, and it has been proposed that precocious puberty occurs when the tumor has specific connections to the median eminence, thus serving as an "accessory hypothalamus" as proposed by Richter.[74] That the tumor may secrete LHRH was proposed by Beirich[9] who found LHRH in the spinal fluid of three such patients. Neurosecretory cells that contained LHRH demonstrable by immunohistochemical study have recently been described in a hamartoma.

The clinical presentation in patients with hamartoma is not different from other known cerebral causes of precocity. Hamartomas occur in either sex, have been seen as early as 3 months of age, and are usually fatal before age 20. Early in the illness, precocity is the only sign; later, progressive pressure on the hypothalamus causes severe local disturbances. These tumors are said to be radioresistant.

HYPOTHYROIDISM. The association of sexual precocity with juvenile hypothyroidism, though rare, is well known and is reversed by treatment with thyroxine.[100, 104] In a small proportion of cases, the precocity is associated with galactorrhea. Van der Werff ten Bosch[100] compiled a series of 14 girls and 3 boys with a combination of thyroid deficiency and precocious puberty. In the case reported by Sadeghi-Nejad and Senior,[80] the disorder was induced by propylthiouracil treatment of hyperthyroidism. Recently, it has been shown that some patients with hypothyroidism (with or without galactorrhea) may have elevated plasma prolactin levels,[28] and some patients with hypothyroidism may also show elevation of plasma gonadotropins. The syndrome of hypothyroidism, galactorrhea, and precocious puberty must require a special susceptibility, since it is an uncommon manifestation of the hypothyroid state. Rarely, the pituitary fossa is enlarged, and hyperpigmentation occurs. Pituitary enlargement is probably due to hyperplasia and hypertrophy of thyrotrope cells. The cause of the pigmentation is unknown.

Various theories of pathogenesis have been proposed to explain the association between sexual maturation and hypothyroidism. That proposed by Van Wyck and Grumbach[102] suggests that there is cross-specificity in feedback control of TSH, LH, and FSH, all glycoprotein hormones secreted by basophil cells. An alternative theory has been proposed that hypothyroidism causes hypothalamic encephalopathy, which in turn interferes with brain regions that normally suppress LHRH secretion. The high prolactin levels sometimes seen in this syndrome might be due to a similarly produced deficiency of PIF. However, increased sensitivity of the pituitary to PRF may also be the cause, since it has been shown that patients with hypothyroidism have higher-than-normal prolactin responses to TRH injection.

The importance of early recognition of this disease lies in the fact that it is completely benign and readily treated by thyroid hormone replacement. Occasionally an ovarian cyst may mimic an estrogen-secreting ovarian tumor. Treatment with thyroid hormone leads to a regression of the ovarian mass.

SEXUAL PRECOCITY WITH POLYOSTOTIC FIBROUS DYSPLASIA. A number of endocrine disturbances are noted in association with the bone lesion *polyostotic fibrous dysplasia*. This disorder, called the Weil-Albright-McCune-Sternberg syndrome (more commonly the Albright syndrome) includes precocious puberty in one third of the cases and smooth-margined pigmented skin areas in most.[29, 33, 87] Other endocrine disturbances seen in this condition include the rare occurrence of thyrotoxicosis, Cushing's syndrome, acromegaly, and gynecomastia. This syndrome is commonly listed as a cause of true precocious puberty because in at least one case, a 6½-year-old boy showed testes development to the point of spermatogenesis and in at least one female patient ovulatory levels of LH have been observed. Another clue to a hypothalamic-pituitary etiology is the occasional thickening of the basal skull. On theoretic grounds Hall and Warrick[29] have proposed that there may be hypersecretion of the hypothalamic releasing hormones in this condition.

However, the bulk of evidence now available indicates that this condition is not true precocity, but rather a primary endocrine disease. Ovulation has not been demonstrated in any of the female patients. In three patients whose ovaries were explored, luteinized corpora were not found, which is evidence that ovulation had not taken place. In four patients with sexual precocity studied at the Massachusetts General Hospital by Danon and Crawford,[20] plasma estrogens were elevated and gonadotropin levels depressed, findings that point to primary hypersecretion of the ovary. In a similar case the patient, in addition, had a prepubertal rather than pubertal type of response to injections of LHRH. Uterine bleeding is of the characteristic breakthrough type. The patients ultimately pass through a normal puberty in which cyclic ovulation occurs. The ovaries are usually cystic (multiple, or single on each side) and removal of the cysts leads to a temporary decrease in estrogen secretion. These considerations make it reasonable to conclude that most of such patients do not have true precocious puberty as defined in this chapter. The true cause of the illness is unknown.

THE PINEAL GLAND AND PRECOCIOUS PUBERTY. In 1898 Huebner[32] reported a case of precocious puberty in a boy with a tumor of the pineal gland. This clinical observation, subsequently reported in a number of other patients, has stimulated much investigation of the role of the pineal gland in sexual maturation, but has led to an exaggerated view of the importance of pineal tumors as the cause of true sexual precocity.[18] In the three large series of patients with cerebral precocious puberty assembled by Wilkins,[110] Jolly,[37] and Thamdrup[96] no cases of pineal disease were identified, and Van der Werff ten Bosch estimated in 1975[100] that only about 50 cases altogether had been described in the literature. Although both precocity and delayed puberty have been recorded in pineal tumors, such sexual disturbance is not a common finding. In a series of 65 pineal tumors recorded by Ringertz[75] only seven occurred in children under age 11, and in none did sexual precocity occur. In Bing and associates'[10] series of 177 patients, 56 were under age 15 and of these one third had sexual precocity. In their series, precocious puberty occurred only when the tumor had extended well beyond the pineal region. Clinical evidence of hypothalamic involvement such as diabetes insipidus, hyperphagia, somnolence, obesity, or behavioral disturbance was found in 71 per cent of the cases.

These compilations have led some workers to the view that when pineal tumors produce precocious puberty they do so by the same mechanism that other brain tumors do, i.e., by physical destruction of the regions of the brain that tonically inhibit gonadotropin secretion.[105, 106] This view is further supported by a consideration of the histologic nature of pineal neoplasms. Most tumors arising from the pineal gland are probably not derived from pineal cells.[79] In one series of 56 cases only nine could be classified as probable pinealocytomas and pinealoblastomas, 18 were histologically unidentifiable lesions assumed to be pineal neoplasms on clinical and roentgenographic grounds, 13 were germinomas, 13 were glial tumors, and 3 were teratomas. The pathologic nature of these tumors of the pineal gland is discussed in Chapter 10.

On the other hand, there is some evidence that at least a proportion of pineal tumors have endocrine function. Kitay,[44] in an extensive review of all published cases of pineal tumor, noted that nonparenchymal tumors were three times as likely to produce precocity as were parenchymal tumors. He therefore postulated that the high incidence was due to pineal destruction; the loss of a pineal secretion was believed to inhibit development of sexual maturity. At least one pineal parenchymal tumor has been reported to contain hydroxyindole-O-methyltransferase (HIOMT) enzyme activity, a marker enzyme which signifies the presence of a biochemical mechanism for the formation of melatonin from its precursor N-acetylserotonin, a characteristic pineal function.

From a theoretic point of view, it is reasonable to predict that some pineal tumors would cause disease by excessive secretion of the puberty-delaying pineal hormone melatonin or another, as yet unidentified, hormone. Although delayed puberty or hypogonadism has been reported by Puschett and Goldberg[67] to occur in cases of pineal tumor, all have been teratomas rather than true pinealomas, and most have had anatomic evidence of invasion of the third ventricle and damage to surrounding structures, including vision loss and diabetes insipidus.[24, 31] In two of Puschett and Goldberg's cases, there was no clinical evidence of basal hypothalamic destruction, but they correctly emphasize the observation of Horrax[31] that "in some cases in which gross evidence of hypothalamic involvement is absent, careful sectioning of the pathologic specimen may reveal microscopic infiltration by tumor in the floor of the third ventricle."

A final opinion as to the mechanism of precocious puberty in pineal tumors cannot be given at this time, but we believe that most likely the bulk of such cases are due to direct hypothalamic damage, and not to pineal hormonal effects.

It should be recognized that in a few rare cases, choriocarcinomas of the pineal region, arising as teratomas, have secreted sufficient amounts of chorionic gonadotropic hormones to stimulate testes growth and mimic true puberty.

Clinical Approach to the Diagnosis of Precocious Puberty

In the child with precocious development of secondary sex characteristics, the first requirement is to determine whether mature germ cells are being formed. If spermatogenesis and ovulation are taking place, the diagnosis of true precocity is evident, and the problem than becomes a neurologic one in evaluating the presence of anatomic damage to the hypothalamus. Polyostotic fibrous dysplasia, a rare cause of pseudoprecocity in boys but more common in girls, can be considered on the basis of characteristic bone cysts on roentgenograms of the long bones, pelvis, and skull, and by the finding of smoothly-marginated brown-pigmented spots on the skin. Factitious precocious development caused by ingestion of hormone pills may cause precocity, but is much more likely to be seen in girls than boys.

MALES. Clues to normal testes development in boys include testes enlargement to adult size, the appearance of sperm in overnight voided urine specimens and after seminal vesicle and prostate massage, and if necessary biopsy of the testicle. Excessive secretion of androgenic hormone by adrenal or other tumors usually leads to *small* prepubertal-size testes. Rarely, however, they may appear to be of normal adult size because they contain adrenal rest tumors. Other reasons why testes size may appear normal in pseudoprecocious puberty are tumors producing testosterone, and testes growth due to excessive chorionic gonadotropic hormone arising from a teratoma located elsewhere (mediastinum, pineal region). The laboratory is helpful in distinguishing these forms of abnormality. The precocious boy with true cerebral precocity will show hormonal values similar to those of a normal adult male. In cases due to excessive adrenal androgens, urinary 17-ketosteroid excretion will be markedly and diagnostically elevated; if due to excessive HCG secretion, plasma radioimmuno-assays of HCG or the specific β-chain of HCG will be grossly abnormal. If due to a testosterone-producing testicular or adrenal tumor, plasma testosterone will be elevated to or above the normal adult male level, unaccompanied by evidence of spermato-genesis.

Once the diagnosis of cerebral precocity is made in the male, the high frequency with which intracranial disease is found requires full neurologic evaluation. Even in the face of normal conventional roentgenogram study, tomography, and CAT scan, we recommend pneumoencephalography. It is important to recognize that in pineal teratomas, pineal calcification occurs earlier than normal. Pineal lesions occur almost exclusively in males.

FEMALES. The appearance of regular menses is evidence for a normal gonadotropin-ovarian axis. The best confirmation of normal ovulatory function by noninvasive methods is the demonstration of a midcycle elevation of plasma LH and FSH by immunoassay. However, more or less regular periods may result from "breakthrough" due to sustained estrogen effect. This can be due to intrinsic ovarian disease, or to estrogen secretion by an adrenal tumor or by a teratoma, but in all such cases, plasma estradiol levels will be persistently elevated to the normal adult range, and plasma gonadotropin concentrations will be in the adult normal range[36] and will not show the characteristic elevation at 12, 13, or 14 days prior to the menses. One possible source of confusion is the occurrence, even in normal puberty, of anovulatory cycles so that irregular and scanty periods may appear for one to three years before periods become normal. Hence, there may be some confusion in differentiating a mild hyperestrogenic state from the early pubertal state accompanying precocious puberty. It may take a period of observation or even colposcopy to evaluate the state of ovarian function. Demonstration of a corpus luteum is adequate evidence that ovulation has taken place. Plasma progesterone measurements or aspiration endometrial biopsy can indicate the presence of a luteinized ovary. Since a relatively conservative neurologic approach is indicated in true precocity, the main condition to identify early is an estrogen-secreting tumor. This can be done readily by measurement of plasma estradiol and gonadotropins by immunoassay. In estrogen hypersecretion, estradiol is adult normal or higher and gonadotropins (LH and FSH) are decreased.

In girls with true precocity, neurologic evaluation should include conventional skull roentgenograms, CAT scan if available, and electroencephalogram. If there are no abnormal neurologic findings, and if pituitary function is otherwise normal, including tests for diabetes insipidus and growth hormone secretory reserve (see Chapter 14), invasive neurologic diagnostic procedures are usually not indicated.

Management

In true precocity with demonstrable neurologic lesions, management usually requires biopsy since many lesions which surgically are not curable may respond to roentgen-otherapy. In the absence of demonstrable disease, hormone therapy may be useful. Injection of medroxyprogesterone acetate (MPGA) reduces secretion of gonadotropic hormones.[76] [81] In girls, this drug usually inhibits ovulation and causes a regression of breast hypertrophy and menses. However, this therapy does not delay the progressive skeletal maturation; the child shows accelerated growth when young, but ultimately becomes a short adult because of early closure of the epiphyses of the long bones.

Psychologic management is of great importance in precocious puberty. This aspect of management has been emphasized by Money and collaborators[55, 56] because, in some cases, there is little else that the physician can do but help the child and parents cope with premature sexual development. Fortunately, almost all girls and most boys do not show precocious sex drive and interests. From experience with MPGA in men with excessive sex drive, it is to be anticipated that treatment with MPGA would also be valuable in children with this condition. The works of Money and of Ehrhardt[22] give valuable guidance to parents of precocious children.

REFERENCES

1. ABRAHAM, G. E., ET AL.: *Simultaneous radioimmunoassay of plasma FSH, LH, progesterone, 17-hydroxyprogesterone, and estradiol-17β during the menstrual cycle.* J. Clin. Endocrinol. Metab. 34:312, 1972.

2. AIYER, M. S., CHIAPPA, S. A. AND FINK, G.: *A priming effect of luteinizing hormone releasing factor on the anterior pituitary gland in the female rat.* J. Endocrinol. 62:573, 1974.

3. ANDERSON, E. AND HAYMAKER, W.: *Breakthroughs in hypothalamic and pituitary research. In* Swaab, D. F. and Schade, J. P. (eds.): *Progress in Brain Research, 41: Integrative Hypothalamic Activity.* Elsevier, Amsterdam, 1974, p.1.

4. ANTAKI, A., ET AL.: *Hypothalamic-pituitary function in the olfactogenital syndrome.* J. Clin. Endocrinol. Metab. 38:1083, 1974.

5. BAKER, B. L., DERMODY, W. C. AND REEL, J. R.: *Distribution of gonadotropin-releasing hormone in the rat brain as observed with immunocytochemistry.* Endocrinology 97:125, 1975.

6. BARKER, H. M., ET AL.: *Radioimmunoassay of luteinizing hormone releasing hormone.* Nature 242: 527, 1973.

7. BARRY, J. AND DUBOIS, M. P.: *Immunofluorescent study of LRF-producing neurones in the cat and dog.* Neuroendocrinology 18:290, 1975.

8. BESSER, G. M., ET AL.: *Hormonal responses to synthetic luteinizing hormone and follicle stimulating hormone-releasing hormone in man.* Br. Med. J. 3:267, 1972.

9. BIERICH, J. R.: *Sexual precocity. In* Bierich, J. R. (ed.): *Clinics in Endocrinology and Metabolism,* vol. 4, no. 1. W. B. Saunders, Philadelphia, 1975, p. 107.

10. BING, J. F., ET AL.: *Pubertas praecox: a survey of the reported cases and verified anatomical findings.* J. Mt. Sinai Hosp. N.Y. 4:935, 1938.

11. BOGUMIL, R. J., ET AL: *Mathematical studies of the human menstrual cycle. I. Formulation of a mathematical model.* J. Clin. Endocrinol. Metab. 35:126, 1972.

12. BOYAR, R. M., ET AL.: *Twenty-four hour luteinizing hormone and follicle-stimulating hormone secretory patterns in gonadal dysgenesis.* J. Clin. Endocrinol. Metab. 37:521, 1973.

13. BOYAR, R. M., ET AL.: *Anorexia nervosa: immaturity of 24-hour luteinizing hormone secretory pattern.* N. Engl. J. Med. 291:861, 1974.

14. BOYAR R., ET AL.: *Synchronization of augmented luteinizing hormone secretion with sleep during puberty.* New Engl. J. Med. 287:582, 1972.

15. BOYAR, R., ET AL.: *Twenty-four hour pattern of luteinizing hormone secretion in normal men with sleep stage.* J. Clin. Endocrinol. Metab. 35:73, 1972.

16. CASTLEMAN, B. AND MCNELLY, B. U.: *Case 25-1971 (germinoma). Case Records of the Massachusetts General Hospital.* N. Eng. J. Med. 284:1427, 1971.

17. CLEMENS, J. A., ET AL.: *Areas of the brain stimulatory to LH and FSH secretion.* Endocrinology 88: 180, 1971.

18. COHEN, R. A. (moderator); WURTMAN, R. J., AXELROD, J. AND SNYDEK, S. H. (discussants): *Combined Clinical Staff Conference at the National Institutes of Health. Some clinical, biochemical and physiological actions of the pineal gland.* Ann. Intern. Med. 61:1144, 1964.

19. CRAMER, O. M. AND BARRACLOUGH, C. A.: *Effects of preoptic electrical stimulation on pituitary LH release following interruption of components of the preoptico-tuberal pathway in rats.* Endocrinology 93:369, 1973.

20. DANON, M. AND CRAWFORD, J. D.: *Peripheral endocrinopathy causing sexual precocity in Albright's syndrome.* Pediatr. Res. 8:368, 1964.

21. DYRENFURTH, I., ET AL.: *Temporal relationships of hormonal variables in the menstrual cycle. In* Ferin, M., et al. (eds.): *Biorhythms and Human Reproduction.* John Wiley & Sons, New York, 1974, p. 171.

22. EHRHARDT, A. A. AND MEYER-BAHLBURG, J. F. L.: *Psychological correlates of abnormal pubertal development. In* Bierich, J. R. (ed.): *Clinics in Endocrinology and Metabolism,* vol. 4, no. l. W. B. Saunders, Philadelphia, 1975, p. 207.

23. FAGLIA, B., ET AL.: *Elevations in plasma growth hormone concentration after luteinizing hormone-releasing hormone (LRH) in patients with active acromegaly.* J. Clin. Endocrinol. Metab. 37:338, 1973.

24. FOWLER, F. D., ALEXANDER, E., JR., AND DAVIS, C. J., JR.: *Pinealoma with metastases in the central nervous system: A rationale of treatment.* J. Neurosurg. 13:271, 1956.

25. FRISCH, R. E. AND REVELLE, R.: *Height and weight at menarche and a hypothesis of critical body weights and adolescent events.* Science 169:397, 1970.

26. FRISCH, R. E. AND REVELLE, R.: *Height and weight at menarche and a hypothesis of menarche.* Arch. Dis. Child. 46:695, 1971.

27. FRANCHIMONT, P., ET AL.: *Effect of hypothalamic luteinizing hormone-releasing hormone (LH-RH) on plasma gonadotropin levels in normal subjects.* Clin. Endocrinol. (Oxf.) 3:27, 1974.

28. FUTTERWEIT, W. AND GOODSELL, C. H.: *Galactorrhea in primary hypothyroidism: Report of two cases and review of the literature.* Mt. Sinai J. Med. N.Y. 37:584, 1970.

29. HALL, R. AND WARRICK, C.: *Hypersecretion of hypothalamic releasing hormones: A possible explanation of the endocrine manifestations of polyostotic fibrous displasia (Albright's syndrome).* Lancet 1: 1313, 1972.

30. HAMPSON, J. G. AND MONEY, J.: *Idiopathic sexual precocity in the female. Report of 3 cases.* Psychosom. Med. 17:16, 1955.

31. HORRAX, G.: *The role of pinealomas in the causation of diabetes insipidus.* Ann. Surg. 126:725, 1947.

32. HUEBNER, O.: *Tumor der Glandula Pinealis.* Dtsch. Med. Wochenschr. 24:214, 1898.

33. HUSBAND, P. AND SNODGRASS, J. A. I.: *McCune-Albright syndrome with endocrinological investigations. Report of a case.* Am. J. Dis. Child. 119:164, 1970.

34. HUTCHINSON, J. S. M., ET AL.: *Sexual precocity due to an intracranial tumor causing unusual testicular secretion of testosterone.* Arch. Dis. Child. 44:732, 1969.

35. ISURUGI, K., ET AL.: *Responses of serum luteinizing hormone and follicle-stimulating hormone levels to synthetic luteinizing hormone-releasing hormone (LH-RH) in various forms of testicular disorders.* J. Clin. Endocrinol. Metab. 37:533, 1973.

36. JENNER, M. R., ET AL.: *Hormonal changes in puberty. IV. Plasma estradiol, LH and FSH in prepubertal children, pubertal females and in precocious puberty, premature thelarche, hypogonadism and in a child with a feminizing ovarian tumor.* J. Clin. Endocrinol. Metab. 34:521, 1972.

37. JOLLY, H.: *Sexual Precocity.* Charles C Thomas, Springfield, 1955.

38. KASTIN, A. J., GUAL, C. AND SCHALLY, A. V.: *Clinical experience with hypothalamic releasing hormones. Part 2. Luteinizing hormone-releasing hormone and other hypophysiotropic releasing hormones.* Recent Prog. Horm. Res. 28:201, 1972.

39. KAWAKAMI, M., ET AL.: *Nature of the hippocampal function in relation to gonadotropin secretion. In* Yogi, K. and Yoshia, S. (eds.): *Neuroendocrine Control.* John Wiley & Sons, New York, 1973, p. 229.

40. KELCH, R. P., KAPLAN, S. L. AND GRUMBACH, M. M.: *Suppression of urinary and plasma follicle-stimulating hormone by exogenous estrogens in prepubertal and pubertal children.* J. Clin. Invest. 52:1122, 1973.

41. KELCH, R. P., GRUMBACH, M. M. AND KAPLAN, S. L.: *Studies on the mechanism of puberty in man. In* Mack, H. C. and Sherman, A. I. (eds.): *The Neuroendocrinology of Human Reproduction.* Charles C Thomas, Springfield, 1971, p. 524.

42. KEYE, W. R., JR. AND JAFFE, R. B.: *Modulation of pituitary gonadotropin response to gonadotropin-releasing hormone by estradiol.* J. Clin. Endocrinol. Metab. 38:805, 1974.

43. KIRSCHNER, M. A. AND BARDIN, C. W.: *Androgen production and metabolism in normal and virilized women.* Metabolism 21:667, 1972.

44. KITAY, J. I.: *Pineal lesions and precocious puberty, a review.* J. Clin. Endocrinol. Metab. 14:622, 1957.

45. KNOBIL, E.: *On the control of gonadotropin secretion in the rhesus monkey.* Recent Prog. Horm. Res. 30:1, 1974.

46. KRAFFT-EBBING: *Psychopathia Sexualis.* (1st English edition of the 7th German edition) Physicians and Surgeons Book Company, New York, 1927, p. 32.

47. KREUS, L. E., ROSE, R. M. AND JENNINGS, J. R.: *Suppression of plasma testosterone levels and psychological stress.* Arch. Gen. Psychiat. 26:479, 1972.

48. KULIN, H. E. AND REITER, E. O.: *Gonadotropins during childhood and adolescence: A review.* Pediatrics 51:260, 1973.

49. Liu, N., et al.: *Prevalence of electroencephalographic abnormalities in idiopathic precocious puberty and premature pubarche: Bearing on pathogenesis and neuroendocrine regulation of puberty.* J. Clin. Endocrinol. Metab. 25:1296, 1965.

50. Males, J. L., Townsend, J. L. and Schneider, R. A.: *Hypogonadotropic hypogonadism with anosmia — Kallmann's syndrome. A disorder of olfactory and hypothalamic function.* Arch. Intern. Med. 131:501, 1973.

51. Marshall, J. C., et al.: *Isolated pituitary gonadotrophin deficiency: gonadotrophin secretion after synthetic luteinizing hormone and follicle stimulating hormone releasing hormone.* Br. Med. J. 4:643, 1972.

52. Marshall, W. A.: *Growth and sexual maturation in normal puberty. In* Bierich, J. R. (ed.): *Clinics in Endocrinology and Metabolism,* vol. 4, no. 1. W. B. Saunders, Philadelphia, 1975, p. 3.

53. McCann, S. M.: *Regulation of secretion of follicle-stimulating hormone and luteinizing hormone. In* Greep, R. O. and Astwood, E. B. (eds.): *Handbook of Physiology, Section 7: Endocrinology,* vol. 4, part 1. American Physiological Society. Williams & Wilkins, Baltimore, 1974, p. 489.

54. Mecklenburg, R. S., et al.: *Hypothalamic dysfunction in patients with anorexia nervosa.* Medicine 53:147, 1974.

55. Money, J. and Hampson, J. G.: *Idiopathic sexual precocity in the male: Management: Report of a case.* Psychosom. Med. 17:1, 1955.

56. Money, J. and Alexander, D.: *Psychosexual development and absence of homosexuality in males with precocious puberty. Review of 18 cases.* J. Nerv. Ment. Dis. 148:111, 1969.

57. Mortimer, C. H., et al.: *Intravenous, intramuscular, subcutaneous and intranasal administration of LH/FSH-RH: The duration of effect and occurrence of asynchronous pulsatile release of LH and FSH.* Clin. Endocrinol. (Oxf.) 3:19 – 25, 1974.

58. Mortimer, C. H., et al.: *Luteinizing hormone and follicle stimulating hormone releasing hormone test in patients with hypothalamic-pituitary-gonadal dysfunction.* Br. Med. J. 4:73, 1973.

59. Naftolin, F., et al.: *Nocturnal patterns of serum gonadotropins during the menstrual cycle.* J. Clin. Endocrinol. Metab. 37:6, 1973.

60. Naftolin, F., Yen, S. S. C. and Tsai, C. C.: *Rapid cycling of plasma gonadotrophins in normal man as demonstrated by frequent sampling.* Nature [New Biol.] 236:92, 1972.

61. Nillius D. J. and Wide, L.: *Gonadotrophin-releasing hormone treatment for induction of follicular maturation and ovulation in amenorrhoeic women with anorexia nervosa.* Br. Med. J. 3:405, 1975.

62. Odell, W. D. and Meyer, D. L.: *Physiology of Reproduction.* C. V. Mosby, St. Louis, 1971.

63. Papkoff, H., et al.: *Studies on the structure and function of interstitial cell-stimulating hormone. In* Greep, R. O. (ed.): *Recent Progress in Hormone Research: Proceedings,* vol. 29. Academic Press, New York, 1973, p. 563.

64. Parks, G. A., et al.: *Variation in pituitary-gonadal function in adolescent male homosexuals and heterosexuals.* J. Clin. Endocrinol. Metab. 39:796, 1974.

65. Pfaff, D. W.: *Luteinizing hormone-releasing factor potentiates lordosis behavior in hypophysectomized ovariectomized female rats.* Science 182:1148, 1973.

66. Prader, A.: *Delayed adolescence. In* Beirich, J. R. (ed.): *Clinics in Endocrinology and Metabolism,* vol. 4, no. 1. W. B. Saunders, Philadelphia, 1975, p. 143.

67. Puschett, J. B. and Golberg, M.: *Endocrinopathy associated with pineal tumor.* Ann. Int. Med. 69:203, 1968.

68. Rabin, D. et al.: *Isolated deficiency of follicle-stimulating hormone.* N. Engl. J. Med. 287:1313, 1972.

69. Raisman, G. and Field, P. M.: *Sexual dimorphism in the preoptic area of the rat.* Science 173:731, 1971.

70. Relkin, R.: *Precocious puberty in Tay-Sachs Disease. In* Volk, B. W. and Aronson, S. M. (eds.): *Sphingolipids, Sphingolipidosis and Allied Disorders.* Plenum, New York, 1972, p. 671.

71. Reichlin, S.: *Neuroendocrinology. In* Williams, R. H. (ed.): *Endocrinology.* W. B. Saunders, Philadelphia, 1974.

72. Reichlin, S.: *The control of anterior pituitary secretion. In* Beeson, P. B. and McDermott, W. (eds.): *Textbook of Medicine.* W. B. Saunders, Philadelphia, 1975, p. 1670.

73. Reichlin, S.: *Regulation of the hypophysiotropic secretions of the brain.* Arch. Int. Med. 135:1350, 1975.

74. Richter, R. B.: *True hamartoma of the hypothalamus associated with pubertas praecox.* J. Neuropath. Exp. Neurol. 10:368, 1951.

75. Ringertz, N., et al.: *Tumors of the pineal region.* J. Neuropath. Exp. Neurol. 13:540, 1954.

76. RITKIND, A. B., ET AL.: *Suppression of urinary excretion of luteinizing hormone (LH) and follicle stimulating hormone (FSH) by medroxygesterone acetate*. J. Clin. Endocrinol. Metab. 29:506, 1969.

77. ROTH, J. C., ET AL.: *FSH and LH response to luteinizing hormone-releasing factor in prepubertal and pubertal children, adult males and patients with hypogonadotropic and hypergonadotropic hypogonadism*. J. Clin. Endocrinol. Metab. 35:926, 1972.

78. ROTHCHILD, I. M.: *Functional amenorrhea. In* Mack, H. C. and Sherman, A. I. (eds.): *The Neuroendocrinology of Human Reproduction*. Charles C Thomas, Springfield, 1971, p. 171.

79. RUSSELL, D. S. AND RUBINSTEIN, L. J.: *Pathology of Tumors of the Nervous System*. Edward Arnold, London, 1963, p. 173.

80. SADEGHI-NEJAD, A. AND SENIOR, B.: *Sexual precocity: An unusual complication of propylthiouracil therapy*. J. Pediatr. 79:833, 1971.

81. SADEGHI-NEJAD, S. L. AND GRUMBACH, M. M.: *The effect of medroxyprogesterone acetate on adrenocortical function in children with precocious puberty*. J. Pediatr. 78:616, 1971.

82. SCHALCH, D. S.: *Gonadotropin secretion in the human. In* Mack, H. C. and Sherman, A. I. (eds.): *Neuroendocrinology of Human Reproduction*. Charles C Thomas, Springfield, 1971, p. 185.

83. SCHALLY, A. V., KASTIN, A. J. AND ARIMURA, A.: *Hypothalamic regulatory hormones*. Science 179: 341, 1973.

84. SCHALLY, A. V., KASTIN, A. J. AND ARIMURA, A.: *FSH releasing hormone and LH releasing hormone*. Vitam. Horm. 30:83, 1972.

85. SCHNEIDER, H. P. G. AND McCANN, S. M.: *Possible role of dopamine as transmitter to promote discharge of LH-releasing factor*. Endocrinology 85:121, 1969.

86. SCHONBERG, D. K.: *Dynamics of hypothalamic-pituitary function during puberty. In* Beirich, J. R. (ed.): *Clinics in Endocrinology and Metabolism*. vol. 4, no. 1. W. B. Saunders, Philadelphia, 1975, p. 57.

87. SCULLY, R. E.: *Case records of the Massachusetts General Hospital. Albright's syndrome*. N. Eng. J. Med. 292:199, 1975.

88. SEYLER, L. E., JR. AND REICHLIN, S.: *Luteinizing hormone-releasing factor (LRF) in plasma of postmenopausal women*. J. Clin. Endocrinol. Metab. 37:197, 1973.

89. SEYLER, L. E., JR. AND REICHLIN, S.: *Feedback regulation of circulating LRF concentrations in men*. *Endocrinology and Metabolism,* vol. 4, no. 1. W. B. Saunders, Philadelphia, 1975, p. 3.

90. SEYLER, L. E., JR., ET AL.: *Sexual dimorphism of human pituitary responses to LRH after sex steroid treatment*. Proceedings of the Fifth International Congress of Endocrinology, Hamburg, July, 1976, p. 301.

91. SHERMAN, B. M. HALMI, K. A. AND ZAMUDIO, R.: *LH and FSH response to gonadotropin-releasing hormone in anorexia nervosa: Effect of nutritional rehabilitation*. J. Clin. Endocrinol. Metab. 41:135, 1975.

92. SILVERMAN, J. A.: *Anorexia nervosa: Clinical observations in successful treatment plan.* J. Pediatr. 86: 68, 1974.

93. SIZONENKO, P. A.: *Endocrine laboratory findings in pubertal disturbances. In* Bierich, J. R. (ed.): *Clinics in Endocrinology and Metabolism,* vol. 4, no. 1. W. B. Saunders, Philadelphia, 1975, p. 173.

94. STOTJIN, C. P. J. AND NAUTA, W. J. H.: *Precocious puberty and tumor of the hypothalamus*. J. Nerv. Ment. Dis. 111:207, 1950.

95. TAMADA, T., ET AL.: *Interrelationships between the levels of ovarian steroids and luteinizing hormone. In* Yagi K. and Yoshida, S. (eds.): *Neuroendocrine Control*. John Wiley & Sons, New York, 1973, p. 271.

96. THAMDRUP, E.: *Precocious sexual development, a clinical study of 100 children*. Dan. Med. Bull. 8: 140, 1961.

97. TANNER, J. M.: *Growth and endocrinology of the adolescent. In* Gardner, L. I. (ed.): *Endocrine and Genetic Diseases of Childhood and Adolescence,* ed. 2. W. B. Saunders, Philadelphia, 1975, p. 14.

98. VALE, W., GRANT, G. AND GUILLEMIN, R.: *Chemistry of the hypothalamic releasing factors — studies on structure-function relationships. In* Ganong, W. F. and Martini, L. (eds.): *Frontiers in Neuroendocrinology*. Oxford University Press, New York, 1973, p. 375.

99. VANDENBERG, G., DeVANE, G. AND YEN, S. S. C.: *Effects of exogenous estrogen and progestin on pituitary responsiveness to synthetic luteinizing hormone-releasing factor*. J. Clin. Invest. 53:1750, 1974.

100. VAN DER WERFF TEN BOSCH, J. J.: *Isosexual precocity. In* Gardner, L. I. (ed.): *Endocrine and Genetic Diseases of Childhood and Adolescence,* ed. 2. W. B. Saunders, Philadelphia, 1975, p. 619.

101. VAN LOON, G. R. AND BROWN, G. M.: *Secondary drug failure occurring during chronic treatment with LHRH: Appearance of an antibody*. J. Clin. Endocrinol. Metab. 41:64, 1975.

102. VAN WYCK, J. J. AND GRUMBACH, M. M.: *Syndrome of precocious menstruation and galactorrhea in juvenile hypothyroidism: an example of hormonal overlap in pituitary feedback.* J. Pediatr. 57:416, 1960.

103. WEINBERGER, L. M. AND GRANT, F. C.: *Precocious puberty and tumors of the hypothalamus. Report of a case and review of the literature with pathophysiological explanation of precocious sexual syndrome.* Arch. Intern. Med. 67:762, 1941.

104. WOOD, L. C., ET AL.: *Syndrome of juvenile hypothyroidism associated with advanced sexual development: report of two new cases and comment of the management of an associated ovarian mass.* J. Clin. Endocrinol. Metab. 25:1289, 1965.

105. WURTMAN, R. J. AND CARDINALI, D. P.: *The pineal organ. In* Williams, R. H. (ed.): *Textbook of Endocrinology,* ed. 5. W. B. Saunders, Philadelphia, 1974, p. 832.

106. WURTMAN, R. J. AND KAMMER, H.: *Melatonin synthesis by ectopic pinealoma.* N. Engl. J. Med. 244:1233, 1966.

107. YAGI, K. AND SAWAKI, Y.: *Feedback of estrogen in the hypothalamic control of gonadotrophin secretion. In* Yagi, K. and Yoshida, S. (eds.): *Neuroendocrine Control.* John Wiley & Sons, New York, 1973, p. 297.

108. YEN, S. S. C., ET AL.: *Causal relationships between the hormonal variables in the menstrual cycle. In* Ferin, M., et al. (eds.): *Biorhythms and Human Reproduction.* John Wiley & Sons, New York, 1974, p. 219.

109. YEN, S. S. C., ET AL.: *Hypothalamic amenorrhea and hypogonadotropinism: Responses to synthetic LRF.* J. Clin. Endocrinol. Metab. 36:811, 1973.

110. WILKINS, L.: *The Diagnosis and Treatment of Endocrine Disorders in Childhood and Adolescence.* Charles C Thomas, Springfield, 1965.

BIBLIOGRAPHY

BIERICH, J. R. (ed.): *Clinics in Endocrinology and Metabolism,* vol. 4, no. 1. W. B. Saunders, Philadelphia, 1975.

DONOVAN, B. T. AND VAN DER WERFF TEN BOSCH, J. J.: *Physiology of Puberty.* Williams & Wilkins, Baltimore, 1965.

FERIN, M., ET AL. (EDS.): *Biorhythms and Human Reproduction,* John Wiley & Sons, New York, 1974.

GARDNER, L. J. (ED.): *Edocrine and Genetic Diseases of Childhood and Adolescence,* ed. 2. W B. Saunders, Philadelphia, 1975.

JOLLY, H.: *Sexual Precocity.* Charles C Thomas, Springfield, 1955.

KNOBIL, E.: *On the control of gonadotropin secretion in the rhesus monkey. In* Greep, R. O. (ed.): *Recent Progress in Hormone Research: Proceedings,* vol. 30. Academic Press, New York, 1974, p. 1.

MACK, H. C. AND SHERMAN, A. I. (EDS.): *The Neuroendocrinology of Human Reproduction.* Charles C Thomas, Springfield, 1971.

McCANN, S. M.: *Regulation of secretion of follicle-stimulating hormone and luteinizing hormone. In* Greep, R. O. and Astwood, E. B. (eds.): *Handbook of Physiology, Section 7: Endocrinology,* vol. 4, part 2. American Physiological Society. Williams & Wilkins, Baltimore, 1974, p. 489.

MECKLENBURG, S., ET AL.: *Hypothalamic dysfunction in patients with anorexia nervosa.* Medicine 53:147, 1974.

ODELL, W. D. AND MEYER, D. L.: *Physiology of Reproduction.* C. V. Mosby, St. Louis, 1971.

SPEROFF, L., GLASS, R. H. AND KASE, N. G.: *Clinical Gynecologic Endocrinology and Infertility.* Williams & Wilkins, Baltimore, 1973.

WARREN, M. P. AND VANDEWIELE, R. L.: *Clinical and metabolic features of anorexia nervosa.* Am. J. Obstet. Gynecol. 117:435, 1973.

WILLIAMS, R. H. (ED.): *Endocrinology.* W. B. Saunders, Philadelphia, 1974.

WURTMAN, R. J. AND CARDINALI, D. P.: *The pineal organ. In* Williams, R. H. (ed.): *Textbook of Endocrinology,* ed. 5. W. B. Saunders, Philadelphia, 1974

YOGI, K. AND YOSHIA, S. (EDS.): *Neuroendocrine Control.* John Wiley & Sons, New York, 1973.

CHAPTER 6

Regulation of Prolactin Secretion and Its Disorders

Long recognized as an important hormone in lower vertebrates, it was not until 1970 that prolactin (PRL) was shown to be a distinct hormone in primates.[7, 9, 27] Until then, many workers considered that GH was responsible for PRL effects in man. The problem in isolating PRL by chemical means stemmed from the fact that the normal pituitary contains 50 to 100 times more GH than PRL and the two hormones are chemically similar.[8] Moreover, GH has intrinsic PRL-like activity. Eventually, by use of immunologic methods highly purified human material was prepared and used to develop a sensitive radioimmunoassay.[12] The introduction of radioimmunoassay has led to the rapid acquisition of knowledge about neuroendocrine control of PRL secretion in man.

It is now evident that the secretion of PRL is influenced by a multiplicity of stimuli. In addition to suckling (Fig. 1), PRL is released in response to physical and emotional stress,[24] arginine infusion,[7] hypoglycemia,[7] and estrogen administration.[21] Sleep-related rhythms also bring about stimulation of PRL secretion.[26, 29, 30] In its lability, PRL secretion thus resembles the secretion of GH and of ACTH. Although many neural stimuli can *induce* PRL release, secretion is tonically inhibited by the hypothalamus. Thus, PRL secretion is increased by any process that interferes with hypothalamic-pituitary continuity. This peculiarity of control has important implications in terms of the neural mechanism involved, in providing a sensitive index of functional disorders of the hypothalamic-pituitary axis, and in understanding the pathogenesis of hypersecretory states.

PITUITARY PROLACTIN SECRETION

Prolactin is a protein hormone synthesized and secreted by specific acidophilic staining cells of the anterior pituitary. These cells have been distinguished from those that secrete GH by histochemical, electron-microscopic, and immunofluorescent methods.[50] The amino acid structure of human PRL has been partially elucidated; its molecular weight is approximately 21,000 daltons.[23] Basal (resting or nonstressed) levels of immunoassayable PRL in the human adult show considerable individual variability and range up to 15 to 25 ng./ml.[34, 35] There are no consistent differences between plasma levels of men and nonpregnant women. Plasma levels are higher in the newborn; amniotic fluid contains enormous amounts of PRL (up to 2000 ng./ml.).[9] Because PRL is known to be involved in regulation of osmolarity in euryhaline fish (e.g., salmon) that migrate from salt to fresh water, it has been postulated that PRL may be important

129

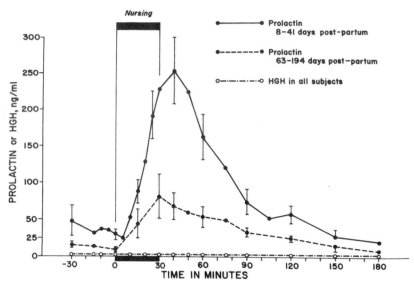

Figure 1. Prolactin and growth hormone release during nursing, showing effect of time postpartum. Growth hormone is not released during suckling. (From Noel, G. L., Suh, H. K. and Frantz, A. G.: *Prolactin release during nursing and breast stimulation in postpartum and non-postpartum subjects.* J. Clin. Endocrinol. Metab. 38:413, 1974, with permission.)

in regulation of fluid homeostasis in the fetus. Elevated serum PRL levels are also found in the last two thirds of pregnancy,[9] during the postpartum period,[5, 9] and reflexly following stimulation of the breast during either normal suckling or accompanying sexual caresses.[10, 17] Such reflex secretion of PRL has also been demonstrated in men in whom milk production has been induced by suckling. Kolodny and collaborators[17] recently found that self-stimulation of the breast was without effect, whereas stimula-

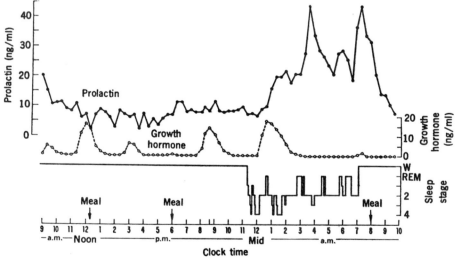

Figure 2. Prolactin and growth hormone secretion during a 24-hour period. Blood samples were taken every 20 minutes. There is an episodic rise in plasma prolactin between 3 and 8 A.M. with a fall to low values after awakening. (From Sassin, J. F., et al.: *Human prolactin: 24 hour pattern with increased release during sleep.* Science 177:1205, 1972, with permission.)

tion by the wife was effective. This means that the psychologic setting can partially determine the PRL response to peripheral stimulation.

Serum PRL levels are increased episodically during sleep (Fig. 2), with peak elevations occurring during the latter part (usually 2:00 to 8:00 A.M.).[28, 29] This late nocturnal rise in plasma PRL levels is followed by a decline immediately after wakening.

HYPOTHALAMIC CONTROL OF PROLACTIN SECRETION (FIG. 3)

It has been repeatedly demonstrated that the control of pituitary PRL secretion by the hypothalamus is predominantly inhibitory; disruption of hypothalamic-pituitary connection by stalk section,[36] pituitary transplantation, or placement of hypothalamic lesions all result in an increase in PRL secretion while secretion of other tropic hormones is reduced.[22] This effect has been reproduced in vitro; the incubated pituitary gland synthesizes and releases large quantities of PRL, while secretion of other hormones steadily declines.[7] The isolated pituitary of the rat incubated in vitro secretes three times as much PRL per day as the pituitary in situ, and human pituitaries behave similarly. These results illustrate the powerful restraint normally imposed by the hypothalamus on PRL secretion.

Prolactin-Inhibiting and Prolactin-Releasing Factors

The physiologic finding that the hypothalamus inhibits PRL secretion led to isolation of prolactin-inhibitory factors (PIF) from hypothalamic extracts and in pituitary-portal

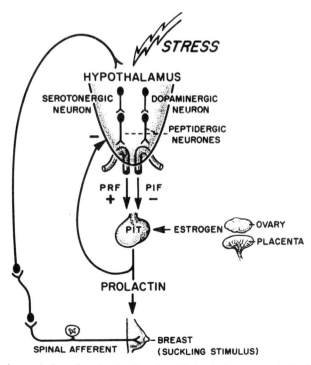

Figure 3. Hypothalamic regulation of prolactin. Two hypothalamic factors, prolactin-inhibiting factor (PIF) and prolactin-releasing factor (PRF) regulate pituitary (PIT) prolactin secretion. Neural inputs such as stress and suckling act upon the hypothalamus. Estrogen from ovary and placenta regulate pituitary sensitivity to hypothalamic factors.

131

vessel blood. The chemical nature of PIF is not known. Because dopamine (as well as other catecholamines) has a direct inhibitory effect on release of PRL in vitro in a concentration that can be regarded as physiologic, it has recently been proposed that this substance, which is found in hypothalamic extracts, may act as the primary PIF.[21] Moreover, L-dopa, the precursor of dopamine, inhibits PRL release in humans.[16] Dopamine has recently been shown to be present in portal-vessel plasma. Kamberi and colleagues[15] claim that dopamine is effective in the intact animal only when injected into the third ventricle of the brain, and not after direct perfusion into pituitary portal vessels. Other workers state that when precautions are taken to prevent oxidation of dopamine, it is effective when placed directly into the portal system.[32] Furthermore, dopaminergic nerve terminals end on median eminence capillaries and could thus release dopamine into the portal system. Current findings suggest that PIF activity in hypothalamic tissue is largely accounted for by dopamine since treatments that eliminate catecholamines also abolish PIF activity.[21, 43] Moreover, it has been shown that stereospecific dopamine-neuroleptic receptors are present in pituitary but not in the basal hypothalamus, indicating that dopaminergic effects on the pituitary are direct rather than mediated by release of a separate PIF from hypothalamus.[37]

Because physiologic studies anticipated the identification of PIF, it came as a surprise when a number of workers noted that hypothalamic extracts contain at least two factors which *release* PRL, both in isolated pituitary assay systems and in whole animals. One of the prolacin-releasing factors (PRF) has been shown to be TRH, administration of which brings about a rise in plasma PRL levels in man and several other species.[10, 13] Prolactin and TSH responses to TRH (Fig. 4) share many similarities. The threshold dose for the PRL response to TRH is similar to the threshold dose for the TSH response, and like the TSH response, PRL release is inhibited by thyroxine excess and enhanced by thyroxine deficiency. The mechanisms whereby TRH stimulates PRL secretion resemble effects on TSH secretion, since radiolabeled TRH binds to membrane receptors on lactotrope as well as thyrotrope cells. On the other hand, the PRL response to TRH is only partially reduced after thyroxine treatment, while that for TSH release is completely abolished.[7, 9] Because TRH influences PRL secretion in the same range of doses that control TSH secretion, it seems reasonable that TRH may function as a PRL regulatory factor. Several lines of evidence, however, argue against TRH being the only PRF, or the one involved in reflex PRL release. The acute burst of PRL release caused by suckling or by stress, or the rise associated

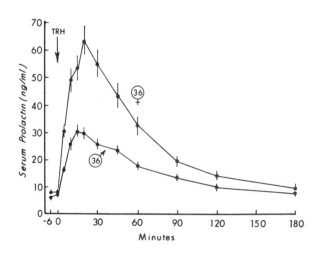

Figure 4. TRH-stimulated prolactin release in 36 men and 36 women. The response is greater and more rapid in women. (From Jacobs, L. S., et al.: *Prolactin response to thyrotropin-releasing hormone in normal subjects.* J. Clin. Endocrinol. Metab. 36:1069, 1973, with permission.)

with certain stages of sleep is not associated with the change in plasma TSH levels which would be anticipated if TRH secretion was activated. But this line of reasoning can be partially refuted. Release of PRL may be due to acute inhibition of PIF. Also, the newly discovered hypothalamic hormone, somatostatin, has been shown to inhibit TSH responses to TRH without altering PRL responses to TRH. Therefore, the concomitant secretion of somatostatin and TRH could theoretically bring about PRL release unaccompanied by TSH release. In specific types of stress, PRL release may be due to inhibition of PIF secretion.

The best evidence that TRH is not the sole PRF comes from studies of hypothalamic extracts. Fractions with PRF activity have been separated from TRH chromatographically, and plasma enzymes which degrade TRH reduce, but do not abolish, PRF activity in crude hypothalamic extracts.[2]

Role of Monoamines

Extensive evidence indicates that the monoamines dopamine and serotonin are important in the control of PRL secretion in animals and man.[4, 21, 22] The morphologic and histochemical evidence of a monoamine neural control system in the basal hypothalamus has been reviewed (see Chapter 3). Dopamine agonists inhibit, and serotonin agonists stimulate PRL secretion.[4, 22] Administration of L-dopa, the precursor of both dopamine and norepinephrine, causes an acute lowering of plasma prolactin levels in man.[16] Pretreatment with L-dopa is effective in blocking the PRL response to TRH,[25] suggesting an effect at the pituitary level (Fig. 5). That this effect is mediated by dopaminergic receptors is indicated by the observation that apomorphine, a specific

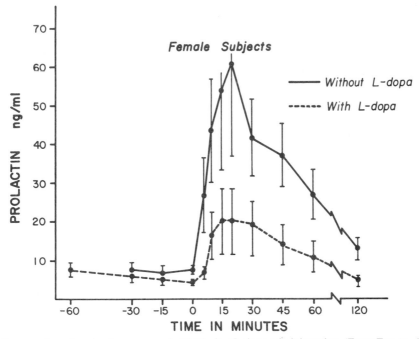

Figure 5. Suppression of prolactin response to TRH after L-dopa administration. (From Frantz, A. G.: *The regulation of prolactin secretion in humans. In* Ganong, W. F. and Martini, L. (eds.): *Frontiers in Neuroendocrinology: 1973.* Oxford University Press, New York, 1973, with permission.)

133

dopamine receptor-stimulating agent, also causes acute suppression of PRL (Fig. 6).[20]

Intraventricular administration of dopamine, but not of norepinephrine, causes inhibition of PRL secretion in the rat together with an increase in bioassayable hypothalamic PIF activity.[15] Since dopamine and apomorphine can inhibit PRL secretion from pituitaries incubated in vitro (an effect blocked by dopamine antagonists such as haloperidol and pimozide), it appears that there are dopamine receptor sites on pituitary PRL cells.[21] Further studies are necessary to determine the extent to which dopamine acts through its effects on the hypothalamus or pituitary.

Additional support for the idea that dopamine plays a role in PRL control comes from observations of effects of several drugs (e.g., the phenothiazines) which affect monoamine transmission in brain. Such drugs, which block dopaminergic receptor sites, cause an acute increase in plasma PRL levels in man.[16] This action of phenothiazines in blocking dopaminergic neuron effects is also believed to be the mechanism by which these agents induce parkinsonism. The administration of α-methyldopa or reserpine (agents that interfere with central catecholamine synthesis or storage) also can cause increased PRL secretion and may result in the production of abnormal lactation (galactorrhea). Serotonin, in contrast to dopamine, causes PRL release when administered into the third ventricle of the rat.[22] Systemic administration of 5-hydroxytryptophan, a serotonin precursor which readily crosses the blood-brain barrier, also causes PRL release in man.

These observations indicate that PRL, like GH, is under a complex double regulatory system that involves both specific hypothalamic regulatory factors (releasing and inhibiting) and a dual monoaminergic control system. Several recent studies in rats suggest that PIF activity is regulated by catecholaminergic neurons and PRF activity by serotonergic neurons. Catecholamine depletion brought out by reserpine or by α-methyl-p-tyrosine treatment of rats leads to a marked increase in plasma PRL levels, believed to be due to inhibition of PIF secretion. Such animals respond to ether stress with the usual increase in plasma PRL, which in this instance is clearly not due to inhibition of PIF. Treatment of reserpinized animals with serotonin antagonists such as methysergide blocks the stress-induced PRL release, a finding that suggests serotonergic control of PRF release.

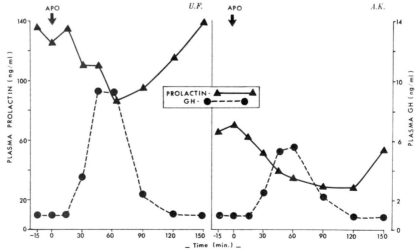

Figure 6. Suppression of prolactin by apomorphine (APO) in two patients with hyperprolactinemia. Both subjects show a normal release of GH after apomorphine.

NEURAL PATHWAYS IN REGULATION OF PROLACTIN RELEASE

Three different types of environmental stimuli are recognized to bring about release of prolactin in the rat.[41] These are the suckling stimulus (a reflex abolished by nipple denervation), mechanical stimulation of the uterine cervix which brings about the hyperprolactinemic state of pseudopregnancy, and physical and emotional stress. In addition, in the female rat, but not the male rat, administration of estrogen brings about the acute release of PRL.[40, 41] The emotional and suckling reflex release of PRL are also readily demonstrated in other species. Attempts to trace the neural pathways mediating these responses have utilized electric stimulation experiments,[19, 39, 45] circumscribed electrolytic lesions,[38, 41] and deafferentation of the hypothalamus by the Halasz technique.[47] All forms of stimuli known to elicit PRL release appear to converge upon the hypothalamus via an anterior route since most responses can be abolished by lesions in the preoptic region. The importance of this region is further demonstrated by electric stimulation or even mechanical stimulation which also brings about increased PRL release. This route within the hypothalamus thus resembles pathways that are comparable to the LHRH and somatostatinergic peptide pathways. In view of numerous recent studies indicating that there is a hypothalamic prolactin-releasing factor, it may be suggested that this pathway is a PRF pathway. In addition to the acute release pathway, a prolactin inhibitory pathway can be demonstrated by sectioning the pituitary stalk,[41] or by electrolytic lesions[38] of the median eminence or the arcuate nucleus. Since systemic estrogen administration[41] or direct intrahypothalamic estrogen implants[42] can induce PRL release, it is possible that the PRF pathway is also estrogen sensitive, in addition to the better established influence of estrogen directly on the pituitary. Although estrogens increase basal levels of plasma PRL in both sexes, only in the female does estrogen cause acute PRL release. This sexually dimorphic response depends upon the early steroid milieu in the perinatal period (see Chapters 5 and 12). Female rats given androgens lose the ability to respond to estrogens as adults.

The course of the prolactin-release pathway has been traced in goats, guinea pigs, and rabbits. Tindal and collaborators report that the pathway for milk ejection and prolactin release are similar:

> In the midbrain, the afferent path of the reflex is compact, lying in the lateral tegmentum of each side and passing forwards to lie medio-ventral to the medial geniculate body. On entering the diencephalon, the pathway on each side bifurcates: a dorsal path passing forwards in association with the extreme rostal central grey and periventricular region, and a ventral path ascending through the subthalamus.[44]
>
> The prolactin-release pathway follows the course of the dorsal path for oxytocin release and then, like the dorsal path, swings laterally into the far-lateral hypothalamus to ascend in the medial forebrain bundle. However, whereas the oxytocin-release path moves dorsally and then medially by means of medial forebrain bundle collaterals at the level of the paraventricular nucleus, the prolactin-release pathway continues forward in the medial forebrain bundle and then spreads out in the preoptic region.[45]

FEEDBACK REGULATION OF PROLACTIN SECRETION

Short-Loop Feedback

Prolactin, like GH, and unlike other tropic pituitary hormones, lacks a specific target gland with which to interact in a negative-feedback loop. Instead, PRL secretion appears to be self-regulated by a short-loop mechanism. Implants of prolactin in the hypothalamus of the rat cause a decrease in pituitary PRL concentration and a fall in plasma PRL levels. In suckling rats, intrahypothalamic PRL inhibits lactation. This effect may be mediated through the effects of PRL on hypothalamic dopaminergic neurons, since there is a rapid and significant increase in dopamine turnover in the hypothalamus following PRL administration. In hypophysectomized animals, the introduction of pituitary transplants, with the consequent elevation of circulating levels of PRL, also leads to increased dopamine levels in the hypothalamus. Feedback effects of PRL on the hypothalamus probably inhibit LHRH secretion as well. This view is supported by the finding that removal of a PRL-secreting microadenoma, or treatment with bromergocryptine in women with galactorrhea-amenorrhea syndromes, generally restores normal menses without changing the responsiveness of the pituitaries of such patients to test doses of LHRH.[2, 35, 46] In the rhesus monkey (but not women) TRH-induced PRL release inhibits ovulation.

Effects of Sex Steroids

Estrogenic hormones have striking effects on lactotrope cells. In rodents and monkeys, estrogen administration increases the number of cells and the rate of PRL synthesis.[21] In the rat, this striking stimulation commonly induces tumor formation. The hyperplasia of the pituitary seen in pregnant women is mainly due to increased numbers and size of lactotrope cells formed under the influence of placental estrogens. This stimulating effect explains the vulnerability of the pituitary of the pregnant woman to infarction, and the tendency of chromophobe PRL-secreting adenomas to grow during pregnancy.[31, 33] The effects of progesterone have not been as thoroughly explored. In rats, progesterone inhibits the estrogen-induced increase in PRL secretion, but its effects in humans are not known. Also unknown is the effect of androgenic hormones on PRL secretion in humans.

FACTORS THAT INFLUENCE PRL SECRETION IN MAN

A number of stimuli that cause acute changes in PRL secretion, such as stress and sleep-associated release, are probably mediated by extrahypothalamic inputs to the medial basal hypothalamus.[24] The precise areas involved have not been determined, but involvement of the limbic system would seem almost certain. A summary of factors that influence PRL secretion is presented in Table 1.

Stress-Associated Release

A variety of stresses cause significant elevation of plasma PRL levels. Prolactin is released during anesthesia and surgical procedures. In one study, mean plasma PRL levels increased from 38.8 ng./ml. to 173.8 ng./ml. in 19 women undergoing surgical explorations under general anesthesia.[24] The increase in PRL was maintained during the entire operation and remained elevated for 20 minutes after completion of surgery. Prolactin levels had returned to preoperative levels the following day. Slightly less marked increases were observed in men. The rise in plasma GH was considerably less. Less stressful procedures such as gastroscopy and proctoscopy also cause a rise in PRL, without significant rise in GH. Acute myocardial infarction also causes PRL release. The effects of psychologic stress on PRL release have not been systematically tested. In an unpublished study,[1] PRL levels were undistinguishable from normal in depressed patients. Prolactin levels and prolactin responses to phenothiazines are normal in schizophrenic patients.[51]

A teleologically satisfactory rationale for stress-induced PRL release in man is not

Table 1. Factors That Influence Serum Prolactin Levels in Man

Physiologic	Pathologic	Pharmacologic
Increase in Serum Prolactin		
1. Pregnancy	1. Prolactin-secreting	1. TRH
2. Postpartum	pituitary tumors	2. Psychotropic drugs
a. Non-nursing mothers	a. With galactorrhea	a. phenothiazines
days 1–7	b. Without galactorrhea	b. reserpine
b. Nursing mothers	2. Hypothalamic-pituitary	3. Oral contraceptives
after suckling	disorders:	4. Estrogen therapy
3. Nipple stimulation	a. Chiari-Frommel	5. α-methyl-dopa
(males and females)	b. Tumors (cranio-	
4. Coitus (some subjects)	pharyngioma)	
5. Stress	metastases	
6. Exercise	c. Histiocytosis X	
7. Neonatal period	d. Inflammation–	
(2–3 months)	sarcoidosis	
8. Sleep	3. Pituitary stalk section	
	4. Hypothyroidism	
	5. Renal failure	
	6. Ectopic production by	
	malignant tumors	
Decrease in Serum Prolactin		
1. Water loading	1. Isolated prolactin	1. L-dopa
	deficiency	2. Apomorphine
		3. 2-α-bromergo
		cryptine

readily apparent. General metabolic effects of PRL have not been described except for possible electrolyte and water-retaining effects (see below). In fact, patients with PRL-secreting pituitary tumors may have plasma levels as high as 5,000 to 10,000 ng./ml. without manifesting any apparent metabolic change that could be interpreted as being helpful in stress.[33, 35]

Sleep-Associated Release

Sleep-related rise in plasma PRL levels has now been demonstrated consistently. The increase in PRL occurs as a series of episodic bursts of secretion, the first of which occurs within 60 to 90 minutes after sleep.[26, 28] Subsequent pulses carry the plasma level to a peak at approximately 4:00 to 6:00 A.M. (see Fig. 2). Values reached rarely exceed 15 to 30 ng./ml. The rise in PRL is not related to a specific phase of the sleep cycle as is the case in GH release which is associated with Stage III or IV sleep. Soon after morning awakening, plasma PRL levels begin to fall and the lowest levels of the 24-hour period are reached one to three hours later. Sassin and coworkers[28] have recently shown that this nocturnal rise in PRL is not simply a circadian rhythm but is related to sleep itself; delay in sleep onset or sleep reversal results in concurrent delay in the response, which is consistently entrained to the episode of sleep. In this respect, sleep-associated PRL release resembles GH release and differs from ACTH release, which although also occurring in an episodic pulsatile manner during the night, is only loosely entrained to sleep. Sleep reversal studies have shown that the ACTH rhythm remains circadian for several days before gradually changing to a reverse pattern in relation to the sleep-wake cycle. The function or significance of sleep-associated PRL release (which occurs in both males and females) is unknown.

The pineal gland may be involved in the regulation of the diurnal variations in PRL secretion. Melatonin, which is synthesized in the pineal gland, has been shown to enhance PRL secretion in the rat, perhaps by stimulation of hypothalamic-serotonergic neurons.[18] Since in this species, activity of the pineal is increased during darkness, it was hypothesized that the pineal gland affected PRL secretion and that this effect might be related to light-dark cycles. In confirmation of this hypothesis, plasma PRL levels in the rat were found to be significantly increased at 6:00 A.M. compared with levels obtained at 6:30 P.M. This rise was completely abolished by pinealectomy.[18]

Episodic Release

In addition to the nocturnal rise, continual or frequent blood sampling has shown that PRL, like other pituitary hormones, is secreted in a pulsatile manner throughout the day and night (see Fig. 2).[29]

Release of PRL occurs during short daytime naps.[26] The physiologic significance of such pulsatile hormone release is of great current interest in neuroendocrinology. The original concept of steady-state feedback regulation of pituitary hormone secretion no longer explains the observed facts. It is probable that episodic neural drive is responsible for these patterned responses. Whether such secretory bursts have physiologic importance remains to be demonstrated.

LACTATION

The sequence of hormonal events responsible for growth of the breast and for lactation are as complex as those of the ovarian cycle. As shown in rat experiments, duct growth requires the combined action of glucocorticoids, GH, and estrogen; growth of the alveolar lobules requires progesterone and PRL in addition. During human pregnancy, placental lactogen (human placental lactogen, HPL) and pituitary PRL are secreted in increased amounts. Delivery of the child initiates lactation mainly because of the sudden withdrawal of placental estrogen and progesterone. Experimental work in rats indicates that secretion of PRL, insulin, and glucocorticoids is required for milk production. Once lactation has developed, its maintenance depends on PRL released after mechanical stimulation of the nipples by suckling. Reflex discharge of PRL from the pituitary gland is abolished by denervation of the nipples or by lesions in the spinal cord and brain stem. Impulses carried over these pathways ultimately impinge upon the hypothalamus, where they bring about the release of PRL. Release of PRL has usually been attributed to an inhibition of the secretion of PIF, which led to an "unleashing" of prolactin secretion. Although this may be the case, the recent demonstration of PRF makes it more tenable to postulate that such acute reflex PRL release is due to secretion of a releasing hormone.

Suckling brings about two additional neurogenic responses: milk let-down and gonadotropic hormone inhibition. Milk let-down refers to the appearance of milk in the nipple ducts a few seconds after nipple stimulation begins. Contraction of the myoepithelial cells of the parenchymal acini is responsible for the appearance of milk in the larger ducts, a response due to the direct effects of oxytocin, in turn released by neural stimuli reaching the hypothalamus. This reflex can be blocked by stress or by epinephrine administration.

The effect of suckling in blocking ovulation is highly interesting and biologically important because it is one of the mechanisms by which pregnancies are spaced in societies that do not practice birth control. Pregnancy is delayed by approximately six months in suckling women, but ovulation may begin earlier than this time, so that the contraceptive effect is only partial. It has seemed reasonable in the past to postulate that suckling inhibits the LH ovulatory surge through neurogenic action on the hypothalamus. More recently, as the inhibitory effects of PRL on LH secretion have been disclosed, it now seems more reasonable to suppose that the anti-ovulatory effects of suckling are mediated by PRL.[28] Prolactin also appears to interfere with the action of gonadotropins on the ovaries and of LHRH on the pituitary.

In addition to stimulation of milk production, PRL in certain species has an important supporting role in initiating and maintaining the corpus luteum of the ovary. For this reason it is also termed luteotropic hormone (LTH). Recent evidence also suggests (contrary to prior belief) that in the primate as well as the rat, PRL may be luteotropic, but this study has not been extended to man as yet.

CLINICAL ABNORMALITIES OF PRL SECRETION

Before sensitive immunoassays for PRL became available, the only indication of disordered prolactin secretion apparent to the clinician was the appearance of inappropriate milk secretion. While this manifestation remains in many cases the clinical hallmark of abnormal PRL secretion, it is now known that PRL secretion may be increased in both men and women without recognizable clinical symptoms. In fact, only one in six patients with elevated PRL levels has galactorrhea, and in long-standing galactorrhea, PRL levels may fall into the normal range.[35, 48]

Transient elevation in serum PRL levels is normal in the newborn and may contribute to the appearance of "witches' milk," milk secreted by the newborn's breast.

Nonpuerperal Galactorrhea

Abnormal lactation occurs in a number of clinical disorders, due usually to excessive secretion of PRL (Fig. 7).[14] There is considerable variability in the expression of this condition, as only a small proportion of individuals with hyperprolactinemia show lactation. In order for galactorrhea to develop in the presence of high PRL, the breast parenchyma must have been properly primed by normal amounts of insulin, GH, glucocorticoids, estrogens, and progesterone, and estrogen secretion must be low or relatively low. In the normal sequence of development of lactation at the time of delivery, the crucial initiating signal is the sudden decline in placental estrogen-progesterone secretion which, though necessary for breast growth and development, inhibits milk secretion. It is not known with certainty whether a similar sequence of ovarian steroid withdrawal is needed for the development of nonpuerperal galactorrhea, but most patients with severe galactorrhea have amenorrhea and variable degrees of estrogen deficiency. In a few cases, treatment with estrogens will inhibit the lactational effects of PRL on the breast. In one galactorrhea syndrome, so-called post-pill amenorrhea, lactation begins when contraceptive therapy is stopped. Because many hormones besides PRL, including glucocorticoids and GH, have milk-stimulating effects, lactation may rarely occur in patients with Cushing's disease or acromegaly. In some cases of acromegaly both GH and prolactin are secreted in excess.

Understanding the nature of hyperprolactinemic states has unfolded gradually with the description of a number of clinical syndromes which bear eponymic descriptions of historic interest. It is now possible to classify these conditions according to pathophysiologic principles.

The first category of nonpuerperal galactorrhea to be recognized, the Chiari-Frommel syndrome, is recognized as the persistence of postpartum lactation accompanied by amenorrhea, ovarian deficiency, and mental disturbance, including schizophrenia-like illness.[33] A somewhat similar illness, but independent of pregnancy, was later described as the Argonz del Castillo syndrome and the Forbes-Albright syndrome. The latter investigators recognized that approximately one half of their patients had

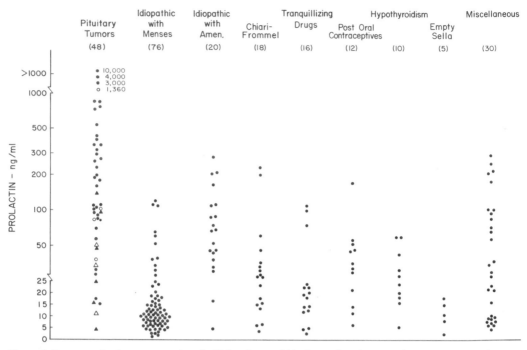

Figure 7. Serum prolactin concentrations in 235 patients with galactorrhea due to various causes. Usual upper limit of normal for serum prolactin is 20 to 25 ng/ml. (From Kleinberg, D. L., Noel, G. L. and Frantz, A. G.: *Galactorrhea: A study of 235 patients.* N. Engl. J. Med., in press, 1976, with permission.)

chromophobe tumors of the pituitary and suggested that occult tumors might be the cause of the disease in the others. Subsequently, pituitary stalk section in women was found to cause lactation, indicating that the syndrome could also occur as a hypothalamic deficiency disorder. These findings, together with the observation that certain neuroleptic drugs such as reserpine and chlorpromazine could induce lactation, provide the clinical basis for basic neuroendocrine insights into the mechanism of regulation of PRL secretion, and a classification of lactational disorders.

Galactorrhea (and PRL hypersecretion) occurs either as primary hypersecretion of a pituitary adenoma, or as a disorder secondary to hypothalamic dysfunction thought to be a deficiency of PIF secretion.[2, 3] Some cases of unknown etiology are believed to be of psychosomatic origin, or due to occult pituitary tumor.

Prolactin-Secreting Adenomas

The most common pituitary tumors are chromophobe adenomas. These were believed for many years to be nonfunctional, but radioimmunoassay methods now show that approximately one third of such tumors secrete PRL into the blood and that the removed tumors contain PRL.[14, 33, 50] Acidophilic staining in these tumors is difficult to demonstrate due to their relatively small hormone storage pool, but characteristic secretory granules are demonstrable by electron microscopy, and explants grown in organ culture synthesize PRL actively. A proportion (up to 4 per cent in one series) of the tumors of acromegaly secrete both GH and PRL. In the studies of Zimmerman and collaborators,[50] acromegalic tumor cells were shown to contain either GH or PRL but not both.

It is obvious that large PRL-secreting adenomas must at one time have been small adenomas; the development of pituitary microsurgery has confirmed this supposition. In a series of over 70 women with galactorrhea operated on by Hardy,[11] all but four had radiologically demonstrable enlargement of the sella turcica; tomography was, however, often necessary to demonstrate slight asymmetry of the sellar floor. In twenty of the latter cases, an intrapituitary microadenoma less than 1 cm. in diameter was identified in the lateral wing of the pituitary gland. Galactorrhea ceased in all cases after removal. Incidentally, two of the patients with tumors had cystic lesions (Rathke pouch cyst or craniopharyngioma) that may be presumed to have caused galactorrhea by interrupting hypothalamic-pituitary connections.

With increasing experience it has become apparent that galactorrheic patients with PRL levels above 150 to 200 ng./ml. almost always have PRL-secreting microadenomas (over 90 per cent in the series of Tolis and Friesen[33]), even when radiologic findings are normal. Several patients desirous of becoming pregnant who failed to respond to treatment with bromergocryptine or had marked elevation of PRL have been explored by the transsphenoidal route and have been cured by removal of a microadenoma. This kind of clinical experience raises the important suggestion that a substantial proportion of the idiopathic cases seen with this disorder, even those with a superficially plausible etiology such as contraceptive use or after pregnancy, may have occult tumors. Clear-cut techniques for differentiating these tumors clinically have not yet been developed. Details of testing methods are reviewed in Chapters 13 and 14 and management is discussed in Chapter 15.

Structural Damage of Hypothalamic-Pituitary Connections

Galactorrhea or hyperprolactinemia may also occur after damage to the ventral hypothalamus or to the pituitary stalk. The syndrome has been reported in patients with craniopharyngioma, granulomas (including sarcoidosis), histiocytosis X, and other destructive lesions.

External head trauma and pituitary stalk section may rarely cause galactorrhea. In the series reported by Turkington and colleagues,[36] plasma PRL levels (by bioassay) were elevated in nine of the eleven patients, but galactorrhea was not observed in any of the cases. Gynecomastia is never seen as a manifestation of PRL excess in men, but galactorrhea does rarely occur.

Abnormalities in Peripheral Receptor Control

Prolonged irritative lesions of the anterior chest wall, notably after thoracotomy or herpes zoster, may cause galactorrhea. Even prolonged mechanical stimulation of the nipples as by suckling has been known to initiate lactation in nonpregnant or even virgin women. A foster mother may thus be enabled to suckle her adopted child.

Galactorrhea with hyperprolactinemia has been observed in women with neurologic lesions of the thoracic spinal cord. The mechanism by which a lesion of ascending pathways could cause PRL hypersecretion is not known. Presumably this is a stimulatory effect of some type.

Neuroleptic Drugs

Large doses of drugs which interfere with central catecholamine metabolism may induce excessive PRL secretion, presumably by interfering with hypothalamic dopaminergic mechanisms that normally inhibit PIF secretion. Drugs commonly implicated are the phenothiazines (expecially chlorpromazine and thioridazine), reserpine, and α-methyldopa (see Table 1).[34] Amenorrhea usually occurs also. This is a practical problem in the long-term management of chronic schizophrenia. It would be of interest to determine the effects of dopamine receptor-stimulating drugs on this type of disorder, but we are not aware that this has been done.

Hyperprolactinemia, occasionally with galactorrhea, is common in advanced renal insufficiency. The underlying mechanism is unknown. Although delayed clearance of PRL may be a factor, it is also possible that there is a disturbance in central catecholamine metabolism, or a form of metabolic encephalopathy. Some of the cases are due to concurrent administration of α-methyldopa for hypertension.

Hypothyroidism

Somewhat less than half of severely hypothyroid patients have elevated plasma PRL levels, and in this group, a small proportion have galactorrhea, usually with amenorrhea. The pathogenesis of this syndrome is a matter of controversy. One theory is that increased TRH secretion in hypothyroidism leads to increased release of both TSH and PRL. There is, however, no evidence that TRH secretion is enhanced in hypothyroidism. It has also been postulated that PRL hypersecretion comes about through TRH stimulation of PRL secretion by the pituitary which is known to be more sensitive in the hypothyroid state. Also, the hypothyroid state may cause a deficit of PIF biosynthesis, with resultant PRL hypersecretion. The last suggestion seems most reasonable to the authors, because of the clinical observation that precocious puberty may result from hypothyroidism in young girls. Since true precocious puberty is always a neurologic deficit syndrome, its occurrence in hypothyroidism is evidence for impaired hypothalamic function.

Post-Pill Amenorrhea-Galactorrhea

A small but significant proportion of women (less than 1 per cent) fail to resume normal menses after taking contraceptive pills, and show hyperprolactinemia. Although early work suggested that these women had an abnormally high incidence of menstrual disturbance prior to use of the contraceptive agents, more recent studies indicate that this is not true. The duration of therapy is not important either. The disturbance is often transient but may become permanent. The underlying pathophysiology is not known, nor is it known whether the progesterone or the estrogen component of the pill is more important. The syndrome is increasingly recognized to be associated with PRL-secreting microadenomas. Whether the oral contraceptives result in adenoma formation is unknown.

DIAGNOSIS AND MANAGEMENT OF HYPERPROLACTINEMIA

Dynamic Tests of Prolactin Secretion

The most difficult problem in differential diagnosis of the etiology of hyperprolactinemic states is the detection of microadenoma before distinctive roentgenographic changes have occurred. Even in cases which appear to be "functional" and unrelated to any obvious etiology, an occult adenoma may be present. A number of workers have tried to develop dynamic secretory tests based on physiologic principles, but none are entirely satisfactory. Perhaps the best guide is the basal level of prolactin. In the series of Tolis and coworkers,[35] PRL levels in excess of 200 ng./ml. were associated with adenomas in over 80 per cent of cases. In another series, six of seven adenomas had PRL levels in excess of 150. However, in both series, several patients had values in this range without evidence of tumor. Prolonged followup may be needed for diagnosis. In one case, an adenoma was removed from a patient whose sella was completely normal roentgenographically. Dynamic tests introduced to differentiate the tumor group have included water loading (which reduces PRL levels in some patients), and L-dopa administration. Responses to water loading are too inconstent to be of diagnostic value, and L-dopa will inhibit both functional and tumor cases of hyperprolactinemia. In one series, the only stimulatory test procedure which appeared to have promise in differentiating adenomas from functional cases was the use of chlorpromazine and TRH tests. Four of seven patients with tumors had brisk responses to TRH, presumably due to direct effects of the releasing factor on the tumor, whereas none had an equivalent response to chropromazine, an agent thought to act by decreasing the secretion of PIF. Most patients with functional disease show similar responses to TRH and chlorpromazine.

Bromergocryptine Therapy

Following the early observation that ergotamine inhibited luteotropic function in the rat, a number of derivatives were tested as inhibitors of lactation. The most potent of these, bromergocryptine, has been evaluated extensively in Europe and North America.[2, 5, 6, 33] This agent appears to act as a dopamine receptor stimulator and will lower plasma PRL levels within one to two months in almost all cases, including many patients with pituitary tumors. In the majority of nontumor cases, values are reduced markedly, lactation stops, and normal menses return. Pregnancies have been reported in women previously incapable of ovulation. Results with tumors are less satisfactory, but have occasionally been striking. Drug therapy may cause morphologic involution as well as functional suppression of pituitary adenomas, but this possibility remains to be explored.

One potentially important application of bromergocryptine has been its use in other pituitary tumors, particularly in acromegaly. Several authors report that elevated GH levels are suppressed partially or markedly by the drug, leading to clinical remission. Curiously, bromergocryptine does not lower GH levels in normal individuals.

Indications for bromergocryptine and specific details about its use are given in Chapter 15.

REFERENCES

1. ARANA, BOYD AND REICHLIN. Unpublished study, 1975.
2. BESSER, G. M., ET AL.: *Galactorrhoea: Successful treatment with reduction of plasma prolactin levels by bromergocryptine.* Br. Med. J. 3:669, 1972.
3. BUCKMAN, M. T., ET AL.: *Utility of L-dopa and water loading in evaluation of hyperprolactinemia.* J. Clin. Endocrinol. Metab. 36:911, 1973.
4. CLEMENS, J. A., ET AL.: *Inhibition of prolactin secretion by ergolines.* Endocrinology 94:1171, 1974.
5. DEL POZO, E., ET AL.: *The inhibition of prolactin secretion in man by CB-154 (2 Br-a-ergocryptine).* J. Clin. Endocr. 35:768, 1972.
6. DEL POZO, E., ET AL.: *Clinical and hormonal response to bromocriptine (CB-154) in the galactorrhea syndromes.* J. Clin. Endocrinol. Metab. 39:18, 1974.
7. FRANTZ, A. G.: *The regulation of prolactin secretion in humans. In* Ganong, W. F. and Martini, L. (eds.): *Frontiers in Neuroendocrinology: 1973.* Oxford University Press, New York, 1973, p. 337.
8. FRANTZ, A. G. AND KLEINBERG, K. L.: *Prolactin: Evidence that it is separate from growth hormone in human blood.* Science 170:745, 1970.
9. FRIESEN, H. AND HWANG, P.: *Human prolactin.* Annu. Rev. Med. 24:251, 1973.
10. GAUTVIK, K. M., ET AL.: *Serum prolactin and TSH: Effects of nursing and pyroGlu-His-ProNH$_2$ administration in postpartum women.* J. Clin. Endocrinol. Metab. 37:135, 1973.
11. HARDY, J.: Personal communication.

12. HWANG, P., GUYDA, H. AND FRIESEN, H.: *A radioimmunoassay for human prolactin.* Proc. Natl. Acad. Sci. U.S.A. 68:1902, 1971.

13. JACOBS, L. S., ET AL.: *Prolactin response to thyrotropin-releasing hormone in normal subjects.* J. Clin. Endocrinol. Metab. 36:1069, 1973.

14. JAFFE, R. B., ET AL.: *Physiologic and pathologic profiles of circulating human prolactin.* Am. J. Obstet. Gynecol. 117:757, 1973.

15. KAMBERI, I. A., MICAL, R. S. AND PORTER, J. C.: *Effect of anterior pituitary perfusion and intraventricular infection of catecholamines on prolactin release.* Endocrinology 88:1012, 1971.

16. KLEINBERG, D. L., NOEL, G. L. AND FRANTZ, A. G.: *Chlorpromazine stimulation and L-dopa suppression of plasma prolactin in man.* J. Clin. Endocrinol. Metab. 33:873, 1971.

17. KOLODNY, R. C., JACOBS, L. S. AND DAUGHADAY, W. H.: *Mammary stimulation causes prolactin secretion in non-lactating women.* Nature 238:284, 1972.

18. LU, K. H. AND MEITES, J.: *Effects of serotonin precursors and melatonin on serum prolactin release in rats.* Endocrinology 93:152, 1973.

19. MALVEN, P. V.: *Prolactin release induced by electrical stimulation of the hypothalamic preoptic area in unanesthetized sheep.* Neuroendocrinology 18:65, 1975.

20. MARTIN, J. B., ET AL.: *Inhibition by apomorphine of prolactin secretion in patients with elevated serum prolactin.* J. Clin. Endocrinol. Metab. 39:180, 1974.

21. MACLEOD, R. M.: *Regulation of prolactin secretion. In* Martini, L. and Ganong, W. F. (eds.): *Frontiers in Neuroendocrinology,* vol. 4. Raven Press, New York, 1975, p. 169.

22. MEITES, J., ET AL.: *Recent studies on functions and control of prolactin secretion in rats.* Recent Progr. Horm. Res. 28:471, 1972.

23. NIALL, H. D., ET AL.: *The chemistry of growth hormone and the lactogenic hormones.* Recent Progr. Horm. Res. 29:387, 1973.

24. NOEL, G. L., ET AL.: *Human prolactin and growth hormone release during surgery and other conditions of stress.* J. Clin. Endocrinol. Metab. 35:840, 1972.

25. NOEL, G. L., SUH, H. K. AND FRANTZ, A. G.: *L-dopa suppression of TRH-stimulated prolactin release in man.* J. Clin. Endocrinol. Metab. 36:1255, 1973.

26. PARKER, D. C., ROSSMAN, L. G. AND VANDERLAAN, E. F.: *Sleep-related, nyctohemeral and briefly episodic variation in human plasma prolactin concentrations.* J. Clin. Endocrinol. Metab. 36:1119, 1973.

27. PASTEELS, J. L. AND ROBYN, C. (EDS.): *Human Prolactin.* Excerpta Medica, Amsterdam, 1973.

28. SASSIN, J. F., ET AL.: *The nocturnal rise of human prolactin is dependent on sleep.* J. Clin. Endocrinol. Metab. 37:436, 1973.

29. SASSIN, J. F., ET AL.: *Human prolactin: 24-hour pattern with increased release during sleep.* Science 177:1205, 1972.

30. SINHA, Y. N., SELBY, F. W. AND VANDERLAAN, W. P.: *Effects of ergot drugs on prolactin and growth hormone secretion, and on mammary nucleic acid content in C3H/Bi mice.* J. Natl. Cancer Inst. 52:189, 1974.

31. SMITHLINE, F., SHERMAN, L. AND KOLODNY, H. D.: *Prolactin and breast carcinoma.* N. Engl. J. Med. 292:784, 1975.

32. TAKAHARA, J., ARIMURA, A. AND SCHALLY, A. V.: *Suppression of prolactin release by a purified porcine PIF preparation and catecholamines infused into a rat hypophysial portal vessel.* Endocrinology 95:462, 1974.

33. TOLIS, G. AND FRIESEN, H. G.: *Studies on the use of bromocriptine in hyperprolactinemia.* Clin. Endocrinol. (Oxf.) (in press).

34. TOLIS, G., GOLDSTEIN, M. AND FRIESEN, H. G.: *Functional evaluation of prolactin secretion in patients with hypothalamic-pituitary disorders.* J. Clin. Invest. 52:783, 1973.

35. TOLIS, G., ET AL.: *Prolactin secretion in sixty-five patients with galactorrhea.* Am. J. Obstet. Gynecol. 118:91, 1974.

36. TURKINGTON, R. W., UNDERWOOD, L. E. AND VAN WYK, J. J.: *Elevated serum prolactin levels after pituitary-stalk section in man.* N. Engl. J. Med. 285:707, 1971.

37. BROWN, G. M.: SEEMAN, P. AND LEE, T.: *Dopamine/neuroleptic receptors in pituitary and basal hypothalamus.* Endocrinology (in press).

38. CHEN, C. L., ET AL.: *Serum prolactin levels in rats with pituitary transplants or hypothalamic lesions.* Neuroendocrinology 6:220, 1970.

39. KNAGGS, G. S., MCNEILLY, A. S. AND TINDAL, J. S.: *The afferent pathway of the milk-ejection reflex in the mid-brain of the goat.* J. Endocrinol. 52:333, 1972.

40. NEILL, J. D.: *Sexual differences in the hypothalamic regulation of prolactin secretion.* Endocrinology 90:1154, 1972.

41. NEILL, J. D.: *Prolactin: its secretion and control. In* Greep, R. O., et al. (eds.): *Handbook of Physiology, Section 7: The pituitary gland and its neuroendocrine control, vol. 4, part 2.* American Physiological Society. Williams & Wilkins, Baltimore, 1974.

42. RAMIREZ, V. D. and McCANN, S. M.: *Induction of prolactin secretion by implants of estrogen into the hypothalamo-hypophysial region of female rats.* Endocrinology 75:206, 1964.

43. SHAAR, C. J. AND CLEMENS, J. A.: *The role of catecholamines in the release of anterior pituitary prolactin in vitro.* Endocrinology 95:1202, 1974.

44. TINDAL, J. S., KNAGGS, G. S. AND TURVEY, A.: *The afferent path of the milk-ejection reflex in the brain of the rabbit.* J. Endocrinol. 43:663, 1969.

45. TINDAL, J. S. AND KNAGGS, G. S.: *Pathways in the forebrain of the rabbit concerned with the release of prolactin.* J. Endocrinol. 52:253, 1972.

46. VARGA, L., WENNER, R. AND DEL POZO, E.: *Treatment of galactorrhea-amenorrhea syndrome with Br-ergocrytpine (CB-154): restoration of ovulatory function and fertility.* Am. J. Obstet. Gynecol. 117:75, 1973.

47. WEINER, R. I., BLAKE, C. A. AND SAWYER, C. H.: *Integrated levels of plasma LH and prolactin following hypothalamic deafferentation in the rat.* Neuroendocrinology 10:349, 1972.

48. YUEN, B. H., KEYE, W. R., JR. AND JAFFE, R. B.: *Human prolactin: secretion, regulation and pathophysiology.* Obstet. Gynecol. Surv. 28:527, 1973.

49. ZARATE, A., ET AL.: *Functional evaluation of pituitary reserve in patients with the amenorrhea-galactorrhea syndrome utilizing luteinizing hormone-releasing hormone (LH-RH), L-dopa and chlorpromazine.* J. Clin. Endocrinol. Metab. 37:855, 1973.

50. ZIMMERMAN, E. A., DEFENDINI, R., AND FRANTZ, A. G.: *Prolactin and growth hormone in patients with pituitary adenomas: a correlative study of hormone in tumor and plasma by immunoperoxidase technique and radioimmunoassay.* J. Clin. Endocrinol. Metab. 38:577, 1974.

51. MELTZER, H. Y. AND FANG, V. S.: *The effect of neuroleptics on serum prolactin in schizophrenic patients.* Arch. Gen. Psychiatry 33:279, 1976.

52. BOYD, A. E., III, ET AL.: *Prolactin releasing factor (PRF) in porcine hypothalamic extract distinct from TRH.* Endocrinology 99:861, 1976.

BIBLIOGRAPHY

Frantz, A. G.: *The regulation of prolactin secretion in humans. In* Ganong, W. F. and Martini, L. (eds.): *Frontiers in Neuroendocrinology: 1973.* Oxford University Press, New York, 1973, p. 337.

FRANTZ, A. G., LEINBERG, K. L. AND NOEL, G. L.: *Studies on prolactin in man.* Recent Progr. Horm. Res. 28:527, 1972.

FRIESEN, H. AND HWANG, P.: *Human prolactin.* Annu. Rev. Med. 24:251, 1973.

MACLEOD, R. M.: *Regulation of prolactin secretion. In* Martini, L. and Ganong, W. F. (eds.): *Frontiers in Neuroendocrinology,* vol. 4. Raven Press, New York, 1976, p. 169.

MEITES, J., ET AL.: *Recent studies on functions and control of prolactin secretion in rats.* Recent Progr. Horm. Res. 28:471, 1972.

PASTEELS, J. L. AND ROBYN, C. (EDS.): *Human Prolactin.* Excerpta Medica, Amsterdam, 1973.

145

CHAPTER 7

Regulation of Growth Hormone Secretion and Its Disorders

The secretion of growth hormone (GH), like that of prolactin, is precisely regulated by a complex interaction of stimulatory and inhibitory neural influences.[31, 38] This control is achieved by at least two hypothalamic hormones, GH-releasing hormone (GRH), the structure of which is still unknown, and GH-inhibiting hormone (GIH) or somatostatin,* which has been isolated and structurally identified.[10] These hormones are synthesized in and released from neurons of the medial basal hypothalamus *(peptidergic neurons)*. In turn, the secretions of these peptidergic neurons are regulated by complex monaminergic neuron systems in which dopamine (DA), norepinephrine (NE) and serotonin all play a role. The GH regulatory system is shown in Figure 1.

PITUITARY GROWTH HORMONE SECRETION

Human growth hormone (HGH) is a single-chain polypeptide (molecular weight 21,500) containing 190 amino acid residues, the sequence of which has been fully elucidated.[14] GH from other primates resembles HGH in many physical properties and crossreacts with it in radioimmunoassay systems. GH accounts for 4 to 10 per cent of the wet weight of the anterior pituitary in the adult human (5 to 15 mg./gland) and gland GH content does not change significantly with age. GH is synthesized and secreted by specific anterior pituitary cells *(somatotropes)*, the majority of which are eosinophilic by conventional staining techniques.[38] Histochemical and immunofluorescence methods have shown that these cells are distinct from those which synthesize other pituitary tropic hormones, including prolactin. Morphologically distinct secretory granules containing GH can be demonstrated in these cells by electron microscopy, which thus provides a tool for identification of the somatotrope and its secretory product.

PHYSIOLOGIC REGULATION OF GROWTH HORMONE SECRETION

GH circulates unbound in plasma. The half-life of disappearance is between 17 and 45 minutes and estimated secretion rate in normal adults is approximately 400 μg./day.[3] There are no significant differences between men and women. It acts at many sites and in this respect is similar to insulin and thyroid hormone and differs from other pituitary hormones such as TSH, LH, and ACTH that have specific target organs. The actions of GH are numerous and include stimulation of growth, regulation of lipolysis, and

---

*The terms GIH and somatostatin are used interchangeably in this text.

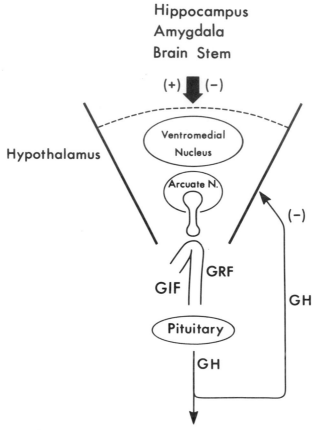

Figure 1. Diagram of growth hormone (GH) regulatory system. Hypothalamic control of pituitary GH secretion is achieved by two hypothalamic hormones, growth-releasing factor (GRF, as yet unidentified) and GIF growth-inhibiting factor (somatostatin). Extrahypothalamic inputs from limbic system relay stress, and sleep-related effects which alter GH secretory patterns. GH may regulate its own secretion by a short-loop feedback system.

promotion of cellular uptake of amino acids.[14] GH is diabetogenic (anti-insulin). The effects of GH on growth are mediated indirectly by a group of low-molecular-weight substances, the *somatomedins*, that are formed in the liver (and perhaps the kidney). Three such substances have now been identified. Although their precise chemical structure is not known,[14] each is a peptide of relatively small molecular weight (2,000 to 7,000). This group of substances has been shown to stimulate sulfate incorporation into cartilage (sulfation factor), to stimulate thymidine uptake in liver (thymidine factor), and to have insulin-like effects. The latter activity is not suppressed after glucose administration and probably represents the same material as that previously named for its nonsuppressible insulin-like activity (NSILA).

Secretory Patterns

Spontaneous Secretion

Basal (resting or nonstressed) levels of immunoassayable GH in plasma in the adult are 1 to 5 ng./ml. However, frequent determinations of GH throughout the day and.

148

night show striking variations in plasma concentration in both man and experimental animals.[18, 24, 40, 57] In man, plasma GH levels may surge as high as 20 to 40 ng./ml., the largest bursts often occurring during the first part of night sleep.[46, 47]

The number and the magnitude of the spontaneous bursts of GH secretion in man are in part age-dependent. Finkelstein and coworkers[18] showed that the transition from early puberty to adolescence is associated with an increased number of GH surges, occurring as frequently as 8 times per 24-hour period (Fig. 2). The surges in GH during the first few hours of night sleep were the largest, reaching plasma levels over 60 ng./ml. in some subjects. This study indicated a close correlation between age and total 24-hour GH secretory rates. Prepubertal children had a mean 24-hour secretory rate of 91 μg., adolescents 690 μg., and young adults 385 μg. Daytime pulses occur more frequently during adolescence, suggesting that bursts of GH secretion account for the increase in total daily GH release during the maximal-growth period in adolescence. Such bursts of secretion occur with sufficient frequency at all ages to cause some difficulty in assessing effects of various stimulatory agents on GH release.[40] Particularly high plasma levels of GH, ranging from 30 to 180 ng./ml., are present at birth. These decline during the first two to three months to reach the basal levels characteristic of the prepubertal child.

The profile of secretory bursts of GH in man, and their nonsuppressibility by potential metabolic regulators of GH secretion, suggest that the surges are the result of primary neural activation of GH release.[43, 57, 58] The pulses often show a strikingly acute profile, with rapid rises in plasma GH followed by a decline consistent with the known half-life of the hormone. Active secretion, therefore, may be quite brief. In this respect, the GH secretory pattern resembles the episodic secretion of ACTH, prolactin, TSH, and the gonadotropins. The surges of GH secretion in man continue during long-term anesthesia.

Similar profiles of GH secretion have been documented in experimental animals. Chair-adapted rhesus monkeys show episodic secretion of GH unrelated to feeding,

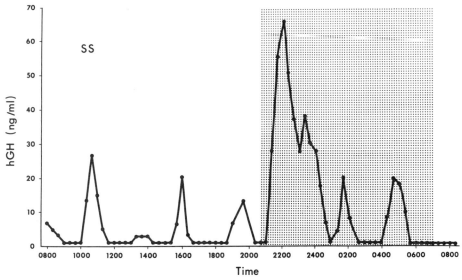

Figure 2. Episodic secretion of growth hormone (GH) in a normal adolescent male. Eight distinct secretory episodes are evident with a large surge of secretion shortly after onset of sleep (shaded area). (Adapted from Finklestein, et al.: *Age-related change in the 24-hour spontaneous secretion of growth hormone.* J. Clin. Endocrinol. Metab. 35:665, 1972.)

stress, or blood glucose levels. The baboon, like man, shows a prominent rise during sleep.[40] Unanesthetized rabbits also show surges of GH secretion.

With random sampling in the rat, particularly marked variations in plasma GH occur which are due to prominent, high-amplitude bursts of GH secretion that may reach levels of 300 to 600 ng./ml. (Fig. 3).[43, 57, 58] The pulses of GH secretion in this species show a regular 3- to 4-hour pattern, often with complex double or triple secretory peaks that are entrained to the light-dark cycle. The bursts of GH release are independent of fluctuations in cortiscosterone, prolactin, or TSH and are not related to stress.

Pulsatile GH secretion in the rat is significantly reduced by bilateral lesions of the hypothalamic ventromedial nuclei,[42] indicating a probable hypothalamic regulatory mechanism. As in man, episodic secretion of GH in the rat is not primarily regulated by glucose requirements, since it is not affected by fasting, feeding, or glucose infusions.[58] The timing of the bursts shows no correlation with either slow-wave or rapid-eye-movement sleep; it was concluded that this secretory GH pattern is regulated by an intrinsic CNS rhythm, cued by the light-dark cycle but unaffected by sleep-wake rhythms.[61]

Metabolic Regulation

All three of the major classes of metabolic substrate (carbohydrate, protein, and fat) affect GH secretion. The first to be recognized was the effect of altered glucose concentration. Glick and associates in 1963 observed, soon after they had developed their immunoassay method, that hypoglycemia produced by insulin administration triggered GH secretion, and glucose administration lowered basal levels of GH.[49] They also found that GH levels rose during the falling phase of the standard glucose tolerance test, and that 2-deoxyglucose, an analogue of glucose that causes intracellular glucose deficiency, also triggered GH release. These responses were not observed in a patient with section of the pituitary stalk. On this basis they proposed that glucoreceptors within the nervous system sensed plasma glucose levels and modulated homeostatic GH regulatory responses.[26] This hypothesis appeared reasonable in view of the fact that GH has anti-insulin effects and is a potent lipolytic substance. Further studies of this control system, reviewed in detail by Reichlin,[49] indicate a far greater degree of complexity than was initially conceived. It is now recognized that GH secre-

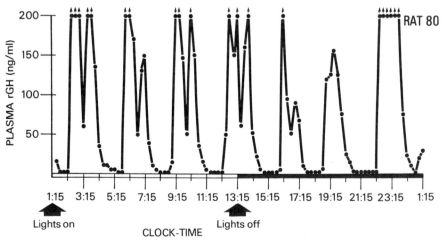

Figure 3. Twenty-four hour secretory pattern of growth hormone (GH) release in the rat. (From Tannen baum, G. S. and Martin, J. B.: *Evidence for an endogenous ultradian rhythm of growth hormone secretio. in the rat.* Endocrinology 98:562, 1976, with permission.)

tion is not regulated in relation to an absolute blood glucose level, but rather is responsive to change in glucose levels, rising levels suppressing and falling levels exciting GH release. The GH response to hypoglycemia is not truly homeostatic since normal blood sugar levels are restored before the GH response has affected carbohydrate metabolism; also, GH secretion is not related to an absolute level of glucose. In part, response to hypoglycemia can be viewed as a stress response. On the other hand, there is a glucoreceptor mechanism unrelated to the stress response, since glucose administration inhibits GH secretion in the basal state or after exercise. Although these observations indicate that glucose affects GH secretion, after review of the available data, Reichlin concluded that:

> These observations provide relatively weak evidence to support the thesis that reflex alterations in GH secretion are important in glucose homeostasis except possibly as an emergency mechanism, as in immature organisms. Even if it could be shown that minor degrees of hypoglycemia induced greater GH responses, the effects of excercise, sleep, psychological stress, random GH bursts, and post-prandial glucose decline, are so much more important in determining the secretion rate of GH that these factors, and not the demands of glucose homeostasis, dominate the controlling mechanisms of GH secretion.[49]

Growth hormone secretion is also linked to protein metabolism. Ingestion of a high-protein meal or the intravenous injection of a number of amino acids leads to release of GH, a response which may be blunted by hyperglycemia. The response to amino acids is not as regularly observed as is the response to hypoglycemia. Since amino acids are ineffective in releasing GH in patients with hypothalamic disease, it has been assumed that this amino acid acts on a neural site in the hypothalamus. There may in fact be specific amino acid receptors in the brain. Recent findings in the monkey have, however, put these findings in doubt. Infusion of a volume of saline equivalent to that used as an infusion vehicle for the amino acid arginine was equally effective in causing rebound secretion of GH. These findings suggest that a plasma volume-sensitive mechanism may exist for GH regulation.[66] Paradoxically, severe protein-calorie malnutrition is associated with an elevation in plasma GH levels. Until recently, the mechanism underlying this response was unknown, but it now seems reasonable to postulate that this effect is due to somatomedin deficiency, which in turn is related to deficiency of substrate for somatomedin synthesis in the depleted individual. In accordance with this view, GH exerts its short feedback effects on the hypothalamus via the somatomedin mechanism.[14, 40]

The alterations in GH secretion that follow changes in blood fatty acids were not apparent to the earlier workers in the field, largely because the administration of fat by mouth causes no significant change in basal plasma GH levels. However, it now appears that elevated levels of fatty acids suppress GH secretion in response to certain provocative stimuli including arginine, hypoglycemia, and sleep-related surges of secretion.

Species may vary in metabolic control with respect to the role of free fatty acids (FFA) in GH regulation. Ruminants, such as the sheep and cow, that depend primarily on FFA for energy requirements, show prominent physiologic GH fluctuations in relation to changes in these plasma metabolites.[40] On the other hand, the available evidence does not indicate any major acute role of glucose, proteins, or lipids in GH secretion in the pig, cat, rabbit, or rat.

In fasting, plasma GH levels also rise, usually within two days, commonly with increased numbers and amplitude of GH peaks.[24] The response is blunted in the obese. On the basis of known effects of GH in stimulating lipolysis, it was postulated that the elevated GH levels of fasting have a homeostatic effect in mobilizing stored calories as free fatty acids. However, the bulk of reported work, exemplified in the studies of Cahill and of Kipnis, indicates that the major influence in the control of lipolysis is the level of insulin secretion, insulin being the most powerful antilipolytic hormone.[49] To be sure, changes in GH may play a complementary role, but they are not essential to the response.

Effects of Activity

GH levels are usually unmeasurable in normal subjects on bedrest after an overnight fast, but spontaneous surges of GH secretion occur in these subjects throughout the day and night.[18, 56] Exercise causes GH release in both men and women.[38, 53] Even minor activity such as getting out of bed in the morning (particularly in women or in estrogen-treated men) causes an elevation in plasma GH levels.

This lability is utilized in provocative screening for GH deficiency in children. Vigorous stair-climbing will raise GH plasma levels in about 70 to 80 per cent of normal children.

Responses to Stress

Stimulation

Most stressful stimuli stimulate GH secretion in a manner analogous to the release of ACTH and of catecholamines under similar circumstances.[10, 11] Surgical operations cause a rise in GH, as does electroshock therapy, even when carried out with neuromuscular blockade. GH levels are also increased following pyrogen administration, acute trauma, and arterial puncture. A stress effect may explain the GH response to insulin hypoglycemia, since GH elevation correlates to some degree with the severity of side effects.

In contrast to the situation with regard to physical stimuli, little is known of the psychophysiologic regulation of GH secretion. In one study, a systematic investigation was undertaken of the psychologic factors involved in the release of both GH and cortisol.[9] Patients undergoing diagnostic cardiac catheterization were rated psychologically by two independent observers. Cortisol elevations were seen in all patients who showed overt manifestations of anxiety. In contrast, only those anxious patients who did not engage in conversation showed GH elevation. In the same study, low GH levels were observed in "depressed" patients who appeared uninvolved and withdrawn. Sadness induced by viewing a documentary film was found in one study to be associated with an elevation in plasma GH levels.

Further evidence of depression-related abnormalities in GH secretion is the finding of Sachar and colleagues[52] that in many such cases the usual stimulating effects of L-dopa on GH secretion are blunted. This finding has been interpreted to indicate an abnormality in central catecholamine metabolism, reflected in disturbance in both affect and hormonal regulation. GH secretion in the nonhuman primate is also markedly stress-responsive, with dramatic elevation occurring following a variety of stressful stimuli including noise, pain, pinching of the abdomen, aversive conditioning, capture from the cage and ether anesthesia. Paradoxically, GH release in the rat is inhibited by stress.[59]

Inhibition

A group of children have been described with growth failure secondary to gross emotional deprivation who showed remarkable growth acceleration when the environment was altered.[40] Some of these children had a significantly impaired GH response to hypoglycemia (and also ACTH deficiency) which became normal after they were restored to a supportive, loving environment. These children have normal sleep patterns, so the GH deficiency is not secondary to a sleep disturbance.

> James Barrie, the English playwright and novelist who wrote *Peter Pan,* may be a case in point. The seventh of eight children, he was subjected to severe maternal deprivation when his mother, after the accidental death of James' elder brother, 'got into bed and stayed there for over a year.' The emotionally deprived James never grew up, remaining less than 5 feet tall and sexually underdeveloped. Like Peter Pan, he may have chosen not to grow up.

As noted above, in the rat, stress lowers and "gentling" (systematic fondling) raises GH levels.

Sleep-Associated Release

Following the introduction of techniques permitting frequent sampling of plasma over a 24 hour period without disturbing the subject, it soon became apparent that most GH secretion takes place at night.[56] Later work has shown that the nocturnal secretion is age-dependent, older individuals gradually losing sleep-related GH secretion.[38] Because nocturnal GH secretion is so important, it has received much study. Evidence that the nocturnal rise is related to sleep onset and not simply to diurnal variations can be summarized thus: 1) the major burst of GH secretion occurs within two hours of sleep (Fig. 4);[56] 2) if onset of sleep is postponed, the onset of GH secretion is postponed; 3) if awakened and permitted to fall asleep again, subjects show a second GH secretory peak within two hours of sleep; and 4) daytime naps may be associated with GH secretory peaks.

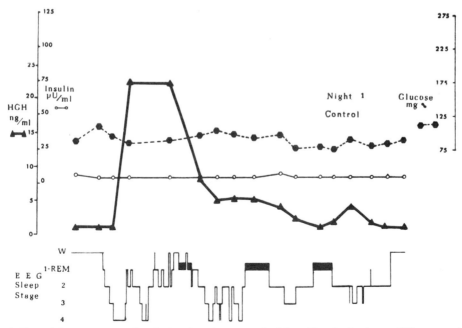

Figure 4. Growth hormone secretion during sleep in a normal subject. The rise in plasma GH occurs shortly after sleep onset and is not associated with any change in glucose or insulin levels. (From Lucke, C. and Glick, S. M.: *Experimental modification of the sleep-induced peak of growth hormone secretion.* J. Clin. Endocrinol. Metab. 32:729, 1971, with permission.)

Attempts have been made to determine whether sleep-related GH secretion is correlated with characteristic EEG changes of slow-wave sleep (SWS, Stages III and IV). Earlier investigators believed that the two phenomena were correlated,[45, 46] but later studies indicate that the association may only be fortuitous.[40] Evidence for correlation of SWS with nocturnal GH secretion came initially from the experiments of Takahashi and coworkers[56] who found that many, but not all, GH surges were correlated with SWS. Subsequently it was found that blind persons, who have less SWS, have less sleep-associated GH release, that ontogenetic development of nocturnal GH secretory patterns correlates somewhat with the appearance of SWS, and that narcoleptic patients, who frequently enter directly into rapid-eye-movement (REM) sleep without an intervening period of SWS, may fail to secrete GH early in sleep.[38]

On the other hand, a number of observations indicate that the two phenomena are not connected. If there were a common neural mechanism that simultaneously triggers SWS and release of GH, the two events would coincide uniformly, in some constant temporal relationship. Several reports of nocturnal GH secretion have been published which permit a test of this hypothesis. In one experiment, seven subjects were studied for two nights.[40] In two episodes, GH was released before sleep onset. In 10 episodes, the first occurrence of SWS preceded GH secretion by 0 to 60 minutes, but in four of these, scrutiny of the data suggests that GH release preceded the onset of SWS on four occasions. Therefore, there appears to be a frequent but not consistent temporal relationship between SWS and GH release. A number of investigators have also pointed out the lack of concurrence of these two phenomena in some normal persons and in the blind.[18, 30] Dissociation between SWS and GH secretion has also been described in a number of disease states in which both abnormal SWS and abnormal GH secretion occur. These include Cushing's disease (both active and in the early stages of recovery), Nelson's syndrome, hypothalamic tumors, Addison's disease, cerebral lupus erythematosus (on steroids), and in patients with the maternal deprivation syndrome. In addition, several pharmacologic agents can cause dissociation of SWS and GH secretion: imipramine, chlorpromazine, phenobarbital, fluorazepam, medroxyprogesterone, acute high-dose glucose infusion, Zn-tetracosactrin (ACTH), and free fatty acids.

A current conservative viewpoint is that nocturnal GH release is a sleep-related event which probably should not be considered to be closely linked to or caused by the neural processes which subserve SWS. The EEG characteristics of SWS relate to cortical electrical activity and need not accurately reflect changes in the subcortical mechanisms involved in neuroendocrine control. The two phenomenon (SWS and GH release) might therefore be dissociated by effects mediated at a number of neural-axis levels.

PHARMACOLOGIC STIMULI FOR GROWTH HORMONE RELEASE

Innumerable neuropharmacologic studies have been carried out in man and in experimental animals to analyze the nature of central control of the hypophysiotrophic neurons involved in GH regulation. These are summarized in Table 1. These indicate that at least three monoaminergic pathways are involved: noradrenergic, dopaminergic, and serotonergic. Factors that inhibit GH secretion are listed in Table 2.

NEURAL MECHANISMS CONTROLLING GROWTH HORMONE SECRETION

Clinically, disturbance in body growth as a result of lesions of the hypothalamus was recognized early in this century, but the pathogenesis of this abnormality was not understood. Growth failure in hypothalamic disease can occur because of inanition, or

Table 1. Factors That Stimulate GH Secretion in Primates

Physiologic	Pharmacologic	Pathologic
1. Episodic, spontaneous	1. Insulin hypoglycemia	1. Acromegaly
2. Exercise	a. 2-deoxyglucose	a. TRH
3. Stress	2. Amino acid infusions	b. LHRH
a. Physical	a. Arginine	c. Glucose
b. Psychologic	b. Leucine	d. Arginine
4. Sleep	c. Lysine, etc.	2. Pyrogens
5. Postprandial glucose decline	3. Small peptides	3. Protein depletion
	a. ADH	4. Fasting and
	b. α-MSH	starvation
	c. ACTH (1–24)	5. Anorexia nervosa
	d. Glucagon	
	4. Monoaminergic Stimuli	
	a. Epinephrine,	
	α-receptor stimulation	
	b. L-dopa	
	c. Apomorphine	
	d. 2-bromo-α-ergocryptine	
	e. Clonidine	
	f. 5-hydroxytryptophan	
	g. Fusaric acid (dopa-β-hydroxylase	
	inhibitor)	
	h. Propranolol	
	i. Melatonin	
	5. Nonpeptide Hormones	
	a. Estrogens	
	b. Diethylstilbestrol	
	6. Potassium infusion	
	7. Dibutyryl-CAMP	

through deficiencies of ADH, ACTH, TSH, or gonadotropins, as well as through GH deficiency. Modern knowledge of the neural control of GH regulation has relied heavily on the development of immunoassay, in conjunction with experiments on the effects of hypothalamic lesions, electric stimulation of the hypothalamus, isolation of GH-releasing and -inhibiting factors, and the effects of provocative testing. The early history of our knowledge of neural control of GH release, in the pre-immunoassay era, is summarized in several recent reviews.[10, 40, 49]

Table 2. Factors That Inhibit GH Secretion in Primates*

Physiologic	Pharmacologic	Pathologic
1. Postprandial hyperglycemia	1. Melatonin	1. Acromegaly
2. Elevated free fatty acids	2. Serotonin antagonists	a. L-dopa
(? pharmacologic)	a. Methysergide	b. Apomorphine
3. Elevated GH levels	b. Cyproheptadine	c. Phentolamine
	3. Phentolamine	d. 2-bromo-α-ergocryptine
	4. Chlorpromazine	2. Hyperthyroidism
	5. Morphine	3. Hypothyroidism
	6. Zn-tetracosactin	
	7. Progesterone	
	8. Theophylline	

*In many instances, the inhibition can only be demonstrated as a suppression of GH release induced by a pharmacologic stimulus.

Hypothalamic Regulation

Hypothalamic Lesions and Deafferentation

Lesion studies in the rat implicate the ventromedial nucleus (VMN)-median eminence region as the final common pathway of control of GH release.[19, 37] Destruction of the VMN area blocks pulsatile GH release[42] and impairs growth, without interfering with the vascular supply of the pituitary. In the squirrel monkey, Brown and coworkers[11] showed that lesions of the anterior lip of the median eminence blocked the release of GH that normally follows stressful stimuli such as restraint or ether anesthesia. GH regulatory functions in man have not been precisely localized, but it is important to emphasize that this neural function is extremely susceptible to even minor damage, reflex GH release being among the earliest signs of hypothalamic failure in man. In the work of Brown and colleagues,[11] stress-induced GH discharge in squirrel monkeys was blocked by only a small lesion in the upper stalk region, which left intact more than 70 per cent of the connecting neurons. On the basis of these observations (together with the positive effects of electric stimulation, and bioassays of releasing hormone [see below]), it appears reasonable to conclude that the VMN and adjacent arcuate nucleus control secretion of the growth hormone-releasing factor.

Recently accumulated data indicates that there is also an inhibitory pathway for GH regulation. Lesions of the anterior hypothalamus, removal of the brain anterior to the septum, or anterior (coronal) deafferentation by the Halasz technique at the level of the optic chiasm, are all followed by evidence of increased GH secretion, including more rapid growth in the rat.[40] In the squirrel monkey, anterior hypothalamic lesions were found to be associated with exaggerated responses to ether anesthesia (suggesting loss of an inhibitory component), and recent immunohistochemical work indicates that in the rat there is an anterior somatostatinergic pathway extending from the preoptic area to the median eminence (see below). These data suggest that GH secretion is regulated by the interaction of excitatory (VMN-basal hypothalamic) and inhibitory (preoptic-basal hypothalamic) pathways.

Hypothalamic Stimulation

Electric stimulation has given far more convincing evidence of specific neural control regions. A rise in GH is produced by electric stimulation of the basal hypothalamus in the monkey, and of the ventromedial nucleus and the adjacent arcuate nucleus in the rat (Fig 5).[20, 37, 41] Either unilateral or bilateral stimulation of the medial basal hypothalamus in the rat elicits GH secretion within 5 to 15 minutes after the onset of pulsed square waves. The effective stimulation sites are strictly confined to the VMN-arcuate complex. Stimulation of the lateral or anterior hypothalamus, or of the supraoptic or paraventricular nuclei has no effect on plasma GH. Stimulation of the preoptic area causes significant inhibition of GH,[40] an interesting observation in view of speculation that there is an anterior hypothalamic or parachiasmatic inhibitory area for GH regulation, and of recent studies demonstrating GIH in this region of brain.

Careful analysis of the time-course of GH release after VMN stimulation permits delineation of both excitatory and inhibitory components of response. The rise of plasma GH levels induced by hypothalamic stimulation invariably occurs *after* termination of the stimulus, as a post-inhibitory rebound surge of secretion.[39] The response peak usually occurs 10 to 15 minutes after cessation of stimulation. Before the discovery of

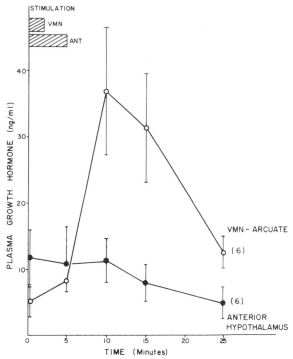

Figure 5. Growth hormone response to electrical stimulation of the ventromedial (VMN)-arcuate region in the rat. Stimulation of other hypothalamic sites is ineffective. (From Martin, J. B.: *Plasma growth hormone (GH) response to hypothalamic or extrahypothalamic electrical stimulation.* Endocrinology 91:107, 1972, with permission.)

somatostatin it was difficult to interpret these findings. It now seems reasonable to speculate that hypothalamic stimulation elicits somatostatin release, resulting in temporary cessation of GH secretion, followed by a post-inhibitory rebound surge of GH secretion, perhaps secondary to release of GH-releasing factor, the latter initially prevented from exerting its stimulatory effect by the inhibitory action of somatostatin. A similar post-inhibitory GH surge has been described after hypothalamic stimulation in sheep. Growth hormone release can be induced also by stimulation of the VMN in the unanesthetized rabbit.[40]

It is likely that stimulation of these hypothalamic sites causes GH release by direct excitation of tuberohypophyseal (also called tuberoinfundibular, TI) peptidergic neurons. Several investigators have now successfully identified such cells by antidromic activation of axon terminals in the median eminence (see Chapter 2). Tuberoinfundibular neurons are not restricted to the arcuate nucleus but are located throughout the medial basal hypothalamus, extending as a rim of cells along the entire wall of the third ventricle to include the periventricular nucleus and the VMN. It can be argued from hypothalamic electric stimulation experiments that regulation of individual anterior pituitary hormones shows some anatomic specificity. Effective sites for TSH release and LH release are much more widespread in the hypothalamus than those for GH release, presumably because these stimuli excite selective populations of peptidergic neurons.

These data indicate a selective neural regulatory system for GH involving a specific group of hypothalamic neurons.

Growth Hormone-Releasing Factors

GROWTH HORMONE-RELEASING HORMONE. Despite the compelling evidence, through physiologic studies of lesions or electrical stimulation, of neural control of GH secretion, attempts to isolate and chemically identify growth hormone-releasing factor (GRF) have been disappointing. Several years ago, Schally and collaborators isolated a decapeptide from porcine hypothalamic extracts which could lower the GH content of pituitaries in vivo, and release GH into the medium in a pituitary incubation system.[49, 54] This material, given the name growth hormone-releasing hormone (GRH), was then synthesized by these workers and found to be ineffective in causing a rise in plasma radioimmunoassayable GH in the rat or man. So-called GRH was almost identical to a portion of the β-chain of porcine hemoglobin, and hence may be an artifact of the extraction procedure. Despite this disappointing denouement, many studies have shown that crude and semipurified extracts of hypothalamic tissue can stimulate the release of radioimmunoassayable GH in both the rat and monkey, both in vivo and in vitro. Although under certain conditions ADH and TRH can act like GRH, GRF activity can be separated from these contaminants, and appears to be a distinct entity.[36] Unlike TRH and ADH, it is relatively stable in blood and is most effective in the estrogen-sensitized rat. On Sephadex column chromatography, Boyd and coworkers[8] have found that GRH moves with TRH, but is not destroyed by incubation with plasma.

OTHER PEPTIDES. A number of structurally unrelated peptides have been shown to be effective in releasing GH in various species, including man. It is well known that several individual amino acids (including arginine, histidine, leucine, phenylalanine, and lysine) can cause GH release, although the site and mechanism of action are unknown.[49] Several small polypeptide hormones also are effective in this regard.

TRH. Although ineffective in inducing GH release in normal human subjects, TRH is a remarkably potent stimulant for GH release in acromegaly[17, 35] and in patients with renal failure. TRH is potent also in stimulating GH release in the cow and in pituitaries incubated in vitro. Interestingly, TRH-induced GH release in acromegaly (unlike basal GH secretion) is not inhibited by somatostatin.[22] LHRH is also reported to cause GH release in some, but not all acromegalic subjects, and this effect also is not prevented by somatostatin.[22]

ADH. ADH in pharmacologic doses releases GH in man, monkey, and rat. This effect was considered to be of little or no physiologic significance until Zimmerman and coworkers[63] found in the rhesus monkey that ADH (and neurophysin) are present in extremely high concentrations in the pituitary portal blood of surgically-stressed monkeys. This has resurrected the possibility that ADH might act as a "GRH" in stimulating GH release during stress. It can be argued convincingly, however, that ADH cannot be the only GRH, since rats with hereditary ADH deficiency have normal plasma levels of GH. These rats also show normal GH release after electric stimulation of the VMN. Further evidence against a role of ADH as a GRH in the rat is the finding that stimulation of the supraoptic nuclei, which is effective in releasing neurophysin (and presumably ADH) has no effect on GH release. It is more likely that ADH acts as a stressor in releasing GH.

α-MSH. Several papers have appeared which suggest that an active peptide sequence of ACTH may be effective in releasing GH in man.[40] Recently, it has been reported that α-MSH, which contains an amino acid sequence identical to the first 13 residues of ACTH, causes a marked rise in GH 30 to 45 minutes after intravenous administration. The physiologic significance of this response requires further study.

Glucagon. Glucagon, which contains 29 amino acids, is well known for its capacity to release GH in man. Its site of action is unknown but it is not likely to be secondary to changes in plasma glucose, although this is still debated by some investigators. The effect of glucagon is potentiated by β-receptor blockade, suggesting that it may act upon neural monoaminergic systems (see below).

Cholera Enterotoxin. A material with potent GRF activity has been isolated from cholera enterotoxin and elicits GH release in vitro by stimulation of cyclic AMP. Its molecular weight is approximately 84,000. Its effects are blocked by somatostatin. These observations are of great interest and may result in identification of structure-activity relationships which will assist in the elucidation of native hypothalamic GRH.

GRH activity has also been reported in human lung tumor tissue, indicating the possibility that the peptide may be synthesized in neoplastic tissue (as has been documented for other peptide hormones).

It remains to be demonstrated whether these polypeptide substances act via specific receptors, or whether their effects are due to individual amino acids which form after breakdown of the parent molecule.

Growth Hormone-Inhibiting Factor: Somatostatin

In efforts to identify and isolate GRF in hypothalamic extracts, materials have been isolated that inhibit pituitary GH release in vitro. Krulich and coworkers[31] were the first to identify such growth hormone-inhibiting factors (GIF), and partially purified the material by chromatography. Using an in vitro pituitary assay system, the anatomic sites of GIF and GRF activities were identified in rat brain and the theory was proposed that GH secretion might be regulated by interaction between excitatory and inhibitory factors. The claims of Krulich and collaborators[31] were not widely accepted, largely because there appeared to be no theoretic rationale for the existence of a GIH, and because inhibitory effects in the assay system used could be attributed to nonspecific toxic effects. Brazeau and collaborators[9] later rediscovered growth hormone-inhibiting factor in ovine hypothalamic tissue, isolated it, identified it chemically, and finally achieved its total chemical synthesis (Fig. 6). Their work was facilitated by the development of a sensitive bioassay system that utilized pituitary cell cultures, and by a highly sophisticated approach to polypeptide analysis and synthesis that had grown out of earlier work on the isolation of TRH and LHRH. The substance finally characterized was named *somatostatin,* and in the short interval since its discovery in 1973, a tremendous amount of investigation has led to new insights into the regulation of the pituitary, and unexpectedly into the function of several other secretory systems, including the islets of the pancreas and the gastrin-producing cells of the stomach. The discovery of somatostatin also has given indication of promising new developments in our understanding of diabetes mellitus.[15, 16, 21, 29] The tetradecapeptide described by Brazeau's group is not the only hypothalamic substance with growth hormone-inhibiting activity; they have isolated several other active GIF fractions which have been partially separated from extracts, and Schally and collaborators have reported similar results.[54]

ACTIONS ON THE PITUITARY. Somatostatin exerts striking inhibitory action on GH secretion, both in vitro and in vivo, in all species of animals in which it has been used, including rat, baboon, dog, sheep, and man.[5, 40] It is effective regardless of the

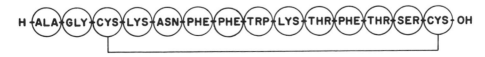

SOMATOSTATIN

Figure 6. Structure of somatostatin.

159

stimulus used to induce secretion. For example, in man, somatostatin blocks the GH secretory response to insulin-induced hypoglycemia, arginine infusion, L-dopa ingestion,[55] and that associated with sleep.[46] It effectively lowers GH plasma levels in most acromegalic patients.[5, 62]

Effects of somatostatin on the pituitary are not limited to inhibition of GH release. The hormone also blocks TRH-induced TSH release but, paradoxically, does not block TRH-induced prolactin release. Somatostatin has no effect on basal levels of TSH, prolactin, FSH, LH, or ACTH, and does not block LHRH-induced LH or FSH release.

Inhibitory action is very prompt after intravenous injection — changes in plasma GH level occurring within five minutes — but the effect wears off quickly as soon as somatostatin infusion is stopped.[5] The major factor in the briefness of action is the extreme rapidity with which stomatostatin disappears from the blood, presumably due to enzymatic inactivation. A striking rebound secretion is observed when treatment is discontinued in man, monkey, dog, and rat, and has also been reported in isolated rat pituitary perfusion systems. Martin[40] has shown that such inhibition is not seen in the rat following damage to the ventromedial nucleus, a finding indicating that rebound may be due to unmasking of GRH effects. Terry and coworkers[59] have recently reported that administration of antiserum to somatostatin blocks stress-induced suppression of GH in the rat. This finding suggests that somatostatin is released physiologically during stress and acts to inhibit GH secretion.

EXTRAPITUITARY EFFECTS. Within a few months after synthetic somatostatin had been made available for studies in laboratory primates, Gale and colleagues reported that this agent caused a lowering of blood glucose and inhibition of secretion of both glucagon and insulin (Fig. 7).[51] These findings have been confirmed repeatedly in many laboratory species and in man. It has been further shown that somatostatin does not influence peripheral glucose metabolism, and that the hypoglycemic effects of the agent are mediated through the inhibition of glucagon release at the level of the islet cell.

More recently it has been shown that somatostatin inhibits the secretion of gastrin, and secondarily of gastric acid, as well as the secretion of vasoactive inhibitory peptide (VIP) and renin. Because at first relatively large amounts of somatostatin were injected, it may well be asked whether the effects are physiologically significant. Using new immunoassay methods, Patel and colleagues[47] have found somatostatin in isolated islet cells of the rat, and this group as well as Arimura and coworkers[4] have found somatostatin in gastric and duodenal mucosa and in islets by immunohistochemical techniques. Except for these tissues, somatostatin is not demonstrable outside the brain; it has a specific distribution. These observations suggest that somatostatin formed in situ may be involved in the normal regulation of secretion in stomach and pancreas, and blood-borne somatostatin of brain origin also may affect the function of these organs. Since perturbations of brain function and psychosomatic factors are known to influence the secretion of gastrin and of the pancreas, a novel neuroendocrine pathway of control via somatostatin must be considered as a possibility.

CLINICAL USE. Because of somatostatin's short action and rebound effects on GH secretion, most work has been done with short-term intravenous injection. A long-acting preparation would be of enormous value in therapeutic trials, but there have been only modest developments in this direction. The most promising preparation is that of Brazeau and collaborators which has utilized a protamine-zinc (Pz) complex that in the rat may act for as long as 12 hours, and in man for 4 to 6 hours.[5, 40] A number of analogues have been studied as well, but none have been shown to have a prolonged action except in combination with Pz.

Despite these limitations of available preparations, a number of striking conclusions already have been drawn. Infusions of somatostatin inhibit stress- and exercise-induced GH release in diabetics. Single subcutaneous injections inhibit glucagon secretion in the

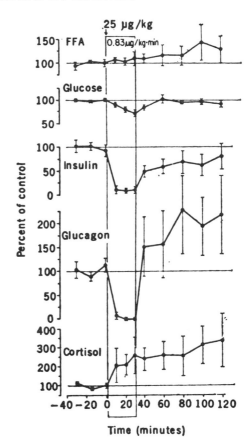

Figure 7. Effects of somatostatin on plasma free fatty acids (FFA), glucose, insulin, glucagon and cortisol. Somatostatin causes immediate suppression of insulin and glucose which is followed by a decline in glucose. (From Koerker, D. J., et al.: *Somatostatin: Hypothalamic inhibitor of the endocrine pancreas.* Science 184:482, 1974, with permission.)

diabetic,[21] prevent reactive hyperglycemia for the most part, and decrease the total insulin requirement. When given early in the course of diabetic ketoacidosis, somatostatin-induced glucagon suppression led to a marked amelioration of ketosis, and this observation has established the importance of glucagon in the pathogenesis of this condition. These observations have created much excitement as a potential means of treating the brittle diabetic, on a short-term basis, and in preventing the long-term degenerative vascular lesions of diabetes which are believed to require GH for their development.

Widespread clinical trials in diabetes, anticipated in 1975, were called to a halt by the unexpected and unexplained high mortality in a group of experimental baboons being infused chronically with large intravenous doses of somatostatin. At autopsy, pulmonary hemorrhage appeared to be the cause of death. No similar cases had been reported in man, or in rodents, and it was not established whether the hemorrhagic lesions were due to another cause, or were related to the long-term somatostatin administration together with some other idiosyncratic factor such as prolonged chairing, which, in the baboon, is an unphysiologic circumstance. The finding of pulmonary hemorrhage in test animals led to the study of somatostatin effects on blood coagulation processes. Several groups now report that this agent in usual therapeutic doses over a six-hour period impairs platelet aggregation in vitro, an effect lasting as long as 24 hours in a few cases, but no abnormality of bleeding time was detected. Similar findings after somatostatin administration were observed in baboons and in rabbits. In the human, direct addition of somatostatin in vitro was without effect on platelet aggregation. It has been

161

stated that the effects are not great, and resemble those seen after the administration of aspirin. However, it has been urged that caution be exercised when using somatostatin over prolonged periods. It has been reported that hitherto-intractable bleeding from a duodenal ulcer ceased upon administration of somatostatin (presumably due to inhibition of gastrin-induced acid secretion); at least in this case somatostatin effects on platelets did not interfere with hemostasis.

DISTRIBUTION IN BRAIN. The results of bioassay and radioimmunoassay agree that somatostatin is localized to a number of neural regions outside the hypothalamus (Table 3).[12, 47] Highest concentrations have been reported in the preoptic area and in the amygdala, and significant amounts are found also in the cerebral cortex, thalamus, cerebellum, brain stem, spinal cord, and the pineal gland. Somatostatin is also present in the CSF and is found in high concentrations in association with certain CNS tumors and degenerative disorders. This intriguing observation may provide new information concerning peptide synthesizing function of brain structures and tissues.

It is possible, given the information available, that the regions of the hypothalamus that contain GIH are those known to contain tuberoinfundibular (releasing factor) neurons. Recent electrophysiologic studies have provided evidence that certain of these cells have branching axon collaterals, one of which terminates on the portal vessels while the other ends in various other regions of the hypothalamus, the preoptic area, or the limbic system. By use of antidromic activation from the median eminence, accompanied by similar concurrent activation from other brain sites, Renaud and Martin[50] defined a population of such cells in the VMN. These observations permit speculation that TI peptidergic neurons (like dopaminergic, noradrenergic, and serotonergic neurons) may give rise to complex neural pathways which terminate in widespread areas of the neural axis. Do such collaterals represent recurrent feedback loops which might function, for example, in the mediation of pulsatile secretion? Do collateral terminals which end in such regions as the preoptic area, brain stem and amygdala—all regions which contain somatostatin—account for the widespread distribution of this peptide in extrahypothalamic tissues? Is somatostatin released from such terminals to have important biologic effects on other neurons by influencing both electrophysiologic and behavioral aspects of brain function? The answers to these and other intriguing questions must await further evidence. Supporting a possible role of hypothalamic peptides in neuron function is the observation that direct application of these peptides by iontophoresis onto single neurons results in significant depression of firing rates. Somatostatin as well as TRH and LHRH depressed a certain population of central neurons, both in the hypothalamus and in other areas such as the cerebral and cerebellar cortex and the spinal cord. There is preliminary evidence that somatostatin, like TRH and LHRH, has behavioral effects, al-

Table 3. Distribution of Somatostatin in Hypothalamic Nuclei and Other Regions of the Brain

Nucleus or Region	ng./mg. Protein ± S.E.M.
Median eminence	309.1 ± 60.8
Arcuate nucleus	44.6 ± 6.1
Periventricular nucleus	23.7 ± 9.0
Ventromedial nucleus	14.6 ± 2.1
Medial preoptic nucleus	10.4 ± 2.5
Paraventricular nucleus	4.4 ± 1.8
Supraoptic nucleus	3.2 ± 0.6
Amygdala	3.9 ± 0.4
Hippocampus	1.1 ± 0.2
Central gray	3.3 ± 0.4

(Adapted from Brownstein, M., et al.: *The regional distribution of somatostatin in the rat brain.* Endrocrinology 96:1456, 1975.)

though the significance of these early reports of behavioral effects of GIH are difficult to assess.[40]

It is apparent that further investigation of the neural effects of somatostatin may have profound significance, not only in terms of our understanding of the role of hypothalamic peptides in anterior pituitary regulation, but also regarding the function of such peptides in regulation of brain mechanisms. Some theoretic aspects are discussed in detail by Martin and associates.[65]

Extrahypothalamic Regulation

Physiologic studies demonstrating the effects of stress and sleep on GH secretion point to a probable role of extrahypothalamic structures in GH control. The isolated hypothalamus appears capable of maintaining near-normal basal secretion of GH, including pulsatile release, but selective hypothalamic cuts indicate that disconnection of specific inputs to the medial basal hypothalamus can have differential excitatory or inhibitory effects on GH secretion, at least in the rat.

The anatomic pathways connecting the limbic system to the medial basal hypothalamus, in general, and the VMN-arcuate complex, in partiuclar, have been most clearly defined in the rat[37] (Fig. 8).

Direct monosynaptic inputs from a portion of the hippocampus reach the arcuate nucleus via the medial corticohypothalamic tract. The amygdala has a large monosynaptic connection from its corticomedial subdivision which reaches the VMN via the stria terminalis. The connection(s) of the basolateral amygdala to the medial basal hypothalamus has not been as clearly defined. Electrophysiologic studies in the cat have indicated an inhibitory pathway from the corticomedial amygdala via the stria terminalis to the VMN and a complementary

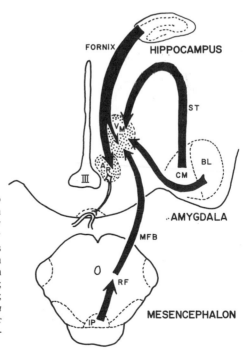

Figure 8. Diagram of major afferent pathways to the ventromedial (VM) and arcuate (AR) nuclei in the rat. A large direct hippocampal-arcuate pathway has been described. Amygdaloid inputs arise by two separate pathways. Interpeduncular (IP) inputs to the hypothalamus ascend in the medial forebrain bundle (MFB) after relay in the reticular formation (RF). *Abbreviations:* BL, basolateral amygdala; CM, corticomedial amygdala; ST, stria terminalis; III, third ventricle. (From Martin, J. B.: *Plasma growth hormone (GH) response to hypothalamic or extrahypothalamic electrical stimulation.* Endocrinology 91:107, 1972, with permission.)

163

excitatory pathway from the basolateral amygdaloid complex to the hypothalamic VMN. It is postulated that this latter pathway is carried in the ventral amygdalohypothalamic tract.

A possible role of extrahypothalamic structure in GH control was first suggested when amygdaloid lesions in the deermouse resulted in an increase in pituitary GH. Lesions of the amygdala and pyriform cortex also have been reported to reduce plasma GH levels in the rat, as determined by radioimmunoassay.

Martin and coworkers[37, 39, 41] have shown that electric stimulation of the hippocampal formation causes GH release, whereas stimulation of the amygdala can elicit either a rise or a fall in plasma GH depending upon the precise site stimulated. Thus, stimulation of the basolateral amygdala causes prompt GH release which appears to be entrained to the stimulus, plasma levels increasing within 5 minutes of the onset of stimulation and declining immediately after its termination (Fig. 9). This response is blocked by placement of bilateral hypothalamic VMN lesions, indicating that the GH release effects are mediated through the medial basal hypothalamus. Stimulation of the cortico-medial amygdala, on the other hand, causes a fall in plasma GH levels comparable to that observed with preoptic stimulation. Since an important component of the efferent system of the corticomedial amygdala travels in the stria terminalis to end in the septum and preoptic area, it remains to be shown whether the corticomedial inhibitory response is mediated via connections in these areas. It is significant, perhaps, that coronal cuts through the anterior hypothalamus cause an increase in growth in the rat and an elevation in plasma GH levels, in some but not all studies. Such cuts would interrupt the stria terminalis, but might also disconnect inhibitory effects of the preoptic area. Complete medial basal hypothalamic deafferentation, in which the VMN and arcuate are isolated from the overlying brain, is reported to result in an increased growth rate and elevated plasma GH levels. It has recently been reported that preoptic lesions block stress-induced inhibition of GH secretion in the rat; such lesions permit emergence of a stress GH-release mechanism in this species. These observations suggest that extrahypothalamic inhibitory inputs to the medial basal hypothalamus are important in maintaining a degree of tonic inhibition of GH in the mediation of stress-induced

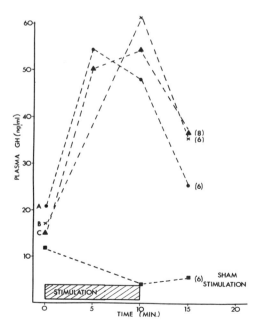

Figure 9. Plasma growth hormone (GH) responses to stimulation of the basolateral amygdala in three separate groups of animals. Sham stimulation had no effect on GH. Number of animals in each group is shown in parentheses. (From Martin, J. B.: *Advances in Human Growth Hormone Release*. NIH publication #74-612, 1974.)

164

GH suppression. Histochemical demonstration of an anterior somatostatinergic pathway supports this hypothesis.

Stimulation of other brain regions also can cause a rise in plasma GH. One effective site is the ventral tegmental area of Tsai surrounding the interpeduncular nucleus, a region giving rise to dopaminergic inputs to higher brain regions. Electric stimulation of the locus ceruleus also resulted in GH release in some, but not all animals. Stimulation of the raphe nucleus, the site of serotonergic neurons in the brain stem, results in GH release.[40] Further investigation of these brain areas will be required to elucidate their role, now a potential one, in GH regulation. The results of locus ceruleus and raphe nucleus stimulation are of interest because both NE and serotonin have been implicated in the regulation of GH secretion (see below).

> The functions of the limbic regions that affect GH secretion are complex. Experimental evidence indicates that the hippocampus is involved in several aspects of behavior, such as the alerting response, and in the recording of new information, as in learning or memory storage.[2] The amygdala, on the other hand, is important in establishing emotionality and in the mediation of aggressive behavior.[44] The amygdala is also important in regulation of feeding and drinking. The locus ceruleus is the origin of the ascending noradrenergic fiber system, lesions of which have been implicated in the "sham rage" associated with the "VMH syndrome."[23] The raphe nuclei have been shown to have a role in induction of sleep. Lesions of the raphe nuclei lead to insomnia, as does inhibition of serotonin synthesis by p-chlorophenylalanine.

Pineal Influences

Significant depressions of body weight, tibia length, and pituitary GH content are caused in rats by combined blinding and olfactory-lobe removal. These effects are partially reversed by pinealectomy, an indication that the pineal exerts tonic inhibitory effects on GH secretion in this species. The mechanism by which this effect is exerted has not been established, but Patel and Reichlin[47] have found that the pineal gland is rich in somatostatin, and in a single patient with ectopic pinealoma, cerebrospinal fluid somatostatin levels were elevated, and pituitary GH secretion reduced. These observations permit the hypothesis that pineal effects on GH secretion may be exerted by way of somatostatin which reaches the pituitary via CSF and transmedian eminence transport.

Monoamines

Growth hormone is regulated by a dual system of hypothalamic hypophysiotrophic hormones, one inhibitory and the other excitatory. Release of these hormones is, in turn, regulated by aminergic neurons. The finding that many stimuli affect GH secretion in man has led to extensive investigations of the role of monoamines, in particular NE, DA, and serotonin, in normal and abnormal GH secretory states. Recent studies have also examined the effects of melatonin and of specific receptor agonists and antagonists on GH secretion. Such studies have led to the development of important insights into both basic control mechanisms, and to the discovery of new therapeutic approaches to disorders of GH secretion.

Each of the three biogenic amines, NE, DA, and serotonin, has a distinct and separate stimulatory role in GH regulation in the primate. Oral administration of L-dopa, the precursor of both NE and DA, which readily crosses the blood-brain barrier, causes release of GH in man[7] (Fig. 10). Evidence that the dopa effect is mediated through its conversion to NE is derived from experiments showing that L-dopa-induced GH release is blocked by phentolamine, an α-receptor blocking agent.[38]

165

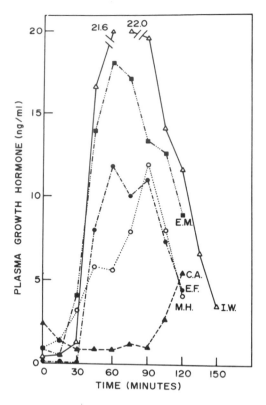

Figure 10. Plasma GH response to L-dopa administered orally. The peak of the response occurs 60 to 90 minutes after L-dopa administration. (From Boyd, A.: *Stimulation of human-growth-hormone secretion by L-dopa.* N. Engl. J. Med. 283:1425, 1970, with permission).

Subemetic doses of apomorphine, a centrally-active, dopamine receptor-stimulating agent, also release GH; evidently there may be an additional dopaminergic control mechanism independent of NE conversion.[32] GH release induced by L-dopa and apomorphine is attenuated by prior glucose administration, the glucoreceptor stimulation partially over-riding catecholaminergic stimuli for GH release.

A role of α-adrenergic receptors in GH control is supported further by the report by Lal and coworkers[33] that clonidine, a central α-agonist, stimulated GH release in man, although not as strongly as apomorphine.

Most stimuli that cause GH release appear to act via central α-adrenergic receptors. In man, GH release induced by insulin hypoglycemia, arginine, exercise, ADH, L-dopa, and certain stresses are all prevented by phentolamine[38] (Fig. 11). On the other hand, propranolol, a β-adrenergic blocker, enhances GH release induced by glucagon, ADH, and L-dopa. The β-agonist isoproterenol is reported to inhibit GH release.[25] These studies indicate that GH secretion is facilitated by both dopaminergic and noradrenergic α-receptor stimulation, and inhibited by noradrenergic β-receptor stimulation. Pharmacologic blockade of GH release by drugs like chlorpromazine, pimozide, and haloperidol is thought to occur at a hypothalamic level, probably by competitive blockade of dopaminergic receptor sites.

Serotonin may also be involved in GH release in primates. Oral administration of L-tryptophan or 5-hydroxytryptophan (5-HTP) in man causes GH release, although the response is not great.[28] The release of GH in response to hypoglycemia is blocked by the serotonin antagonists methysergide and cyproheptadine.[6] Melatonin is reported both to facilitate GH release and to block release in response to insulin hypoglycemia; these apparently conflicting effects were explained by differences in the time course of melatonin action.[40]

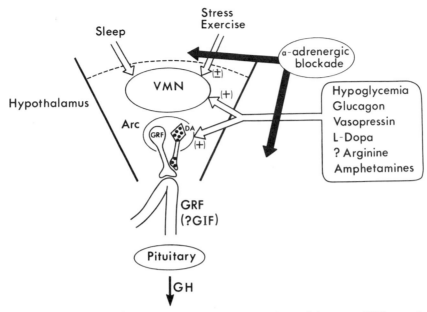

Figure 11. Diagram of hypothalamic mechanisms for regulation of growth hormone (GH) secretion. Alpha-adrenergic blockade (with phentolamine) partially or completely blocks GH release to the stimuli shown. Sleep-release of GH is not affected. (Modified from Martin, J. B.: *Neural regulation of growth hormone secretion.* N. Engl. J. Med. 228:1384, 1973.)

Physiologic GH release, as in sleep, may be regulated by yet another mechanism. Neither α- nor β-adrenergic receptor blockade nor dopaminergic blockade with chlorpromazine affects nocturnal sleep-associated GH release.[38] Blockade of serotonin receptors with methysergide has resulted in an increase in GH release during sleep.

Species seem to differ with respect to GH responses to pharmacologic stimuli. In the rhesus monkey, intravenous clonidine and 5-hydroxytryptophan are potent stimulants for GH release, whereas apomorphine is ineffective except at doses that induce vomiting (and therefore act as a nonspecific stress effect). In these studies by Chambers and Brown,[67] the administration of dihydroxyphenylserine, a precursor of norepinephrine but not dopamine, also was effective in releasing GH. Similarly, in the dog, systemic administration of L-dopa and clonidine released GH, but apomorphine had no effect. These findings suggest that there may be no animal model available that precisely duplicates GH control in man.

It is probable that biogenic amine agonists and antagonists act at a hypothalamic level to modulate GRF or somatostatin release. Intrahypothalamic infusions of norepinephrine are effective in releasing GH in the baboon.[60] Moreover, cerebral intraventricular or hypothalamic injections of systemically ineffective doses of phentolamine prevent hypoglycemic-induced GH release in this species. There is *no* compelling experimental evidence to indicate that catecholamines act at the pituitary somatotrope level, either directly or in synergism with hypothalamic hormones. A hypothetical construct of the hypothalamic sites of action of several agents known to affect GH secretion can now be proposed and is illustrated in Fig. 12.

Experimental studies in the rat have indicated that catecholamines are involved in the relay of GH release induced by stimulation of extrahypothalamic structures. Depletion of central catecholamines by administration of α-methyl-*p*-tyrosine, an inhibitor of catechol-

167

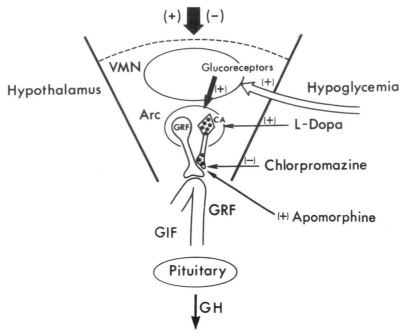

Figure 12. Diagram of hypothalamic mechanisms for regulation of growth hormone (GH) secretion. Hypoglycemia acts on glucoreceptors to trigger GH release. L-dopa, by increasing substrate for formation of catecholamines stimulates growth-releasing factor (GRF) release. Chlorpromazine blocks catecholaminergic receptors to inhibit GH secretion, and apomorphine, a dopamine receptor agonist, stimulates GH release. (Modified from Martin, J. B.: *Neural regulation of growth hormone secretion.* N. Engl. J. Med. 228:1384, 1973.)

amine synthesis, has no effect on GH release induced by hypothalamic stimulation, but prevents GH release after stimulation of the hippocampus or basolateral amygdala. Depletion of serotonin with *p*-chlorophenylalanine also prevented GH release after amygdaloid stimulation, but did not affect GH release induced by hypothalamic stimulation.[39]

Electric stimulation studies in the rat have also shown that direct stimulation of monoaminergic neurons in the brain stem causes GH release. Stimulation of dopaminergic, noradrenergic, and serotonergic neurons were all effective.[40] These observations are consistent with a role of both catecholamines and serotonin acting as neurotransmitters in the relay of responses from higher brain regions to tuberoinfundibular neurons. They also make it seem unlikely that these monoamines function directly at the pituitary level.

Short-Loop Feedback Control

Current evidence indicates that under certain defined conditions, GH is capable of inhibiting its own secretion.[2, 14] Systemic administration of GH, direct hypothalamic placement of GH pellets, or implantation of a GH-secreting tumor in rats has been shown to reduce pituitary GH levels.

Acute experiments have also shown that pharmacologically-stimulated GH secretion can partially block a subsequent GH response to a second stimulus. Elevation of serum GH levels by exercise in man prevented a further rise in response to arginine. Prior GH administration to man and monkeys partially blocks GH release induced by arginine or by insulin hypoglycemia.[40] Although these results support a role for GH in regulation of its own secretion, they do not provide an explanation of the mechanism. Since GH induces formation of somatomedin in peripheral tissue, it is relevant to ask whether the feedback might be mediated via this second "hormone." Direct evidence to support this mechanism is not available, but the Laron dwarf, who seems to lack normal periph-eral-tissue production of somatomedin, has strikingly elevated levels of GH, consistent with a failure in normal feedback regulation. Similarly the high GH levels of kwashior-kor are associated with low plasma somatomedin.

Experiments in rats infested with the tapeworm *Spirometra mansonoides* have pro-vided further evidence for a short-loop feedback control of GH, mediated by soma-tomedin.[14] This tapeworm produces a substance(s) which is not immunoreactive in GH assays, but which does compete with GH in radioreceptor assays and is capable of stimulating somatomedin production. Infestation with the worm leads to depletion of radioimmunoassayable GH in the pituitary, indicating a feedback effect either via the tapeworm substance or via somatomedin.

In summary, it is probable that acute fluctuations in GH secretion result from acute neural effects, but basal levels and the degree of GH secretory response to neural stim-uli may be determined by the previous circulating levels of GH and/or somatomedin. With further purification of somatomedin it should be possible to test this hypothesis directly.

DISORDERS OF GROWTH HORMONE SECRETION

It appears that plasma GH levels fluctuate widely during the day and night, and that these changes are mediated by neural mechanisms. The extent to which autonomous pituitary GH secretion can occur in the absence of hypothalamic drive is unknown. Studies in stalk-sectioned patients indicate that basal GH levels are low and that reflex release in response to stimuli such as insulin hypoglycemia is blocked.

Hyposecretion

Growth hormone deficiency in childhood results in growth failure and dwarfism. In the adult, unmeasurable or reduced basal GH levels may occur as the result of either primary pituitary disturbances or hypothalamic disorders in which no pathologic in-volvement of the pituitary is evident. In individual cases, often one cannot distinguish whether the deficiency in GH is due to pituitary or hypothalamic disease. Several forms of hyposomatotropic dwarfism are recognized.

Organic Lesions of Pituitary or Hypothalamus

Lesions within the sella turcica, either primary or secondary to surgical manipula-tion, may induce GH deficiency. Hypothalamic lesions due to inflammatory conditions, malformations, histiocytosis X, tumors, trauma, or roentgenotherapy are recognized causes of GH deficiency. These disorders are generally characterized by undetectable basal GH levels and failure of GH release after insulin-induced hypoglycemia, L-dopa administration, or arginine infusion. Developmental abnormalities associated with anatomic malformations of midline cerebral structures have been documented in which associated disturbances in GH secretion occur. Patients have been described with a clinical syndrome of hypopituitarism, optic-nerve dysplasia, and midline prosen-cephalic malformations including absence of the septum pellucidum and an abnormal third ventricle and lamina terminalis. In one series of six patients, all had GH deficiency and four of the six had more than one pituitary disturbance, all presumably due to ab-sence of the appropriate hypothalamic hypophysiotropic hormone.[38]

Idiopathic Hypopituitarism

Complete hypopituitarism (panhypopituitarism) or partial hypopituitarism may occur in either a sporadic or a familial form. Several recent studies of the response to TRH and LHRH in such patients with secondary hypothyroidism or hypogonadotropism have indicated that the pituitary is responsive to these hypothalamic hormones. These studies provide convincing evidence that many patients with idiopathic hypopituitarism actually have a primary deficiency in hypophysiotropic hormone synthesis or release, occurring in either a multiple or monotropic form. Monotropic GH deficiency may occur in either a sporadic or a familial form. Intrauterine growth is normal in many such cases and GH deficiency is not recognized until early childhood. A deficiency of GRF is the most likely cause of the disease in such cases, but proof of the primary site of pathophysiologic disturbance in these patients must await the availability of purified or synthetic GRF. The possibility that release mechanisms mediated by catecholamines play a role in this disorder has been suggested. Beta-adrenergic blockade with propranolol can restore normal GH responses to insulin hypoglycemia in certain hypopituitary patients. This observation has not been confirmed, but it does introduce the interesting possibility that certain GH deficiency states might result from GRF release defects.

Laron Dwarfism

A form of dwarfism associated with high levels of circulating GH was first described by Laron and colleagues.[14] The GH in the pituitary and plasma of such patients is immunologically indistinguishable from that of normal subjects and they fail to grow when given exogenous GH. Recently it has been shown that somatomedin levels are reduced in the Laron dwarf; hepatic GH receptors may be defective. This interesting pathophysiologic disorder provides indirect evidence for a negative-feedback regulation of GH, perhaps involving somatomedin (see above). Deficiency of somatomedin leads to excessive GH secretion, which is ineffective in producing normal growth. There is no treatment for these patients. Isolation and purification of somatomedin may provide an effective treatment, but this prospect is remote.

Maternal Deprivation Syndrome (Psychosocial Deprivation Syndrome)

Many reports have documented impairment of GH secretion apparently due to emotional factors.[10] This disorder, which occurs in children, is characterized by growth failure in the context of severe emotional deprivation. These children have deficient GH release in response to stimuli such as insulin-induced hypoglycemia or arginine infusion and, in a smaller proportion, deficiency in release of ACTH and gonadotropins. This disorder is rapidly reversed by placing a child in a supportive hospital milieu; growth and neuroendocrine GH responses return rapidly. Excessive β-adrenergic inhibitory effects may be one of the causative factors in the syndrome. In one such patient, normal GH secretion could be restored immediately by acute treatment with propranolol. If confirmed, this observation has important implications in the understanding of the physiologic significance of adrenergic systems in the control of GH secretion. It is important in each individual case to exclude malnutrition as a causative or contributory factor to poor growth.

Hyposecretion in the Adult

In the adult, a deficiency of GH does not produce readily recognizable clinical symptoms or signs. Laboratory data are therefore essential. Decreased basal levels of GH may accompany any hypothalamic-pituitary lesion. Of more importance is the recognition that neuroendocrine reflexes for GH release may be lost in patients with widely differing intracranial disorders, and such loss may be an early sign of disturbance of the hypothalamic-pituitary axis. For example, following cranial radiation, GH hyposecretion is the first and almost always the only pituitary deficit.

Hypersecretion

Gigantism and Acromegaly

Hypersecretion of GH in childhood results in gigantism, and in adults, acromegaly. In addition, GH levels may be above the normal range, unaccompanied by clinical signs of hypersomatotropism, in a number of other conditions, many of which appear in the context of nutritional deficiencies of one kind or another. It has long been recognized that excessive GH secretion from pituitary tumors is the cause of acromegaly and gigantism in the majority of cases. In cases with normal pituitary fossae on roentgenography, undoubtedly some have small adenomas; in a few, there may be only hyperplasia of the growth hormone-producing cells. The true incidence of microadenomas as opposed to hyperplasia as the cause of acromegaly is unknown; most patients with normal appearing fossae and normal pneumoencephalograms, now recognized early because of the availability of immunoassay methods for GH detection, are treated nonsurgically. Although the tinctorial properties of the GH-secreting adenomas have classically been viewed as acidophilic, many are chromophobic by conventional stains. Recent histochemical staining methods, as used for example by Zimmerman and colleagues,[64] indicate a high degree of correlation between GH hypersecretion as determined by blood hormone measurements, and GH staining in the adenoma regardless of its conventional tinctorial properties. Only three of eight cases in their series had eosinophilia, but all stained with the antibody technique.

It is now recognized that the signs and symptoms of GH hypersecretion, accompanied by elevated plasma GH levels, may precede the clinical appearance of pituitary adenoma. On the basis of cases of this type it has been postulated that acromegaly might be of hypothalamic origin. The suggestion that the primary disturbance in these cases is at the hypothalamic level, due to increased or inappropriate secretion of GRF, or alternatively to somatostatin deficiency, has been echoed by many workers. It has been proposed further that some or all cases with established adenomas may have been caused by sustained hypothalamic dysfunction. Several lines of evidence support this contention. Episodic release of GH, such as is found in normal subjects, may persist in acromegalics, suggesting that secretory bursts of GH release, presumably driven by GRF, still occur. In addition, although plasma GH levels are elevated, most patients continue to show some response to the stimuli which usually affect GH release. Thus, glucose may depress plasma GH levels, and hypoglycemia and arginine infusion may cause further elevation. These results indicate that in acromegaly, pituitary secretion of GH is not entirely autonomous but is still influenced by factors which are known to act at a hypothalamic level.

Evidence for a direct hypothalamic role in some instances of GH hypersecretion has been provided in cases of primary hypothalamic involvement. There have been several cases of hypothalamic tumors in which GH levels are elevated. In one of these, a child with an optic glioma and assumed anterior hypothalamic compression had markedly elevated GH levels.[38] Increased plasma GH levels are commonly found in the "diencephalic syndrome" of early infancy, a condition characterized clinically by malnutrition and emaciation and almost invariably associated with anterior hypothalamic gliomas.

Such anterior hypothalamic lesions could alter normal inhibitory mechanisms for GH control, perhaps through disruption of somatostatin release from the preoptic area.

Two reports give direct support to the hypothesis of excessive GRF secretion. In both instances, a material with GH-releasing activity in vitro was shown to be present in the peripheral plasma of acromegalics.[37] An error in GH or somatomedin feedback has been suggested as the primary disturbance in such cases.

On the other hand, acromegalic patients show a number of aberrant or "paradoxic" regulatory responses, indicating that GH hypersecretion is not due simply to a "reset" of the normal feedback control mechanism, as has been established, say, for Cushing's disease. Inhibition by glucose administration is only partial in most acromegalics; it may not occur at all; and in as many as 15 to 20 per cent, there may be a paradoxic *increase* in GH levels. Other paradoxic effects include a fall in plasma GH after administration of L-dopa or apomorphine,[35] and hypersecretion of GH after the administration of TRH.[17] These effects suggest that altered hypothalamic control of GRF (or somatostatin) may be of pathophysiologic significance in acromegaly.

Since α-adrenergic stimulation is normally stimulatory for GH control and β-stimulation is inhibitory, it is of interest to speculate whether these receptors might be abnormal in acromegaly. In a study of 10 acromegalic subjects, Cryer and Daughaday[13] found a significant decline in GH after α-adrenergic blockade induced by phentolamine infusion. A further fall was induced by combining isoproteronol (a β-receptor agonist) with phentolamine. In these same subjects, L-dopa (500 mg., p.o.) produced a comparable decline in GH. Variation in response led the authors to suggest that acromegaly may represent a homogeneous disorder and that patients with the disease may be divided into responders and nonresponders.

These observations have resulted in a great deal of current interest with respect to the possibility that dopaminergic drugs may find use in acromegaly. At present, bromergocryptine, which has long-acting dopaminergic effects, is being investigated in several centers[34, 35] (see Chapter 15) and the early results are encouraging. Responders appear to have a sustained inhibitory effect after several months of administration of bromergocryptine. Administration of pimozide, an α-dopamine blocking agent, is effective in counteracting the suppression of GH induced by bromergocryptine, pointing to mediation of the effect by dopamine receptors.

The main argument against the primary-hypothalamic-abnormality hypothesis comes from the detailed study of individual cases treated by resection of small adenomas. An illustrative case has been reported by Hoyte and Martin.[27] In their studies, removal of a microadenoma was followed by restoration of normal regulatory responses. Treatment by roentgenotherapy or heavy particles, though it may reduce baseline levels of GH, nevertheless usually leads to a retention of the abnormal and paradoxic responses. It has also been shown that in some acromegalics GH circulates in an abnormal form that is immunologically active but biologically less active. It is not known whether this is due to abnormal secretion by a neoplasm or to hypersecretion of normal cells with premature delivery of a prohormone form, as has been shown to occur normally in the rat. Further evidence that the primary lesion in acromegaly is an intrinsic lesion of the pituitary is the finding of mixed prolactin and GH secreting tumors. In the series of Zimmerman and collaborators,[64] four of eight patients had prolactin-containing as well as GH-containing cells in their pituitaries. It is unlikely that hypersecretion of a GRF could cause prolactin cell stimulation as well. Finally, in experimental pituitary tumors, it has been shown repeatedly that treatment of the rat with estrogens in high dosage induces GH-secreting tumors that also secrete large amounts of prolactin. In these animals, the primary lesion does in fact appear to lie in the pituitary, although an effect of estrogens on hypophysiotrophic-hormone secretion cannot be excluded.

The most reasonable hypothesis to explain these findings is that acromegaly arises as a neoplastic change in the pituitary, but the adenoma retains to a degree its dependence on normal GH-secretory-controlling hormones. The significance of GRF-like materials in acromegalic plasma or spinal fluid remains a matter for continuing study.

Several attempts at medical treatment of acromegaly have been based on the hypothesis that GRF suppression may reduce GH secretion. In early reports, chlorpromazine was said to lower GH levels in acromegaly, both acutely after a single administration and chronically after several months of treatment. However, subsequent studies have failed to confirm this initial observation.

Elevated Growth Hormone Levels Unrelated to Acromegaly

Increased basal GH levels have now been described in several conditions in addition to acromegaly which have in common a disturbance in nutrition. Thus, elevations in GH have been reported in anorexia nervosa, starvation, kwashiorkor, renal failure, mucoviscidosis, and hepatic cirrhosis.[38] The most likely mechanism of this effect is a secondary deficiency of somatomedin (postulated to be the functional link between GH and feedback control).

Anorexia Nervosa

In a significant percentage of cases of anorexia nervosa, GH levels are markedly elevated, as they are in a number of other states of starvation or malnutrition. We have observed levels as high as 50 to 70 ng./ml. The elevation in GH correlates closely with the degree of malnutrition. Recently, Garfinkel and coworkers[68] have shown that the GH elevation is related directly to deficient caloric intake. Refeeding rapidly led to normalization of plasma GH levels and of GH responses. The disturbance in GH is distinct from the alteration in menstrual function. The gonadotropin deficiency is more closely related to reduction in body weight and is usually only reversed after increase in body weight occurs (see Chapter 5). The possibility has not been excluded, however, that the disorder in food intake might be due in part to abnormalities in adrenergic control of appetite mechanisms. Concurrent anomalies of adrenergic control of GH might also be present.

Paradoxic Release

In many clinical conditions associated with GH hypersecretion, the responses of GH to provocative stimuli are, on occasion, paradoxic. Thus there is a rise, rather than the expected fall, in plasma GH levels after glucose administration, or suppression after administration of dopaminergic agents. Such paradoxic responses occur normally in the neonatal period. It is commonly noted in acromegaly (see above), and was present in a child with an optic glioma. Paradoxic GH responses to glucose have also been described in renal failure, breast carcinoma, anorexia nervosa, and Turner's syndrome. Paradoxic responses in Huntington's chorea, Wilson's disease, and acute intermittent porphyria suggest that neuroendocrine abnormalities may exist in such cases. The mechanism of these effects is unknown.

Non-GH-Related Growth

A number of clinical instances have been described in which a normal or exaggerated growth pattern occcurs in the absence of elevated radioimmunoassayable GH levels. Intrauterine and early prenatal growth do not require GH. Cerebral gigantism, a condition associated with an increased growth rate in early childhood, mental retardation, and cerebral ventricular dilatation, is not accompanied by measurable elevation in plasma GH levels. Studies to determine whether the total 24-hour secretion of GH may be elevated in such cases have not yet been reported. A similarly perplexing group of disorders are the postoperative hypothalamic or pituitary tumor cases which often show remarkable "catch-up" growth in the absence of measurable GH in plasma. These observations raise the possibility that a biologically active but immunologically inactive material may be present in such cases, or that other hormones such as prolactin may have a growth-stimulating effect. A recent report suggests that somatomedin is detectable in the plasma of such patients. The reverse situation has now been described in some dwarfs in whom elevated plasma levels of immunoassayable GH fail to stimulate normal growth. In such cases, the primary abnormality appears to be an inability to generate somatomedin.[14]

Abnormalities of Nocturnal Release

Growth hormone release during the first 90 minutes of nocturnal sleep is sufficiently reproducible in normal subjects to be useful as a physiologic test for pituitary GH reserve. A number of conditions have now been described in which such release is absent or diminished. Elevation of GH levels, either endogenously as in acromegaly or following exogenous GH administration, prevents nocturnal GH release. Cushing's disease (bilateral adrenal hyperplasia) or chronic steroid administration also is reported to block sleep-related GH secretion, whereas acute steroid administration has no effect. Interestingly, the disturbance in Cushing's disease may persist for months following effective treatment. The recovery of nocturnal GH responses appears to precede the return of GH release in response to other provocative stimuli. Other metabolic factors which suppress nocturnal GH release include elevated plasma free fatty acid levels and obesity.

Several central nervous system disorders have been described in which SWS-related GH release is abnormal. Blindness, whether congenital or acquired, is associated with lack of nocturnal GH responses, a disturbance which was found to correlate with the decrease in percentage of time spent in the third and fourth stages of sleep. Narcoleptics, who have a sleep disorder typified by direct transition from waking to REM sleep without an intervening period of SWS, have been noted in a single report to lack GH release during sleep (see above).

Pharmacologic blockade of SWS-related GH release has been reported after administration of both imipramine, a tricyclic antidepressant that blocks postsynaptic uptake of both norepinephrine and serotonin, and medroxyprogesterone. The site of action of the latter is unknown. The magnitude of the SWS-induced GH response appears to decrease with advancing age and it is frequently absent in normal subjects beyond age 50.

MANAGEMENT OF PATIENTS WITH ABNORMAL GROWTH HORMONE SECRETION

Hyposecretion During Growth: Pituitary Dwarfism

Growth failure due to GH deficiency may be apparent as early as 6 months, but is usually not diagnosed until age 1 to 3 years when the child is observed to fall behind his peers in body size. After demonstration of GH deficiency by failure of GH responses to two or more provocative stimuli (see Chapter 14), treatment with GH is begun. The usual protocol consists of administration of purified human GH, 2 to 3 mg. twice weekly. Responses are detectable within a few weeks. Increases in height of 4 to 6 inches are often achieved within the first year. Treatment is continued until a satisfactory height is achieved or until no further effects are observable. Detailed methods of treatment and evaluation of deficiency can be found in *Advances in Human Growth Hormone Research,* edited by S. Raiti and published by the Department of Health, Education and Welfare (publication no. NIH74-612).

Hyposecretion in the Adult

No definitive or diagnostic symptoms or signs are attributable to GH deficiency in the adult. There has been some speculation that a degree of the lassitude and lethargy of panhypopituitarism may be due to GH deficiency. However, proof of this is lacking, and most patients show near-normal recovery after replacement with thyroid hormones and cortisol.

Hypersecretion: Acromegaly and Gigantism

The management of patients with GH excess has evolved considerably since the advent of transsphenoidal hypophysectomy. The choice of treatment in a given patient depends upon several factors including age, size of tumor, general medical condition, neurologic manifestations, need for preservation of other pituitary hormone functions, and the local availability of specialized radiotherapeutic and neurosurgical facilities. These are detailed in Chapter 15, on management of pituitary tumors.

Hypersecretion in Diabetes Mellitus

A majority of patients with diabetes show hyper-responsiveness of GH release to stimuli such as exercise, and this response is blocked by phentolamine. Careful clinical control of the diabetic reduces this excessive GH responsivity. Further characterization of this anomaly might be important, as GH has been implicated (although a role for it is not proven) in the vascular complications arising in diabetes. The use of hypophysectomy in severe diabetics with retinopathy has generally been attributed to removal of GH effects.

REFERENCES

1. ABRAMS, R. L., GRUMBACH, M. M. AND KAPLAN, S. L.: *The effect of administration of human growth hormone on the plasma growth hormone, cortisol, glucose, and free fatty acid response to insulin: Evidence for growth hormone autoregulation in man.* J. Clin. Invest. 50:940, 1971.

2. ADEY, W. R.: *Intensive organization of cerebral tissue in alert, orienting and discriminative response. In* Quarton, G. C., Melnechuk, T. and Schmitt, F. O. (eds.): *The Neurosciences—A Study Program.* Rockefeller University Press, New York, 1967, p. 615.

3. ALFORD, F. P., BAKER, H. W. AND BURGER, H. G.: *The secretion rate of human growth hormone. I. Daily secretion rates, effect of posture and sleep.* J. Clin. Endocrinol. Metab. 37:515, 1973.

4. ARIMURA, A., ET AL.: *Somatostatin: Abundance of immunoreactive hormone in rat stomach and pancreas.* Science 189:1007, 1975.

5. BESSER, G. M., ET AL.: *Long-term infusion of growth hormone release inhibiting hormone in acromegaly: Effects on pituitary and pancreatic hormones.* Br. Med. J. 4:622, 1974.

6. BIVENS, C. H., LEBOVITZ, H. E. AND FELDMAN, J. M.: *Inhibition of hypoglycemia-induced growth hormone secretion by the serotonin antagonists cyproheptadine and methysergide.* N Engl. J. Med. 289: 236, 1973.

7. BOYD, A. E., LEBOVITZ, H. E. AND PFEIFFER, J. B.: *Stimulation of human-growth-hormone secretion by L-DOPA.* N. Engl. J. Med. 283:1425, 1970.

8. BOYD, C., PATEL, Y. AND REICHLIN, S.: Unpublished study, 1975.

9. BRAZEAU, P., ET AL.: *Hypothalamic polypeptide that inhibits the secretion of immunoreactive pituitary growth hormone*. Science 179:77, 1973.

10. BROWN, G. M. AND REICHLIN, S.: *Psychologic and neural regulation of growth hormone secretion*. Psychosom. Med. 34:45, 1972.

11. BROWN, G. M., SCHALCH, D. S. AND REICHLIN, S.: *Hypothalamic mediation of growth hormone and adrenal stress response in the squirrel monkey*. Endocrinology 89:694, 1971.

12. BROWNSTEIN, M., ET AL.: *The regional distribution of somatostatin in the rat brain*. Endocrinology 96: 1456, 1975.

13. CRYER, P. E. AND DAUGHADAY, W. H.: *Adrenergic modulation of growth hormone secretion in acromegaly: Suppression during phentolamine and phentoxamine-isoproterenol administration*. J. Clin. Endocrinol. Metab. 39:658, 1974.

14. DAUGHADAY, W. H., HERINGTON, A. C. AND PHILLIPS, L. S.: *The regulation of growth by endocrines*. Annu. Rev. Physiol. 37:211, 1975.

15. DEVANE, G. W., SILER, T. M. AND YEN, S. S. C.: *Acute suppression of insulin and glucose levels by synthetic somatostatin in normal human subjects*. J. Clin. Endocrinol. Metab. 38:913, 1974.

16. DOBBS, R., ET AL.: *Glucagon: role in the hyperglycemia of diabetes mellitus*. Science 187:544, 1975.

17. FAGLIA, G., ET AL.: *Plasma growth hormone response to thyrotropin-releasing hormone in patients with active acromegaly*. J. Clin. Endocrinol. Metab. 36:1259, 1973.

18. FINKLESTEIN, J. W., ET AL.: *Age-related change in the twenty-four-hour spontaneous secretion of growth hormone*. J. Clin. Endocrinol. Metab. 35:665, 1972.

19. FROHMAN, L. A. AND BERNARDIS, L. L.: *Growth hormone and insulin levels in weanling rats with ventromedial hypothalamic lesions*. Endocrinology 82:1125, 1968.

20. FROHMAN, L. A., BERNARDIS, L. L. AND KANT, K. J.: *Hypothalamic stimulation of growth hormone secretion*. Science 162:580, 1968.

21. GERICH, J. E., ET AL.: *Effects of somatostatin on plasma glucose and glucagon levels in human diabetes mellitus. Pathophysiologic and therapeutic implications*. N. Engl. J. Med. 291:544, 1974.

22. GIUSTINA, G., ET AL.: *Failure of somatostatin to suppress thyrotropin releasing factor and luteinizing hormone releasing factor-induced growth hormone release in acromegaly*. J. Clin. Endocrinol. Metab. 38: 906, 1974.

23. GOLD, R. M.: *Hypothalamic obesity: The myth of the ventromedial nucleus*. Science 182:488, 1973.

24. GOLDSMITH, S. J. AND GLICK, S. M.: *Rhythmlcity of human growth hormone secretion*. Mt. Sinai J. Med. N.Y. 37:501, 1970.

25. HEIDINGSFELDER, S. A. AND BLACKARD, W. G.: *Adrenergic control mechanism for vasopressin-induced plasma growth hormone response*. Metabolism 17:1019, 1968.

26. HIMSWORTH, R. L., CARMEL, P. W. AND FRANTZ, A. G.: *The location of the chemoreceptor controlling growth hormone secretion during hypoglycemia in primates*. Endocrinology 91:217, 1972.

27. HOYTE, K. M. AND MARTIN, J. B.: *Recovery from paradoxical growth hormone responses in acromegaly after transsphenoidal selective adenonectomy*. J. Clin. Endocrinol. Metab. 41:656, 1975.

28. IMURA, H., NAKAI, Y. AND YOSHIMI, T.: *Effect of 5-hydroxytryptophan (5-HTP) on growth hormone and ACTH release in man*. J. Clin. Endocrinol. Metab. 36:204, 1973.

29. KOERKER, D. J., GOODNER, C. J. AND RUCH, W.: *Somatostatin action on pancreas*. N. Engl. J. Med. 291:262, 1974.

30. KRIEGER, D. T. AND GEWIRTZ, G. P.: *Recovery of hypothalamic-pituitary-adrenal function, growth hormone responsiveness and sleep EEG pattern in a patient following removal of an adrenal cortical adenoma*. J. Clin. Endocrinol. Metab. 38:1075, 1974.

31. KRULICH, L., ET AL.: *Dual hypothalamic regulation of growth hormone secretion*. *In* Pecile, A. and Muller, E. E. (eds.): *Growth and Growth Hormone*. Excerpta Medica Foundation, Amsterdam, 1972, p. 306.

32. LAL, S., ET AL.: *Comparison of the effect of apomorphine and L-DOPA on serum growth hormone levels in normal men*. Clin. Endocrinol. (Oxf.) 4:277, 1975.

33. LAL, S., ET AL.: *Effect of clonidine on growth hormone, prolactin, luteinizing hormone, follicle-stimulating hormone, and thyroid-stimulating hormone in the serum of normal men*. J. Clin. Endocrinol. Metab. 41:827, 1975.

34. LIUZZI, A., ET AL.: *Decreased plasma growth hormone (GH) levels in acromegalies following CB 154 (2-Br-alpha-ergocryptine) administration*. J. Clin. Endocrinol. Metab. 38:910, 1974.

35. LIUZZI, A., ET AL.: *Growth Hormone (GH)-releasing activity of TRH and GH-lowering effect of dopamine drugs in acromegaly: Homogeneity in the two responses*. J. Clin. Endocrinol. Metab. 39:871, 1974.

36. MALACARA, J. M., VALVERDE, C. AND REICHLIN, S.: *Elevation of plasma radioimmunoassayable growth hormone in the rat induced by porcine hypothalamic extract.* Endocrinology 91:1189, 1972.

37. MARTIN, J. B.: *Plasma growth hormone (GH) response to hypothalamic or extrahypothalamic electrical stimulation.* Endocrinology 91:107, 1972.

38. MARTIN, J. B.: *Neural regulation of growth hormone secretion. Medical Progress Report.* New Engl. J. Med. 228:1384, 1973.

39. MARTIN, J. B.: *The role of hypothalamic and extrahypothalamic structures in the control of GH secretion. In* Raiti, S. (ed.): *Advances in Human Growth Hormone Research.* DHEW publication no. (NIH)74-612, Washington, D.C., 1974.

40. MARTIN, J. B.: *Brain regulation of growth hormone secretion. In* Martini, L. and Ganong, W. F. (eds.): *Frontiers in Neuroendocrinology,* vol. 4. Raven Press, New York, 1976 p. 129.

41. MARTIN, J. B., KONTOR, J. AND MEAD, P.: *Plasma GH responses to hypothalamic, hippocampal and amygdaloid electrical stimulation: Effects of variation in stimulus parameters and treatment with α-methyl-p-tyrosine (α-MT).* Endocrinology 92:1354, 1973.

42. MARTIN, J. B., RENAUD, L. P. AND BRAZEAU, P., JR.: *Pulsatile growth hormone secretion: Suppression by hypothalamic ventromedial lesions and by long-acting somatostatin.* Science 186:538, 1974.

43. MARTIN, J. B., WILLOUGHBY, J. O. AND TANNENBAUM, G. S.: *Evidence for an intrinsic central nervous system rhythm governing episodic GH secretion in the rat.* Proceedings 57th Annual Meeting Endocrine Society, 1975b, p. 254.

44. MOGENSON C. J. AND HUANG, Y. H.: *The neurobiology of motivated behaviour. In* Kerkut, G. A. and Phillis, J. H. (eds.): *Progress in Neurobiology.* Pergamon Press, Oxford, 1973, p. 53.

45. PARKER, D. C. AND ROSSMAN, L. G.: *Human growth hormone release in sleep: nonsuppression by acute hyperglycemia.* J. Clin. Endocrinol. Metab. 32:65, 1971.

46. PARKER, D. C., ET AL.: *Inhibition of the sleep-related peak in physiologic human growth hormone release by somatostatin.* J. Clin. Endocrinol. Metab. 38:496, 1974.

47. PATEL, Y. C., WEIR, G. C. AND REICHLIN, S.: *Anatomic distribution of somatostatin (SRIF) in brain and pancreatic islets as studied by radioimmunoassay (RIA).* Proceedings 57th Annual Meeting Endocrine Society, 1975, p. 154.

48. REICHLIN, S.: *Regulation of somatotrophic hormone secretion. In* Harris, G. W. and Donovan, B. T. (eds.): *The Pituitary Gland.* Butterworth, London, 1966, p. 270.

49. REICHLIN, S.: *Regulation of somatotrophic hormone secretion. In* Greep, R. O. and Astwood, E. B. (eds.): *Handbook of Physiology, Section 7: Endocrinology,* vol. 4, part 2. American Physiological Society. Williams & Wilkins, Baltimore, 1975, p. 405.

50. RENAUD, L. P., MARTIN, J. B. AND BRAZEAU, P.: *Depressant action of TRH, LH-RH and somatostatin on activity of central neurones.* Nature, 255:233, 1975.

51. RUCH, W., ET AL.: *Studies on somatostatin (somatotropin release inhibiting factor) in conscious baboons. In* Raiti, S. (ed.): *Advances in Human Growth Hormone Research.* DHEW publication no. (NIH)74-612, Washington, D.C. 1974.

52. SACHAR, E. J., et al.: *Growth hormone response to L-dopa in depressed patients.* Science 178:1304, 1972.

53. SCHALCH, D. S. AND REICHLIN, S.: *Stress and growth hormone release. In* Pecile, A. and Muller, E. E. (eds.): *Growth Hormone.* Excerpta Medica Foundation, Amsterdam, 1968, p. 211.

54. SCHALLY, A. V., ARIMURA, A. AND KASTIN, A. J.: *Hypothalamic regulatory hormones: At least nine substances from the hypothalamus control the secretion of pituitary hormones.* Science 179:341, 1973.

55. SILER, T. M., VANDENBERG, G. AND YEN. S. S. C.: *Inhibition of growth hormone release in humans by somatostatin.* J. Clin. Endocrinol. Metab. 37:632, 1973.

56. TAKAHASHI, Y., KIPNIS, D. M. AND DAUGHADAY, W. H.: *Growth hormone secretion during sleep.* J. Clin. Invest. 47:2079, 1968.

57. TANNENBAUM, G. S., MARTIN. J. B. AND COLLE, E.: *Evidence for an endogenous ultradian rhythm governing growth hormone secretion in the rat.* Endocrinology 98:562, 1976.

58. TANNENBAUM, G., MARTIN, J. B. AND COLLE, E.: *Ultradian growth hormone rhythm in the rat: Effects of feeding, hyperglycemia and insulin-induced hypoglycemia.* Endocrinology 99:720, 1976.

59. TERRY, L. C., ET AL.: *Antiserum to somatostatin prevents stress-induced inhibition of growth hormone secretion in the rat.* Science 192:565, 1976.

60. TOIVOLA, P. T. K. AND GALE, C. C.: *Stimulation of growth release by microinjection of norepinephrine into hypothalamus of baboons.* Endocrinology 90:895, 1972.

61. WILLOUGHBY, J. O., ET AL.: *Pulsatile growth hormone release in the rat: failure to demonstrate a correlation with sleep phases.* Endocrinology 98:991, 1976.

62. Yen, S. S. C., Silver, T. M. and DeVane, G. W.: *Effect of somatostatin in patients with acromegaly. Suppression of growth hormone, prolactin, insulin and glucose levels.* N. Engl. J. Med. 290:935, 1974.

63. Zimmerman, E. A., et al.: *Vasopressin and neurophysin: High concentrations in monkey hypophyseal portal blood.* Science 182:925, 1973.

64. Zimmerman, E. A., Defendini, R. and Frantz, A. G.: *Prolactin and growth hormone in patients with pituitary adenomas: A correlative study of hormone in tumor and plasma by immunoperoxidase technique and radioimmunoassay.* J. Clin. Endocrinol. Metab. 38:577, 1974.

65. Martin, J. B., Renaud, L. P. and Brazeau, P.: *Hypothalamic peptides: New evidence for peptidergic pathways in the CNS.* Lancet 2:393, 1975.

66. Chambers, J. W. and Brown, G. M.: *Stimulation of rhesus monkey GH release: arginine versus plasma volume expansion.* J. Clin. Endocrinol. Metab. 42:169, 1976.

67. Chambers, J. W. and Brown, G. M.: *Neurotransmitter regulation of growth hormone and ACTH in the rhesus monkey: Effects of biogenic amines.* Endocrinology 98:420, 1976.

68. Garfinkel, P. E., et. al.: *Hypothalamic-pituitary function in anorexia nervosa.* Arch. Gen. Psychiatry 32:739, 1975.

BIBLIOGRAPHY

Brown, G. M. and Reichlin, S.: *Psychologic and neural regulation of growth hormone secretion.* Psychosom. Med. 34:45, 1972.

Daughaday, W. H., Herington, A. C. and Phillips, L. S.: *The regulation of growth by endocrines.* Annu. Rev. Physiol. 37:211, 1975.

Martin, J. B.: *Neural regulation of growth hormone secretion. Medical progress report.* N. Engl. J. Med. 288:1384, 1973.

Martin, J. B.: *Brain regulation of growth hormone secretion. In* Martini, L. and Ganong, W. F. (eds.): *Frontiers in Neuroendocrinology,* vol. 4. Raven Press, New York, 1976, p. 129.

Muller, E. E.: *Nervous control of growth hormone secretion.* Neuroendocrinology 11:338, 1973.

Reichlin, S.: *Regulation of somatrophic hormone secretion. In* Harris, G. W. and Donovan, B. T. (eds.): *The Pituitary Gland.* Butterworth, London, 1966, p. 270.

Reichlin, S.: *Regulation of somatotrophic hormone secretion. In* Greep, R. O. and Astwood, E. B. (eds.): *Handbook of Physiology, Section 7: Endocrinology,* vol. 4, part 2. American Physiological Society. Williams & Wilkins, Baltimore, 1975, p. 405.

Raiti, S. (ed.): *Advances in Human Growth Hormone Research.* DHEW publication no. (NIH)74-612, 1974.

CHAPTER 8

Regulation of ACTH Secretion and Its Disorders

A quarter of a century has passed since hypothalamic control of the pituitary-adrenal axis was recognized. This regulation is essential for the characteristic changes in secretion of glucocorticoids in phase with the daily-activity cycle, and the increased output that occurs during emergencies. Moreover, neural control is responsible for the specific pattern of secretion in sleep.

Although the adrenal and pituitary hormones have long since been identified, the nature of the hypothalamic factor(s) involved in pituitary-adrenal regulation remains elusive. The availability of sensitive assay procedures for the pituitary and adrenal hormones however, has led to a detailed understanding of many aspects of neural control of the hypothalamic-pituitary-adrenal system (Fig. 1).

HORMONES INVOLVED IN PITUITARY-ADRENAL REGULATION

Corticotropin-Releasing Factor

Although corticotropin-releasing factor (CRF) was the first releasing factor recognized, its identity is still unknown.[8, 54, 55] CRF activity, measured in the hypothalamus, is at least partly granule-bound in nerve endings, shows diurnal variation, and increases in response to stress. ADH was once thought to be CRF because under certain conditions it can cause release of ACTH.[8, 31] It now appears that ADH is not CRF, since humans or animals with diabetes insipidus lack ADH but can release ACTH in response to stress.

Adrenocorticotropic Hormone

The secretion of the cortex of the adrenal gland is largely governed by circulating adrenocorticotropic hormone (ACTH) from the anterior lobe of the pituitary gland. ACTH is the primary regulator of glucocorticoid and sex-hormone secretion by the adrenal cortex.[27]

Human ACTH is a basic 39-residue peptide that differs in structure from that of other known species by only three amino acids (Fig. 2). The N-terminal sequence of ACTH (residues 1–19) has nearly full steroidogenic activity, while smaller peptide fragments require concentrations several orders of magnitude greater. Synthetic ACTH 1–24, widely available for clinical testing, is highly active. Alpha-melanotropin (α-melanocyte-stimulating hormone, α-MSH) is a peptide consisting of 13 amino acids

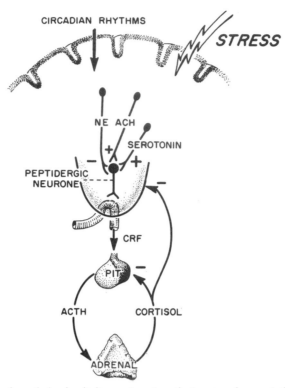

Figure 1. Elements of the hypothalamic-pituitary-adrenal cortical system for regulation of cortisol secretion. Secretion of adrenocorticotropic hormone (ACTH) is stimulated by corticotropin releasing factor (CRF) and inhibited at the pituitary level by cortisol. The secretion of CRF is regulated by a complex set of neurotransmitter neurons which include two stimulatory components (cholinergic and serotonergic), and an adrenergic inhibitory pathway. These pathways mediate stress-induced and circadian ACTH secretory changes. Feedback effects of cortisol may be exerted on the nervous system as well as on the pituitary. *Abbreviations:* NE, norepinephrine; ACH, acetylcholine.

with N-terminal acylserine and C-terminal valineamide, which is identical to the 1–13 sequence of ACTH. A peptide that appears to be ACTH 18–39 has been isolated from an MSH-producing human tumor as well as from other species.

It has been suggested that α-MSH and this peptide are produced from ACTH by proteolysis. It has also been suggested that ACTH itself is synthesized from a larger peptide. A 20,000-dalton precursor found in both plasma and pituitary can be converted by trypsin to an immunoreactive form having ACTH-like characteristics. Together these findings suggest that biosynthesis of α-MSH occurs in the order: procorticotropin → corticotropin → α-MSH, although biosynthesis studies are still required to establish these relationships. β-MSH and other lipotropins (LPH) are structurally related to ACTH and α-MSH, as all contain an identical seven-amino-acid sequence. The entire structure of β-MSH occurs within that of β-LPH, suggesting that β-LPH may be the precursor of β-MSH. The roles of α-MSH, β-MSH, and the lipotropins in human physiology and pathology remain to be established. Most studies indicate that α-MSH secretion parallels that of ACTH in man, and α-MSH may be produced in the same pituitary cells as ACTH or may be a breakdown product of ACTH secreted from the pituitary.

The half-life of ACTH in blood after a "bolus" injection is short (about 10 minutes) and effects on adrenal function are transient. To elicit a prolonged effect, frequent IV

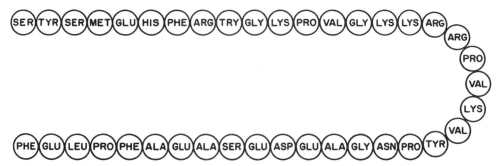

Figure 2. Structure of ACTH. ACTH is a linear peptide, 39 amino acids in length. Counting from the free amino end (SER), biologic activity requires a chain 13 amino acids long and full biologic activity is reached with 20 amino acids. Synthetic ACTH 1–24 is available for clinical use. Segments 1 to 13 of ACTH bear close resemblance to the peptide hormones α- and β-MSH.

injections, IV infusion, or the administration of long-acting, slowly absorbable forms is necessary. In response to severe stress, ACTH concentration in blood is often well above the amount necessary to produce maximal glucocorticoid output. This maximum secretion of glucocorticoids occurs with relatively low doses of intravenously administered ACTH. These observations indicate a "ceiling" rate of glucocorticoid secretory response to ACTH.[55] ACTH stimulation of the adrenal cortex is necessary for maintainance of the responsiveness of the gland to subsequent exposure to ACTH. In patients with hypopituitarism, several hours or days of treatment with ACTH are necessary before steroid output returns to normal. Conversely, prolonged exposure to high ACTH increases the responsiveness of the adrenal cortex to a given dose of ACTH, so that in Cushing's disease due to hypersecretion of ACTH adrenocorticoid response to exogenously administered ACTH is increased. ACTH is necessary for normal structural integrity of the inner two zones of the adrenal cortex, the zona fasciculata and zona reticularis, the primary zones that secrete glucocorticoids and sex steroids, respectively.

ACTH is one of many hormones known to act through the mediation of cyclic 3',5'-adenosine monophosphate (cyclic AMP). ACTH binds to specific receptor sites on the surface of the membrane of sensitive adrenocortical cells and activates the enzyme adenyl cyclase that converts adenosine triphosphate to cyclic AMP.

A sensitive radioimmunoassay and, more recently, an even more sensitive "redox" assay, have become available for examining plasma ACTH levels in a variety of conditions. Resting morning plasma levels of ACTH are in the range of 0.1 to 1.0 mU./100 ml. (10 to 100 pg./ml.) while evening levels are only one tenth of these values.[53] After stress, levels of ACTH may increase tenfold.

Adrenal Hormones

The principal hormones of the adrenal cortex are of three classes: *glucocorticoids, mineralocorticoids,* and *androcorticoids* (Figs. 3 and 4).[27, 29, 54] The principal natural glucocorticoid in man is *cortisol* (hydrocortisone), the archetypical glucocorticoid. Cortisol is largely responsible for the clinical manifestations of Cushing's syndrome and its actions include effects on metabolism of carbohydrate, fat, and protein. Cortisol also has weak mineralocorticoid activity (defined as promoting potassium excretion and sodium retention), and weak androcorticoid activity (defined as causing masculinizing effects). The principal mineralocorticoid in humans is *aldosterone,* more than two hundred times as active as cortisol in promoting sodium retention, and the principal androcorticoids are *androsterone* and *androstenedione.* The latter compounds, though

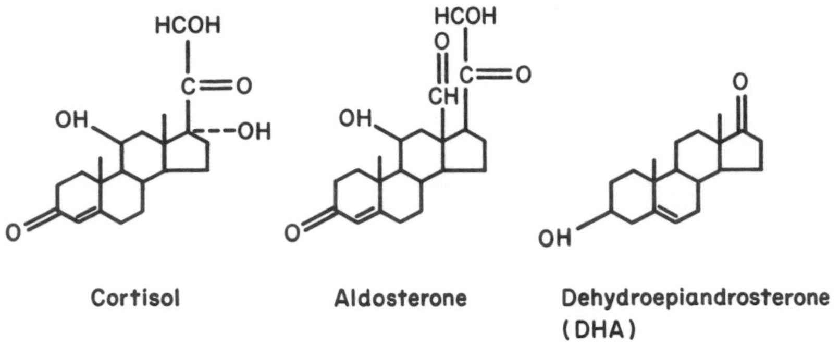

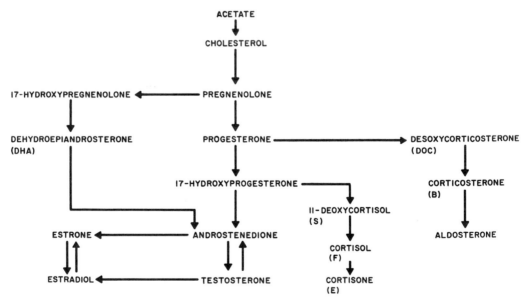

Cortisol   **Aldosterone**   **Dehydroepiandrosterone**
                                       (DHA)

Figure 3. Structures of major adrenal steroid hormones. The three principal classes of adrenal steroids are the glucocorticoids of which cortisol is the most important, mineralocorticoids of which aldosterone is the most important, and androgenic hormones of which dehydroepiandrosterone (DHA) is the most important; small amounts of dehydroisoandrosterone, Δ^4-adrostenedione and testosterone are also secreted. Trace amounts of 17β-estradiol are also synthesized. In pathologic states, the various androgenic and estrogenic hormones may be secreted in excess.

far more androgenic than cortisol, are extremely weak compared with testosterone. As a consequence, masculinization due to androcorticoids is accompanied by high rates of excretion of the principal metabolites as 17-ketosteroids.

The secretion of cortisol, androsterone, and androstenedione is under moment-to-moment control by ACTH.[27, 29] On the other hand, although aldosterone release may be triggered by ACTH administration and continued aldosterone secretion requires a certain level of ACTH secretion, the principal regulating factor for aldosterone is the renin-angiotensin system (see Chapter 4).

Figure 4. Diagram of major biosynthetic pathways for adrenal steroidogenesis. These pathways are mediated by specific enzymes localized either to the cytosol or the mitochondria. Congenital deficiency of specific enzymes leads to underproduction of certain steroids and may give rise to deficiency of aldosterone or cortisol. Loss of cortisol synthesis leads to overproduction of other steroids due to activation of ACTH production by the negative-feedback loop. Drugs also can interfere with biosynthesis of adrenal hormones. Metyrapone, used for the diagnosis of pituitary-adrenal insufficiency, blocks the formation of cortisol from 11-deoxycortisol, leading to an increase in the secretion of this compound.

182

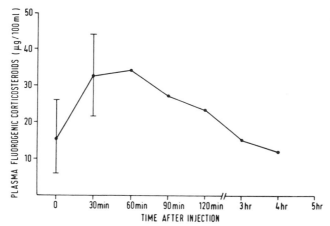

Figure 5. Effect of an intramuscular injection of synthetic ACTH 1–24 on plasma cortisol levels in the human. Results shown are means and ranges in 45 patients and 5 normals. (From Irvine, W. J. and Barnes, E. W.: *Adrenocortical insufficiency. In* Mason, A. S. (ed.): *Clinics in Endocrinology and Metabolism,* vol. 1. W. B. Saunders Co. Ltd., London, 1972, p. 562, with permission.)

The glucocorticoid response to a pulse of ACTH begins rapidly, the earliest change in peripheral blood being observed within three minutes. The blood level peaks at about ten minutes and then declines over a further ten minutes if the dose is small. With a larger dose IM, the peak response is prolonged and the decline more gradual (Fig. 5). The half-life of cortisol in blood is about 60 to 90 minutes.

Glucocorticoids circulate in blood in both bound and free forms. Under physiologic conditions, about 75 per cent of cortisol is bound to transcortin (cortisol-binding globulin), about 15 per cent to albumin, and only about 10 per cent is free. It is principally the free fraction that is available to cells. Transcortin levels are elevated in pregnancy and during treatment with estrogen, giving rise to increased total plasma cortisol levels; the concentration of free hormone remains constant. Contrariwise, transcortin levels may be low in liver disease, but free-hormone concentrations remain normal.

Steroids exert their biologic effects after passage into the cytosol of cells, where they bind to specific receptor proteins that have high affinity for the steroid hormone.[30] The steroid-receptor complex migrates into the nucleus, where it becomes attached to chromatin and acts to de-repress or activate genes. New RNA formed in response to this action controls the formation of new proteins some of which are enzymes that regulate cell function. Target tissues for a steroid contain cytoplasmic receptors for that steroid, while other tissues do not.

PITUITARY-ADRENAL RHYTHMS AND THE SLEEP-WAKE CYCLE

Glucocorticoid levels in plasma exhibit diurnal variation, with the highest levels at about 6 A.M. in an individual who sleeps from 11 P.M. to 7:30 A.M., and the lowest levels in late evening (Fig. 6).[2, 24, 52] Studies using indwelling cannulas and frequent sampling have shown that ACTH is secreted episodically for very brief periods of time and that cortisol secretion occurs within 5 to 10 minutes after the ACTH rise (Fig. 7). The latter half of the night's sleep is characterized largely by alternating REM (rapid-eye-movement) and Stage II sleep, while early sleep contains greater amounts of Stages III and IV. ACTH and cortisol secretory bursts occur predominately during the latter half of the sleep cycle. Secretory activity is not related to REM episodes. The rise in ACTH and cortisol occurs even when subjects are sleep-deprived; established patterns persist

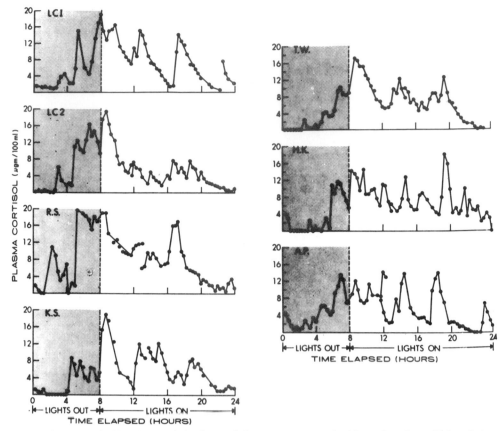

Figure 6. Plasma cortisol levels sampled at intervals in seven unstressed subjects. Levels are highest between 4 and 9 A.M., lowest around midnight, and fluctuate during the day without obvious relationship to external events. (From Weitzman, E. D., et al.: *Twenty-four hour pattern of the episodic secretion of cortisol in normal subjects.* J. Clin. Endocrinol. Metab. 33:14, 1971, with permission.)

with little change for several days when the sleep-wake cycle is phase-shifted. ACTH is secreted in bursts throughout the day, an average of 8 to 9 major secretory episodes occurring in a 24-hour period, even in the absence of stressful stimuli. Most normal persons secrete cortisol only 25 per cent of the time, to achieve normal secretion rates of about 16 mg. per day. The episodic release of ACTH is independent of circulating cortisol levels; the magnitude of an individual ACTH secretory episode bears no relation to preceding plasma cortisol levels. Moreover, the ACTH rhythm persists in patients with Addison's disease, in whom insufficient adrenal glucocorticoids are released. In such patients, baseline ACTH levels are elevated, and fluctuate around this higher level.

Episodic and rhythmic release of ACTH is under neural control. The diurnal rhythm is impaired in patients with certain brain disorders including localized hypothalamic disease, general paresis, Wernicke's encephalopathy, and lesions that result in impaired consciousness.[24] A diurnal rhythm in hypothalamic CRF content has been reported in both normal and adrenalectomized rats, and lesion of the anterior hypothalamus, or treatment with p-chlorophenylalanine, a brain serotonin depletor, abolishes the diurnal changes in plasma cortisol.[15, 23, 51] In man, cyproheptadine inhibits nocturnal cortisol secretion.

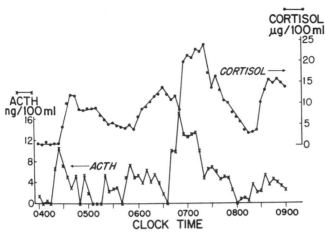

Figure 7. Relationship between plasma ACTH and cortisol. ACTH is secreted in bursts. Each major spurt in cortisol release follows a burst of ACTH secretion. (From Weitzman, E. D., et al.: *Twenty-four hour pattern of the episodic secretion of cortisol in normal subjects.* J. Clin. Endocrinol. Metab. 33:14, 1971, with permission.)

STRESS

The pituitary-adrenal axis is activated by a wide variety of stressful stimuli ranging from the psychologic, such as apprehension or fear, to the physical, such as severe cold exposure, hemorrhage, and electroshock therapy (Fig. 8).[33, 40] Although the meaning of the word "stress" would appear to be instinctively clear to most people, an attempt to define stress soon leads to crucial and difficult questions as to the nature of homeostasis and of disease. In a purely technical sense, the term as derived from physics means "the physical pressure, pull, or other force exerted by one thing on another" *(Random House Dictionary of English Usage)*. In accord with this definition, it is easy to see how cold exposure, trauma, or sensory stimulation might be considered a stress. On the other hand, many stimuli cause physiologic distress through their symbolic impact, and environmental changes may be distressing to some and pleasing to others, depending on circumstances. For this reason, it becomes difficult to define stressful stimuli in objective terms, the ultimate determinant of the stress state being the response of the stressed organism. Physiologists and psychiatrists therefore commonly smudge the physicist's meaning of stress to include both the environmental and the perturbed psychologic state. Thus, excessive cold may be a stress, and the psychologic state resulting from an actual or symbolic threat also constitutes a stress. Obviously, this kind of definition tends to confuse the stimulus and the response, a problem that still plagues those attempting to do objective studies of the role of stress in disease.

Mason[33] has pointed out that most stimuli that give rise to adrenal activation have in common a significant psychologic component. He has suggested that factors such as emotional arousal, novelty, or uncertainty may be the common stimulus for the adrenocortical hormonal response. He points out, however, that certain physical stimuli, notably cold, hypoxia, or hemorrhage, also can produce pituitary-adrenal activation, even when measures are taken to minimize psychologic stress.

Various attempts have been made to differentiate the type or severity of stress in terms of the hypothalamic-pituitary-adrenal system.[5] One classification, based on differences in capacity to stimulate ACTH release, divides stresses into those whose responses are suppressible by dexamethasone pretreatment and those that are nonsup-

185

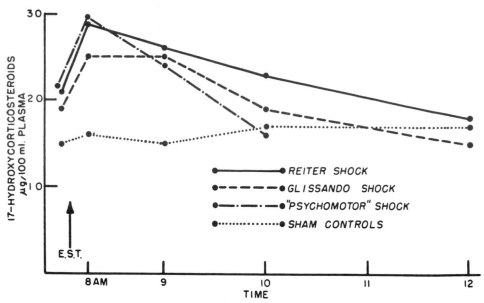

Figure 8. Effect of electroconvulsive therapy on level of 17-hydroxycorticosteroids in plasma. An example of stress-induced pituitary-adrenal activation. (From Bliss, E. L., et al.: *Influence of ECT and insulin coma on level of adrenocortical steroids in peripheral circulation.* Arch. Neurol Psych. 72:352, 1954, with permission.)

pressible.[13, 31] The failure of adrenal steroid pretreatment to inhibit a given response suggests a more potent neural mechanism.[8]

Another principle that is becoming clear is that there are several hormones which characteristically respond to many stimuli. In man, epinephrine, norepinephrine, cortisol, GH, and prolactin are commonly released in response to "nonspecific" stress. In addition, however, a single stimulus may give rise to a multihormonal response that at least in some instances is specific to the stimulus in question. For example, during physical exercise produced by climbing, cortisol elevation can occur without a rise in GH secretion. In contrast, during exposure to heat, GH elevation is observed in the absence of a cortisol rise. It would appear, therefore, that stress evokes a multihormonal patterned response that may be stressor-specific.

NEURAL CONTROL OF ACTH SECRETION

Role of the Hypothalamus

The median eminence of the tuber cinereum is the final common pathway through which neural control of ACTH is exerted.[8, 31, 50, 55] An intact median eminence is essential for normal endocrine responses to stress, although some basal ACTH secretion remains after complete destruction of the median eminence. The hypothalamic region controlling ACTH release apparently involves a large part of the basal hypothalamus. In addition to this excitatory control, there may be an inhibitory area in the posterior hypothalamus close to the mammillary bodies. Lesions in the anterior hypothalamus can abolish the adrenal diurnal rhythm while leaving stress responses unaffected; evidently the neural pathways involved in stress responses and diurnal rhythms are separate. Total disconnection of the hypothalamus from the rest of the brain results in elimination of the adrenal diurnal rhythm and elimination of adrenal responses following a variety of stimuli including severe cold, surgical trauma, and acoustic or photic stimuli.

Since, in contrast, the response to ether requires only an intact hypothalamus, this agent must act directly on the hypothalamus.[19]

Certain severely stressful stimuli, mainly systemic, appear to bypass the hypothalamus, perhaps acting directly on the pituitary, or perhaps causing release of a postulated "tissue-CRF."[19] These include *E. coli* endotoxin, a large dose of formaldehyde, lysine ADH, hemorrhage, and laparotomy.

Feedback Regulation

The non-episodic secretion of ACTH is controlled by the negative-feedback effects of cortisol (see Fig. 1). Removal or spontaneous disease of the adrenal glands leads to a marked rise in plasma ACTH concentration, and the administration of cortisol depresses ACTH secretion (Fig. 9).[19, 48] The site of glucocorticoid feedback effect is still a matter of dispute; there is evidence for a direct pituitary action, for a direct effect on the hypothalamus, and for an effect on mesencephalic and limbic-system structures. All three loci may be involved, and their relative importance in physiologic control is still uncertain. In vitro studies show that cortisol acts directly on pituitary cells to inhibit ACTH release.[19] The effects of CRF are inhibited by cortisol and inhibition is prevented by prior treatment with inhibitors of protein synthesis. This mechanism is similar to that postulated for feedback control of TSH secretion (see Chapter 9). On the other hand, local implantation of cortisol into the hypothalamus or midbrain is also reported to inhibit ACTH release, and corticoid administration depresses hypothalamic CRF concentration, although these effects have been criticized as pharmacologic. Results of implantation studies may be explained by the distribution of the glucocorticoid to the pituitary by way of cerebrospinal fluid and the median eminence, a route demonstrated experimentally by Kendall[19] using labeled glucocorticoids. Thus, the relative importance of pituitary and neural feedback sites is still incompletely defined.

Isolation of the hypothalamus by cutting fiber connections from the overlying brain results in sustained high plasma corticosterone levels in the rat, providing strong evidence that areas outside the hypothalamus have a tonic inhibitory influence on the hypothalamic secretion of CRF.[8, 55] Increased blood levels of ACTH decrease the release of ACTH from the pituitary, an effect that does not require altered glucocorticoid levels, as has been demonstrated in adrenalectomized animals maintained on a constant replacement dose of glucocorticoids. These observations are interpreted to mean that there is "short-loop" feedback of ACTH release. An "ultra-short-loop" feedback in which CRF inhibits the release of CRF has also been postulated.

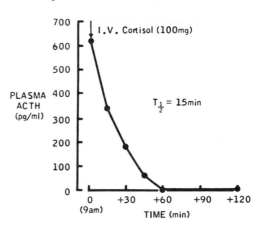

Figure 9. Response of plasma ACTH to the intravenous injection of cortisol in a patient with adrenocortical insufficiency. The initially elevated levels fall rapidly, illustrating the negative-feedback regulation and the short half-life of ACTH in plasma. (From W. J. Irvine, W. J. and Barnes, E. W.: *Adrenal insufficiency. In* Mason, A. S. (ed.): *Clinics in Endocrinology and Metabolism,* vol. 1. W. B. Saunders Co., Ltd., London, 1972, p. 549, with permission.)

187

Role of Nervous Structures Outside the Hypothalamus

A number of suprahypothalamic structures also are involved in ACTH regulation.[13, 31] Both activating and inhibitory functions have been described for midbrain structures. Responses to a variety of stressful stimuli depend on the integrity of afferents from the brain stem. This is so for stimuli such as fracture of the leg and surgical trauma that involve a crossed afferent pathway from the periphery. However, it is also the case for responses to a variety of other stimuli, such as acoustic or photic stimuli and cold stress, for which posterior inputs to the hypothalamus are essential. This has been demonstrated by posterior deafferentation of the hypothalamus. A variety of lesioning and stimulation experiments indicate that the midbrain also inhibits ACTH release, and it has been proposed that these inputs may be one of the factors that influence the diurnal variation in adrenal function. However, there is evidence that the sleep-wake cycle and the adrenal diurnal rhythm can be dissociated (see above), and other neural structures appear to influence the diurnal rhythm.

Several limbic structures are also important in ACTH regulation. The amygdala has a predominantly facilitatory effect on ACTH release, as shown by ACTH release following electric stimulation (Fig. 10, Table 1).[34, 41] Studies in which the whole amygdala is lesioned demonstrate in the rat that the amygdaloid complex is essential in ACTH release in response to neurogenic stresses such as fracture of the leg, but not in response to systemic stresses such as tourniquet or ether.[56] Available evidence indicates that this effect is mediated by a direct ventral pathway from the lateral amygdala to the hypothalamus, rather than by the more indirect stria terminalis.

The hippocampus and septum appear to function in reciprocal relationship with the amygdala in regulating ACTH secretion.[31, 56] Electric stimulation of these regions diminishes stress-induced ACTH release, while lesions facilitate release. Normal resting levels and diurnal rhythm of adrenal hormones are maintained after septal lesions. The septal region has a more general role in determining stress responses, not only with respect to ACTH release but also involving GH and behavioral responses. Destruction of the medial and lateral septal nuclei produces hyper-reactivity of both hormonal and behavioral responses to stress stimuli, a finding that led Uhlir and coworkers[47] to suggest that this region is involved in the "coping" responses to stress.

Neurotransmitter Regulation

The analysis of central neurotransmitter control of CRF-ACTH secretion by neuropharmacologic means has proven to be the most difficult of all of the anterior pituitary

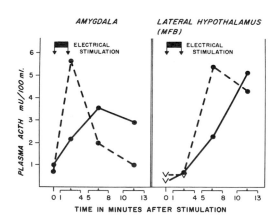

Figure 10. Effect of electric stimulation of the amygdala and lateral hypothalamus (MFB, medial forebrain bundle) on plasma bioassayable ACTH in the cat, showing activation of release. Each line shows a different experiment. Electrical stimulation of the median eminence was without effect. (Plotted from data of Redgate, E. S.: *ACTH release evoked by electrical stimulation of brain stem and limbic system sites in the cat: The absence of ACTH release upon infundibular area stimulation.* Endocrinology 86:806, 1970.)

Table 1. Summary of ACTH Stimulation Experiments

Site of Stimulation	Increment in ACTH, mU/100 ml ± S.E.	
	Early Response (1–4 min)	Delayed Response (10–13 min)
Control	<0.3	<0.3
Hemorrhage	4.5	6.2
Scrotic nerve	8.8	2.7
Medullary reticular formation	0.1	0.5
Medial midbrain	<0.3	0.8
Lateral midbrain	0.1	1.7
Medial forebrain bundle	0.2	2.2
Infundibular hypothalamus	<0.3	0.4
Amygdala-septal complex	2.3	0.8

(Adapted from Redgate, E. S.: *ACTH release evoked by electrical stimulation of brain stem and limbic sites in the cat: The absence of ACTH release upon infundibular area stimulation.* Endocrinology 86:806, 1970.)

hormone systems. This is because both excitatory and inhibitory catecholaminergic neural pathways appear to exert an influence on ACTH release; and both serotonin and acetylcholine also have important effects on ACTH secretion.[15, 51]

Catecholamines—Epinephrine or norepinephrine infused directly into the basal hypothalamus causes prompt release of ACTH from the pituitary, indicating an agonist effect of these hormones. On the other hand, blockade of catecholamine effects brought about by reserpine (a depletor) by chlorpromazine (a receptor blocker), or by α-methyl-p-tyrosine (a catecholamine-synthesis inhibitor) also result in elevated ACTH and cortisol in rat and dog.[51] The inhibitory catecholaminergic pathway is probably noradrenergic, as indicated by the finding that inhibitors of the enzyme dopamine-β-oxidase, that deplete hypothalamic content of norepinephrine, but not of dopamine, cause a rise in plasma corticosterone in the rat. This inhibitory effect appears to be related to stress responses rather to resting (basal) output.

In man, evidence concerning the role of catecholamines in ACTH regulation is inconclusive. Acute administration of L-dopa has no effect on ACTH release in most studies. L-dopa is ineffective in treatment of Cushing's disease due to excess ACTH secretion.[22] Alpha-adrenergic stimulating agents cause a rise in plasma ACTH and cortisol in man, while β-adrenergic blockade enhances the ACTH response to hypoglycemia. These studies suggest a stimulatory effect of α-receptors and an inhibitory effect of β-receptors in ACTH regulation. The issue of the role of catecholamines in the control of ACTH remains unresolved; conflicting evidence points to an inhibitory, an excitatory, or no role.

Serotonin—Serotonin has also been implicated in ACTH regulation. In one report there was a rise in ACTH after administration of 5-hydroxytryptophan in man. Insulin hypoglycemia-induced ACTH secretion is inhibited by cyproheptadine, but not by methysergide.[7] The ACTH response to metyrapone is also blunted by prior administration of metergoline, a specific, potent, and long-acting antiserotonergic agent. These drugs do not alter basal secretion of ACTH but do interfere with pharmacologic responses. Recently, Krieger[23] has reported that Cushing's disease can be successfully treated by cyproheptadine. Nocturnal ACTH release is blocked in normal subjects by this drug.

Acetylcholine—A cholinergic component has also been suggested in ACTH regulation. In the rat, implantation of atropine in the hypothalamus blocks the activation of the pituitary adrenal axis after various stress stimuli including ether, laparotomy, histamine, and carbachol, as well as after adrenalectomy. It thus appears that cholinergic synapses in the hypo-thalamus are involved in the activation of the pituitary adrenal system after stressful stimuli.

NEUROENDOCRINE DISEASE OF THE ADRENAL GLAND

Cushing's Syndrome

Cushing's description in 1932 of the manifestations of excessive secretion of cortisol included virtually all of the features now recognized in florid cases. As summarized by Ross,[43] Cushing's first case was a 23-year-old woman who had gained 25 pounds in two years and who complained of headaches, nausea, shortness of breath, bruising, bald-ness, excessive facial hair, and amenorrhea. She had become round-shouldered and had lost four inches in height. On clinical examination, she is described by Cushing as being of most extraordinary appearance: a kyphotic, under-sized young woman whose round face was dusky, cyanosed, and abnormally hairy. Her abdomen had the appearance of a full-term pregnancy, her breasts were pendulous, and there were pads of fat over the supraclavicular and posterior cervical regions. Purple striae were present over the ab-domen, breasts, shoulders, and hips. Her skin was cyanotic, especially over the trunk and lower extremities, and of marbled appearance, rough and pigmented. The tense and painful adiposity of the trunk contrasted markedly with her thin extremities. The skin bruised easily and often spontaneously, without apparent trauma. Hypertension and glucosuria completed the clinical picture.

Cushing's syndrome is predominantly a condition of females (female to male ratio 9:1) and when it occurs in males is much more difficult to detect clinically because most of the symptoms are attenuated. The term *Cushing's syndrome* refers to all patients with excessive amounts of cortisol, whether due to spontaneous disease of pituitary or adrenal, or secondary to steroid therapy. The term *Cushing's disease* is reserved for patients with bilateral adrenal hyperplasia due to excessive secretion of pituitary ACTH.

The modern clinician, armed with a high index of suspicion and improved laboratory tests for the diagnosis of hypercortisolism, need not wait for the entire array of serious disturbances; and only moderate changes may be noted at any time in patients with clear-cut disease.[36] Today, moreover, the most common cause of Cushing's syndrome by far is the administration of corticoids for their beneficial effects in inflammatory or allergic disease. Because of duration of disease, degree of steroid hypersecretion, and the variability of the time at which the disorder comes to the attention of physicians, the relative frequencies of the various manifestations in Cushing's syndrome cannot be given precisely.

The clinical presentation is diagnostic of Cushing's syndrome in only 50 per cent of mild or early cases, and most frequently the clinician must differentiate between au-thentic hypercortisolism, and the "pseudo-cushingoid" patient who has primary obesity with hormonal changes secondary to the obesity.[49] These aspects are considered below.

Etiology

Spontaneous Cushing's syndrome is due either to excessive ACTH secretion from the pituitary or from nonpituitary tumors, or to primary hypersecretion of cortisol from the adrenals with suppressed ACTH levels.

The most common pathologic finding in spontaneous Cushing's syndrome (approxi-mately 75 per cent of cases) is bilateral hyperplasia of the adrenal cortex secondary to excessive ACTH secretion by the pituitary.[44] This disease properly fits the designa-tion of Cushing's disease (which Cushing called pituitary basophilism). The other causes, in more or less equal proportions, are adenoma of the adrenal, carcinoma of the adrenal, and the "ectopic" production of ACTH by a malignant neoplasm of an organ such as lung or pancreas.

PITUITARY HYPERSECRETION OF ACTH. The cases of Cushing's disease with increased pituitary ACTH secretion have the greatest interest to the neuroendocrinologist. Cushing believed that most arose from basophil adenomas of the pituitary gland, but studies by others suggested that only a minority of cases had tumors, and for some years it was considered that the basophilic changes in the pituitary (Crooke's hyaline changes) were in fact secondary to excessive cortisol secretion. But the pendulum of thought about the etiology of Cushing's disease swung back to the pituitary when it was recognized that these patients had high plasma ACTH levels, had an elevated set-point for feedback inhibition of ACTH-cortisol secretion, and developed pituitary ACTH-secreting tumors following adrenalectomy in about 15 per cent of cases (Nelson's syndrome). Approximately 5 to 10 per cent of cases of Cushing's disease have roentgenographic evidence of sellar abnormality. Most recently, the application of microsurgical approaches to the pituitary has led to the claim that a high proportion of Cushing's disease patients have microadenomas.[14] For example, 8 of 10 patients were cured by microsurgical removal of an adenoma, including 6 cases with apparently normal sella turcica. It can be fairly stated that current ideas about the etiology of Cushing's disease are in flux, but Cushing's original idea that the disease was due to ACTH-producing adenoma (and hence analogous to acromegaly due to GH-secreting adenoma) may be close to true in most cases. This viewpoint has important implications for ideas of pathogenesis and therapy.

The idea that ACTH hypersecretion could arise from hypothalamic dysfunction was put forth by Heinbecker, who was the first to point out that patients dying of Cushing's disease had histologic abnormalities in the hypothalamus.[24, 25] Subsequently, it was found that similar changes could be produced in rat hypothalamus by giving high doses of cortisone, but the idea of central nervous system abnormality as the root cause of Cushing's disease remained strong. In part this was because emotional and physical stress cause ACTH hypersecretion, and because in Cushing's disease, adrenal responses to stress and to suppressive doses of exogenous steroids are qualitatively normal, but quantitatively abnormal, suggesting retention of the normal physiologic regulating mechanisms, but at a new set-point of control. In support of a central nervous system etiology it has been pointed out that GH secretory rhythms are also abnormal, and that patients with depressive illness have adrenal hypersecretion poorly suppressed by exogenous steroid administration. Most recently, Krieger's group[23] have shown that treatment with the drug cyproheptadine, a serotonin-receptor blocker, lowered adrenal cortical function to normal in three cases. Subsequently, twelve additional cases have been sucessfully treated with the drug. The neuroendocrine hypothesis of Cushing's disease is that there is excessive secretion of CRF, which in time may lead to adenoma formation. When the adrenal gland is removed the feedback loop is opened, causing excessive unapposed pituitary hyperfunction which may lead ultimately to true tumor formation and the appearance of serious locally invasive and potentially fatal "malignant" growth of the adenoma. Further evidence that Cushing's disease can arise as a central nervous system disorder is the rare occurrence of hypercortisolism in conjunction with central nervous system disease, including hypothalamic tumors[25] and hydrocephalus.[4] Like Cushing's disease of the usual type, these patients may show suppression with high doses of exogenous steroids. A single case has been reported with paroxysmal release of cortisol, responsive to therapy with chlorpromazine (see Chapter 11).

Another viewpoint, equally harmonious with clinical observations is that Cushing's disease begins as a pituitary microadenoma which retains normal responsiveness to CRF. This might arise because of the loss of feedback receptors for cortisol on ACTH-producing cells. Loss of feedback inhibition after adrenalectomy leads to de-differentiation of the adenoma to the point where it cannot be suppressed by cortisol. The crucial observation required to establish which of these two hypotheses is correct will require the measurement of CRF concentration in either portal-vessel blood or other body fluids such as blood or cerebrospinal fluid.

Whether due to the hypothalamus or the pituitary, the form of hypercortisolism due to excessive secretion of pituitary ACTH can often be controlled by measures directed at the pituitary, such as proton-beam therapy[21] or transsphenoidal microsurgery.[14]

TUMORS. Benign and malignant tumors of the adrenals themselves make up most of the remaining causes of hypercortisolism.[10, 11, 17, 20] Differential diagnosis will be dealt with below. In such cases, the treatment is obviously directed at the adrenal gland. A third type of tumor-induced Cushing's syndrome is now being recognized with increasing frequency, and that is the form of disease caused by ACTH-producing neoplasms. The first of these associations to be recognized was that of oat-cell carcinoma of the lung, although the etiologic relationship was not appreciated at the time. The case, reported by Brown in 1928, was that of a 45-year old woman who (as quoted by Friedman and collaborators[11]) developed the clinical picture of Cushing's syndrome, and died within five months of onset of her illness. At postmortem examination she was found to have oat-cell carcinoma of the lung and bilateral adrenal hyperplasia. A number of such cases, due to a variety of neoplasms, were reported sporadically in the literature but only in 1961 did three groups of investigators (Liddle, Christy and Holub and their respective collaborators) recognize that the plasma or tumors of such patients contained an ACTH-like material indistinguishable by usual tests from pituitary ACTH.[37, 42] It was therefore proposed that ACTH was secreted by the tumor due to its de-differentiation. Detailed studies of the chemical properties of the ACTH secreted by tumors have been carried out. Like ACTH in pituitaries, there are large and small forms both recognizable by anti-ACTH antibodies, but only the small form is biologically active. Tumors generally contain and secrete a larger proportion of the large (inactive) than the small form of ACTH. In fact, virtually all bronchogenic carcinomas secrete large ACTH, which produces no clinical manifestations because it is biologically inactive. It may prove to be a tumor marker.

The most common tumor associated with the ectopic-ACTH syndrome is carcinoma of the lung, mainly oat-cell tumor but also bronchial adenoma. Less common carcinomas, in decreasing frequency, as summarized by Odell,[37] are thymus, pancreas (including islet-cell tumors), carcinoid, neoplasms of neural-crest tissues (pheochromocytoma, neuroblastoma, paraganglioma, ganglioma, medullary carcinoma of the thyroid), and isolated cases of tumor of the ovary, prostate, breast, thyroid, kidney, salivary glands, testis, stomach, colon, gallbladder, esophagus, and appendix.

The presentation of Cushing's syndrome due to ectopic ACTH production usually occurs atypically. Marked hypercortisolism may develop almost explosively, either at the beginning or late in the course of tumor growth, so that many of the usual features (such as obesity and striae) do not have time to develop.[28] Instead, electrolyte abnormalities (notably severe hypokalemic alkalosis), hypertension, and diabetes mellitus may dominate the picture. The electrolyte abnormalities are due to excessive secretion of the mineralocorticoids, desoxycorticosterone (DOC) and, as shown by Melby,[35] 18-hydroxy-DOC. Usually other manifestations of tumor are evident, but in some the differentiation from Cushing's disease is not readily apparent because the primary tumor is occult. Such cases are extremely difficult to distinguish from Cushing's disease and, fortunately, are uncommon. A striking feature of the ectopic ACTH syndrome is marked pigmentation due to excess MSH secretion;[45] the production of cortisol is usually much higher than in Cushing's disease. Plasma cortisol levels over 50 μg./100 ml. are virtually pathognomonic of the disorder.

Several types of tumors producing ACTH are of particular interest from a neuroendocrine point of view. These are tumors arising from neural-crest cells, and include medullary carcinoma of the thyroid, islet-cell tumors, gangliomas, and pheochromocytomas. According to Pearse,[39] ACTH-producing cells of the pituitary belong to the APUD series (*A*mine *P*recursor *U*ptake *D*ecarboxylase cells) as do the other cells of neural-crest origin, and it is not surprising, therefore, that these other cells might share the primitive capacity to form ACTH. However, other tumors not having similar embryologic origin may form ACTH, suggesting a still more primitive differentiation of protein synthesis and secretion.

Differential Diagnosis

Details of the metabolic aspects of Cushing's disease are dealt with in standard endocrinology texts, and in Chapter 12 the important neural and psychologic aspects of this condition are reviewed. This section summarizes the physiologic basis of tests for the differential diagnosis of cortisol hypersecretion.

From a clinical point of view it is first essential to exclude iatrogenic hypercortisolism. A history of ingestion of glucocorticoids such as prednisone and cortisone may be readily disclosed, but less obvious would be the long-term use of topical steroids (cortisol analogues) which in patients with severe skin disease may be absorbed in amounts sufficient to cause systemic toxicity. Such patients present with evidence of hypercortisolism with suppressed adrenal cortical function, as indicated by the low excretion of cortisol and its metabolites and low plasma ACTH. Factitious hypercortisolism should also be considered.

The ectopic ACTH syndrome is associated (as in Cushing's disease) with evidence of atypically high cortisol secretion and high ACTH levels in blood (over 200 pg./ml. and usually greater than 500 pg./ml.). Most ectopic-tumor cases have evident systemic disease, more than half showing lung tumor, but rarely, occult tumors may cause the syndrome. Extremely high cortisol excretion and severe electrolyte abnormality, particularly if it appears over a short period, strongly favor the existence of a tumor. Hypokalemic alkalosis is uncommon in Cushing's disease.

Plasma ACTH measurements permit differentiation of the main forms of Cushing's syndrome into two main groups, the hypersecretors and the hyposecretors of ACTH.[53] High ACTH is due to pituitary overactivity or ectopic production of hormone. On the other hand, primary overactivity of the adrenal causes suppression of the secretion of ACTH. ACTH measurements are now available in commercial laboratories and are useful in differential diagnosis when the diagnosis is not clearly apparent by the older tests. Skull roentgenograms including tomograms should be taken.

The measurement of cortisol in blood and its degradation products in urine, and the use of the adrenal "suppression" tests as pioneered by Liddle[29] revolutionized the diagnosis of adrenal disease (Fig. 11). In normal individuals, plasma cortisol follows a diurnal pattern, maximum values up to 25 μg./100 ml. occurring between 4:00 A.M. and 8:00 A.M. and minimum values, usually not exceeding 8 μg., in late afternoon and evening. In psychically and physically stressed patients, particularly during the first day or two of hospitalization, it is not uncommon for values to run even higher (up to 40 μg./100 ml.) and to see loss of normal diurnal variation. Loss of the diurnal variation is not decisive in differential diagnosis of excessive adrenal cortical function.[32] On the other hand, marked and invariable elevation of plasma cortisol throughout the day (15 μg./100 ml. late afternoon, 35 μg./100 ml. in A.M.) is strong evidence for hypersecretion. Increased cortisol secretion is reflected in increased excretion in the urine of cortisol and its metabolites.[3, 6, 18] Normal values for adult corticoid excretion (17-hydroxycorticoids) is 4 to 12 mg. per 24 hours and is a function of muscle mass. Marked eleva-

193

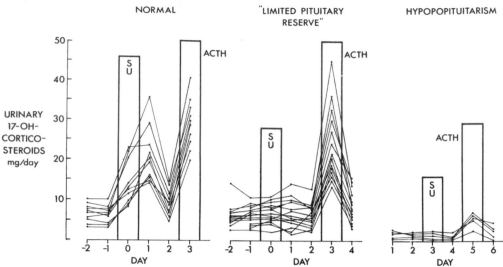

Figure 11. Stimulation tests in diagnosis of impared ACTH secretory reserve. In the normal urinary excretion of 17-hydroxycorticoids is increased by injection of ACTH, and by the administration of the drug metyrapone (SU) which inhibits the formation of cortisol. Low cortisol levels, in turn, lead to increased ACTH release and an increase in production of 11-deoxycortisol, the precursor of cortisol. In hypopituitarism no ACTH is released in response to metyrapone and the response to ACTH is itself impaired because the chronically unstimulated adrenal has decreased response to ACTH. In patients with "limited pituitary reserve" baseline secretion is normal, there is no further response to metyrapone (because endogenous ACTH secretion is already maximal) and the adrenal responds normally because it has been stimulated by ACTH. (From Liddle, G. W., Island, D. and Meador, C. K.: *Normal and abnormal regulation of corticotropin secretion in man.* Recent Progr. Horm. Res. 18:125, 1962, with permission.)

tion of urinary corticoid excretion is seen in well-established Cushing's disease, but there is an overlap with the normal; some very obese patients who have a form of secondary hypercortisolism and a number of patients with Cushing's syndrome may have total corticoid secretion that falls within the normal range. Streeten and coworkers[49] have found that the excretion of corticoids in the urine gives a far more accurate diagnosis of Cushing's syndrome when corrected for body mass using creatinine measurements. In normal persons, urinary 17-hydroxycorticoids/g. creatinine was 3.99 ± 0.12 (S.E.M.) in patients over the age of 3 years, but in all Cushing's cases tested, values were in excess of the upper limit of normal, 6.5. The use of such techniques compensates for the difference in size between women and men and for the effects of androgens. In a critical study of criteria for diagnosis, Eddy and collaborators[6] found that the best single technique was the measurement of free cortisol in urine. Normal values were 36 to 297 μg. per 24 hours in females and 75 to 378 μg. per 24 hours in males. In a series of 24 patients with Cushing's disease values were above 552 μg. per 24 hours in all. Other studies of this method have reported a 90 per cent accuracy.

Given clinical evidence of hypercortisolism and laboratory evidence of increased cortisol secretion — such as high plasma cortisol, loss of diurnal rhythm, increased corticoid excretion, or increased free cortisol excretion in urine — the use of the adrenal suppression tests provides the best confirmatory evidence of adrenal abnormality and gives great assistance in classifying the nature of the defect.[18, 29] In normal persons, the administration of dexamethasone 2 mg. per day for two days (equivalent to approximately three to four times the normal daily requirement of cortisol) uniformly suppresses urinary corticoid excretion to 3 mg. or less in 24 hours. In most (but not all) patients with Cushing's syndrome, of whatever cause, this dosage level of dexamethasone will *not* inhibit endogenous corticoid secretion, a finding that indicates an elevation of set-point control (Fig. 12). The main exceptions to this generalization are patients with severe depression who may not show suppression, some patients with obesity who may suppress only after a longer period of administration (up to four days), and a few patients with Cushing's disease secondary to hypothalamic tumor or to ectopic ACTH production. In the patient who fails to suppress corticoid secretion with the 2 mg. per day dexamethasone dose, it is recommended that 8 mg. per day be administered. In most but not all cases of Cushing's disease, this dose will suppress corticoid excretion into the normal range, whereas it usually will not suppress the corticoid excretion in patients with adenomas, carcinomas of the adrenal, or the ectopic-ACTH syndrome. Although this conclusion is generally correct, several rare instances have been reported in which this differentiation was not valid. These cases included patients with adrenal carcinoma and adrenal adenoma. Paradoxic responses (i.e., increased cortisol excretion after dexamethasone) have been observed in one patient who otherwise showed typical Cushing's disease.[10] The metyrapone test is useful in differentiating Cushing's disease from other forms of Cushing's syndrome.

The exceptions to the rule, though uncommon, re-emphasize the importance of the clinical evaluation and the recognition that no one test is infallible for proper diagnosis of Cushing's disease.

Patients with adrenal tumors usually do not show adrenal response to the administration of ACTH, while patients with Cushing's disease are hyper-responsive. On the other hand, a few patients with adrenal carcinoma are ACTH-responsive.

Obesity with secondary hypercortisolism is a special problem, particularly important because many very obese women develop purple striae, hirsutism, and amenorrhea.

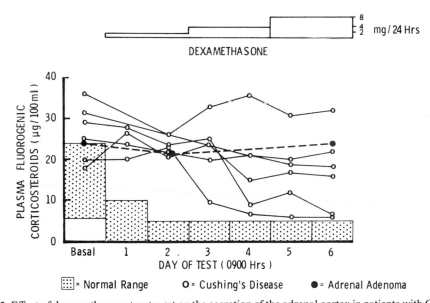

Figure 12. Effect of dexamethasone treatment on the secretion of the adrenal cortex in patients with Cushing's disease and adrenal hyperfunction due to adrenal adenoma. In five of the six patients with Cushing's disease (open circles), plasma cortisol gradually decreased but the dose required for suppression was much greater than that required in normal individuals. In the patient with adenoma, there were no changes in plasma cortisol. Responses in the patient with Cushing's disease indicate an "elevated setpoint" for feedback control of ACTH secretion, whereas the response in the patient with adenoma indicates completely autonomous function. (From Besser, G. M. and Edwards, C. R. W.: *Cushing's syndrome. In* Mason, A. S. (ed.): *Clinics in Endocrinology and Metabolism*, vol. 1. W. B. Saunders Co., Ltd., London, 1972, p. 451, with permission.)

Also, uniform obesity rather than the classic, central type is relatively common in Cushing's disease. Most obese patients will show suppression of plasma cortisol to less than 5 μg./100 ml. after the administration of a single dose of 0.5 mg. dexamethasone at bedtime (screening suppression test) but a few require 2 mg. per day for more than four days. Urinary free cortisol is rarely elevated in obesity.

PHYSICAL METHODS FOR DIAGNOSIS OF ADRENAL DISEASE. Local disease of the adrenal can be diagnosed by modern angiographic methods. Large adrenal tumors may be detected by intravenous pyelography (in association with tomography) or by echo scans. Retroperitoneal air injection to provide better contrast is no longer used, angiography having supplanted this procedure. Small tumors may be detected by the characteristic blush and typical vascular pattern. The extent of large tumors can also be outlined by arteriography. In many cases of bilateral hyperplasia, angiography shows widening of the cortex. Selective venous catheterization demonstrates elevated cortisol levels. New adrenal-cortical radioisotope imaging techniques using iodinated cholesterol analogues or blockers of adrenal steroid synthesis, such as metyrapone, have also been introduced.

Treatment

If the syndrome is due to tumor of the adrenal, excision is the treatment of choice. In ectopic ACTH production, the culprit tumor is removed if possible or treated by chemotherapy or roentgenotherapy. If the condition is due to an operable lesion, cure may result. The excess cortisol secretion can be controlled by drugs that act on the adrenal cortex to suppress steroid formation. These drugs include metyrapone, aminoglutethemide and the adrenocortolytic drug o,p'-DDD.[38] Metyrapone blocks the formation of cortisol by blocking the 11-hydroxylase step. Aminoglutethemide, a drug that is selectively concentrated in the adrenal cortex and interferes with corticoid biosynthesis with damage to the cell, is a better choice and effects are evident within a few days. It is so effective that replacement cortisol therapy is usually required. At this writing, this agent is still an investigational drug in the United States and Canada. o,p'-DDD, another adrenal cortical toxin, is widely used for treatment of inoperable and metastatic adrenal carcinoma.

Unlike the situation in tumor-induced Cushing's syndrome, whether of adrenal or extra-adrenal origin, in which the course of therapy is usually straightforward, the treatment of Cushing's disease has passed through many fashions and is still subject to continuing revisions. Before synthetic corticoids were developed, these patients were treated by adrenalectomy on one side and subtotal adrenalectomy on the other, the idea being that sufficient adrenal tissue would be left to maintain health. However, this procedure in most cases led either to adrenal insufficiency or to relapse, and is no longer used. Instead, bilateral total adrenalectomy is widely practiced, the patient then being maintained on regular replacement therapy with the equivalent of 25 to 37.5 mg. of cortisone per day and 9-α-fluorohydrocortisone, a mineralocorticoid, at a dose of 0.1 to 0.2 mg. per day. However, such patients almost invariably show increasing pigmentation, increasingly high ACTH levels in blood (over 500 to 750 pg./ml.), and in 10 to 15 per cent, evidence of pituitary tumor. This occurrence, now called *Nelson's syndrome*, requires either radiotherapy or neurosurgical removal because this type of tumor is especially likely to behave like a carcinoma by invading the base of the skull, and to cause optic and cranial nerve damage.

Because bilateral adrenalectomy is followed by the lifetime requirement for adrenal cortical replacement, and in a few cases by pituitary tumors, there has been continuing study of effective ways of directing therapy at the pituitary. In many centers, conventional roentgenotherapy (5,000 rads) is used and will cause a remission in about 50 per cent of cases and virtually completely prevent the late occurrence of Nelson's syndrome. Because the response is quite slow, this approach is not advised in severe cases unless direct therapy of the adrenals with drugs, such as aminoglutethemide, or (as in some series) unilateral adrenalectomy is carried out. Proton-beam irradiation[21] is said to cause amelioration of Cushing's disease in a much higher proportion of cases (60 per cent or more) but this procedure is new and not fully explored. The use of pituitary microsurgery in cases with tomographic evidence of abnormality in the sella is recommended if the proper surgical support is available.[14, 26] The role of microsurgery in treatment of cases without evident adenomas by roentgenography is under active investigation in several centers, but experience is insufficient to support a broad generalization. The problem of maintaining normal pituitary function after either microsurgery or proton-beam irradiation must be considered. Only a small proportion (about 10 per cent) are reported to develop hypopituitarism, but this is a consideration, especially in patients who want to have children.

In our opinion, in the future, all patients with Cushing's disease will be best treated by either pituitary microsurgery or by proton-beam irradiation. If the hypercortisolism is severe, medical measures directed against adrenal steroidogenesis are available until the pituitary disorder can be attacked directly. Proper choice of treatment now depends on access to treatment resources such as radiation therapy, skilled abdominal surgeons, and skilled neurosurgeons. Most centers now recommend unilateral or bilateral adrenalectomy plus conventional pituitary radiotherapy, but this recommendation must be subject to continuing review. Recently Krieger[23] has reported that cyproheptadine, a serotonin-receptor blocker, induced partial or full remission in three cases. Withdrawal of cyproheptadine was followed by return of cortisol secretory excess. Whether this might be used as the only therapy or as an adjunct to other modalities awaits further study. Subsequent experience indicates that about 40 per cent of patients respond to this therapy.

Adrenal Cortical Insufficiency: Addison's Disease

Acute or chronic adrenal insufficiency poses a severe threat to the life of the patient.[9] Insufficiency may be primary (adrenal failure) or secondary due to pituitary hypofunction. The disease described by Addison and which bears his name is a chronic, primary disease of adrenal glands of diverse causes. In Addison's disease, hypothalamic-pituitary regulation of the adrenal is qualitatively normal. ACTH levels are elevated in response to the low plasma corticosteroids. Negative feedback of plasma corticosteroids is intact, with normal or slightly diminished sensitivity as assessed by the response to exogenously administered glucocorticoids. Circadian periodicity of plasma ACTH is retained despite the overall elevation in circulating levels.

Adrenal insufficiency secondary to pituitary disease may occur with pituitary tumors, infarction, granulomas, or other pituitary lesions. Defects in pituitary function are usually multiple and lead to panhypopituitarism (Simmonds' disease). There is often a sequential development of failure of gonadotropins, thyrotropin, and ACTH. In the absence of ACTH, cortisol secretion is markedly reduced but aldosterone secretion is less affected. In chronic hypopituitarism the response to ACTH may be delayed, due to atrophy of the adrenal cortex. The adrenal medulla is spared. The clinical presentation of glucocorticoid deficiency in secondary adrenal failure is less severe than in Addison's disease. The clinical findings and management of patients with panhypopituitarism are discussed in Chapter 15.

Hypothalamic Hypoadrenalism

Disturbance of adrenal function secondary to hypothalamic or other brain lesions occurs less frequently than alteration of gonadotropin, GH, or prolactin secretion. As Krieger and coworkers[23, 24] have emphasized, however, disturbances of diurnal rhythms of pituitary-adrenal secretion are common with intracranial disease, and provide an early, sensitive index to disturbance of neuroendocrine control. Structural lesions of the hypothalamus (tumors, inflammation, hydrocephalus) rarely result in serious adrenal insufficiency. The reason for this is not clear; as in the case of the thyroid, perhaps a large reserve of hypophysiotrophic hormone influence is not readily completely destroyed. In fact, anencephalic infants without histologic evidence of any hypothalamic tissue secrete measurable concentrations of cortisol into the blood, and in some cases respond to insulin hypoglycemia or ADH with further cortisol release. Isolated ACTH deficiency is rare but has been reported in a few cases.[1, 2, 16] One may speculate that congenital absence of CRF can occur in a situation analagous to hypothalamic hypothyroidism and hypogonadism.

Adrenoleukodystrophy

The association of adrenal insufficiency with demyelination of the brain has recently been extensively investigated by Schaumberg and collaborators.[46] This condition, called adrenoleukodystrophy, is sex-linked, occurring exclusively in males. It is now recognized that most cases of so-called Schilder's disease fit nosologically into this group. The adrenals become atrophic and show specific cytoplasmic inclusions. Extensive demyelination occurs in the cerebrum and results in hemianopia or blindness, and dementia. Adrenal failure and central demyelination are believed to be due to an enzymatic defect in lipid (myelin) metabolism, but the precise abnormality has not been identified. Lesions have also been described in peripheral nerve and in the testis.

REFERENCES

1. ABRAMSON, E. A. AND ARKY, R. A.: *Coexistent diabetes mellitus and isolated ACTH deficiency: Report of a case.* Metabolism 17:492, 1968.

2. BURGHEN, G. A., CAMACHO, A. M. AND ETTELDOR, P.: *Isolated ACTH deficiency with ketotic hypoglycemia and hypoalanemia.* Clin. Res. 21:126, 1973.

3. BURKE, C. W. AND BEARDWELL, C. G.: *Cushing's syndrome: An evaluation of the clinical usefulness of urinary free cortisol and other urinary steriod measurements in diagnosis.* Q. J. Med. 42:175, 1973.

4. CRISPELL, K. R. AND PARSON, W.: *Coexistence of Cushing's syndrome and internal hydrocephalus produced by a cerebellar tumor.* Am. J. Med. 13:247, 1952.

5. DEWIED, D. AND WEIJNEN, J. A. W. M. (EDS.): *Pituitary, adrenal and the brain.* Prog. Brain Res. 32:125, 1970.

6. EDDY, R. L., ET AL.: *Cushing's syndrome: A prospective study of diagnostic methods.* Am. J. Med. 55: 621, 1973.

7. FELDMAN, J. M.: *Cushing's disease: A hypothalamic flush?* N. Engl. J. Med. 293:930, 1975.

8. FORTIER, C.: *Nervous control of ACTH secretion. In* Harris, G. W. and Donovan, B. T. (eds.): *The Pituitary Gland.* Butterworth, London, 1966, p. 195.

9. FRAWLEY, T. F.: *Adrenal cortical insufficiency. In* Eisenstein, A. B. (ed.): *The Adrenal Cortex.* Little, Brown and Co., Boston, 1967, p. 439.

10. FRENCH, F. S., ET AL.: *Cushing's syndrome with a paradoxical response to dexamethasone.* Am. J. Med. 47:619, 1969.

11. FRIEDMAN, M., MARSHALL-JONES, P. AND ROSS, E. J.: *Cushing's syndrome: Adrencortical hyperactivity secondary to neoplasms arising outside the pituitary-adrenal system.* Q. J. Med. 34:193, 1966.

12. GALLAGHER, T. F., ET AL.: *ACTH and cortisol secretory patterns in man.* J. Clin. Endocrinol. Metab. 36:1058, 1973.

13. GANONG, W. R., ALPERT, L. C. AND LEE, T. C.: *ACTH and the regulation of adrenocortical secretion.* N. Engl. J. Med. 290:1006, 1974.

14. HARDY, J.: *Transsphenoidal surgery of hypersecreting pituitary tumors. In* Kohler, P.O. and Ross, G. T. (eds.): *Diagnosis and Treatment of Pituitary Tumors.* Excerpta Medica, Amsterdam, 1973, p. 179.

15. HIROSHIGE, T. AND ABE, K.: *Role of brain biogenic amines in the regulation of ACTH secretion. In* Yagi, K. and Yoshida, S. (eds.): *Neuroendocrine Control.* John Wiley & Sons, New York, 1973, p. 205.

16. HUNG, W. AND MIGEON, C. J.: *Hypoglycemia in a two-year-old boy with adrenocorticotrophic hormone (ACTH) deficiency (probably isolated) and adrenal medullary unresponsiveness to insulin induced hypoglycemia.* J. Clin. Endocrinol. Metab. 28:146, 1968.

17. HUTTER, A. M. AND KAYHOE, D. E.: *Adrenal cortical carcinoma.* Am. J. Med. 41:572, 1966.

18. JAMES, V. H. T. AND LANDON, J. (EDS.): *The Investigation of Hypothalamic-Pituitary-Adrenal Function, Memoirs of the Society for Endocrinology 17.* Cambridge University Press, Cambridge, 1968.

19. KENDALL, J. W.: *Feedback control of adrenocorticotropic hormone secretion. In* Martini, L. and Ganong, W. F. (eds.): *Frontiers in Neuroendocrinology.* Oxford University Press, New York; 1971, p. 177.

20. KENDALL, J. W. AND SLOOP, JR., P. R.: *Dexamethasone-suppressible adrenocortical tumor.* N. Engl. J. Med. 279:532, 1968.

21. KJELLBERG, R. N. AND KLIMAN, B.: *A system for therapy of pituitary tumors. In* Kohler, P. O. and Ross, G. T. (eds.): *Diagnosis and Treatment of Pituitary Tumors.* Excerpta Medica, Amsterdam, 1973.

22. KRIEGER, D. T.: *Lack of responsiveness to L-dopa in Cushing's disease.* J. Clin. Endocrinol. Metab. 36: 277, 1973.

23. KRIEGER, D. T., AMOROSA, L. AND LINICK, F.: *Cyproheptadine-induced remission of Cushing's disease.* N. Engl. J. Med. 293:893, 1975.

24. KRIEGER, D. T. AND GLICK, S. M.: *Growth hormone and cortisol responsiveness in Cushing's syndrome; relation to a possible central nervous system etiology.* Am. J. Med. 52:25, 1972.

25. KRIEGER, D. T., KRIEGER, H. P. AND SOFFER, L. J.: *Cushing's syndrome associated with a suprasellar tumor.* Acta Endocrinol. 47:185, 1964.

26. LAGERQUIST, L. G., ET AL.: *Cushing's disease with cure by resection of a pituitary adenoma; evidence against a primary hypothalamic defect.* Am. J. Med. 57:826, 1974.

27. LIDDLE, G. W.: *The adrenals, part 1: The adrenal cortex. In* Williams, R. H. (ed.): *Textbook of Endocrinology,* ed. 5. W. B. Saunders, Philadelphia, 1974, p. 233.

28. LIDDLE, G. W., ET AL.: *The ectopic ACTH syndrome.* Cancer Res. 25:1057, 1965.

29. LIDDLE, G. W., ISLAND, D. AND MEADOR, C. K.: *Normal and abnormal regulation of corticotropin secretion in man.* Recent Progr. Horm. Res. 18:125, 1962.

30. LIDDLE, G. W.: *Pathogenesis of glucocorticiod disorders.* Am. J. Med. 53:638, 1972.

31. MANGILI, G., MOTTA, M. AND MARTINI, L.: *Control of adrenocorticotropic hormone secretion. In* Martini, L. and Ganong, W. F. (eds.): *Neuroendocrinology.* Academic Press, New York, 1966, p. 297.

32. MAROJI, T., ET AL.: *Circadian rhythm of glucocorticoid secretion. In* Yagi, K. and Yoshida, S. (eds.): *Neuroendocrine Control.* John Wiley & Sons, New York, 1973, p. 57.

33. MASON, J. W.: *A historical view of the stress field.* J. Hum. Stress 1(1):6, and 1(2):22, 1975.

34. MATHESON, G. K., BRAUCH, B. J. AND TAYLOR, A. N.: *Effects of amygdaloid stimulation on pituitary-adrenal activity in conscious cats.* Brain Res. 32:151, 1971.

35. MELBY, J. C.: *Therapeutic possibilities in Cushing's syndrome.* N. Engl. J. Med. 285:288, 1971.

36. NUGENT, C. A., ET AL.: *Probability theory in the diagnosis of Cushing's syndrome.* J. Clin. Endocrinol. Metab. 24:621, 1964.

37. ODELL, W. D.: *Humoral manifestations of norendocrine neoplasms—ectopic hormone production. In* Williams, R. H. (ed.): *Textbook of Endocrinology,* ed. 5. W. B. Saunders, Philadelphia, 1974, p. 1105.

38. ORTH, D. N. AND LIDDLE, G. W.: *Results of treatment in 108 patients with Cushing's syndrome.* N. Engl. J. Med. 285:243, 1971.

39. PEARCE, A. G.: *The APUD cell concept and its implications in pathology.* Pathol. Annu. 9:27, 1974.

40. PERSKY, H.: *Adrenocortical function and anxiety.* Psychoneuroendocrinology 1:37, 1975.

41. REDGATE, E. S.: *ACTH release evoked by electrical stimulation of brain stem and limbic system sites in the cat: The absence of ACTH release upon infundibular area stimulation.* Endocrinology 86:806, 1970.

42. REES, L. H. AND RATCLIFFE, J. G.: *Ectopic hormone production by nonendocrine tumors.* Clin. Endocrinol. (Oxf.) 3:263, 1974.

43. ROSS, E. J., MARSHALL-JONES, P. AND FRIEDMAN, M.: *Cushing's syndrome: Diagnostic criteria.* Q. J. Med. 35:149, 1966.

44. ROVIT, R. L. AND DUANE, T. D.: *Cushing's syndrome and pituitary tumors. Pathophysiology and ocular manifestation of ACTH-secreting pituitary adenomas.* Am. J. Med. 46:416, 1969.

45. SAWIN, C. T., ABE, K. AND ORTH, D. N.: *Hyperpigmentation due solely to increased plasma β-melanotropin.* Arch. Int. Med. 125:708, 1970.

46. SCHAUMBERG, H. H., ET AL.: *Adrenoleukodystrophy: A clinical and pathological study of 17 cases.* Arch. Neurol. 32:577, 1975.

47. UHLIR, I., SEGGIE, J. AND BROWN, G. M.: *The effect of septal lesions on the threshold of adrenal stress response.* Neuroendocrinology 14:351, 1974.

48. SMELIK, P. G.: *The regulation of ACTH secretion.* Acta Physiol. Pharmacol. Neurol. 15:123, 1969.

49. STREETEN, D. H. P., ET AL.: *The diagnosis of hypercortisolism. Biochemical criteria differentiating patients from lean and obese normal subjects and from females on oral contraceptives.* J. Clin. Endocrinol. Metab. 29:1191, 1969.

50. SZENTHAGATHAI, J., ET AL.: *Hypothalamic Control of the Anterior Pituitary,* ed. 3. Akademiai Kiado, Budapest, 1968.

51. VAN LOON, G. R.: *Brain catecholamines in the regulation of ACTH secretion. In* Lederis, K. and Cooper, K. E. (eds.): *Recent Studies of Hypothalamic Function.* S. Karger, Basel, 1974, p. 100.

52. WEITZMAN, E. D.: *Temporal organization of neuroendocrine function in relation to the sleep-waking cycle in man. In* Lederis, K. and Cooper, K. E.: (eds.): *Recent Studies of Hypothalamic Function.* S. Karger, Basel, 1974, p. 26.

53. YALOW, R. S. AND BERSON, S. A.: *Size heterogeneity of immunoreactive human ACTH in plasma and in extracts of pituitary glands and ACTH-producing thymoma.* Biochem. Biophys. Res. Commun. 44:439, 1971.

54. YATES, F. E.: *Physiological control of adrenal cortical hormone secretion. In* Eisenstein, A. B. (ed.): *The Adrenal Cortex.* Little, Brown and Co., Boston, 1967, p. 133.

55. YATES, F. E., ET AL.: *The pituitary-adrenal cortical system: Stimulation and inhibition of secretion of corticotrophin. In* McCann, S. M. (ed.): *Endocrine Physiology. M.T.P. International Review of Science, Physiol. Ser. 1, vol. 5.* Butterworth, London, 1974, p. 109.

56. ZOLOVICK, A. J.: *Effects of lesions and electrical stimulation of the amygdala on hypothalamic-hypophyseal-regulation. In* Eleftheriou, B. E. (ed.): *Advances in Behavioural Biology, vol. 2, The Neurobiology of the Amygdala.* Plenum Press, New York, 1972, p. 643.

BIBLIOGRAPHY

DEWIED, D. AND WEIJNEN, J. A. W. M. (EDS.): *Pituitary, adrenal and the brain.* Progr. Brain Res. 32:125, 1970.

FORTIER, C.: *Nervous control of ACTH secretion. In* Harris, G. W. and Donovan, B. T. (eds.): *The Pituitary Gland.* Butterworth, London, 1966, p. 195.

FRAWLEY, T. F.: *Adrenal cortical insufficiency. In* Eisenstein, A. B. (ed.): *The Adrenal Cortex.* Little, Brown and Co., Boston, 1967, p. 439.

KENDALL, J. W.: *Feedback control of adrenocorticotropic hormone secretion. In* Martini, L. and Ganong, W. F. (eds.): *Frontiers in Neuroendocrinology.* Oxford University Press, New York, 1971, p. 177.

LIDDLE, G. W.: *The adrenals, part 1: The adrenal cortex. In* Williams, R. H. (ed.): *Textbook of Endocrinology,* ed. 5. W. B. Saunders, Philadelphia, 1974, p. 233.

MANGILI, G., MOTTA, M. AND MARTINI, L.: *Control of adrenocorticotropic hormone secretion. In* Martini, L. and Ganong, W. F. (eds.): *Neuroendocrinology.* Academic Press, New York, 1966, p. 297.

SZENTHAGATHAI, J., ET AL.: *Hypothalamic Control of the Anterior Pituitary,* ed. 3. Akademiai Kiado, Budapest, 1968.

YATES, F. E.: *Physiological control of adrenal cortical hormone secretion. In* Eisenstein, A. B. (ed.): *The Adrenal Cortex.* Little, Brown and Co., Boston, 1967, p. 133.

YATES, F. E., ET AL.: *The pituitary-adrenal cortical system: Stimulation and inhibition of secretion of corticotrophin. In* McCann, S. M. (ed.): *Endocrine Physiology. M. T. P. International Review of Science.* Butterworth, London, 1974, p. 109.

CHAPTER 9

Regulation of TSH Secretion and Its Disorders

The pituitary-thyroid axis has served neuroendocrinology as the example par excellence of a negative-feedback self-regulatory system.[19, 35] This regulation is achieved by the interaction of at least three groups of hormones. Hypothalamic thyrotropin-releasing hormone (TRH) stimulates the synthesis and release of thyrotropin (thyroid-stimulating hormone, TSH) by the pituitary thyrotrope. TSH, in turn, activates iodide uptake, hormonogenesis, and release of the thyroid hormones thyroxine (T_4) and tri-iodothyronine (T_3). The circulating thyroid hormones exert feedback effects on the pituitary to regulate TSH secretion. Interaction between the negative-feedback effects of T_4 and T_3 at the pituitary level and the stimulatory effects of TRH appears to be the primary control of TSH secretion (Fig. 1).

Although this simple model describes most of the regulatory factors in pituitary-thyroid function, other mechanisms influence the rate of TSH secretion. These include peripheral degradation of TSH, of thyroid hormones, and of TRH, and the physical state of thyroid hormones in the blood. An inhibitory hypothalamic hormone (somatostatin) which affects TSH secretion also has been described. This chapter outlines these mechanisms of control and describes the disorders of TSH secretion in man.

PITUITARY TSH SECRETION

Human pituitary thyrotropin is a glycoprotein, molecular weight 28,000, secreted by specific basophilic cells of the anterior pituitary (thyrotrope cells) distinct from the basophils that secrete the gonadotropins and ACTH. TSH is made up of two chemical subunits, α and β.[17] The α subunit, identical to and interchangeable with the α subunit of LH and FSH, is devoid of biologic activity. Determinants of the immunologic and biologic actions of TSH are located in the β subunit. Circulating TSH is identical to pituitary TSH; small amounts of the β subunit also are normally secreted into the blood.[17]

The development of radioimmunoassays for TSH in man has advanced the study of TSH regulation. Such assays are sufficiently sensitive to permit measurement of basal plasma TSH levels in most normal individuals. Normal serum levels of TSH in man are 1 to 10 μU./ml. TSH circulates unbound in the blood and has a half-life of 50 to 60 minutes. It is estimated that 10 to 30 per cent of total pituitary TSH content is secreted daily.[17]

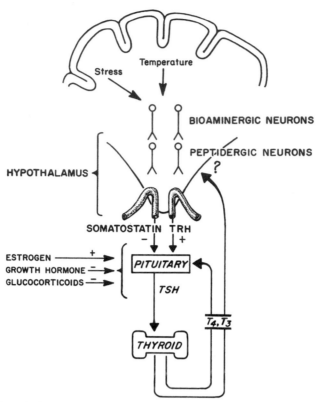

Figure 1. Diagram of regulation of the hypothalamic-pituitary-thyroid axis. Pituitary TSH secretion is stimulated by TRH and inhibited by somatostatin. The release of the hypothalamic hormones from peptidergic neurons are in turn regulated by bioaminergic neurons. Higher brain centers are involved in relay of stress- and temperature-mediated influences on hypothalamic centers. Thyroid hormones (T_4, T_3) feedback predominantly at pituitary level but may also have effects on hypothalamus. Estrogen facilitates, and growth hormone and glucocorticoids inhibit, pituitary responsiveness to TRH.

SECRETORY PATTERNS OF TSH

Sequential blood sampling has shown that basal TSH levels in man fluctuate considerably throughout the day and night. Episodic or pulsatile TSH release has been demonstrated, and highest levels are usually observed during the morning hours from 4 to 8 A.M. (Fig. 2).[41]

Serum TSH levels rise transiently in the infant immediately after birth, a peak occurring within the first half hour of life.[7] TSH levels return to baseline adult values within 48 to 72 hours.

PITUITARY-THYROID FEEDBACK

Administration of increasing doses of T_4 to hypothyroid individuals produces a graded suppression of plasma TSH levels. When data relating TSH to T_4 concentration are plotted to show TSH as a function of plasma T_4, a curvilinear relationship is evident (Fig. 3).[36] In extensive studies of this phenomenon it has been shown that plasma TSH is a function of the negative log of plasma T_4. In terms of servosystems analysis, the thyroid hormone concentration in the blood can be viewed as the "controlled vari-

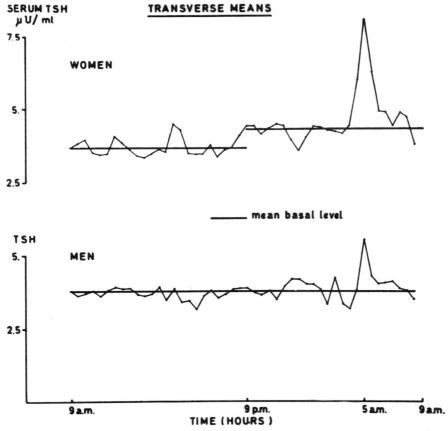

Figure 2. Mean basal levels of plasma TSH throughout the day in women and men. Concentration in blood rises during the night, reaching highest levels in morning hours before awaking. (From Vanhaelst, L., et al.: *Circadian variations of serum thyrotropin levels in man.* J. Clin. Endocrinol. Metab. 35:479, 1972, with permission.)

able." The normal "setpoint" of pituitary-thyroid function is the resting concentration of plasma thyroid hormone maintained by a specific concentration of TSH. The secretion of TSH is inversely regulated by the concentration of thyroid hormones in such a way that deviations from the control setpoint lead to appropriate changes in the rate of TSH secretion. Inhibition of TSH secretion follows 15 to 45 minutes after T_4 and T_3 administration.

The precise setpoint, or level at which TSH secretion is maintained, is determined by the amount of TRH secreted by the hypothalamus. The TSH-releasing effects of hypothalamic TRH are immediate; increases in plasma TSH levels follow IV administration of TRH within two minutes.[8, 15, 16, 17, 43] The effects of TRH administration can be blocked by pretreatment with either T_4 or T_3.[42] Moderate inhibition however, can be overcome by subsequent administration of larger doses of TRH. These studies indicate that competitive interaction exists at the pituitary level between TRH and thyroid hormones to determine TSH secretion.[11] TRH stimulation does not depend on new protein synthesis, whereas T_4- and T_3-induced effects on the pituitary do require new protein synthesis. This finding has led some to postulate that thyroid hormone causes the thyrotrope to produce an inhibitory protein that subsequently interferes with the TSH-

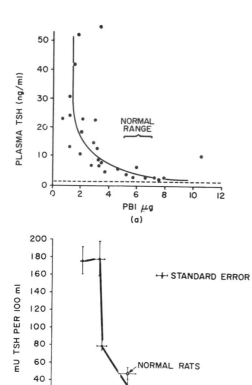

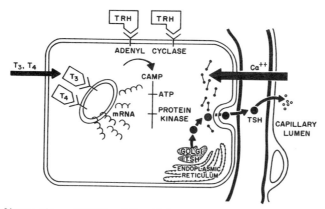

Figure 3. Relationship of plasma TSH to plasma thyroid hormone levels in the human (*a*) and rat (*b*). Studies in humans were carried out by replacing six myxedematous patients with successive increments of thyroxine (T₄) at approximately 10-day intervals. Each point represents simultaneous measurement of plasma T₄ and plasma TSH at various times. The studies in rats were done by treating thyroidectomized rats with various doses of thyroxine for two weeks. (*a* from Reichlin, S. and Utiger, R. D.: *Regulation of the pituitary-thyroid axis in man: The relationship of TSH concentration to free and total thyroid thyroxine level in plasma.* J. Clin. Endocrinol. 27:251, 1967; *b* from Reichlin, S. et al.: *Measurement of TSH in plasma and pituitary of the rat by a radioimmunoassay utilizing bovine TSH: Effect of thyroidectomy on thyroxine replacement.* Endocrinology 87:1022, 1970, with permission.)

releasing effects of TRH (Fig. 4). TRH probably acts through the cyclic AMP mechanism after interacting with cell-membrane receptors.

The remarkable sensitivity of the thyroid hormone feedback system to small changes in plasma levels of thyroid hormones is well documented. Snyder and Utiger[42] showed

Figure 4. Diagram of interactions of TRH and thyroid hormones (T₄ and T₃) in regulation of TSH secretion. TRH acts at a membrane site via adenyl cyclase and cyclic AMP (CAMP) to stimulate TSH release. Thyroid hormones act via nucleus and messenger RNA (mRNA) to inhibit TSH synthesis and release.

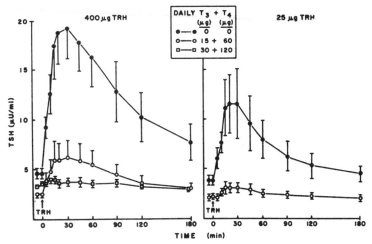

Figure 5. Plasma TSH responses to two doses of TRH (400 μg. *left* and 25 μg. *right*) in normal subjects before and after oral administration of small doses of T_3 and T_4. Administration of 15 μg. T_3 and 60 μg. T_4 for two weeks markedly suppressed the TSH response to TRH. (From Snyder, P. J. and Utiger, R. D.: *Inhibition of thyrotropin response to thyrotropin-releasing hormone by small quantities of thyroid hormones.* J. Clin. Invest. 51:2077, 1972, with permission.)

that the daily administration to normal human volunteers of small doses of T_4 and T_3 (15 μg. T_3 and 60 μg. T_4 daily for three to four weeks) substantially reduced plasma TSH responses to intravenous TRH, without measurable increases in plasma T_3 or T_4 levels (Fig. 5). These data suggest that the setpoint of control between TRH and thyroid hormones is exquisitely sensitive and responsive to thyroid hormone feedback effects within the physiologic range.[26, 36] This delicate setting can be overcome by pharmacologic doses of TRH. Increases in plasma T_4 and T_3 levels, as occur in hyperthyroidism, result in refractoriness of the pituitary to TRH administration. Even subclinical hyperthyroidism can reduce responsiveness to TRH.

NEURAL REGULATION OF TSH SECRETION

Hypothalamic Control

Hypothalamic input is essential to normal pituitary-thyroid function.[25, 27] Since disconnection of the pituitary from the hypothalamus by stalk section or transplantation decreases pituitary TSH secretion and results in hypothyroidism, it can be concluded that the hypothalamus tonically drives TSH secretion under basal conditions. Nearly normal TSH secretion continues in animals in which a hypothalamic island has been prepared by surgical isolation methods, indicating that only the hypophysiotrophic area is essential for maintaining basal secretion.[14] On the other hand, cold-induced thyroid activation is blocked in the deafferented preparation, indicating that there is control by remote sites as well (see below).

Effects of Hypothalamic Ablation

Lesions placed in the vicinity of the paraventricular nuclei of the rat result in marked decrease in pituitary-thyroid function without major effects on regulation of other pituitary hormones.[26] Although TSH levels are reduced in such animals, the system remains capable of a compensatory increase in TSH secretion following thyroidectomy. Rats with hypothalamic lesions are also more sensitive than intact controls to the feed-

205

back effects of small doses of T_4.[26, 36] These studies suggest that anterior hypothalamic lesions lower basal TRH secretion and modify, but do not prevent, qualitatively normal secretory responses to alterations in plasma thyroid hormone levels. The hypothalamus thus acts to determine the sensitivity of the pituitary to feedback inhibition, presumably by regulating the quantity of TRH which reaches the pituitary.

Additional evidence for the importance of the anterior hypothalamic-paraventricular region in TSH control has been shown by the effects of coronal hypothalamic cuts which separate this region from the arcuate nucleus-median eminence area. Such cuts also cause a decrease in TSH secretion. Recent immunoassay work indicates that destruction of the anterior hypothalamus leads to a two-thirds reduction in TRH content in the stalk-median eminence area, but the remaining hypothalamus contains some TRH.

TRH-producing neurons are distributed within the medial basal hypothalamus of the rat.[3, 20, 49] TRH-containing areas of the hypothalamus have been analyzed in detail by immunoassay of microdissected material (Fig. 6).[3] TRH is found throughout the classically defined hypophysiotrophic area, with the greatest concentrations in the periventricular areas. Little is found in the mammillary nucleus, and modest amounts in the medial preoptic area. These findings conform generally to earlier bioassay studies and to electrically excitable regions (see below).

Recent studies have localized TRH by immunohistochemical methods.[18] The highest concentration was present in nerve terminals of median eminence; a few scattered nerve cells containing TRH were noted in other brain regions. Anatomic and electrophysiologic studies support the concept that tuberohypophysial neurons are indeed located over this entire region, although restricted to the medial zone which extends 1.0 to 1.5 mm. on either side of the third ventricle (see Chapter 2).

Effects of Electric Stimulation

The TSH regulatory system of the hypothalamus has been identified by electric stimulation techniques in several species. For example, plasma TSH levels rise within five

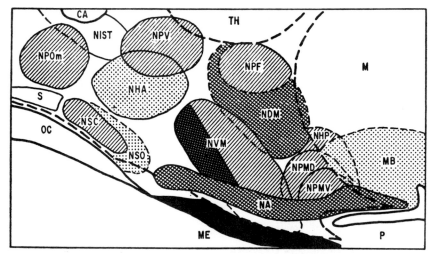

Figure 6. Distribution of TRH in hypothalamic nuclei. Individual punch biopsies of frozen sections (300 μ) of hypothalamus were assayed for TRH content by radioimmunoassay. TRH is widely distributed throughout hypothalamus. Greatest concentrations are shown in black, moderate in diagonal lines and cross-hatch, and least in stippled areas. (From Brownstein, M. J., et al.: *Thyrotropin-releasing hormone in specific nuclei of rat brain.* Science 185:267, 1974, with permission.)

minutes after hypothalamic stimulation in pentobarbital-anesthetized rats (Fig. 7).[28] The area from which positive responses can be obtained is extensive, including the anterior hypothalamus and preoptic area, the paraventricular nuclei, and the dorsomedial, ventromedial, and arcuate nuclei (Fig. 8). The largest responses in the rat occur with stimulation of the anterior hypothalamus in the vicinity of the paraventricular nuclei. Stimulation of the lateral hypothalamus, thalamus, and mammillary bodies is ineffective. The time course of TSH release induced by electric stimulation resembles that occurring after intravenous administration of synthetic TRH. In addition, either electrically-induced or TRH-induced TSH release is blocked by pretreatment with large doses of T_4 (see Fig. 7).[27, 28]

The localizations appear to be specific, since in parallel studies, GH secretory responses are strictly limited to the ventromedial and arcuate regions. These results correspond to the distribution of the respective releasing factor as determined by immunoassay or bioassay.

The similarity of the time course of TSH release following electric stimulation to that following TRH administration suggests that hypothalamic electric stimulation is effective by causing release of stored TRH. Wilber and Porter[47] reported that bioassayable TRH activity appears in the portal blood after electric stimulation of the anterior hypothalamus. Prior T_4 administration had no effect on this response, indicating that the action of T_4 is directly on the pituitary.

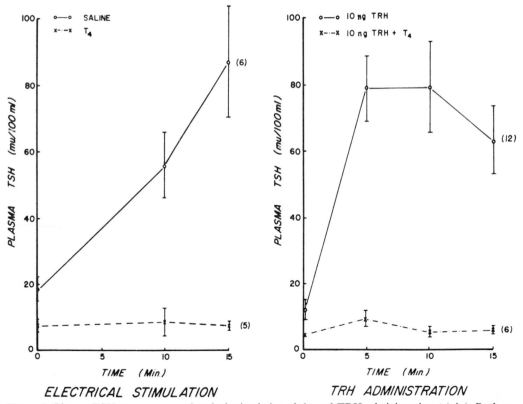

Figure 7. Plasma TSH responses to electrical stimulation *(left)* and TRH administration *(right)*. Both responses are blocked by prior administration of T_4. (From Martin, J. B. and Reichlin, S.: *Plasma thyrotropin (TSH) response to hypothalamic electrical stimulation and to injection of synthetic thyrotropin-releasing hormone.* Endocrinology 90:1079, 1972, with permission.)

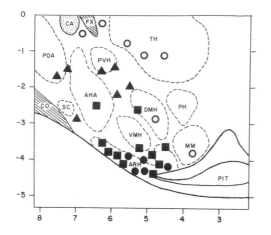

Figure 8. Hypothalamic sites that induced release of TSH after electric stimulation. Solid symbols indicate positive, and open circles negative, responses. The distribution of positive stimulation sites corresponds closely to distribution of TRH (see Fig. 5). (From Martin, J. B. and Reichlin, S.: *Plasma thyrotropin (TSH) response to hypothalamic electrical stimulation and to injection of synthetic thyrotropin-releasing hormone.* Endocrinology 90:1079, 1972, with permission.)

Hypothalamic Inhibition (Thyrotropin-Inhibiting Factor)

A number of stressful stimuli in the rat cause a rapid reduction in plasma TSH levels, a fall similar to that observed in GH in this species.[5] Although adrenal steroids may suppress TSH release by feedback action, it has been convincingly shown that TSH inhibition is independent of the pituitary-adrenal system.[6] Instead, it has seemed reasonable to propose that stress inhibited the tonic secretion of TRH. Several recent observations indicate that the hypothalamus may also exert a direct inhibitory effect on TSH release through a putative thyrotropin-inhibiting factor (TIF) analogous to the growth hormone-inhibiting factor, somatostatin. In the goldfish, tonic hypothalamic inhibition may be the primary mechanism of control.[32] Stalk section in this species causes *increased* TSH secretion and pituitaries from this species incubated in vitro show increased secretory activity resembling that observed in prolactin-producing cells of the mammalian pituitary explant. It was postulated that the hypothalamic inhibition is mediated by a TIF.

In the light of these speculations based on physiologic experiments, recent studies with somatostatin (growth hormone-inhibiting factor, GIF) are particularly relevant. This hypothalamic hormone, identified in 1973 by Guillemin and collaborators on the basis of its ability to inhibit GH secretion both in vitro and in vivo in a variety of assay preparations (see Chapter 7), has also been found to inhibit pituitary TSH secretion. This is true for pituitary cells grown in culture, for studies in the whole rat, and in the human. It is probable that there is a dual hypothalamic control for TSH regulation similar to that for prolactin and for growth hormone regulation. In rats, the TSH response to cold exposure is enhanced by pretreatment with antibody to somatostatin. It may be that somatostatin effects are observed after only certain forms of stress, that this hormone is responsible for stress inhibition of both TSH and GH, and that species differ in the relative importance of this hormone in TSH and GH regulation.

Extrahypothalamic Control

Considering the number of observations concerning the role of extrahypothalamic structures in GH, ACTH, and gonadotropin regulation, it is somewhat surprising that so little data are available with respect to the function of these structures in TSH control. Although the medial basal hypothalamus appears capable of maintaining basal

TSH secretion, phasic release of TSH, such as occurs in diurnal or circadian rhythms, stress-induced inhibition, and cold-induced release are probably mediated via extra-hypothalamic structures and inputs. In this section, evidence indicating a role for extra-hypothalamic structures in TSH secretion is considered.

Habenula and Pineal

Of extrahypothalamic structures, the function of the habenula in thyroid control has received the most attention, particularly by Szentagothai and colleagues.[41] Based on the effects of habenular lesions on thyroid responses to cold exposure, these workers postulated that the habenula functions in an indirect and primarily inhibitory manner, outside the primary thyroid-hormone feedback loop, to integrate neural homeostatic responses with hormonal needs. They proposed that these effects are mediated via the anterior hypothalamic thyrotropic area since lesions in this region of the hypothalamus blocked supranormal thyroid responses which occurred in habenula-lesioned rats. Earlier reports also implicated inhibitory effects of the habenula in thyroid control but there have been no recent reports to either confirm or deny the relevance of these observations. It is of interest that the major efferent pathway from the habenula is the fasciculus retroflexus, which terminates in the medial mesencephalic region (interpeduncular nucleus), an area which forms part of the midbrain limbic system and has important relays to the hypothalamus via the medial forebrain bundle. Thus, significant anatomic inputs do exist from the habenula to the hypothalamus. This problem merits further study.

Of equal uncertainty is the role of the pineal in TSH and thyroid control. Various measures of thyroid secretion have suggested a pineal influence, predominantly inhibitory, and perhaps mediated by melatonin. Thus, melatonin decreases thyroid weight and ^{131}I uptake and causes a reduction in thyroid secretory rate. On the other hand, pinealectomy is reported to cause thyroid hyperactivity in the tadpole and enhanced thyroid secretory rate in the rat. Relkin[37] reported the occurrence of a transient increase in plasma TSH levels during the first few days after pinealectomy in the rat. The mechanism of this transient elevation in TSH levels has not been demonstrated but it would appear to be of minimal physiologic significance since Rowe and collaborators[39] found no effect of pinealectomy on pituitary-thyroid function under a variety of lighting conditions.

Extrapyramidal and Limbic Structures

In 1962, Lupulescu and coworkers[24] reported that bilateral lesions of the globus pallidus and of the septal area cause increased thyroid activity as indicated by increased thyroid weight, ^{131}I uptake, and enhanced goitrogenic responses to propylthiouracil. Chiefetz[4] recently confirmed this finding and suggested that tonic inhibitory influences may arise from extrapyramidal structures.

The role of the limbic system in TSH control has not been adequately defined. It has been reported that electric stimulation of the hippocampal formation causes thyroid activation in the dog,[25] and increased TSH blood levels as measured by bioassay. Stimulation of the orbital frontal cortex and of the amygdaloid nuclear complex did not cause significant change in thyroid secretion. Lesions of the corticomedial amygdala cause thyroid atrophy and decreased plasma TSH.[25]

It is evident at this point that data on the role of extrahypothalamic structures in TSH control are fragmentary and inconclusive. It is interesting that both inhibitory and excitatory inputs have been suggested. However, until the precise role of these structures in pituitary-thyroid control has been more adequately defined, and until it has been clearly shown that none of the effects are secondary to changes in adrenal or other hormonal alterations, conclusions concerning the role of these structures must remain tentative.

OTHER FACTORS THAT AFFECT TSH SECRETION

Cold

In laboratory and domestic animals, exposure to cold is usually followed by thyroid activation. For example, exposure of the rat to a modest decline in ambient temperature usually causes a prompt, albeit transient, increase in plasma TSH.[27] Chronic exposure to cold is followed in most species by evidence of thyroid hypertrophy and increased secretion of thyroid hormone. In adult humans, on the other hand, it has been extremely difficult to demonstrate cold-induced thyroid activation.

Although it has been clearly demonstrated that TSH is essential for survival at lowered environmental temperatures in rats, it has not been established whether changes in thyroid secretion form an important homeostatic mechanism for regulation of metabolism during exposure to cold.[9] It is appropriate for the purpose of considering this literature to divide pituitary-thyroid responses into those which occur in response to acute exposure to cold and those which occur in response to chronic exposure to cold.

Acute Exposure to Cold

In the rat, acute exposure to cold causes an almost immediate burst of TSH release suggesting activation by a neuroendocrine reflex.[6, 27] Abrupt lowering of the ambient temperature by sudden introduction of cold air into a closed cage was shown to elicit a rise in immunoassayable plasma TSH levels within 5 to 10 minutes in unanesthetized rats bearing chronic indwelling jugular cannulas (Fig. 9). This TSH surge proved to be short-lived, with a return to baseline within 40 to 60 minutes. A similar rapid increase in plasma TSH levels, as measured by radioimmunoassay, was reported by Hershman and coworkers[17] in rats transferred to a 2° to 4° C room.

That acute-cold-exposure-induced TSH release is likely triggered by peripheral cold receptors is suggested by the finding that during acute exposure to cold, hypothalamus core temperature shows either no change or a slight rise. On the other hand, TSH release can also be induced by lowering of core temperature, indicating that inputs from either peripheral or central thermoreceptors may trigger TSH secretion.

Exposure of the newborn human infant to cold also elicits a rise in plasma TSH.[7] The effect may in part be due to peripheral circulatory adjustments, but cold-receptor reflexes also appear to play a role in the response.

Chronic Exposure to Cold

There is much less certainty concerning the role of the hypothalamic-pituitary-thyroid system in homeostatic responses to prolonged exposure to cold. The bulk of exper-

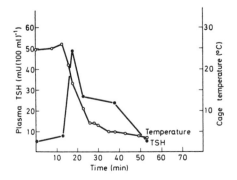

Figure 9. Plasma TSH response (●) to lowered environmental temperature (○) in the rat. Cold air introduced into the sampling cage resulted in a rapid fall in cage temperature which is associated with a prompt increase in circulating TSH. (From Martin, J. B. and Reichlin, S.: *Neural regulation of the pituitary-thyroid axis.* In *Proceedings of the Sixth Midwest Conference on the Thyroid and Endocrinology.* University of Missouri Press, 1970, with permission.)

iments performed in a number of species, including man, have in general failed to show any change in plasma T_4 levels (total or free) during chronic exposure to cold and, in fact, a fall in plasma thyroid-hormone levels has been noted in some studies.[25] It has been demonstrated repeatedly that TSH and thyroid gland secretion is increased during prolonged exposure to cold, despite the evidence of low or normal plasma T_4 in the rat. This response has been attributed to increased utilization, excretion, or degradation of T_4 as part of metabolic adaptation to cold which included increased food intake, and it has been proposed that it may be entirely secondary to a decrease in negative-feedback effects on TSH secretion resulting from falling plasma thyroid hormone levels.

The pituitary-thyroid component of adaptation to chronic cold is but one aspect of the larger homeostatic question as to how the thyroid hormones interact with the catecholamines in the regulation of thermogenesis. In the process of adaptation to chronic exposure to cold, activation of nonshivering thermogenesis plays a significant role. It is generally believed that the increased heat production in cold-adapted men and animals is mainly related to increased catecholamine secretion by both the adrenal medulla and the noradrenergic sympathetic nerve endings. At the target-tissue level, thyroid hormones probably interact to regulate oxygen consumption and heat production. It has now been shown that thyroidectomy leads to an increased catecholamine response to exposure to cold, and thyroxine administration leads to a decreased catecholamine response. These effects fit well the hypothesis of an integrated thyroid-catecholamine mechanism for heat production, increased catecholamine secretion in this instance serving as a compensation for thyroid insufficiency. Conversely, Martin and Reichlin[36] have shown that in animals deprived of sympathetic-adrenal medullary function by a combination of immunosympathectomy and adrenal demedullation, there is a greater increase in thyroid function after chronic exposure to cold than in normal animals.

Recent studies indicate that there is a higher plasma concentration of T_3 (but not of T_4) in cold-exposed animals. Since T_3 is more active metabolically, increased effective thyroid hormone action is likely in exposure to cold.[25] Based on current views of the origin of circulating T_3, one may postulate that the rate of peripheral conversion of T_4 to T_3 is increased in cold-adapted animals. In support of this idea is the demonstration that T_4 disappears from the circulation more rapidly in cold-adapted than in normal cold-exposed animals, and exposure to cold leads to increase in concentration of T_3-binding proteins in a number of parenchymal tissues including kidney and liver.

Final proof of hypothalamic-activated TSH release during chronic exposure to cold requires demonstration that TRH synthesis and secretion are enhanced. Increased TRH levels in the blood and urine have been reported in cold-exposed rats, but this finding has not been confirmed.

Stress

The effects of stress on pituitary-thyroid function have intrigued many generations of investigators.[5, 29] This concern is based in part on the traditional assumption that Graves' disease is a physical response to psychic stress, and in part on analogy with the effects of stress on the pituitary-adrenal system. The study of stress-induced changes in pituitary-thyroid function has produced ambiguous results. Stressful factors may alter hypothalamic-pituitary-thyroid function at many levels of control. These include altered TRH secretion, changes in responsiveness of the pituitary to TRH, altered metabolism of TSH, altered metabolism of the thyroid hormones in peripheral tissue, and alterations in the physical state of thyroid hormone-binding proteins in blood. Other hormones, such as those of the adrenal gland also may influence TSH secretion. Moreover, many types of stressful conditions are not as nonspecific as has been thought. For example, exposure to cold generally increases TSH secretion in small animals, but if the cold is intense enough, TSH secretion is inhibited, a finding generally attributed to the "nonspecific" component of cold stress.[5] Bacterial infection also has been regarded as a nonspecific stress, but recent work indicates that during a severe infection, such as pneumonia in man, the thyroid hormones disappear more rapidly from plasma, and T_4 is degraded more rapidly by leukocytes. The finding that plasma thyroid-hormone levels remain unchanged despite these changes in thyroid-hormone clearance suggests that there is a compensatory increase in pituitary thyroid-hormone secretion, possibly expressing operation of the negative-feedback control system.

Another example of the problem in identifying the site of disturbance when thyroid function is altered by stress is seen in patients suffering from chronic illness. The thyroid hormone-binding blood proteins are decreased in many patients with chronic wasting disease, while the concentration of free thyroxine is increased. Such patients have been shown by Sullivan and collaborators[44] to have a T_3 deficiency in both plasma and tissue, believed to be due to a defect in tissue conversion of T_4 to T_3. These observations emphasize that thyroid changes in stress cannot be simply attributed, without further consideration, to altered TRH secretion.

With these reservations, we can summarize certain observations about the effects of stress. In general, TSH secretion is inhibited during severe stress.[6] Thyroid hormone may be increased after acute stress in man, or after aversive conditioning in the rhesus monkey.[29] A few isolated reports have claimed that emotional stress in man is followed by increased pituitary-thyroid function.

Insulin-induced hypoglycemia also has been reported to cause release of TSH in man, although surgical procedures and electroshock therapy have no effect on pituitary-thyroid function other than the acute change in concentration attributable to blood-volume shifts.

Even if it could be shown that any form of stress increased pituitary-thyroid function, it would still be largely irrelevant to the problem of Graves' disease. With a few rare exceptions (see under Hypothalamic-Pituitary-Thyroid Disease), all patients with thyrotoxicosis have low, even unmeasurable, plasma levels of TSH. This finding has been confirmed using the specific immunoassay for the TSH β-chain. If stress factors play a role in the pathogenesis of Graves' disease, they do not operate through an increase of TSH secretion.

Hormones

A number of hormones other than those of the thyroid interact with the secretion of TSH in the human.

Glucocorticoids

Perhaps the most important nonthyroidal hormones involved in TSH regulation are glucocorticoids.[17] The earlier literature dealing with the effects of the adrenal cortex on thyroid function indicates that most aspects of pituitary-thyroid secretion are inhibited by adrenal corticoids. The advent of immunoassay has now made it possible to show that either brief or chronic exposure to excessively high levels of cortisol inhibits TSH secretion in man. The residual pituitary-thyroid activity observed in patients maximally suppressed with exogenous T_3 is further reduced by treatment with high doses of corticoids. Corticoids apparently act at two loci in bringing about this response. They appear to reduce the sensitivity of the pituitary to TRH, presumably by acting at the pituitary level, and under some circumstances probably act to reduce the secretion of TRH, as indicated in some experiments by the finding of unchanged pituitary sensitivity to TRH in cortisol-suppressed glands.

It is important to note that stress-induced TRH suppression is not mediated by concomitant activation of ACTH-adrenal secretion, since it is observed even in adrenalectomized animals maintained on a constant dose of glucocorticoid.[6]

Estrogenic Hormones

The high incidence of thyroid disease in women as compared with men (4:1 for multinodular goiter, 7:1 for Graves' disease, 9:1 for myxedema) has provoked inquiry as to differences in TSH secretory dynamics in relation to sex-hormone status. The early literature is complex and contradictory, partly because estrogenic hormones modify peripheral metabolism of the thyroid hormone, and partly because in the widely studied rodent model the estrogen doses usually administered cause inanition with secondary effects on thyroid function. From immunoassay work it appears that the basal levels of TSH do not differ among men, women, and prepubertal children.[17] On the other hand, the pituitary TSH secretory response to exogenous TRH is greater in women than in men.[15, 16] This effect may be due to estrogen sensitization, since pituitary responsiveness is greatest in that phase (late follicular) of the menstrual cycle associated with the highest levels of estradiol, and the response of the pituitary in men is enhanced by prior treatment with estrogenic hormone. This is probably due to a direct effect of estrogen on thyrotrope cells analogous to the sensitizing effects on the growth hormone and prolactin-releasing effects of hypothalamic extracts, and the LH release sensitizing responses to LHRH in women. The precise nature of the estrogen effect is unknown, nor is the estrogen effect on the pituitary necessarily related to the increased incidence of thyroid disorder in women. Little is known about the effects of progesterone and testosterone on pituitary-thyroid function.

Growth Hormone

Although it has been known for a long time that the synthesis and secretion of GH is affected markedly by the thyroid hormone, particularly in hypothyroidism, effects of GH on the secretion of TSH have only recently been recognized. In patients with hypopituitarism assumed to be of hypothalamic origin, the administration of GH in therapeutic amounts has been shown to cause hypothyroidism due to a decreased pituitary TSH responsiveness to TRH. This phenomenon may be partly responsible for the reduced TSH secretory responses to TRH observed in patients with acromegaly. To explain this finding it has been proposed that GH administration may bring about the release of somatostatin by a short-loop feedback mechanism. Somatostatin would then in turn inhibit pituitary responsiveness to TRH.

Drugs

Many drugs influence pituitary-thyroid function, most by altering peripheral metabolism of thyroid hormone or by changing the thyroid hormone-binding characteristics of plasma.[17, 35] Secondary changes then occur through activation of normal pituitary-thyroid feedback control. Examples of such phenomena are seen after treatment with phenobarbital, phenytoin, or chlorpromazine, drugs that induce microsomal changes in the liver leading to an increase in the rate of breakdown of T_4. Phenytoin, aspirin, and 2,3-dinitrophenol compete with T_4 for binding sites on T_4 binding globulin and cause an increase in plasma-free T_4 concentration. Compensatory decrease in TSH secretion is then required to maintain constancy of the free thyroid hormone level. The conversion of T_4 to T_3 in peripheral tissue is partially blocked by propylthiouracil, presumably by affecting a peripheral tissue monodeiodinase. Under carefully controlled conditions in hypothyroid patients maintained on constant T_4 replacement, this slight lowering of plasma T_3 is capable of increasing TSH secretory response to TRH.

Most drugs that alter pituitary-thyroid function do so by changing elements in the peripheral control system, as noted above, but some may act more directly on hypothalamic TSH control. Phenytoin which, in addition to its peripheral effects, brings about a decrease in free T_4 concentration, exerts an effect best attributed to a depression in TSH secretion. The site of action of phenytoin in this response is unknown. Morphine is also reported to decrease TSH secretion in man. In experimental animals, phenobarbital in anesthetic doses will cause a lowering of plasma TSH levels. Reserpine has also been reported to cause a decrease in plasma TSH,[36] a response attributed to interference with the central monoaminergic control of TRH excretion (see under Role of Monoamines).

THYROTROPIN-RELEASING HORMONE

As the first of the hypothalamic hormones to be chemically identified, synthesized, and administered to the human, the identification of thyrotropin-releasing hormone (TRH) has been a landmark in neuroendocrinology and has, in a sense, legitimized the entire field. That a thyrotropin hormone-releasing hormone existed was predicted by the studies of Harris and collaborators in the early 1950s, and the name TRH applied by Shibasawa and collaborators to material extracted from dog hypothalamus and human urine as early as 1959.[35] However, the claims of the Shibasawa group could not be substantiated, and acceptable proof of the TRH activity of hypothalamic extracts had to await the development of sensitive and specific assays, the first successful one of which was the preparation of Yamazaki and Guillemin. Others, developed shortly thereafter by Reichlin, by Schally and collaborators, and by Schreiber, led to the proof that the hypothalamus contained materials capable of releasing TSH from the pituitary, and that the effect was blocked by the administration of thyroid hormone.[30, 46] The laboratories of Guillemin and of Schally finally identified this material. The small amount of compound available, even after the extraction of literally hundreds of thousands of hypothalamic fragments, plus the unique structure of the compound led to a number of false starts; but, finally, the compound was found to be a tripeptide pyroglutamyl-histidyl-proline-amide of molecular weight 362 (Fig. 10).

The synthetic material has been shown to have all the biologic and chemical characteristics of the native material. Synthetic TRH is now widely available for both experimental and clinical use. TRH has been shown to be active in every mammalian species to which it has been administered. Hypothalamic fragments cultured in vitro are capable of synthesizing biologically active TRH from precursor amino acids.[31] This capability is demonstrated by ventral, dorsal, and anterior hypothalamic fragments but not by cortex.

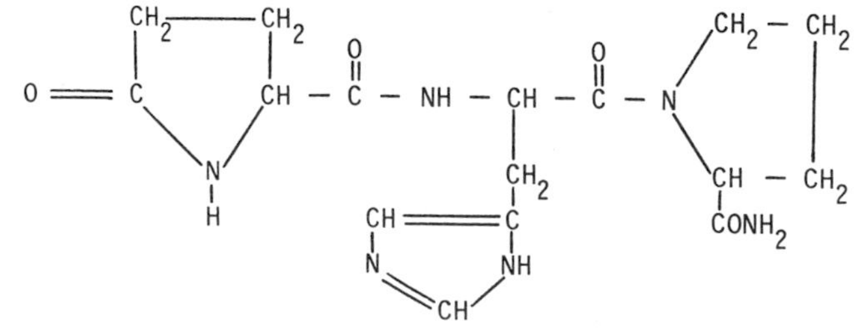

Figure 10. Structure of TRH.

Chemistry and Structure-Activity Relationships

A number of TRH analogues have been synthesized in an effort to delineate the structural requirements for activity, and to devise a molecule that would either be longer-acting or block TRH effects. The presence of both the pyroglutamic acid terminus and the terminal amide is crucial to the activity of the compound. Modifying groups added to either the N-terminus or the C-terminus markedly reduce activity.

As summarized by Wilber,[46] "the central histidine residue is a critical determinant of TRH activity. The TRH distereoisomeric analogue, in which the histidine residue is optically reversed to the D form, has only 3 per cent of the native potency, and photooxidation of the imidazole ring abolished TRH activity completely." All substituted derivatives of TRH have less activity than the parent compound except for the unique compound methylated on the 3 position of histidine, which has eight times the TSH-releasing potency of native TRH. Several analogues have recently been reported which block the effect of TRH. The most potent of these is cyclopentylcarbonyl-histidylpyrolidine.

Although it is reasonable to suppose that resistance to degradation might be a factor in longer activity of a given analogue, it appears that differences in activity are related primarily to differences in binding of the analogue to specific sites in pituitary cells.

Extrahypothalamic Distribution

On the basis of early physiologic study and bioassays, it was reasonable to assume that TRH would be demonstrated in the hypothalamus. This distribution has been confirmed by recently developed immunoassay methods.[1, 3, 20] Beyond the hypothalamic distribution, the introduction of immunoassay has permitted the study of extrahypothalamic TRH, and the phylogenetic aspects of TRH secretion.

Though low in concentration as compared with the hypothalamus, TRH in extrahypothalamic areas of the brain accounts for as much as 80 per cent of the total brain TRH.[20] It is present in rat spinal cord also. The pineal gland of the sheep, cow, and pig is said to contain large quantities of TRH, but only low levels are found in the rat pineal. After lesions of the "thyrotropic" area of the hypothalamus, there is slight or no reduction in cerebral cortical TRH concentration, suggesting that most (though not necessarily all) of the TRH in rat extrahypothalamic brain is not synthesized in the hypothalamus. Surgical isolation of the medial basal hypothalamus causes a lowering of median eminence TRH concentration.

Phylogenetic Distribution

When studied from a phylogenetic point of view, TRH proved to be widely distributed throughout the vertebrates and has even been found in prevertebrates, including the amphioxus, and an invertebrate, the snail.[20] TRH has been found in the hypothalami of chicks, snakes, frogs, tadpoles and salmon, the values being particularly high in amphibia where concentration in frogs may be 3,620 pg./mg. tissue, as compared with whole rat hypothalamus which contains 280 pg./mg. (Table 1). Substantial amounts of TRH are found in the neurohypophyses of rats and chickens, and the "pituitary complex" of lower vertebrates such as snakes and frogs, believed to be analogous to the medial eminence or neurohypophysis, contains large concentrations of TRH. In the larval lamprey, the pituitary contains at least 700 pg./mg. as compared with the whole brain tissue which contains 38 pg./mg. TRH has also been found in the neural ganglia of the snail. That this material is identical with pyro Glu-His-Pro NH_2 is evidenced by

Table 1. Distribution of TRH in Brain Areas of Several Species

Species	Hypothalamus (pg./mg.)	Cortex (pg./mg.)	Brain Stem (pg./mg.)
Rat	280	2	5
Chicken	41	2	9
Snake	564	338	283
Tadpole	947	447	303
Human	300		

(Adapted from Jackson, I. M. D. and Reichlin, S.: *Thyrotropin-releasing hormone (TRH): Distribution in hypothalamic and extrahypothalamic brain tissues of mammalian and submammalian chordates.* Endocrinology 95:854, 1974.)

identical inhibition curves in immunoassay, and by the demonstration of biologic TSH-releasing activity in material extracted from frog and salamander brain.

The functional significance of TRH in lower forms is a matter of conjecture. It is found in the lamprey which is believed to lack TSH, in the amphioxus which has no pituitary, and in ganglia of the snail which lacks any endocrine systems homologous with the vertebrate. It has been proposed by Jackson and Reichlin[20] that TRH is a primitive molecule, which has been "co-opted" by the pituitary for TSH secretory control. The function of TRH has been well shown in mammals, and also is capable of stimulating TSH release in birds. However, in the poikilotherms there is no evidence that TRH is a TSH-stimulating substance. TRH does not induce metamorphosis in frog tadpoles (which are sensitive to TSH or T_4), nor in the Mexican axolotl, and does not stimulate thyroid function in the lungfish.

The estimated half-life of circulating TRH in man is about four minutes. Approximately 15 per cent of injected TRH is rapidly excreted unchanged in the urine. TRH is rapidly inactivated in plasma by one or more heat-labile enzymes capable of splitting NH_2 from the terminal amide and of splitting other peptide bonds in the molecule.

Mechanisms of Action

TRH is effective when administered parenterally and is much less active when given orally. The effects of intravenous TRH are extremely rapid, causing increases in plasma TSH levels within one to two minutes in both man and animals (Fig. 11).[8, 13, 15, 16] This is in contrast to the negative-feedback effects of thyroid hormones on pituitary TSH secretion which require at least 15 minutes to develop in vitro and an even longer period in vivo.[36] The potency of TRH is indicated by the fact that estimations of the "multiplication factor" of TRH-induced TSH release are of the order of 1:100,000; i.e., a single molecule of TRH induces release of more than 100,000 molecules of TSH.[27]

TRH stimulatory effects appear to be the result of activation of cellular secretory processes initiated by attachment of the TRH molecule to specific membrane receptor sites on the thyrotrope cell.[11, 23] Such binding to the cell membrane occurs very rapidly and is reversible. The binding of TRH is not affected by simultaneous presence of other hormones, including LHRH, MIF, ADH, PRL, LH, glucagon, or the thyroid hormones T_4 and T_3.

The sequence of events that are set into motion by the attachment of TRH to the receptor sites appears to involve activation of the adenylate cyclase-cyclic AMP sys-

216

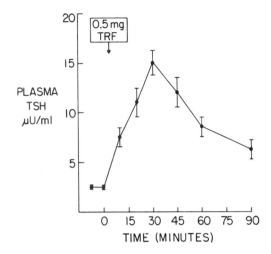

Figure 11. Plasma TSH response to 0.5 mg. TRF in normal subjects. The peak of the response occurs at 30 minutes (see also Fig. 5). (From Fleisher, N., et al.: *Synthetic thyrotropin, recent factors – a test of pituitary thyrotropin reserve.* J. Clin. Endocrinol. Metab. 34:617, 1972, with permission.)

tem. This effect was first reported by Wilber and Utiger[48] in 1968, and has since been confirmed by others. Prolonged pituitary stimulation by TRH apparently leads to increased TSH synthesis as well as release. TSH release in vitro is also stimulated by excessive potassium ions and appears to depend on calcium ions; membrane depolarization may also be important for the secretory process. Unlike the effects of thyroxine, TRH effects on release are not mediated by new protein synthesis.

Specificity of Action

It was shown early that TRH administration had no effect on plasma GH, FSH, LH, or cortisol. Following the development of sensitive radioimmunoassays for prolactin, it was observed that intravenous TRH also elicits prolactin release qualitatively and quantitatively like its stimulation of TSH release[40] (see Chapter 6). The significance of this observation is unclear, but it has been shown that TRH administration is associated with sufficient prolactin release to result in increased milk secretion. TRH administration also induces GH release in acromegaly, in chronic renal failure, and in some patients with depression. A small increase in plasma GH levels has also been observed after TRH in some normal subjects.

TRH in Body Fluids

Blood

TRH was initially detected in hypophysial-portal blood by bioassay.[47] More recently, TRH has been detectable by radioimmunoassay in the peripheral blood in man and in several lower forms including rat, frog, and chicken. Most work has been done with man and rat, and there are several conflicting estimates of TRH levels in plasma of these species. This is due, in part, to the rapid inactivation of TRH in the blood, and also to the low concentrations found. Values have been given ranging from unmeasurable to as high as 700 pg./ml. Estimates by indirect criteria (production rate and urinary secretion) suggest that normal values in the rat and man are less than 5 pg./ml. Because of uncertainty about significance of assays there is controversy about the effects of thyroid status and cold exposure on plasma TRH. Jackson and collaborators[21, 22] have cautioned that plasma levels should not necessarily be taken as a measure of TRH secretion rate, since peripheral turnover shows wide alterations in different thyroid functional states, the turnover being very rapid in hyperthyroidism and low in hypothyroidism.

In contrast to the situation in mammals where circulating TRH levels are quite low, we have found high values in chicken plasma (up to 300 pg./ml.), and in the leopard frog (but not bullfrog) the extraordinary level of 150 ng./ml. was demonstrated. This material releases TSH from rat pituitaries in vivo and is therefore active. The Mexican axolotl also has exceedingly high plasma TRH levels.

Urine

The first report of a TRH-like material in the urine of mammals was that by Shibusawa and associates in 1959.[35] However, subsequent studies by other workers using bioassays failed to confirm these findings. Following the development of radioimmunoassays, TRH was detected in urine of the rat and man.[21]

It should be emphasized that since TRH in the blood or urine probably comes from both hypothalamic and extrahypothalamic brain, it may not be possible to infer hypothalamic-TRH secretion rates from measurements of TRH in blood and urine. The estimation of the precise concentration of TRH in urine is still controversial because of technical problems in the radioimmunoassay.

Cerebrospinal Fluid

TRH has been reported in cerebrospinal fluid with levels ranging between 65 and 290 pg./ml. The relative importance of hypothalamic and extrahypothalamic sources of the TRH has not been determined.

Developmental Aspects

TRH is detectable in fetal rat brain as early as the thirteenth day of gestation. The brain content of TRH increases from 16 pg. at 14 days to 388 pg. at term (23 days), and over the first 10 days following birth rises sharply to adult levels. It is also reported that serum TRH rises markedly between the tenth and thirty-fifth days of postnatal life. In the human fetus, TRH is detectable as early as 4½ weeks after conception; the highest levels in human fetuses were in the hypothalamus, though significant levels were noted in the cerebellum also.

Effects on the Brain

A number of mild side effects are observed in volunteers given TRH by IV bolus injection. These include nausea, flushed feeling, an urge to urinate, taste in mouth, light-headedness, headache, and urge to defecate.[8, 15, 16] Transient mild hypertension is seen in a small fraction of cases. The site of action of the hormone in producing these effects is unknown, but in a single case it has been reported that the urge to urinate was present in a patient with paraplegia, anesthetic from the neck down. Therefore, TRH may act on the central neurons subserving urinary bladder sensations.

Chronic effects of TRH have been reported in patients with depression, a number of investigators claiming a relief of clinical symptoms, but most investigators find that TRH given either by injection or by mouth is without effect on depression symptoms. In the light of conflicting claims, this question cannot be resolved now. One unexplained aspect of studies of TRH in depression is that many patients have subnormal TSH and prolactin secretory responses and, paradoxically, in some studies an increase in plasma GH. This can be interpreted as indicating a pituitary abnormality associated with or due to the depressed state, the nature of which is still unknown. The possibility that this is due to abnormalities of a neurotransmitter control is suggested by the finding that in normals L-dopa inhibits pituitary responses to exogenous TRH as does the IV infusion of dopamine.

Wide distribution of TRH in brain, and evidence for its primitive phylogenetic appearance in the animal kingdom have raised the question whether TRH has functional significance in brain function. Several preliminary lines of evidence suggest that TRH has behavioral and electrophysiologic effects not explainable on the basis of its pituitary-stimulating effects. The most extensive studies of the behavioral effects of TRH in experimental animals have been carried out by Plotnikoff and associates.[33, 34] Administration of pargyline, a monoamine oxidase inhibitor, in combination with L-dopa, causes marked behavioral activation in the mouse. This response, which includes jumping, running, fighting, piloerection, salivation, and marked irritability, is enhanced by the administration of TRH. The TRH effects persist in thyroidectomized and hypophysectomized animals, indicating that TRH has direct stimulatory effects on brain. Large doses of TRH are reported to be tremorogenic, and this response is also mediated by direct effects on the brain, independent of pituitary. Since the doses in these experiments were large, it is difficult to assess the physiologic role of TRH in brain function. TRH in large doses was also reported to enhance cerebral norepinephrine turnover and to cause hypothermia.

Recent electrophysiologic studies indicate that TRH may have potent effects on electric activity of single neurons.[38] Microiontophoretic application of TRH on single hypothalamic neurons resulted in depression of firing in a certain population of cells (Fig. 12). The response in the hypothalamus, observed with small ejection currents, was closely entrained to the application of TRH, and normal cellular firing was restored within a few seconds after TRH application. Subsequent experiments have shown that a proportion of neurons in cerebral cortex, cerebellar cortex, and brain stem cuneate nucleus also are depressed by local application of TRH.

Further evidence supporting the hypothesis that TRH may act as a neurotransmitter or synaptic modulator includes the demonstration of localization in hypothalamic synaptosomes separated by centrifugation, histochemical localization in nerve endings in spinal cord as well as in the hypothalamus, the finding of specific TRH receptor binding sites in the brain, and the demonstration of specific enzymatic degrading systems in hypothalamic and whole brain extracts.

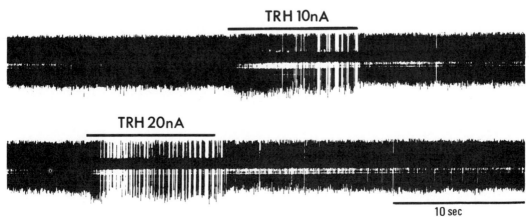

Figure 12. Effects of TRH applied by microiontophoresis on single neurons in the cerebellum. (Courtesy of L. P. Renaud.)

219

Role of Monoamines in Regulation of TRH Secretion

Extensive experimental observations support the hypothesis that central mono-amines (in particular, norepinephrine, dopamine, and serotonin) have important modu-lating effects on hypothalamic secretion of releasing and inhibiting factors for LH, FSH, prolactin, and GH; however, surprisingly few experimental studies have been reported on the effects of these substances on TRH release. Brown and coworkers[2] recently showed that the hypothalamic content of dopamine but not norepinephrine is affected by T_4 treatment.

A more direct approach to the problem of the role of monoamines in hypothalamic TRH synthesis and release has been to study release of pulse-labeled TRH from mouse hypothalamic tissue in vitro.[12] Dopamine and norepinephrine released TRH, and dopa-mine was ineffective when conversion of dopamine to norepinephrine was blocked with disulfiram (Fig. 13). Conversely, serotonin inhibited TRH release, and acetylcholine analogues had no effect. It was concluded from these experiments that catecholaminer-gic neurons or neurotransmitters may function in a regulatory manner to control syn-thesis or release of TRH. The suggestion that serotonergic pathways inhibit TRH se-cretion is further supported by the observation that injection of 5-hydroxytryptophan increases hypothalamic content of serotonin and inhibits TSH release (as well as stim-ulating prolactin release). That this effect is not due to serotonin-induced somato-statin release is shown by the finding that GH levels are unchanged and pituitary sen-sitivity to injected TRH is not altered.

L-dopa administration, which in man causes acute GH release, is not associated with any change in plasma TSH levels; on the contrary, chronic L-dopa administration is reported to interfere with TSH release induced by TRH, suggesting an effect of L-dopa at the pituitary level. This is of interest because L-dopa causes inhibition of pro-lactin secretion in vitro in the rat by direct effects on pituitary prolactin-producing cells. Recent studies suggest that this effect of L-dopa is related to dopamine, IV administra-tion of which has been shown to interfere with TSH release after TRH. In man, neither the administration of phentolamine (an α-adrenergic blocking agent) nor propranolol (a β-adrenergic blocker) has any effect on TRH-induced TSH secretion. In the rat, the TSH response to acute cold exposure is decreased by drugs that interfere with cate-

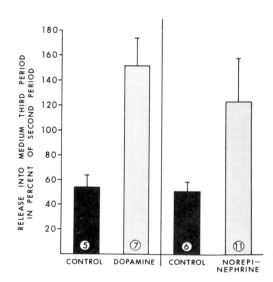

Figure 13. Effects of dopamine and norepinephrine on TRH release in vitro.

cholamine synthesis or action. L-dopa decreased the TSH response to cold, as did apomorphine, a drug that stimulates dopaminergic receptors.

Clinical Uses

The availability of TRH for clinical studies has already resulted in extensive documentation of its potential use in man. Many of the relevant observations have recently been summarized by Hershman and Pittmann.[17]

Normal Response to TRH

Intravenous administration of TRH in doses ranging from 10 to 500 pg. results in a rapid release of TSH with a peak response at 15 to 30 minutes.[8, 15, 17] This response is followed by marked increases in T_3 and marginal increases in T_4 two to four hours later. Women tend to have greater responses than men, an effect which appears to be due to estrogen (Fig. 14). Synthetic TRH is also effective when administered orally, but much larger doses are required. Several acute but minor side effects have been noted after rapid IV administration which do not occur with administration over a three- to five-minute interval. The most common are facial flushing, urinary urgency, and occasionally slight nausea. These are transient effects and no serious short-term or long-term consequences of TSH administration have been reported. Because about 15 per cent of cases develop a transient hypertension (up to 40 mm. diastolic and systolic), and a much smaller proportion have a slight decline in blood pressure, it is advised that the subject lie supine for 15 minutes after the test dose. The degree of the plasma TSH

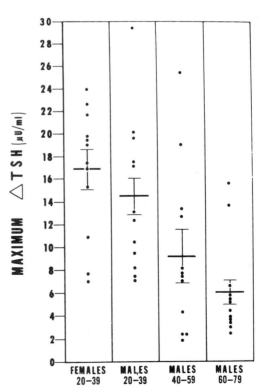

Figure 14. Mean increase in plasma TSH after administration of TRH. The response is greater in females than in males and declines in males with increasing age. (From Snyder, P. J. and Utiger, R. D.: *Response to thyrotropin releasing hormone.* J. Clin. Endocrinol. Metab. 34:380, 1972, with permission.)

response to TRH depends upon thyroid state, as might be predicted from the known interaction of TRH and thyroid hormones at the pituitary level.

Primary hypothyroidism results in an exaggerated TSH response in more than 70 per cent of cases.[8] Subjects with hyperthyroidism, on the other hand, show no, or a markedly attenuated, response in more that 99 per cent of cases (Fig. 15).[13] This suppression lasts for several weeks after adequate treatment of the hyperthyroid state. Even minor degrees of hyperthyroidism will block pituitary response. Many patients with "euthyroid" Graves' disease, for example, also fail to respond to exogenous TRH, presumably because their thyroid function is above the upper limit of normal. It is in the evaluation of mild degrees of thyrotoxicosis that TRH testing has achieved its greatest practical utility. It can be confidently assumed that preservation of TSH responsiveness to TRH will exclude the diagnosis of thyrotoxicosis in 95 per cent of patients.

Administration of TRH has provided a valuable tool for the assessment of TSH secretory reserve in hypothalamic-pituitary disorders. Details of the testing procedure and standards for normal and abnormal patients are given in Chapter 15. It would be anticipated that patients with TSH deficiency due to intrinsic pituitary disease would not respond to TRH, whereas patients with TSH deficiency due to hypothalamic failure would be responsive. This generalization has proved true in some groups of patients, as in children with idiopathic hypopituitarism, but there is a degree of overlap of responses in hypothalamic-pituitary syndromes, and some normal individuals may have quite low TSH secretory responses to TRH without evident pituitary disease. An appreciable number of normals (as much as 15 per cent), particularly older men, have TSH responses to TRH of only 2 or 3 μU. TSH/ml., which is in the same range of response as patients with intrinsic pituitary disease. For this reason, preservation of TSH

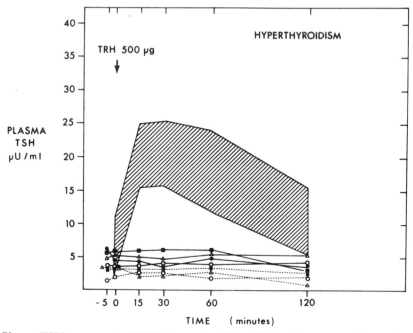

Figure 15. Plasma TSH response to TRH in hyperthyroidism. Each of the seven patients shows failure to release TSH. The shaded area represents the range of responses in a group of normal subjects. (Modified from Gual, C., et al.: *Administration of thyrotropin release hormone (TRH) as a clinical test for pituitary thyrotropin reserve.* Revista de Investagacion Clinica 24:35, 1972.)

Table 2. Factors that Influence TRH-Induced TSH Release

Factors That Increase	Factors That Decrease
1. Sex—greater response in females (during luteal phase of cycle) 2. Hypothyroidism 3. Estrogen Administration to Men 4. Renal Failure	1. Age—decreased response in elderly 2. Hyperthyroidism 3. Euthyroid Graves Disease 4. L-dopa 5. Bromergocryptine 6. Adrenal Steroids—Cushing's Disease 7. Somatostatin

responsiveness in the so-called normal range is not absolute proof of intrinsic pituitary normality. Detailed testing procedures are still under investigation, but at this time, diagnosis of hypothalamic hypothyroidism on the basis of retained TRH responsiveness alone is insufficient. One must consider the entire clinical picture in making this diagnosis. On the other hand, persistent failure of pituitary response in the presence of hypothyroidism is almost certain evidence of intrinsic pituitary failure.

A number of other factors in the plasma TSH response to TRH are summarized in Table 2.

HYPOTHALAMIC-PITUITARY-THYROID DISEASE

Modifications in TSH secretion observed in clinical disease of the pituitary and thyroid generally conform to predictions based on classic formulations of pituitary-thyroid negative-feedback regulation, with a few paradoxic exceptions.

Primary Hypothyroidism

Effects of long-standing thyroid insufficiency on the pituitary were recognized long before the modern concept of pituitary-thyroid feedback or even the understanding of the function of the thyroid gland was developed. Nièpce, in 1847, reported the finding of an enlarged pituitary gland in patients dying with cretinism.[35] More recently, a number of authors have drawn attention to the fact that enlargement of the pituitary fossa may occur in long-standing hypothyroidism, so much so that a patient may appear on superficial study to have a tumor of the pituitary with secondary thyroid failure. The syndrome of primary hypothyroidism, TSH hypersecretion, and pituitary enlargement must be borne in mind in differential diagnosis of pituitary tumor. It has been suggested that pituitary TSH-secreting tumors may rarely arise in man secondary to prolonged hypothyroidism. Such a phenomenon is frequently observed in the hypothyroid mouse (Furth thyrotropic tumor).

All primary diseases of the thyroid gland with thyroid failure usually cause an increase in plasma TSH levels. This is true after thyroidectomy, thyroiditis, and treatment with radioactive iodine. Incipient or subclinical thyroid failure, seen, for example, during the evolution of Hashimoto's disease or postradiation thyroiditis, may be followed by an increase in plasma TSH, and is accentuated when thyroid secretion is reduced further by administration of inorganic iodide in therapeutic doses. Even in normal individuals, the slight lowering of plasma TH caused by iodide administration may sensitize the pituitary to TRH. In patients with marginal thyroid-secretion defects, plasma TSH levels may be elevated disproportionately in relationship to the thyroid-hormone level, suggesting a compensatory stage of thyroid failure in which adequate thyroid function is maintained only by TSH hypersecretion. This phenomenon may

223

account for the disproportionate elevation in TSH levels in thyrotoxic patents after treatment.

Secondary Hypothyroidism

Failure of pituitary TSH secretion causes secondary hypothyroidism. As predicted from the concept of negative-feedback control of the pituitary-thyroid axis, most such patients have low or unmeasurable TSH levels in blood, and usually do not respond to TRH injection (Fig. 16).[8] A few patients with established pituitary lesions demonstrate an exaggerated response to TRH. It is proposed that in such cases both suprasellar and pituitary involvement has led to a reduction in TRH, as well as to thyrotrope-cell damage, but this has not been proved. Euthyroid acromegalic patients frequently fail to show a normal TSH response to TRH. Whether this is a pituitary-depressing effect of high circulating levels of GH or is due to pituitary destruction (or both) has not been determined.

Paradoxically, a few patients with pituitary lesions and hypothyroidism have been found to have TSH in the blood within the normal or even high range. A rational explanation of this phenomenon is not available.

Hypothalamic Hypothyroidism (Tertiary Hypothyroidism)

The introduction of TRH into clinical medicine made it possible to evaluate pituitary secretory reserve in hypothyroid patients with low plasma TSH levels, commonly considered to be due to pituitary insufficiency. A number of patients with secondary hypothyroidism ("thyrotropic failure") have now been shown to have normal or even supranormal responses to exogenous TRH (Fig. 17). Since the pituitary can function normally in these individuals, it has been inferred that the defect is due to failure of stimulation by the hypothalamus.

The importance of hypothalamic hypothyroidism as a cause of thyrotropin failure depends upon the population studied. The majority of children suffering from "idiopathic" partial or total hypopituitarism have TRH-responsive pituitaries. This impor-

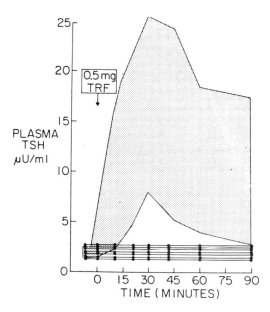

Figure 16. Absence of TSH response to TRF in patients with panhypopituitarism secondary to pituitary infarction (Sheehan's syndrome). The shaded area represents the range of responses in a group of normal subjects. (From Fleisher, N., et al.: *Synthetic thyrotropin, recent factors — a test of pituitary thyrotropin reserve.* J. Clin. Endocrinol. Metab. 34:617, 1972, with permission.)

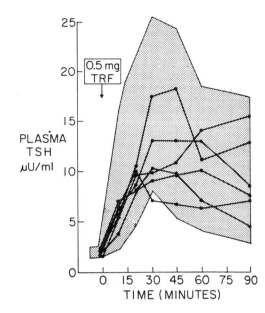

Figure 17. Normal plasma TSH response to TRF in six patients with idiopathic panhypopituitarism. The finding of TSH release to TRF implicates the hypothalamus as the cause of TSH insufficiency due to endogenous TRF deficiency. The shaded area represents the range of responses in a group of normal subjects. (From Fleisher, N., et al.: *Synthetic thyrotropin, recent factors—a test of pituitary thyrotropin reserve.* J. Clin. Endocrinol. Metab. 34:617, 1972, with permission.)

tant observation indicates that idiopathic dwarfism is due in most instances to an intrinsic hypothalamic disorder.

In sporadic cases of "hypothalamic hypothyroidism," hypothalamic failure may be due to hypothalamic tumors, inflammation, pituitary stalk section, rarely in Sheehan's syndrome (then attributed to hypothalamic or stalk infarction), and also occasionally either as a single defect or in association with other pituitary defects. Autopsy findings in the latter group of patients have not been reported. It may be anticipated that a group of such cases will prove to have hypophysiotrophic neuron failure analogous to the atrophy of the supraoptic-hypophysial neurons seen in human cases of idiopathic diabetes insipidus. Although infrequent, such isolated cases have been reported from many clinics. For example, Gantt, of Abbott Laboratories, has collected 35 cases of the syndrome from scientists conducting clinical evaluations of TRH.

Most patients with hypothalamic disease of various types have shown normal or exaggerated TSH responses to administration of TRH, indicating that the primary pathophysiologic mechanism may be a failure to synthesize or release endogenous TRH. It was proposed at one time that hypothalamic hypothyroid patients characteristically showed a delayed peak response (and thus resemble patients with primary hypothyroidism), but in the series reported by Snyder and Utiger,[43] several patients with presumed intrinsic pituitary disease showed a delayed response to TRH. Multiple injections of TRH may correct hyporesponsiveness due to TRH deficiency, but it should be pointed out in a cautionary way that similar results could theoretically be obtained by repeated stimulation of a small number of residual pituitary cells. Criteria for the diagnosis of hypothalamic hypothyroidism are: 1) low thyroid function, 2) inappropriately low or undetectable plasma TSH levels, and 3) a normal or exaggerated response to exogenous TRH. As noted above, a few patients with intrinsic pituitary disease may show TSH responses in the low normal range, and for this reason, the criteria listed above cannot be taken as absolutely diagnostic. The full clinical picture must be considered.

An apparent exception to the rule that TSH secretion is dependent upon an intact hypothalamus is the finding of normal pituitary-thyroid function in anencephalic infants. Recently it has been shown that the minimal brain tissue found in such infants synthesizes TRH when grown in tissue culture, a finding that suggests that some TRH has been available to the developing pituitary.

Isolated thyrotropin deficiency with TRH unresponsiveness has been reported, suggesting that, rarely, there may be a true failure of thyrotropes to develop.

Hyperthyroidism

With a few rare exceptions (discussed below), hyperthyroidism is due to overactivity of the thyroid gland and TSH secretion is inhibited, as is the response to TRH (see Fig. 15). This observation gives overwhelming evidence that Graves' disease is not caused by TSH hypersecretion.

However, a few cases have been reported in which TSH levels were elevated.[10] They differ in the extent to which the secretion of TSH is suppressible by exogenous thyroid hormones. In one patient, a young adolescent with a large goiter and severe hyperthyroidism, the pituitary responded to TRH despite the high levels of circulating T_3 and T_4. Increasingly large amounts of T_3 caused increasing suppression of TRH responsiveness and of thyroid function. It seems highly likely that this case represents a defect in the thyroid feedback-control loop at the pituitary level, leading to an altered control setpoint. In this respect, the disorder is analogous to Cushing's disease in which ACTH hypersecretion is due to an altered control-feedback loop of the pituitary-adrenal axis.

It has also been postulated that TRH hypersecretion might be responsible for TSH hypersecretion, but in the absence of specific measurements of TRH, this hypothesis is only conjectural. Moreover, thyrotoxicosis has not been reported to follow prolonged TRH administration, and it is not certain that this can happen if feedback inhibitory control is normal.

Pituitary Tumors and TSH Secretion

A few reports of primary pituitary adenomas that secrete excessive TSH have appeared, but these are extremely rare. The combination of a pituitary tumor and hyperthyroidism is not sufficient to make this diagnosis, since in most such instances the hyperthyroidism is likely secondary to Graves' disease or autonomous nodular goiter. The demonstration of hyperthyroidism in combination with elevated TSH levels in plasma is essential for this diagnosis.

To reiterate, it must be remembered that excessive TSH secretion secondary to *primary* hypothyroidism may lead to marked hypertrophy of the pituitary, with enlargement of the sella turcica resembling a tumor. In this case, the elevation of plasma TSH levels in combination with *hypo*thyroidism provides the clue to the underlying pathophysiology.

REFERENCES

1. BASSIRI, R. M. AND UTIGER, R. D.: *The preparation and specificity of antibody to thyrotopin releasing hormone.* Endocrinology 90:722, 1972.

2. BROWN, G. M., ET AL.: *Relationship between hypothalamic and median eminence catecholamines and thyroid function.* Neuroendocrinology 10:207, 1972.

3. BROWNSTEIN, M. J., ET AL.: *Thyrotropin-releasing hormone in specific nuclei of rat brain.* Science 185: 267, 1974.

4. CHEIFETZ, P. N.: *Effect of lesions in the globus pallidus upon thyroid function.* J. Endocrinol. 43:36, 1969.

5. DEWHURST, K. E., EL-KABIR, D. J. AND HARRIS, G. W.: *A review of the effect of stress on the activity of the central nervous-pituitary-thyroid axis in animals and man.* Confin. Neurol. 30:161, 1968.

6. DUPONT, A., ET AL.: *Effect of hippocampal stimulation on the plasma thyrotropin (TSH) and corticosterone responses to acute cold exposure in the rat.* Can. J. Physiol. Pharmacol. 50:364, 1972.

7. FISHER, D. A. AND ODELL, W. D.: *Effect of cold on TSH secretion in man.* J. Clin. Endocrinol. Metab. 33:859, 1971.

8. FLEISHER, N., ET AL.: *Synthetic thyrotropin releasing factor as a test of pituitary thyrotropin reserve.* J. Clin. Endocrinol. Metab. 34:617, 1972.

9. GALE, C. C.: *Neuroendocrine aspects of thermoregulation.* Annu. Rev. Physiol. 35:391, 1973.

10. GERSHENGORN, M. C. AND WEINTRAUB, B. D.: *Thyrotropin-induced hyperthyroidism caused by selective pituitary resistance to thyroid hormone: A new syndrome.* J. Clin. Invest. 56:633, 1975.

11. GRANT, G., ET AL.: *Interaction of thyrotropin-releasing factor with membrane receptors of pituitary cells.* Biochem. Biophys. Res. Commun. 46:28, 1972.

12. GRIMM, Y. AND REICHLIN, S.: *Thyrotropin-releasing hormone (TRH): Neurotransmitter regulation of secretion by mouse hypothalamic tissue in vitro.* Endocrinology 93:626, 1973.

13. GUAL, C., ET AL.: *Administration of thyrotropin release hormone (TRH) as a clinical test for pituitary thyrotropin reserve.* Revista de Investigacion Clinica 24:35, 1972.

14. HALASZ, B., ET AL.: *Thyrotrophic hormone secretion in rats after partial or total interruption of neural afferents to the median basal hypothalamus.* Endocrinology 80:1075, 1967.

15. HALL, R., ET AL.: *Thyroid stimulating hormone response to synthetic thyrotrophic releasing hormone in man.* Br. Med. J. 2:274, 1970.

16. HALL, R., ET AL.: *The thyrotropin-releasing hormone test in diseases of the pituitary and hypothalamus.* Lancet 1:759, 1972.

17. HERSHMAN, J. M. AND PITTMANN, J. A., JR.: *Control of thyrotropin secretion in man.* N. Engl. J. Med. 285:997, 1971.

18. HOKFELT, T., ET AL.: *Distribution of thyrotropin-releasing hormone (TRH) in the central nervous system as revealed with immunocytochemistry.* Eur. J. Pharmacol. 34:389, 1975.

19. HOSKINS, R. G.: *The thyroid-pituitary apparatus as a servo (feedback) mechanism.* J. Clin. Endocrinol. 9:1429, 1949.

20. JACKSON, I. M. D. AND REICHLIN, S.: *Thyrotropin-releasing hormone (TRH): Distribution in hypothalamic and extrahypothalamic brain tissues of mammalian and submammalian chordates.* Endocrinology 95:854, 1974.

21. JACKSON, I. M. D., ET AL.: *Pituitary, hypothalamic and urinary thyrotropin releasing hormone (TRH) concentration in altered thyroid states in rat and man.* Clin. Res. 22:342a, 1974.

22. JACKSON, I. M. D., ET AL.: *TRH excretion and metabolism in man.* Clin. Res. 23:238a, 1975.

23. LABRIE, F., ET AL.: *Binding of thyrotropin-releasing hormone to plasma membranes of bovine anterior pituitary gland.* Proc. Nat. Acad. Sci. U.S.A. 69:283, 1972.

24. LUPULESCU, A., ET AL.: *Neural control of the thyroid gland: studies of the role of extrapyramidal and rhinencephalon areas in the development of goiter.* Endocrinology 70:517, 1962.

25. MARTIN, J. B.: *Regulation of the pituitary-thyroid axis.* In McCann, S. M. (ed.): *Endocrine Physiology.* M.T.P. International Review of Science, Physiol. Ser. 1, vol. 5. Butterworth, London, 1974, 67.

26. MARTIN, J. B., ET AL.: *Feedback regulation of TSH secretion in rats with hypothalamic lesions.* Endocrinology 87:1032, 1970.

27. MARTIN, J. B. AND REICHLIN, S.: *Neural regulation of the pituitary-thyroid axis.* In Kenny, A. D. and Anderson, R. R. (eds.): *Proceedings of the Sixth Midwest Conference on the Thyroid.* University of Columbia Press, Columbia, Missouri, 1970, p. 1.

28. MARTIN, J. B. AND REICHLIN, S.: *Plasma thyrotropin (TSH) response to hypothalamic electrical stimulation and to injection of synthetic thyrotropin-releasing hormone (TRH).* Endocrinology 90:1079, 1972.

29. MASON, J. W.: *A review of psychoendocrine research on the pituitary-thyroid system.* Psychosom. Med. 30:666, 1968.

30. MEITES, J.: *Hypophysiotropic Hormones of the Hypothalamus: Assay and Chemistry.* Williams & Wilkins, Baltimore, 1970.

31. MITNICK, M. AND REICHLIN, S.: *Thyrotropin-releasing hormone: Biosynthesis by rat hypothalamic fragments in vitro.* Science 172:1241, 1971.

32. PETER, R. E.: *Feedback effects of thyroxine on the hypothalamus and pituitary of goldfish, Carassius auratus.* J. Endocrinol. 51:31, 1971.

33. PLOTNIKOFF, N. P., ET AL.: *Thyrotropin releasing hormone: Enhancement of DOPA activity by a hypothalamic hormone.* Science 178:417, 1972.

34. PLOTNIKOFF, N. P., ET AL.: *Thyrotropin releasing hormone: Enhancement of DOPA activity in thyroid-ectomized rats.* Life Sci. 14:1271, 1974.

35. REICHLIN, S.: *Control of thyrotropin hormone secretion. In* Martini, L. and Ganong, W. (eds.): *Neuroendocrinology,* vol. 1. Academic Press, New York, 1966, p. 445.

36. REICHLIN, S., ET AL.: *The hypothalamus in pituitary-thyroid regulation.* Recent Prog. Horm. Res. 28: 229, 1972.

37. RELKIN, R.: *Effects of pinealectomy and constant light and darkness on thyrotropin levels in pituitary and plasma of rat.* Neuroendocrinology 10:46, 1972.

38. RENAUD, L. P. AND MARTIN, J. B.: *Thyrotropin releasing hormone (TRH): Depressant action of central neuronal activity.* Brain Res. 86:150, 1972.

39. ROWE, J. W., ET AL.: *Relation of the pituitary gland and environmental lighting to thyroid function in the rat.* Neuroendocrinology 6:247, 1970.

40. SACHSON, R., ET AL.: *Prolactin stimulation by thyrotropin releasing hormone in a patient with isolated thyrotropin deficiency.* N. Engl. J. Med. 287:972, 1972.

41. SZENTAGOTHAI, J., ET AL.: *Hypothalamic Control of the Anterior Pituitary.* Akademiai Kiado, Budapest, 1968.

42. SNYDER, P. J. AND UTIGER, R. D.: *Inhibition of thyrotropin response to thyrotropin-releasing hormone by small quantities of thyroid hormones.* J. Clin. Invest. 51:2077, 1972.

43. SNYDER, P. J. AND UTIGER, R. D.: *Response to thyrotropin releasing hormone.* J. Clin. Endocrinol. Metab. 34:380, 1972.

44. SULLIVAN, P. R., BOLLINGER, J. A. AND REICHLIN, S.: *Selective deficiency of tissue triiodothyronine: A proposed mechanism of elevated free thyroxine in the euthyroid sick.* J. Clin. Invest. 52:83a, 1973.

45. VANHAELST, L., ET AL.: *Circadian variations of serum thyrotropin levels in man.* J. Clin. Endocrinol. Metab. 35:479, 1972.

46. WILBER, J. F.: *Thyrotropin releasing hormone: Secretion and actions.* Annu. Rev. Med. 24:353, 1973.

47. WILBER, J. F. AND PORTER, J. C.: *Thyrotropin and growth hormone releasing activity in hypophysial portal blood.* Endocrinology 87:807, 1970.

48. WILBER, J. F. AND UTIGER, R. D.: *In vitro studies on mechanism of action of thyrotropin releasing factor.* Proc. Soc. Exp. Biol. Med. 127:488, 1968.

49. WINOKUR, A. AND UTIGER, R. D.: *Thyrotropin-releasing hormone: Regional distribution in rat brain.* Science 185:265, 1974.

BIBLIOGRAPHY

BROWN-GRANT, K.: *The control of TSH secretion. In* Harris, G. W. and Donovan, B. T. (eds.): *The Pituitary Gland,* vol. 2, Butterworth, London, 1966, p. 235.

DEWHURST, K. E., EL-KABIR, D. J. AND HARRIS, G. W.: *A review of the effect of stress on the activity of the central nervous-pituitary-thyroid axis in animals and man.* Confin. Neurol. 30:161, 1968.

HARRIS, G. W. AND GEORGE, R.: *Neurohumoral control of the adenohypophysis and the regulation of the secretion of TSH, ACTH and growth hormone. In* Haymaker, W., Anderson, E. and Nauta, W. J. H. (eds.): *The Hypothalamus.* Charles C Thomas, Springfield, p. 326, 1969.

HERSHMAN, J. M. AND PITTMANN, J. A., JR.: *Control of thryotropin secretion in man.* N. Engl. J. Med. 285: 997, 1971.

MARTIN, J. B.: *Regulation of the pituitary-thyroid axis. In* McCann, S. M. (ed.): *Endocrine Physiology.* M.T.P. *International Review of Science, Physiol. Ser. 1, vol. 5,* Butterworth, London, 1974, p. 67.

REICHLIN, S.: *Control of thyrotropin hormone secretion. In* Martini, L. and Ganong, W. (eds.): *Neuroendocrinology,* vol. 1. Academic Press, New York, 1966, p. 445.

REICHLIN, S., ET AL.: *The hypothalamus in pituitary-thyroid regulation.* Recent Prog. Horm. Res. 28:229, 1972.

CHAPTER 10

The Pineal Gland
and Periventricular Organs

Although readily overlooked in dissections of the brain because of its small size (100 to 150 mg.) and its relatively inaccessible position (attached to the posterior roof of the third ventricle, under the corpus callosum), the pineal gland (Latin *pinea,* pine cone) has been recognized for many centuries and its function has been the subject of much speculation. Galen believed that it served as a valve controlling thoughts flowing in the brain ventricles, and Descartes, quite reasonably "observing that the pineal gland is the only part of the brain that is single was determined by this to make that gland the soul's habitation." The function of the pineal gland in man is still unknown, but the vast amount of recent research on the pineal gland in lower mammals makes it virtually certain that it plays a role in neuroendocrine control of the pituitary gland, and may be involved in determination of body functions that are marked by circadian rhythms. In this chapter, the evidence relating the pineal gland to neuroendocrine function in the human is reviewed, and pineal function as known from the experimental literature is summarized.

ANATOMY AND DEVELOPMENT

The pineal gland of man and other vertebrates arises from modified ependymal cells of the epithalamic region of the third ventricle as one of a family of periventricular (or circumventricular) secretory organs which includes the subcommissural organ, the area postrema, the subfornical organ and the median eminence and neurohypophysis.[24, 25, 72] In lower animals (amphibians and certain fishes), the pineal cells have characteristics of photoreceptors, displaying photosensitivity and electric activity suggestive of a "third eye;"[26] in higher vertebrates, the eye-like features of the pineal gland give way to the glandular-secretory characteristics of the pineal cell (pinealocyte), and the primitive afferent nerve connections which are analogous to an optic nerve are lost.[24, 25] Instead, a new efferent (sympathetic secretomotor) nerve supply reaches the pineal gland from the superior cervical ganglia by way of paired nervi conarii, which penetrate the dome of the organ from the tentorium of the cerebellum. Additional sympathetic innervation also may reach the pineal gland within the walls of the veins of the region. There is also evidence that a parasympathetic innervation of unknown significance arises in the greater superficial petrosal nerves.

Despite the fact that the pineal gland is connected by a cord-like stalk to the apex of the epithalamus, there is no direct nerve supply from brain to pineal gland, nor does there appear to be a channel, either real or potential, for pineal secretion into the third ventricle.[24, 25] For this reason, most investigators believe that pineal secretions which alter hypothalamic function do so after entry into the general circulation or into the cerebrospinal fluid (CSF) of the subarachnoid space which surrounds the pineal gland, although some believe that the possibility of direct entry into the third-ventricle CSF has not been fully excluded.[52]

The human pineal gland is about 7 mm. long, 5 mm. wide, and 4 mm. thick. It lies under the posterior portion of the corpus callosum, nestled between the superior colliculi. The gland is invested in pia mater, and its blood supply arises from vessels of the adjacent choroid plexus. The substance of the gland is solid, and divided into lobules by richly vascular connective tissue septa that contain the unmyelinated postganglionic sympathetic nerve fibers.[75] Blood flow in relation to the mass of tissue is very high, exceeding that of most endocrine glands. Pineal circulation, like that of the other circumventricular organs, lacks a blood-brain barrier so that vital dyes and heavy metals enter freely from the circulation. The pineal gland does not contain a portal vasculature like that of the anterior pituitary.

The predominant cell type, the pinealocyte, differs from typical neurons or glia.[5] It has secretory properties and receives a direct innervation from club endings of the sympathetic neurons which form recognizable synapses on the pinealocyte (Fig. 1). The pinealocyte has one or more processes of variable length, a configuration adapted for secretory function, as shown by ultrastructure studies. The club endings of these processes terminate close to the perivascular space, surrounding capillaries that have fenestrations typical of endocrine glands. Other nerve endings are found in the perivascular space.

The other major cell type in the pineal gland, the glial cell, morphologically resembles

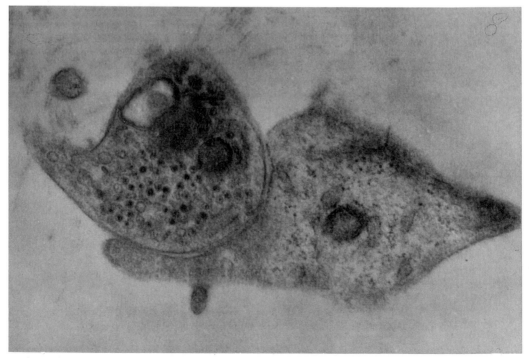

Figure 1. Electron photomicrograph showing synapse of noradrenergic nerve terminal on pinealocyte. (From Wurtman, R. J., et al.: *The Pineal.* Academic Press, New York, 1968, p. 126, with permission.)

an astrocyte.[5, 63] A functional relationship between glial and parenchymal cells has not been established.

NEURAL REGULATION OF PINEAL SECRETION

Impulses carried by the sympathetic nerve supply to the pineal gland are modified by changes in light and dark in the external environment. Although not established for the human, in rodents a nonvisual optic pathway (the inferior accessory optic tract) exists.[35] This arises in the retina, is entirely crossed in the optic chiasm (unlike the visual pathway), and passes via the suprachiasmatic nucleus and the medial forebrain bundle of the hypothalamus to terminate in the nuclei of the inferior accessory tract which are located immediately ventral to the medial geniculate nuclei (Fig. 2). The neural pathway beyond this point by which connections are made to influence sympathetic outflow is unknown.

The best known of the pineal secretions are the biogenic amines serotonin, norepinephrine, and melatonin.[49] Melatonin, like serotonin, belongs to a class of indolealkylamines, and others, such as 5-hydroxytryptophol, may be as important as the better-known melatonin. The pineal gland contains significant concentrations of each of the

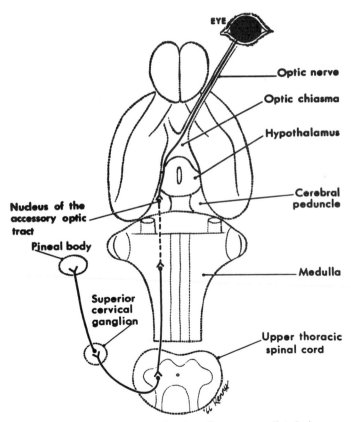

Figure 2. Innervation of the pineal. Photoneuroendocrine effects are mediated via a crossed pathway that descends through brain stem to sympathetic outflow. Postganglionic sympathetic fibers from the superior cervical ganglion end in the pineal body. (From Wurtman, R. J., et al.: *The Pineal.* Academic Press, New York, 1968, p. 81, with permission.)

231

identified hypothalamic peptides TRH, LHRH, and somatostatin. In addition, peptide fractions of unknown nature have been reported in pineal extracts; several of these have biologic activity.

Norepinephrine is synthesized in sympathetic axons which terminate both on pineal parenchymal cells and in the perivascular space.[49] The parenchymal cells synthesize the other amines. Bioassay and radioimmunoassay data have recently shown that melatonin circulates in the blood of humans[4, 68] and is excreted into urine (thus proving that the pineal gland has secretory function), and that there is a diurnal rhythm in this secretion, maximal values being observed during darkness.[33]

Pineal parenchymal cells contain the enzymes that mediate the synthesis of serotonin from tryptophan.[40, 49] This occurs through conversion of 5-hydroxytryptophan to serotonin and subsequently to N-acetylserotonin, the latter regulated by the enzyme N-acetyltransferase (NAT).[28] Melatonin is finally formed by the enzyme hydroxyindole-O-methyltransferase (HIOMT) (Fig. 3). The N-acetyltransferase enzyme is apparently rate-limiting for melatonin formation.[29] The melatonin-forming enzyme, HIOMT, has served as a highly specific marker for the site of formation of melatonin, both in pineal and extrapineal sites, and also as a marker for human pineal tumors.[14] Outside the pineal gland, which is the richest source of the enzyme, small amounts are found in the retina, the harderian gland (a modified lachrymal gland) of rodents, and in the cho-

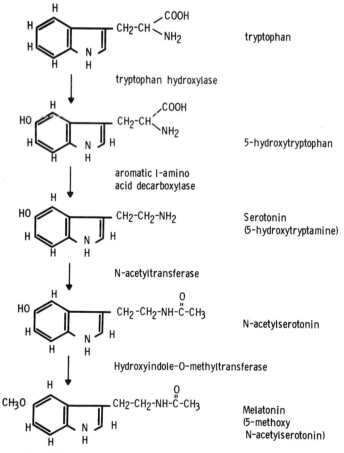

Figure 3. Metabolic pathway for synthesis of serotonin, N-acetylserotonin, and melatonin.

roid plexus, this last presumably reflecting the ependymal-cell origin of both the choroid plexus and pineal gland.[13, 14] One of the most valuable aspects of the study of pineal enzymes is that it has permitted accurate study of the factors which regulate pineal function.

Melatonin has been localized by immunohistologic methods in pinealocytes as well as in the outer nuclear layer of the retina, the optic chiasm and optic nerve, and the suprachiasmatic nucleus (Fig. 4a, b).[9, 10] It has also been found outside the central nervous system in the harderian gland[10, 11] and in secretory cells throughout the gastrointestinal tract, namely, in the esophagus, stomach, duodenum, cecum, colon, and rectum (Fig.

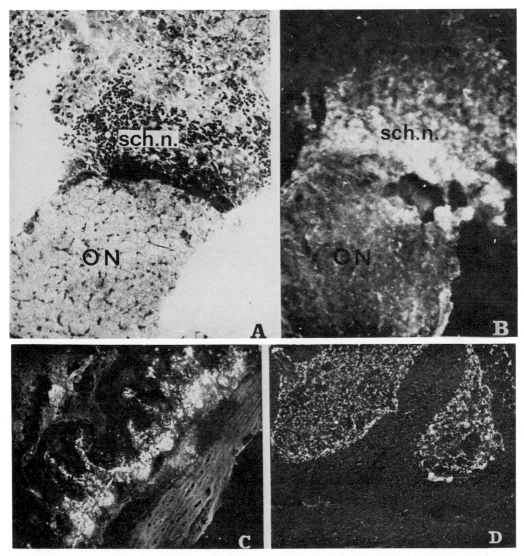

Figure 4. Immunohistologic localization of melatonin and N-acetylserotonin. *A*, Cresyl violet staining of the rat optic nerve (ON) and the suprachiasmatic nucleus (sch. n.). (Reduced 24% from ×100.) *B*, Fluorescein-labeled antibody technique. Fluorescence in sch. n. indicates melatonin. (Reduced 24% from ×100.) *C*, Fluorescence in the Lieberkühn's crypts of the rat rectum. It appears that most of the melatonin is concentrated at the base of the crypts. (Reduced 38% from ×100.) *D*, Fluorescence in the granule layer of the rat cerebellum indicating N-acetylserotonin. (Reduced 38% from ×45.)

4c).[12] Melatonin has also been demonstrated in retina and harderian gland by radioimmunoassay.[44] These findings, together with the presence of the synthesizing enzyme in various nonpineal tissues, suggest that melatonin may have functions separate from its role as a pineal hormone. N-acetylserotonin, but not melatonin, has been found in the granular layer of the cerebellum (Fig. 4d), in the spinal tract of the trigeminal roots, and in the ventral nucleus of the reticular formation.[9] The synthesizing enzyme N-acetylserotonin transferase, but not HIOMT, is also found in high concentration in cerebellum,[21] suggesting that there is a distinct role for N-acetylserotonin in brain, distinct from that of melatonin.

Another pineal substance, arginine vasotocin, has recently become of great interest. This substance, found in the pineal gland of a variety of species including man, has potent antigonadal and antiadrenal actions.[69]

FUNCTION OF THE PINEAL GLAND IN EXPERIMENTAL ANIMALS

The demonstration of pineal regulation by the sympathetic nervous system and the effects of environmental events on this control have been documented chiefly in rodents. These findings are briefly summarized here because they may be important clues to pineal function in higher animals, including man.

Pineal Rhythm

The content of norepinephrine, serotonin, and melatonin in the pineal gland of the rat shows a circadian variation that depends primarily on external lighting and is mediated by diurnal changes in the levels of the enzymes NAT and HIOMT.[49] Normally this rhythm results in high levels of NAT, and hence of melatonin, in the pineal during the night, with a rapid decline when the light part of the cycle begins.[28] When rats are in continuous darkness, levels of both NAT and HIOMT are extremely high and melatonin content increases.[29] Exposure to continuous light has the reverse effect. In contrast, pineal serotonin content is 180° out of phase, with high levels during the day. These rhythms are normally cued by information reaching the pineal gland via the sympathetic fibers arising in the superior cervical ganglion since cervical sympathectomy abolishes the pineal response to light. However, the rhythm of melatonin-synthesizing and secretory activities is not solely dependent on light. The rhythm persists in constant darkness, indicating that there is an intrinsic neural oscillator.[50] Recent studies indicate that the suprachiasmatic nucleus is the central neuronal element in generation of this rhythm.[32, 65] It appears that the suprachiasmatic rhythm is endogenous, but can be cued by light-dark information from the retina (Fig. 5).

The details of this interaction have now been extensively documented. During initial exposure to darkness, sympathetic nerve terminals within the pineal gland presumably liberate more norepinephrine.[49] The released catecholamine acts on β-adrenergic receptors located on the pinealocyte plasma membrane to increase adenyl cyclase activity and the subsequent formation of cyclic AMP.[57] Cyclic AMP, in turn, increases the activity of the rate-limiting enzyme, NAT, which results in increased melatonin synthesis (Fig. 6).[30] The decline in serotonin content during the night probably reflects enhanced synthesis of melatonin.[49] The sympathetic input seems to control virtually all aspects of enzyme function in the pineal gland, including nucleic acid metabolism.

Effects on the Brain

Radioactive melatonin is taken up by brain tissue, particularly by the hypothalamus and brain stem, and these regions may be specific target areas for melatonin action.[3]

234

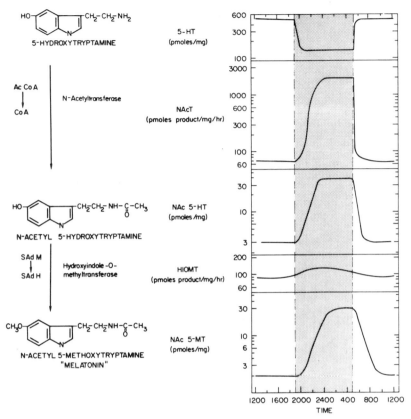

Figure 5. Circadian rhythms in indole metabolism in the rat pineal gland. The graph on the right shows changes in amine content and enzyme activity from light periods to dark periods (shaded area). (From Klein, D. C.: *Circadian rhythms in indole metabolism in the rat pineal gland. In* Schmitt, F. O. and Worden, F. G. (eds.): *The Neurosciences,* Third Study Program. MIT Press, Cambridge, Mass., 1974, p. 509, with permission.)

Melatonin measured in chicken brain by bioassay shows a diurnal rhythm similar to the pineal rhythm and is present at a concentration five times that of serum.[65] The highest levels are in the hypothalamus and brain stem. Melatonin is undetectable following pinealectomy, indicating that most brain melatonin is of pineal origin.[29] Fragmentary data suggest that the pineal gland or its secretion influences the electric activity of the brain.[2] Pineal extracts administered to cats cause an increase in the frequency of spontaneous electric activity of several subcortical nuclear groups, while pinealectomy in rabbits induces convulsive patterns of activity in dorsal hippocampal neurons after contralateral stimulation. In the rat, intermittent paroxysmal outbursts of cortical electric activity occur after pinealectomy, and in parathyroidectomized (hence calcium-deficient) rats, pinealectomy is followed by convulsions which may be fatal and which are not prevented by phenytoin.[51] Although not specifically related to electric activity, it may be significant that pinealectomy appears to retard the development of myelin in rats.

The adventitious movements induced by the administration of L-dopa in mice are also reported to be suppressed by pineal extract. A significant decrease or abolition of reflex sensory activation is observed in cats with experimental epileptic foci in cortical primary sensory areas. In the rat, intraventricular administration of antimelatonin antibody rapidly produces flattening and desynchronization of the EEG together with corti-

235

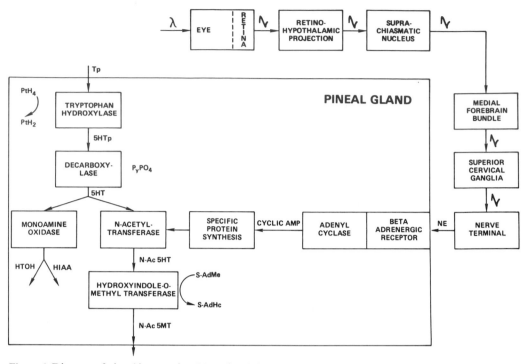

Figure 6. Diagram of pineal innervation. Norepinephrine (NE) released from nerve terminal combines with β-adrenergic receptor to activate adenyl cyclase. Increased cyclic AMP stimulates specific protein synthesis which leads to increase in N-acetyltransferase activity and formation of melatonin. (From Klein, D. C. and Parfitt, A.: *Ouabain blocks the adrenergic-cyclic AMP stimulation of pineal N-acetyltransferase activity. In* Weiss, B. (ed.): *Cyclic AMP in Disease.* University Park Press, Baltimore, 1976, p. 36, with permission.)

cal spikes and ictal events.[18] The potential significance of the peptides TRH, LHRH, and somatostatin, which are present in the pineal, in relation to these electrophysiologic and behavioral effects has not been investigated. Tsang and Martin[80] have shown that TRH, but not LHRH or somatostatin, blocks β-receptor stimulation of cyclic AMP formation in the pineal.

Endocrine Regulation

The best-established endocrine effects of the pineal gland are those on gonad development.[52] When rats were exposed to constant darkness, pubertal females showed delayed development of the ovary, males of the testis; comparable changes are observed in hamsters. All these effects are reversed by pinealectomy, suggesting that when pineal activity is increased, gonadal function is suppressed. The site of inhibitory feedback of melatonin on LH release has not been established with certainty. That it interferes at the pituitary level with LHRH has been shown by in vitro studies, but when given as a microinjection to the rat, melatonin blocked LH release when placed into the third ventricle, but not when placed into a portal vessel going directly to the pituitary.[20, 23] It has been suggested that this hypothalamic effect may be mediated by serotonin, since intraperitoneal injection of melatonin causes a rapid increase in brain serotonin content. Another melatonin-like agent, 5-methoxytryptophol, also found in the pineal, is even more potent than melatonin in this regard.[20] Recent studies in the hamster have complicated this interpretation, however. Low doses of melatonin cause gonadal atrophy in this species, whereas the gonad is stimulated at high doses. Moreover, melatonin implants can *block* darkness-induced involution of the testis.[53] In addition, active immunization of hamsters against melatonin fails to block gonadal atrophy induced by short photoperiod.[79] Recently, arginine vasotocin has become a second candidate as a potential pineal antigonadal hormone.[54, 59] This peptide has been isolated from bovine and human fetal pineal glands and tenatively identified in human CSF.[45]

The relationship of the pineal gland to onset of puberty is of more than passing interest because of the known relationship between precocious puberty and pinealomas in man.[27] After pinealectomy, the immature rat shows a significant advance in the onset of puberty, an effect attributed to removal of an antigonadal influence.[52]

Melatonin may also affect the gonads directly. Melatonin is taken up selectively by the testis, and testicular androgen synthesis is inhibited by its administration.[47]

The effect of the pineal on other endocrine systems is less well established.[76] Melatonin is said to inhibit thyroid function, but pinealectomy had no effect on the pituitary-thyroid axis under various lighting regimens. Recently a transient postpinealectomy depression of TSH secretion was reported. The growth impairment of dark-exposed rats is also reversed by pinealectomy (suggesting an effect on GH secretion).[66] Inconsistencies and contradictions fill the literature on pineal-adrenal relationships. Several reports, however, indicate that pinealectomy causes adrenal hypertrophy and elevation of plasma corticosterone, while blinding or continuous darkness decreases the size of the zona fasciculata (the adrenal cortical region that secretes glucocorticoids) and reduces plasma corticosterone levels. These findings suggest an overall inhibitory effect of the pineal. The role of melatonin in this response is not clear; its administration has variously been reported to depress, have no effect, or increase plasma corticosterone levels. Recent studies have shown that immunization against melatonin produces a lowering of corticosterone rather than an increase, suggesting that the inhibitory pineal substance may not be melatonin.[37] The peptide arginine vasotocin has recently been shown to be highly effective in blocking compensatory adrenal hypertrophy in the mouse, and thus may also be a candidate for the pineal substance that inhibits adrenal function.[46] A central role has been postulated for the suprachiasmatic nucleus in the generation of circadian rhythms of both the pineal gland and the pituitary-adrenal axis. It is still not known to what extent light-dark rhythms mediated by way of the pineal gland influence circadian endocrine rhythms in man.

There is preliminary evidence for a prolactin-release stimulating effect of the pineal gland in the rodent.[55] Blinding, constant darkness, or intraventricular administration of melatonin causes a rise in plasma prolactin levels.[37] Pinealectomy, on the other hand, is reported to block the nocturnal surge of prolactin release in male rats.[58] Immunization of animals so that they produce antibodies capable of binding circulating melatonin causes a lowering of plasma prolactin levels.[23, 55] These findings are consistent with the hypothesis that the pineal gland enhances prolactin release, an effect that may be mediated by melatonin, possibly through a decrease in hypothalamic secretion of prolactin-inhibiting factor.

CLINICAL ASPECTS

The pineal gland has no known normal function in man but becomes important clinically in calcification and tumor formation.

Calcification

Calcific nodules termed *acervuli* form in a matrix of ground substance secreted by pinealocytes. Recent studies indicate that the appearance of calcification may be a consequence of cellular secretory activity, since in the hamster, the normal calcification that develops with aging is prevented by superior cervical ganglionectomy. The nature of the protein matrix is unknown.

The calcified pineal gland is an established landmark widely used by radiologists to determine whether there has been a shift in midline brain structures. Because calcification is first noticeable by roentgenography around the time of puberty, it has been suggested that the pineal may have a role in producing puberty and then cease to function. In fact, this is not the case. Calcification can be detected in autopsy material before puberty, and the ground-substance matrix for calcification is present as early as one year of life. No difference in enzyme activity is found between heavily calcified glands from aged subjects and lightly calcified ones from young subjects.[76] Finally, in the adult, normal structure and weight of the pineal gland are preserved into old age, supporting the concept of a functional role of the gland during one's entire life.[49] The calcified material appears to be hydroxyapatite, the same salt as is found in bones and teeth. A lower incidence of calcification occurs in subjects in Japan and Nigeria than in Europe and America.

Hypoplasia and Aplasia

Hypoplasia and aplasia of the pineal gland are rare. A high proportion of patients with primary hypoplasia are reported to have genital precocity and many of these patients have associated pituitary lesions.

Tumors

Tumors of the pineal gland are rare, making up less than 1 per cent of intracranial neoplasms, and are seen almost exclusively in young males. As defined by Russell,[60, 61] the term *pinealoma* refers to tumor of the pineal parenchymal cell, called pineoblastoma or pineocytoma according to its maturity. In the series of 53 cases classified as tumors of the pineal gland by De Girolami and Schmidek[17] at the Massachusetts General Hospital, only nine fitted this category. Glial tumors of the pineal gland such as astrocytomas and glioblastomas were more common, accounting for 13 cases. The most common tumor of the pineal region is best termed *germinoma* because it apparently arises from undifferentiated germ cells. Approximately one half of the cases in the De Girolami series were classified as germinomas. Germinomas are also called ectopic pinealomas, or seminomatous pinealomas. Although the pineal gland is the site of origin of these tumors, they do not arise from pineal parenchymal cells. Identical types of tumors are found in the testis and the anterior mediastinum. The pathogenesis of the germinomas, as described by Scully, is that "during early embryonic development, germ cells, which arise in the yolk sac and migrate to the gonadal ridges of the male and female embryo, may be aberrant, wandering into atypical sites where the anterior mediastinum and pineal gland eventually lie. Isolated germ cells have been found within the head of the embryo."[62] Scully also points out that "in addition to germinomas, most other types of germ-cell tumor seen in the testis and ovary, including the endodermal sinus tumor, the choriocarcinoma and benign and malignant teratomas have arisen in the pineal gland and anterior mediastinum."[62] Approximately 10 per cent of intracranial germinomas metastasize to the spinal cord. Germinomas of this type commonly arise in the pineal gland and then infiltrate the third ventricle and the floor of the hypothalamus, producing a characteristic triad: diabetes insipidus, hypogonadism, and optic atrophy. Pineal calcification occurs earlier in such cases. Probably germinomas also can arise from midline tissues at the base of the brain and give an identical clinical picture.[22] Although these tumors usually produce severe damage to the hypothalamus before bone is destroyed, at least two rare cases have been observed in which the germinoma grew within the pituitary fossa and mimicked completely an expanding intrasellar tumor. True pinealomas can also spread to the floor of the third ventricle and produce various degrees of compression and destruction of the hypothalamus.

A small porportion of tumors in the pineal region are true teratomas believed also to arise from ectopic germ cells.[60, 61] Teratomas contain cell types originating from each of the three germinal layers that differentiate to form somatic structures. Pineal teratomas are identical with those of testis and mediastinum, and can give rise to choriocarcinoma capable of secreting chorionic gonadotropin. The CSF in one such case had elevated chorionic gonadotropin and somatostatin. In one case of a male patient, the nuclei of a typical pineal teratoma were chromatin-positive, whereas the normal epidermal nuclei were chromatin-negative. Scully suggests "that in that case, the tumor arose from a germ cell that had undergone meiotic division, so that each new cell contained either an X or a Y chromosome, and that after a subsequent division, two haploid cells with an X chromosome reunited to form a cell with female sex chromatin which differentiated to form the tumor."[62]

Other rare tumors in this region are spongioblastomas, ependymomas, choroid-plexus papillomas, and chemodectomas related to the carotid sinus-type cell.

Manifestations

Although pineal tumors have classically been associated with precocious puberty in boys, in some series no patients, and in others less than one third of those under 15 years of age were precocious. The relationship between pineal tumors and precocious puberty has been discussed in Chapter 5. We believe that most pineal tumors cause precocity by damaging hypothalamic structures that normally delay pubertal development. The most important manifestation of pineal neoplasms relates to their propensity for invading the third ventricle and hypothalamus, and producing symptoms through local pressure on the quadrigeminal plate of the midbrain.[16] An enlarging mass in the pineal region compresses the aqueduct of Sylvius and distorts the upper brain stem. Internal hydrocephalus gives rise to characteristic headache, vomiting, papilledema, and disturbed consciousness. Pressure on the superior colliculi causes paralysis of conjugate upward gaze (Parinaud's syndrome). Gait also may be disturbed due to either hydrocephalus or pressure on the cerebellum or brain stem.

Management

Pineal tumors are rarely resectable by the time clinical signs appear, although some centers have successfully treated selected cases by surgery.[16] Fortunately, the germinoma type are radiosensitive, and prolonged survival and even "cure" have been claimed in some cases. Most workers recommend that craniotomy be carried out for diagnostic purposes, that no attempt be made to remove the entire tumor, and that supervoltage roentgenotherapy be given.[7, 15] There is little experience with chemotherapy of these tumors.[6] In emergency situations with hydrocephalus, it may be necessary to carry out a shunt procedure.[7]

Melatonin in Tissue

The human pineal gland obtained at autopsy is capable of forming melatonin and hence contains HIOMT. Human nerve tissue and urine have been shown to contain a skin-lightening material which is presumably melatonin. Melatonin has been identified by bioassay[68] and radioimmunoassay[4] in plasma obtained from human males during darkness, but not during light. The nocturnal rise in blood melatonin continues during 2½ day-night cycle lengths after the onset of constant light, indicating that the cycle is not driven solely by the dark phase of the light-dark cycle.[68] On the other hand, no rise in melatonin is found during daytime sleep after reversal of the sleep-activity cycle or during a daytime nap indicating that the cycle is not driven simply by the sleep cycle.[68] Administration of isoproterenol produces no definite effect on melatonin levels suggesting that β-adrenergic stimulation may be less important in pineal regulation in the human than in the rat.[68] A precedent for such a species difference is the lack of pineal N-acetyltransferase response to β-stimulation in the chicken, hamster and sparrow.[42, 78] Resting morning melatonin levels have been shown to fluctuate during the menstrual cycle with highest levels at the time of menstrual bleeding and lowest levels at the time of ovulation.[73]

Clinical Effects of Melatonin

Although melatonin is an extremely potent skin-lightening agent in amphibians, it has no significant effect on human skin, possibly because in man most melanin pigment is stored outside the melanocyte.

In rodents with transplanted tumors, survival has been inversely related to pineal function. In the human, there are reports that at autopsy, pineal glands from patients with malignancy were larger than those from patients dying of other causes;[56] however, the reverse also has been reported.[67] In a number of patients with malignancy associated with high GH levels, continuous infusion of melatonin for one to two weeks has been reported to cause a fall in GH (after an initial rise) and amelioration of the clinical features of the tumor. These findings, if confirmed, have many implications.

Administration of melatonin has no undesirable side effects. It is rapidly metabolized by the liver, however, and has low solubility. Intravenous administration of melatonin to healthy volunteers induces EEG deactivation, followed by sleep accompanied by vivid dreams.[2] In three patients with temporal-lobe epilepsy, intravenous administration of melatonin was reported to cause a reduction in paroxysmal activity and an elevation of the convulsion threshold. Oral administration of melatonin has been reported to induce improvement in both rigidity and tremor in patients with Parkinson's disease, together with a feeling of well-being.

PERIVENTRICULAR ORGANS OF EPENDYMAL ORIGIN

The ventricles and the central canal of the spinal cord are lined with cuboidal, usually ciliated ependymal cells.[72] In several areas of the brain, the ependymal cells form specialized glandular structures whose function, though obscure, is suspected to be endocrine on the basis of morphologic study.[31] These structures include the pineal gland (derived embryologically from the roof of the third ventricle), the subcommissural organ, the subfornical organ, the organum vasculosum of the lamina terminalis, the lining ependyma of the floor of the third ventricle, and a specialized area in the fourth ventricle, the area postrema (Fig. 7).[71, 72] The choroid plexus, also an ependymal-vascular structure, in addition to its important fluid and electrolyte transport functions, also contains one or more peptide compounds with both melanotropic and lipolytic activity. One of these peptides, as shown by Rudman and collaborators,[59] is similar or identical to a peptide found in the pineal gland. Characteristic of all of these periventricular organs is the presence of fenestrated endothelial cells, a hallmark of a gland of internal secretion. In these regions, even large molecules such as horseradish peroxidase can enter the interstitial space. Most of the periventricular organs show granule-containing nerve endings in contact with ependymal (tanycyte) processes, and a rich blood

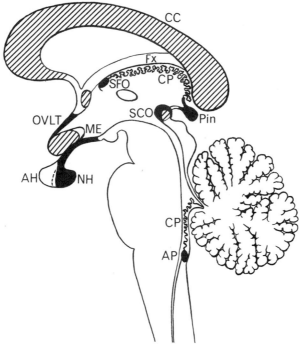

Figure 7. Sagittal section of the human brain illustrating the position of the circumventricular organs shown in black. *Abbreviations:* AH, adenohypophysis; AP, area postrema; CC, corpus callosum; CP, choroid plexus; Fx, fornix; ME, median eminence; NH, neurohypophysis; OVLT, organum vasculosum of the lamina terminalis; Pin, pineal; SCO, subcommisural organ; SFO, subfornical organ.

supply. Tight junctions between ependymal cells prevent the access of substances from the ventricles into the organs, but the tanycytes themselves may have an active transport function.

Subcommissural Organ (SCO)

This periventricular organ is found throughout the vertebrate evolutionary scale. It consists of a group of columnar cells lining the roof of the third ventricle at the caudal end, beneath the habenular commissure and adjacent to the pineal recess.[34, 72] The secretory granules of these cells react with a number of stains.[39] The secretory product of the cells (in all species except man) is condensed to form a strand of proteinaceous material (Reissner's fiber) that extends through the aqueduct, the fourth ventricle, and the caudal spinal canal. The fiber contains mucopolysaccharides and is believed to break down or dissolve in spinal fluid. Because humans do not have an anatomically detectable Reissner's fiber, it is possible that the secretions (if they form) are more soluble. The subcommissural organ has no apparent anatomic or functional connection with the adjacent pineal gland.

The function of the SCO is unknown; attempts to determine its function are thwarted by the difficulty of destroying this structure without producing gross damage to the habenular commissure and to the dynamics of fluid in the third ventricle.[41] Its appearance is believed to change in states of dehydration, suggesting a possible role in water or salt balance, and it has been claimed that the region controls thirst because SCO extracts, injected into rats, reduce water intake.[19] Recently, somatostatin has been identified in this structure.

241

Organum Vasculosum of the Lamina Terminalis (OVLT)

This structure lies in the midline of the lamina terminalis of the third ventricle, its external surface in contact with the CSF of the prechiasmatic cistern, and its internal surface in contact with the CSF of the anterior end of the third ventricle.[72] As outlined by Weindl and collaborators[70] in studies of the rabbit and cat, the ependyma here are flattened so that the vascular spaces of the OVLT closely approach the third ventricle. Blood vessels from the pia covering the external wall of the lamina form arching loops directed toward the ventricular lumen. Nerve endings in the interstitial space of the OVLT conceivably could transmit secretory products to capillaries in this region. There is no evidence for a "portal system" analogous to that for anterior pituitary regulation, nor an anatomic basis for direct transport of secretory product to the pituitary.

The function of the OVLT is unknown, but recent studies have modified speculations as to its function. The use of immunologic techniques has led to the surprising demonstration that nerve fibers and perikarya of the OVLT are rich in LHRH.[74, 77] Since there is no direct relationship to the pituitary, it would appear likely that if LHRH is liberated at nerve endings in the OVLT, the peptide would enter the general circulation via the capillary loops, or be transported by ependyma either into the lumen of the third ventricle, or into the cisternal space. At present, evidence is insufficient to support any of these possibilities. A clue to the function of the OVLT is the finding that destruction of this region in the rat leads to loss of the mechanism for cyclic gonadotropin secretion, but it is not clear whether this function involves the OVLT or adjacent nerve fibers. There is also evidence that perikarya in the region of the OVLT may project to the median eminence. On the basis of the finding by Moss and McCann[36] and Pfaff[48] that intraventricular injection of LHRH stimulates sexual activity in the rat, and previous demonstrations that lesions of the preoptic hypothalamus interfere with sexual function, it is also possible that this structure is involved in some way with sexual behavior, possibly by a hormonal factor borne in CSF. Somatostatin has also been demonstrated in the OVLT.

Subfornical Organ (SFO)

The subfornical organ is a neurohemal structure found at the junction between the lamina terminalis and the tela choroidea of the third ventricle.[1] Its name is derived from its location under the fornices of the hippocampus. It consists of both neurosecretory neurons and modified ependymal cells. Cells are oriented so that secretion into the lumen of the ventricle is at least a theoretic possibility, although it has not been demonstrated. Neurons of the SFO are reported to receive a cholinergic innervation from cells in the midbrain. Morphology of the SFO cells is modified by stress of various kinds, by hypertonic salt injection, and by estrogen administration.

A role for the SFO in salt and water regulation is supported by recent studies of the effects of injection of angiotensin II in the region of the SFO (although the localization of effect cannot be regarded as being entirely specific).[64] Such injections lead to the release of ADH and the stimulation of drinking behavior. The effects are enhanced by the addition of hypertonic saline. The endothelium of this region (as well as most other endothelia of the brain) contains enzymes capable of converting angiotensin I to angiotensin II.

It is clear that the function of the ependymal glands is still uncertain. It is fascinating to consider the possible behavioral effects of the secretion of unknown hormones, especially peptides, into the fluid bathing the cerebral hemispheres.

REFERENCES

1. AKERT, K.: *The mammalian subfornical organ.* J. Neurovisceral Relations Suppl. IX:78, 1969.

2. ANTON-TAY, F.: *Melatonin: Effects on brain function. In* Costa, E., Gessa, G. L. and Sandler, M. (eds.): *Serotonin—New Vistas, Advances in Biochemical Pharmacology,* vol. 11, Raven Press, New York, 1974, p. 315.

3. ANTON-TAY, F. AND WURTMAN, R. J.: *Regional uptake of ³H-melatonin from blood or cerebrospinal fluid by rat brain.* Nature 221:474, 1969.

4. ARENDT, J., PAUNIER, L. AND SIZONENKO, P. C.: *Melatonin radioimmunoassay.* J. Clin. Endocrinol. Metab. 40:347, 1975.

5. ARSTILA, A. U., KALIMO, A. O. AND HYYPPA, M.: *Secretory organelles of the rat pineal gland: Electron microscopic and histochemical studies in vivo and in vitro. In* Wolstenholme, G. E. W. and Knight, J. (eds.): *The Pineal Gland.* Churchill, London, 1971, p. 147.

6. BORDEN, S., ET AL.: *Pineal germinoma. Long-term survival despite tematogenous metastases.* Am. J. Dis. Child. 126:214, 1973.

7. BRADFIELD, J. S. AND PEREZ, C. A.: *Pineal tumors and ectopic pinealomas. Analysis of treatment and failures.* Radiology 103:399, 1972.

8. BROWN, G. M. AND MARTIN, J. B.: *Neuroendocrine relationships. In* Spiegel, E. A. (ed.): *Progress in Neurology and Psychiatry,* vol. 28, Grune and Stratton, New York, 1973, p. 199.

9. BUBENIK, G. A., ET AL.: *Immunohistological localization of N-acetylindolealkylamines in pineal gland, retina and cerebellum.* Brain Res. 81:233, 1974.

10. BUBENIK, G. A., BROWN, G. M. AND GROTA, L. J.: *Differential localization of N-acetylated indoles in CNS and the Harderian gland using immunohistology.* Brain Res., in press.

11. BUBENIK, G. A., BROWN, G. M. AND GROTA, L. J.: *Immunohistochemical localization of melatonin in the rat Harderian gland.* J. Histochem. Cytochem., in press.

12. BUBENIK, G. A., BROWN, G. M. AND GROTA, L. J.: *Immunohistological localization of melatonin in the rat digestive system.* Experienta, in press.

13. CARDINALI, D. P. AND WURTMAN, R. J.: *The pineal organ. In* Marks, N. and Rodnight, R. (eds.): *Research Methods in Neurochemistry,* vol. 2, New York, Plenum Press, 1974, p. 389.

14. CARDINALI, D. P. AND WURTMAN, R. J.: *Hydroxyindole-O-methyl transferases in rat pineal, retina and harderian gland.* Endocrinology 91:247, 1972.

15. COLE, H.: *Tumors in the region of the pineal.* Clin. Radiol. 22:110, 1971.

16. DAVIDOFF, L. M.: *Some considerations in the therapy of pineal tumors.* Proc. Rudolf Virchow Med. Soc., New York, 24:92, 1966.

17. DE GIROLAMI, U. AND SCHMIDEK, H.: *Clinicopathological study of 53 tumors of the pineal region.* J. Neurosurg. 39:455, 1973.

18. FARIELLO, R. G., ET AL.: *Melatonin and experimental epilepsy.* Neurology 26:389, 1976.

19. FOLDVARA, I. P. AND PALKOVITS, M.: *Effect of sodium and potassium restriction on the functional morphology of the subcommissural organ.* Nature 202:905, 1964.

20. FRASCHINI, F., CULLO, R. AND MARTINI, L.: *Mechanisms of inhibitory action of pineal principles on gonadotropin secretion. In* Wolsteinholme, G. E. W. and Knight, J. (eds.): *The Pineal Gland,* Churchill, London, 1971, p. 259.

21. HSU, L. L., GEYER, M. A. AND MANDELL, A. J.: *Extrapineal amine N-acetylation in rat brain.* Biochem. Pharmacol. 25:815, 1976.

22. KAGEYAMA, N.: *Ectopic pinealoma in the region of the optic chiasm.* J. Neurosurg. 35:755, 1971.

23. KAMBERI, I. A., MICAL, R. S. AND PORTER, J. C.: *Effects of melatonin and serotonin on the release of FSH and prolactin.* Endocrinology 88:1288, 1971.

24. KAPPERS, J. A.: *The mammalian pineal organ.* J. Neurovisceral Relations Suppl. IX:140, 1969.

25. KAPPERS, J. A.: *The pineal organ: An introduction. In* Wolstenholme, G. E. W. and Knight, J. (eds.): *The Pineal Gland.* Churchill, London, 1971, p. 3.

26. KELLY, D. E.: *Developmental aspects of amphibian pineal systems. In* Wolstenholme, G. E. W. and Knight, J. (eds.): *The Pineal Gland.* Churchill, London, 1971, p. 53.

27. KITAY, J. I.: *Pineal lesions and precocious puberty: A review.* J. Clin. Endocrinol. Metab. 14:622, 1954.

28. KLEIN, D. C. AND WELLER, J. L.: *Indole metabolism in the pineal gland: A circadian rhythm in N-acetyltransferase.* Science 169:1093, 1970.

29. KLEIN, D. C.: *The role of serotonin N-acetyltransferase in the adrenergic regulation of indole metabo-*

lism in the pineal gland. In Barchas, J. and Usdin, E. (eds.): *Serotonin and Behavior.* Academic Press, New York, 1973, p. 109.

30. KLEIN, D. C. AND PARFITT, A.: *Ouabain blocks the adrenergic-cyclic AMP stimulation of pineal N-acetyltransferase activity. In* Weiss, B. (ed.): *Cyclic AMP in Disease.* in press.

31. KNOWLES, F.: *Ependymal secretion, especially in the hypothalamic region.* J. Neurovisceral Relations Suppl. IX:97, 1969.

32. KOIZUMI, K., NISHINO, H. AND COLMAN, D.: *The suprachiasmatic nuclei and circadian rhythms.* Neuroscience Abstracts, 5th Annual Meeting, Society for Neuroscience, 1975, p. 446.

33. LYNCH, H. J., ET AL.: *Daily rhythm in human urinary melatonin.* Science 187:169, 1975.

34. MAZZI, V.: *L'Organe-Sous-Commissural.* Scientia, Italy, 1960, p. 1.

35. MOORE, R. Y., ET AL.: *Central control of the pineal gland.* Arch. Neurol. 18:208, 1968.

36. MOSS, R. L. AND MCCANN, S. M.: *Induction of mating behavior in rats by luteinizing hormone-releasing factor.* Science 181:177, 1973.

37. NILES, L. P., BROWN, G. M. AND GROTA, L. J.: *Effects of pineal and indoleamines on adrenocortical function.* Clin. Res. 23:617A, 1975.

38. NILES, L. P., BROWN, G. M. AND GROTA, L. J.: *N-acetylindoleamine effects on diurnal plasma prolactin levels.* Proc. Can. Fed. Biol. Soc. 19:112, 1976.

39. OKSCHE, A.: *The subcommissural organ.* J. Neurovisceral Relations Suppl. IX:111, 1969.

40. OTANI, J., GYORKEY, F. AND FARRELL, G.: *Enzymes of the human pineal body.* J. Clin. Endocrinol. Metab. 28:349, 1968.

41. PALKOVITS, M., MONOS, E. AND FACHET, J.: *This effect of subcommissural-organ lesions on aldosterone production in the rat.* Acta Endocrinol. 48:169, 1965.

42. PANG, S. F., RALPH, C. L. AND REILLY, D. P.: *Melatonin in the chicken brain: its origin, diurnal variation and regional distribution.* Gen. Comp. Endocrinol. 22:499, 1974.

43. PANG, S. F. AND RALPH, C. L.: *Mode of secretion of pineal melatonin in the chicken.* Gen. Comp. Endocrinol. 27:125, 1975.

44. PANG, S. F., ET AL.: *Radioimmunoassay of melatonin in pineal glands, Harderian glands, retinas and sera of rats or chickens.* Fed. Proc. 35:691, 1976.

45. PAVEL, S.: *Arginine vasotocin release into cerebrospinal fluid of cats induced by melatonin.* Nature [New Biol.] 246:183, 1973.

46. PAVEL, S., MATRESCU, L. AND PETRESCU, M.: *Central corticotropin inhibition by arginine vasotocin in the mouse.* Neuroendocrinology 12:371, 1973.

47. PEAT, F. AND KINSON, G. A.: *Testicular steroidogenesis in vitro in the rat in response to blinding, pinealectomy and to the addition of melatonin.* Steroids 17:251, 1971.

48. PFAFF, D. W.: *Luteinizing hormone releasing factor potentiates lordosis behavior in hypophysectomized ovariectomized female rats.* Science 182:1148, 1973.

49. QUAY, W. B.: *Pineal Chemistry in the Cellular and Physiological Mechanisms.* Charles C Thomas, Springfield, 1974.

50. RALPH, C. L., ET AL.: *A melatonin rhythm persists in rat pineals in darkness.* Endocrinology 89:1361, 1971.

51. REITER, R. J.: *Comparative physiology: Pineal gland.* Annu. Rev. Physiol. 35:305, 1973.

52. REITER, R. J.: *Pineal regulation of hypothalamicopituitary axis: gonadotrophins. In* Greep, R. O., et al. (eds.): *Handbook of Physiology, Section 7: Endocrinology,* vol. 4, part 2. American Physiological Society, Williams & Wilkins, Baltimore, 1974, p. 519.

53. REITER, R. J., ET AL.: *Melatonin: Its inhibition of pineal antigonadotrophic activity in male hamsters.* Science 185:1169, 1974.

54. REITER, R. J., ET AL.: *New horizons of pineal research.* Am. Zool. 16:93, 1976.

55. RELKIN, R.: *Effects of variations in environmental lighting on pituitary and plasma prolactin levels in the rat.* Neuroendocrinology 9:278, 1973.

56. RODIN, A. E. AND OVERALL, J.: *Statistical relationships of weight of the human pineal to age and malignancy.* Cancer 20:1203, 1967.

57. ROMERO, J. A. AND AXELROD, J.: *Pineal beta-adrenergic receptor: regulation of sensitivity. In* Usdin, E. and Bunney, W. E., Jr. (eds.): *Pre- and Postsynaptic Receptors.* Marcel Dekker, New York, 1975.

58. RONNEKLIEV, O. K. AND MCCANN, S. M.: *Effects of pinealectomy, anosmia and blinding on serum and pituitary prolactin in intact and castrated male rats.* Neuroendocrinology 17:340, 1975.

59. RUDMAN, D., ET AL.: *Comparison of lipolytic and melanotropic factors in bovine choroid plexus and in bovine pineal gland.* Endocrinology 90:1139, 1972.

60. RUSSELL, D. S.: *The pinealoma: Its relationship to teratoma.* J. Pathol. Bacteriol. 56:145, 1944.

61. RUSSELL, D. S. AND RUBINSTEIN, L. J.: *Pathology of tumours of the nervous system.* Edward Arnold, London, 1963.

62. SCULLY, R. E.: *Discussion in case records of the Massachusetts General Hospital.* N. Engl. J. Med. 284:1427, 1971.

63. SHERIDAN, M. N., REITER, R. J. AND JACOBS, J.: *An interesting anatomical relationship between the hamster pineal gland and the ventricular system of the brain.* J. Endocrinol. 45:131, 1969.

64. SIMPSON, J. B. AND ROUTTENBERG, A.: *Subfornical organ: Site of drinking elicitation by angiotensin-II.* Science 173:1172, 1973.

65. SMALSTIG, E. B. AND CLEMENS, J. A.: *The role of the suprachiasmatic nuclei in reproductive cyclicity.* Neuroscience Abstracts, 5th Annual Meeting, Society for Neuroscience, 1975, p. 434.

66. SORRENTINO, S., JR., REITER, R. J. AND SCHALCH, D. S.: *Interactions of the pineal gland blinding and underfeeding on reproductive organ size and radioimmunoassayable growth hormone.* Neuroendocrinology 7:105, 1971.

67. TAPP, E. AND BLUMFIELD, M.: *The weight of the pineal gland in malignancy.* Br. J. Cancer 24:67, 1970.

68. VAUGHAN, G. M., ET AL.: *Nocturnal elevation of plasma melatonin and urinary 5-hydroxyindoleacetic acid in young men: Attempts at modification by brief changes in environmental lighting and sleep and by autonomic drugs.* J. Clin. Endocrinol. Metab. 42:752, 1976.

69. VAUGHAN, M. K., ET AL.: *Arginine vasotocin: structure-activity relationships and influence on gonadal growth and function.* Am. Zool. 16:25, 1976.

70. WEINDL, A., SCHWINK, A. AND WETZSTEIN, R.: *De Feinbau des Gefassorgans der Lamina terminalis beim Kaninchen.* Zeitschrift fur Zellforschung 79:1, 1967.

71. WEINDL, A. AND JOYNT, R. J.: *The median eminence as a circumventricular organ.* In Knigge, K. M., et al. (eds.): *Brain-Endocrine Interaction, Median Eminence: Structure and Function.* Karger, Basel, 1972, p. 280.

72. WEINDL, A.: *Neuroendocrine aspects of circumventricular organs.* In Ganong, W. F. and Martini, L. (eds.): *Frontiers in Neuroendocrinology,* Oxford University Press, London, 1973, p. 3.

73. WETTERBERG, L., ET AL.: *Human serum melatonin changes during the menstrual cycle.* J. Clin. Endocrinol. Metab. 42:185, 1976.

74. WHEATON, J. E., KRULICH, L. AND McCANN, S. M.: *Localization of luteinizing hormone-releasing hormone in the preoptic area and hypothalamus of the rat using radioimmunoassay.* Endocrinology 97:30, 1975.

75. WURTMAN, R. J., AXELROD, J. AND KELLY, D. E.: *The Pineal.* Academic Press, New York, 1968.

76. WURTMAN, R. J. AND CARDINALI, D. P.: *The pineal organ.* In Williams, R. H. (ed.): *Textbook of Endocrinology,* ed. 5. W. B. Saunders, Philadelphia, 1974, p. 832.

77. ZIMMERMAN, E. A.: *Localization of hypothalamic hormones by immunocytochemical techniques.* In Martini, L. and Ganong, W. F. (eds.): *Frontiers in Neuroendocrinology.* Raven Press, New York, 1976, p. 25.

78. BINKLEY, S.: *Comparative biochemistry of the pineal glands of birds and mammals.* Am. Zool. 16:57, 1976.

79. BROWN, G. M., ET AL.: *Gonadal effects of pinealectomy and immunization against N-acetylindolealkylamines in the hamster.* Neuroendocrinology, in press.

80. TSANG, D. AND MARTIN. J. B.: *Effect of hypothalamic hormones on the concentration of adenosine 3',5'.-monophosphate in incubated rat pineal glands.* Life Sci. 19:911, 1976.

BIBLIOGRAPHY

AXELROD, J.: *The pineal gland.* Endeavour 29:144, 1970.

BROWNSTEIN, M. J.: *Minireview, the pineal gland.* Life Sci. 16:1363, 1975.

CARDINALI, D. P. AND WURTMAN, R. J.: *The pineal organ.* In Marks, N. and Rodnight, R. (eds.): *Research Methods in Neurochemistry,* vol. 2. Plenum Press, New York, 1974.

KITAY, J. I. AND ALTSCHULE, M. D.: *The Pineal Gland.* Harvard University Press, Cambridge, 1954.

QUAY, W. B.: *Pineal Chemistry in Cellular and Physiological Mechanisms.* Charles C Thomas, Springfield, 1974.

REITER, R. J. AND FRASCHINI, F.: *Endocrine aspects of the mammalian pineal gland: A review.* Neuroendocrinology 5:219, 1969.

REITER, R. J.: *The role of the pineal in reproduction. In* Balin, H. and Glasser, S. (eds.): *Reproductive Biology.* Excerpta Medica, Amsterdam, 1972.

REITER, R. J.: *Comparative physiology: Pineal gland.* Annu. Rev. Physiol. 35:305, 1973.

SIVAK, J. G.: *Historical note: The vertebrate median eye.* Vision Res. 14:137, 1974.

WEINDL, A.: *Neuroendocrine aspects of circumventricular organs. In* Ganong, W. F. and Martini, L. (eds.): *Frontiers in Neuroendocrinology 1973.* Oxford University Press, London, 1973.

WOLSTENHOLME, G. E. W. AND KNIGHT, J. (EDS.): *The Pineal Gland.* Churchill, London, 1971.

WURTMAN, R. J., AXELROD, J. AND KELLY, D. E. (EDS.): *The Pineal.* Academic Press, New York, 1968.

WURTMAN, R. J. AND ANTON-TAY, F.: *The pineal gland as a neuroendocrine transducer.* Recent Prog. Horm. Res. 25:493, 1969.

WURTMAN, R. J.: *The pineal gland: Endocrine interrelationships.* Adv. Intern. Med. 16:155, 1970.

WURTMAN, R. J. AND CARDINALI, D. P.: *The pineal organ. In* Williams, R. H. (ed.): *Textbook of Endocrinology,* ed. 5. W. B. Saunders, Philadelphia, 1974, p. 832.

CHAPTER 11

Neurologic Manifestations of Hypothalamic Disease

The many functions attributable to the hypothalamus are remarkable. In addition to its role in the regulation of the anterior and posterior pituitary gland, the hypothalamus homeostatically controls water balance[2] and body temperature,[8] and influences consciousness,[54] sleep,[64] emotion, and behavior[23] (Table 1). Many of these insights into hypothalamic function came from the careful observation of patients with diencephalic disease—as detailed, for example, in the classic 1929 review by Fulton and Bailey[19] of the effects of third-ventricle tumors. However, clinical-pathologic correlations have not been very useful in precise analysis of hypothalamic function. The relatively small size of this structure and its inaccessibility make it difficult to analyze deficits except at autopsy, by which time lesions are large and the primary areas of involvement are obscured. Moreover, manifestations of hypothalamic disease depend in part upon the time course of their development. For example, relatively trivial trauma to the anterior hypothalamus, if inflicted acutely at the time of neurosurgery, can cause fatal hyperthermia, while massive destruction of this region is compatible with almost normal function if the disease has developed gradually over many years, as for example in the slowly growing craniopharyngioma. The capacity for compensation of function is rather striking and not fully explained, although it has been shown that certain groups of neurons in the hypothalamus (central catecholaminergic and neurosecretory neurons), unlike other CNS neurons, can regenerate after damage.

Most contemporary insights into hypothalamic mechanisms are therefore based on studies in experimental animals. The earliest methods of study were the use of ablative lesions by the method of Horsley and Clark, and the electric-stimulation methods of Hess.[30] More recent methods include restricted neuropharmacologic manipulation by local microinjection or microiontophoresis, unit cell recording, and self-stimulation.

It is important to recognize that vegetative and affective functions are not mediated solely by the hypothalamus acting as an isolated, distinct functional or anatomic entity.[56] Rather, the hypothalamus forms but one important component of an extensive and complex integrative brain network comprising the limbic system. Because this system functions as an integrated whole, it is frequently difficult or impossible to determine the function localized to the hypothalamus itself as opposed to its involvement as part of a larger integrative nerve-net. Loss or disturbance of function when lesions are placed in the hypothalamus does not prove that these functions reside in the hypothalamus. For example, a lesion in the anterolateral hypothalamus of several species of animals is followed by fatal aphagia.[1] Although this finding suggests that a "feeding center" exists in the lateral hypothalamus, it cannot be taken as final proof that this part of the hypothal-

Table 1. Neurologic Manifestations of Nonendocrine Hypothalamic Disease

Disorders of Temperature Regulation	*Disorders of Psychic Function*
Hyperthermia	Rage behavior
Hypothermia	Hallucinations
Poikilothermia	*Periodic Diseases of Hypothalamic Origin*
Disorders of Food Intake	Diencephalic epilepsy
Hyperphagia (bulimia)	Kleine-Levin syndrome
Anorexia, aphagia	Periodic discharge syndrome of Wolff
Disorders of Water Intake	*Disorders of the Autonomic Nervous System*
Compulsive water drinking	Pulmonary edema
Adipsia	Cardiac arrhythmias
Essential hypernatremia	Sphincter disturbance
Disorders of Sleep and Consciousness	*Hereditary Hypothalamic Disease*
Somnolence	Laurence-Moon-Biedl syndrome
Sleep-rhythm reversal	*Miscellaneous*
Akinetic mutism	Prader-Willi syndrome
Coma	Diencephalic syndrome of infancy
	Cerebral gigantism

amus is the only, or even the primary, region involved in the regulation of feeding. Such a lesion not only destroys neurons located in the lateral hypothalamus, but also interrupts numerous axons which pass through this area in the medial forebrain bundle, the main rostral-caudal pathway of the limbic system connecting the amygdala, hippocampus, and mesencephalon.

Even when the hypothalamus has been shown to be important in the regulation of a particular behavior or homeostatic mechanism, the possibility is not excluded that other areas of the brain can mediate similar functions. An example can be taken from recent experimental work by Chi and coworkers[4, 12] in which hypothalamic islands that disconnected the hypothalamus from the rest of the brain in the cat were shown to permit fully integrated responses to painful stimuli. Aggressive responses (a behavior classically attributed to the hypothalamus) persisted in such animals. Moreover, the animals were able to stalk and kill in a relatively normal manner and to eat and drink when presented with food and water. On the other hand, the animals showed a striking general lethargy and lack of interest in the environment, manifested by a marked diminution in spontaneous activity. In this context, the hypothalamus appeared to act as an amplifier of certain behavioral responses organized elsewhere in the brain, rather than as the "center" for these responses.

Table 2. Symptoms and Signs of Hypothalamic Disease (From a Review of 60 Autopsy Proven Cases)

Symptoms and Signs	Number of Cases
Sexual abnormalities (hypogonadism or precocious puberty)	43
Diabetes insipidus	21
Psychic disturbance	21
Obesity or hyperphagia	20
Somnolence	18
Emaciation, anorexia	15
Thermodysregulation	13
Sphincter disturbance	5

(Adapted from Bauer, H. G.: *Endocrine and other clinical manifestations of hypothalamic disease: A survey of 60 cases with autopsies.* J. Clin. Endocrinol. Metab. 14:13, 1954.)

In a survey of 60 cases of autopsy-proven hypothalamic lesions, Bauer[6] described a number of disorders of endocrine and nonendocrine function. The most common manifestations are summarized in Table 2.

TEMPERATURE REGULATION

Aronsohn and Sachs[3] in 1885 obtained the first evidence of a role of the brain in temperature regulation when they observed that large puncture lesions in the brain of the rabbit resulted in a rise in body temperature. In 1912, Isenschmid and Krehl[33] demonstrated that posterior hypothalamic lesions prevented normal adaptive responses to cold exposure, providing evidence that the hypothalamus functions to protect against cold.

The detailed investigations of Ranson and coworkers[54] in the 1930s and 1940s showed that anterior hypothalamic lesions in cats and monkeys resulted in a tendency to hyperthermia with defective defense against heat, whereas posterior hypothalamic lesions caused hypothermia or poikilothermia. The studies of Ranson were important models for research into the negative functions of the hypothalamus. Poikilothermia is defined as a disorder of temperature regulation in which body core temperature follows that of the environment. Thus, exposure to cold results in hypothermia and exposure to warmth leads to hyperthermia.

The essential components of the temperature regulatory system are diagrammed in Figure 1. The anterior hypothalamus and preoptic area contain a population of specific temperature-sensitive neurons that can alter their firing rates in response to local changes in hypothalamic temperature.[8, 28, 29] The responsivity of such cells varies diurnally with the circadian temperature rhythm, and is altered by afferent impulses from peripheral thermoreceptors. Few, if any, temperature-sensing cells are located in the posterior hypothalamus. Lesions in the anterior hypothalamus and preoptic area interfere with heat-loss mechanisms, including sweating and vasodilatation. Because heat production in normals usually exceeds need, active heat dissipation is required under temperate environmental conditions and such lesions may result in severe hyperthermia. The extent of hyperthermia that occurs in such circumstances depends upon the acuteness, location, and size of the lesion. Acute destruction of the preoptic area may result in severe, even fatal fever.

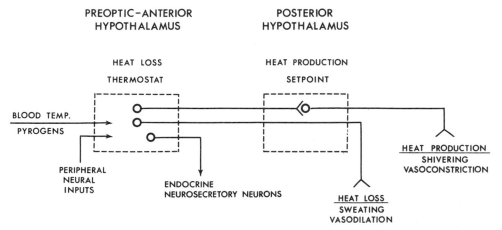

Figure 1. Diagram of hypothalamic temperature regulation mechanisms. The preoptic-anterior hypothalamic area functions as a thermostat and contains mechanisms for regulation of heat loss. The posterior hypothalamus integrates heat production mechanisms. Lesions of the preoptic-anterior hypothalamic area result in hyperthermia; lesions of the posterior hypothalamus cause hypothermia or poikilothermia.

Lesions in the posterior hypothalamus may cause hypothermia by interference with shivering and vasoconstrictive mechanisms. If the lesions are large enough to damage both anterior and posterior hypothalamic efferent systems, poikilothermia results. Anterior hypothalamic lesions have also been shown to interfere with shivering, suggesting that facilitatory inputs may reach the posterior hypothalamus from anterior hypothalamic areas.

The mechanism by which the hypothalamus senses environmental temperature and how this information is transduced into neural signals of a type appropriate to initiate temperature adaptation has been extensively studied.[8, 28, 29] Two major inputs, one central through temperature-sensitive neurons in the anterior hypothalamus and the other peripheral from cold or warmth receptors in the skin and internal organs, control temperature. That the anterior hypothalamus functions as a central thermal receptor is shown by local warming of the anterior hypothalamic-preoptic area which induces sweating and vasodilatation, and by local cooling which has opposite effects: shivering, vasoconstriction, and thyroid activation. The anterior hypothalamic-preoptic area alone appears to subserve this function. Changes in local temperature in the posterior hypothalamus and in other brain areas are without effect. Studies of single-neuron activity have confirmed the concept that nerve cells in this region of the hypothalamus can transduce temperature changes into varying rates of cell firing. Units which show an increased rate of activity with warming have been identified in several species and have been generally labeled as warmth receptors. Units with increasing activity on cooling are less readily demonstrated but also exist. However, data obtained from recording of units in relation to temperature changes must be interpreted with caution, because it is not generally possible to distinguish between primary-receptor neurons and secondary interneurons affected by primary temperature-sensing neurons at a separate site.

The concept of a heat-loss center in the anterior hypothalamus is probably oversimplified. Hypothalamic regulation of temperature is achieved by a complex, multi-integrated system that determines autonomic, behavioral, and hormonal responses to variations in central or environmental temperature. The maintenance of a constant core temperature requires the integration of several inputs, a comparison of this information with a predetermined setpoint, and the coordination of the various effector systems. Substances such as drugs, hormones, and pyrogens act at a hypothalamic level to alter body temperature (Fig. 2).

The relative importance of thermosensitive hypothalamic neurons as compared to peripheral skin receptors in caloric homeostasis also has been extensively investigated. Core-temperature recordings from the hypothalamus show little fluctuation with changes in environmental temperature, and changes in hypothalamic blood flow are probably the result rather than the cause of body temperature regulatory adjustments. Exposure to cold may, in fact, cause a slight rise in hypothalamic temperature in the rat.[40] Peripheral inputs are believed to be of greater physiologic significance than local effects in temperature regulation.

In addition to adjustments in heat-loss and heat-maintenance mechanisms which are mediated via the autonomic nervous system, the hypothalamus also integrates behavioral and neuroendocrine responses appropriate for homeostasis. The behavioral responses include seeking warmer or colder environments, and altered food intake. The neuroendocrine control response includes the sympathoadrenal system, the pituitary-thyroid axis, and the pituitary-adrenal axis.[20] Rats with lesions in the anterior hypothalamic-preoptic area, for example, demonstrate abnormalities of feeding behavior when thermally stressed. Normal rats reduce food intake when the ambient temperature is raised and eat more in the cold. In contrast, anterior hypothalamic-preoptic-lesioned animals fail to reduce food intake in warm environments, and exposure to cold fails to

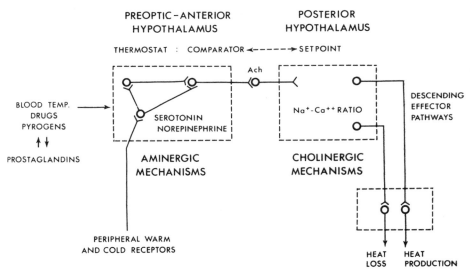

Figure 2. Diagram of the function of central amines in thermoregulation in the primate. The preoptic-anterior hypothalamic area contains thermosensitive neurons whose responses can be altered by: 1) blood temperature, 2) drugs, 3) pyrogens (probably acting via prostaglandins), 4) peripheral-receptor signals, and 5) "comparator" inputs from other brain areas including the posterior hypothalamic setpoint mechanism. Serotonin and norepinephrine may play a role in preoptic-anterior hypothalamic thermoregulation. The setpoint control of the posterior hypothalamus is dependent on the Na^+-Ca^{++} ratio. Cholinergic pathways serve effector systems via the hypothalamus and descending brain stem connections which initiate heat loss and heat production.

increase food intake. Local hypothalamic cooling in goats stimulates food intake. These data would indicate a strong influence of thermoregulatory functions on food intake. These connections are believed to be mediated through descending pathways from the anterior hypothalamic-preoptic region to ventromedial and lateral hypothalamic areas.

As emphasized by Hardy,[28] there is a striking correlation between skin temperature and the sensation of comfort or discomfort (Fig. 3). Two components of the conscious

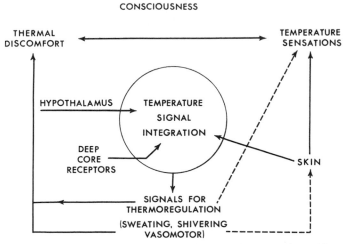

Figure 3. Diagram of relationship of thermal discomfort and temperature sensation. Although both sensations reach consciousness, they result in differing subjective experiences. The emotional feelings do not reflect the activity of peripheral thermoreceptors alone but rather an integrated state of the thermoregulatory system. (Courtesy of J. D. Hardy.)

251

perceptual experience relate to changes in environmental temperature. As skin temperature is reduced during cold exposure, man perceives increasing sensations of both cold and discomfort. It is evident that warm/cold sensation and comfort/discomfort motivation can be consciously distinguished as two separate aspects of thermal experience. When placed in a warm environment, a sense of warmth increases with the rise in skin temperature, while the feeling of thermal discomfort correlates more closely to sweat rate (and evaporative loss). Such studies indicate the importance of peripheral receptors in the control of both autonomic responses for temperature regulation and the perception of discomfort associated with deviations from the norm. In fact, behavioral thermoregulation is of major importance in man, and precedes the mobilization of sympathoadrenal and other endocrine responses.

Behavioral thermoregulation is the most important mechanism of temperature control in lower, poikilothermic animals, such as amphibians and reptiles. Although they lack the physiologic mechanisms for regulating heat production and heat dissipation and hence are called "cold-blooded," these species have sophisticated thermoreceptor systems and regulate their behavior appropriately.

Neuropharmacologic Aspects

Neuropharmacologic studies indicate that central catecholamine and serotonin neurotransmitters are involved in temperature regulation.[16] Fever can be induced in cats and monkeys by intraventricular injection of 5-hydroxytryptophan, and this effect is blocked by intraventricular administration of epinephrine or norepinephrine. Based on such experiments, Feldberg and Myers[16] have posulated a "pharmacologic" theory of temperature regulation. They propose that the elevation of body temperature induced by anterior hypothalamic-preoptic mechanisms involves the release of serotonin (as a neurotransmitter), while the lowering of body temperature (or a counteracting of the elevation in body temperature) is mediated by a catecholaminergic system. Although such data superficially suggest such an interpretation, it is probably an oversimplification, as is the suggested role of biogenic amines in feeding and thirst behavior (see below). It is unlikely that a simple neurotransmitter difference can account for the full effects of such complex responses. Moreover, species differences have been reported.

Core-temperature regulation may be mediated also by prostaglandins (see below) and by cationic influences. In studies directed toward localizing a setpoint control for temperature in the CNS, Myers[46] observed that infusions of Na^+ and Ca^{++} ions into the posterior hypothalamus could raise or lower the body core temperature, respectively (Fig. 4). He proposed that a shift in the $Na^+:Ca^{++}$ ratio might determine core temperature; subsequent temperature alterations induced by pyrogens or drugs were shown to be superimposed upon the new setpoint caused by Na^+ or Ca^{++} perturbations. The animals were also capable of normal thermoregulation at the new level. These observations, although of interest, have not yet been proved to be of physiologic significance.

Mechanism of Pyrogen-Induced Fever

Fever, one of the cardinal signs of infectious disease, is due to a chemically induced alteration in the setpoint of the central thermoregulatory system. The chemicals involved (so-called endogenous pyrogens) are produced mainly in leukocytes and perhaps other tissues as well. Tissue damage, destruction of leukocytes or monocytes (in the case of viral infection), tumor breakdown products, or the injection of foreign (exogenous) pyrogens (such as bacterial polysaccharide capsular materials) release endogenous pyrogen into the blood to act on the brain. The mechanism of this effect is not clear. Prostaglandin E_1 may mediate this form of fever, since aspirin

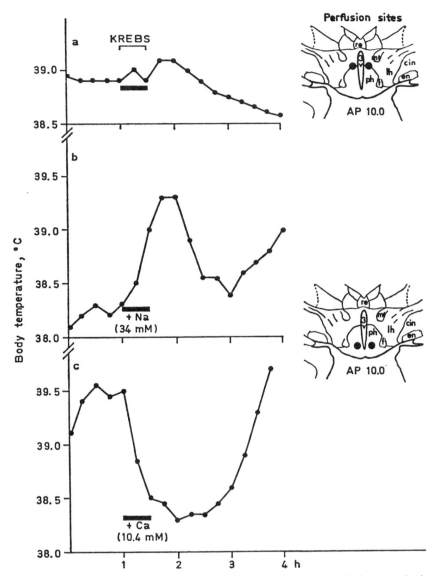

Figure 4. Effects of infusions of Na+ *(middle)* and Ca++ *(lower)* in posterior hypothalamus on body temperature regulation in the cat. Sodium ion caused a rise in body temperature and calcium caused a fall. The sites of the infusions are indicated by filled circles (●). *Abbreviations:* cin, internal capsule; en, endopeduncular nucleus; f, fornix; lh, lateral hypothalamic area; mt, mammillothalamic tract; ph, posterior hypothalamus; re, nucleus reuniens; 3v, third ventricle. (From Myers, R. D.: *Ionic concepts of the set-point for body temperature. In* Lederis, K. and Cooper, K. E. (eds.): *Recent Studies of Hypothalamic Function.* Karger, Basel, 1974, p. 374, with permission.)

and butazolidine (prostaglandin-synthesis and prostaglandin-action blocking agents, respectively) can block pyrogen-induced fever, and when administered intraventricularly, or into the anterior hypothalamus, this prostaglandin can cause fever.[65]

Central fevers can come about through physical destruction of heat regulating areas, but central inflammatory lesions may cause fever by direct effects on the anterior hypothalamic area. For example, in the studies of Veale and Cooper,[65] the direct injection of endogenous pyrogen into the hypothalamus is accompanied by evident cellular response which may in fact be the mediator of the temperature effects. Injections of pyrogen are effective, however, only when placed in the anterior hypothalamic-preoptic area.

Neuroendocrine Aspects

In addition to changes in behavior, skin heat dissipation, heat conserving mechanisms, and shivering, endocrine secretion plays an important role in body temperature homeostasis. Nonshivering thermogenesis, a major factor in maintenance of body temperature in chronic-cold-adapted men, is due in large measure to increased secretion of catecholamines which alters intermediary metabolism of parenchymal organs (mainly liver and kidney) and muscles so as to increase heat production. This response, mediated through the autonomic nervous system, is the most important reflex endocrine element in body temperature control. The thyroid gland is not activated in response to cold in man (unlike most lower animal forms), but its normal function is nevertheless important in body heat regulation.[20, 40] In the absence of thyroid function (as in myxedema), body heat production is reduced, the peripheral vascular system is constricted, and the patient may develop hypothermia. Patients with hyperthyroidism respond poorly to increased environmental temperature and may develop hyperthermia if the mechanisms for heat dissipation fail to work, if the heat load is too great, or if environmental temperatures are too high. This situation is characteristic of thyrotoxic "storm." The possible exception to the generalization that exposure to cold does not activate thyroid function in man is the response of the newborn. Within a few hours of delivery, human babies develop a surge in TSH and thyroid-hormone secretion which can in part be blocked by warming. Peripheral circulatory factors in adjustment to delivery may also be involved in this response. In older humans, cellular conversion of thyroxine to the more potent thyroid hormone analogue triiodothyronine may also play a role in thyroid adaptation to cold.

Exposure to cold also leads to activation of the pituitary-adrenal axis, as evidenced by adrenal hypertrophy and elevated circulating levels of cortisol.[20]

DISORDERS OF THERMOREGULATION IN MAN*

Several normal physiologic fluctuations or rhythms affect temperature control. The most striking of these is the normal diurnal variation in body temperature characterized by a rise in the late afternoon and early evening and a fall during the night to a low point shortly after arising in the morning. This well-defined diurnal rhythm in temperature accounts for the fact that temperature elevation in illness tends to be maximal in late afternoon and that fever tends to be minimal early in the morning. A second rhythm is that of the menstrual cycle. Progesterone secreted during the second half of the menstrual cycle results in an elevation of body temperature that correlates closely with the occurrence of ovulation, and is used as a yardstick of normal pituitary-ovarian function. Progesterone produces this effect by an action on hypothalamic neurons.

Disturbance of temperature regulation in man is a rather common manifestation of hypothalamic disease. The causes, diagnosis, and management have been extensively reviewed by Johnson and Spalding.[35] A few decades ago, it was considered that hyperthermia was the most common manifestation of hypothalamic disorders, since acute lesions or pressure on the anterior hypothalamus may result in intense vasoconstric-

---

*The authors thank Dr. Otto Rorstad for his assistance with this section.

tion, tachycardia, and hypothermia. Careful testing of patients in recent years has demonstrated that hypothermia is perhaps even more common.

On the basis of clinical presentation, central hypothermia may be considered as either chronic or periodic. Shapiro and associates[58] proposed a classification of hypothermia based on "chronic hypothermia associated with structural intracranial abnormalities" and "episodic hypothermia without evidence of intracranial abnormality." The latter group included patients with a distinctive episodic syndrome of autonomic activation accompanied by hypothermia.

Chronic Hypothermia

These patients suffer from a disturbance of thermoregulation that is persistent or demonstrates only slow change. The CNS defect predisposes to hypothermia under conditions in which a subject with intact thermoregulatory function maintains normal body temperature. The lesion usually affects other neurologic functions as well. The majority of such patients have a structural lesion of the posterior or entire hypothalamus, and several pathologic lesions have been described (Table 3). The predominance of lesions involving the posterior hypothalamus is compatible with experimental evidence indicating that this region functions to integrate thermoregulatory cold-defense mechanisms. Paradoxically, in the case reported by Fox and coworkers,[17] scarring and neuronal damage were observed in the anterior hypothalamus; the posterior hypothalamus was intact. Endocrinologic studies in this patient, a 26-year-old man, showed that he had lost normal diurnal variation of plasma cortisol and was hypothyroid, but had preserved cortisol and GH responses to metyrapone, glucose, and insulin.

Periventricular lesions such as those in Wernicke's encephalopathy may lead to severe hypothermia.[66] Several drugs, including barbiturates and alcohol, also contribute to defective heat-maintenance mechanisms. Sustained hypoglycemia may result in hypothermia and this effect can be mimicked by 2-deoxyglucose (which blocks glucose uptake by the cell), suggesting that the hypothermia is induced by intracellular glucopenia. Exclusion of glucose from CNS sites appeared to be the mechanism of this hypothermia, which is present despite markedly increased excretion of catecholamines.

Episodes of hypothermia in elderly, nonalcoholic patients may be more common than usually is appreciated.[35] The evidence for this condition has recently been summarized by Johnson and Spalding.[34] Such patients, it has been suggested, have defective central

Table 3. Neuropathologic Abnormalities in Chronic Disorders of Central Thermoregulation

Neoplasm	*Metabolic*
Craniopharyngioma	Wernicke's encephalopathy
Glioblastoma multiforme	*Degenerative*
Neuroblastoma	Glial scarring, anterior hypothalamus
Angioma, third ventricle	Parkinson's disease with reduction and shrinkage
Facial hemangioma involving the hypothalamus	of neurons in posterior hypothalamus
Infectious	*Developmental*
Poliomyelitis	Hydrocephalus
Syphilitic endarteritis	Encephalocele
Vascular	*Traumatic*
Infarction	Postneurosurgical
Granulomatous	Head trauma
Sarcoidosis	

thermoregulatory mechanisms. Peripheral vasomotor and shivering responses could be demonstrated. Similar defects are seen in anorexia nervosa.

Spontaneous Periodic Hypothermia

In 1907, Gowers[24] described a 28-year-old woman and a 30-year-old man with periodic excessive autonomic activity associated with icy coldness of the extremities. Temperatures were not measured in Gowers' cases but the similarity of their clinical features to later reports suggests that he should receive recognition for first description of the disorder now called spontaneous periodic hypothermia. In 1929, Penfield[51] reported a 41-year-old woman with periodic vasodilatation, sweating, lacrimation, and hypothermia associated with a cholesteatoma of the third ventricle. The periodic symptoms were attributed to seizure activity and the descriptive term "diencephalic autonomic epilepsy" was applied.

Various authors have applied the descriptions "spontaneous periodic hypothermia," "diencephalic epilepsy," or "intermittent hypothermia with disabling hyperhidrosis" to this syndrome.[17, 26, 62] The term spontaneous periodic hypothermia adequately characterizes all these. Because the literature also contains several reports of spontaneous periodic hypothermia in association with intracranial abnormalities, we propose that the requirement of "no evidence of intracranial abnormality" be excluded from the definition.

This syndrome describes periodic hypothermia with normal body temperature regulation present during the intervals. Symptoms of profound autonomic nervous system activity such as sweating, vasodilatation, nausea, vomiting, salivation, lacrimation, and bradycardia may occur. Often dulling of mentation occurs, and shivering may coincide with return of the body temperature to normal. Neurologic deficits are usually absent between paroxysms. The episodes are short-lived, lasting minutes or hours. The rectal temperature may drop below 30° C.

Thirteen cases of spontaneous periodic hypothermia have been reported in the literature. Agenesis of the corpus callosum has been detected by pneumoencephalography in four of these patients. Noel and coworkers[48] reported autopsy findings of gliosis of the arcuate nucleus and premammillary area in a patient with agenesis of the corpus callosum associated with spontaneous periodic hypothermia. Their study supports the concept that associated lesions of the hypothalamus may coexist with agenesis of the corpus callosum and cause the manifestations of spontaneous periodic hypothermia. The majority of patients with agenesis of the corpus callosum, however, do not develop spontaneous periodic hypothermia.

Few endocrine disorders have been reported to occur in patients with spontaneous periodic hypothermia. Guihard and associates[26] described a 9-year-old boy with precocious puberty, diabetes insipidus, and GH deficiency associated with agenesis of the corpus callosum. Noel and coworkers[48] noted hypogonadism but did not measure gonadotropins. Assays of serum T_4 and GH were normal, as was the cortisol response to metyrapone administration in this patient. Biochemical assessments of anterior pituitary function in five other patients (including one with agenesis of the corpus callosum) were normal.

Spontaneous Periodic Hyperthermia

A single case of an interesting periodic discharge syndrome has been described by Wolff and colleagues.[68] The patient presented with recurrent episodes of fever, hyper-

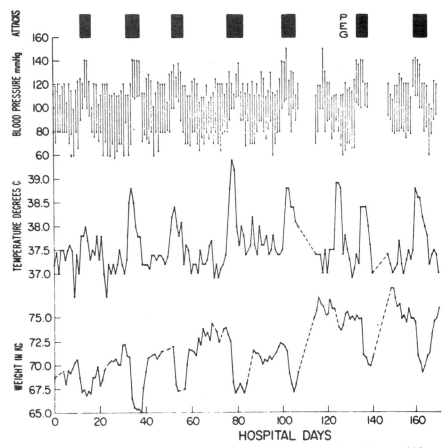

Figure 5. Recurrent episodes of hypertension, hyperthermia, and weight loss in a 14-year-old boy. Clinical attacks occurred at approximately 3-week intervals. Pneumoencephalogram (PEG) was associated with fever only. (From Wolff, S. M., et al.: *A syndrome of periodic hypothalamic discharge.* Am. J. Med. 36:956, 1964, with permission.)

tension, vomiting, and weight loss, associated with increased excretion of corticoids (Fig. 5). Treatment with chlorpromazine was successful.

CARDIOVASCULAR MANIFESTATIONS OF HYPOTHALAMIC DISEASE

Anterior hypothalamic lesions, particularly if sudden in onset, may be associated with cardiovascular disturbances ranging from mild ECG alterations to pulmonary edema. Such changes are frequently observed in patients with ruptured aneurysm of the anterior communicating artery and intracerebral hemorrhages in the region of the anterior hypothalamic-preoptic area. Acute head injury in man may be accompanied by pulmonary edema. The mechanisms of pulmonary edema induced by hypothalamic lesions have been investigated and it appears that such lesions produce vasoconstriction with attendant left heart strain and a failure of the left heart to relax adequately in diastole. Blood may also be redistributed from abdominal venous pools. A combination of these two events can lead to pulmonary edema. In experimental animals, administration of phenoxybenzamine, an α-adrenergic blocking agent, can prevent

257

such pulmonary edema. Hypothalamic mechanisms for cardiovascular regulation have been recently reviewed by Hilton[31] and Smith and coworkers.[61]

NEURAL CONTROL OF FOOD INTAKE

In 1901, Fröhlich[18] described a case of hypogonadism with obesity in a 14-year-old boy with a pituitary tumor. Although he originally attributed the disorder to pituitary dysfunction, he later recognized that involvement of the hypothalamus was the primary cause. The association of obesity with hypogonadism in hypothalamic disease is now a commonly recognized, although not invariable, association; hypogonadism of hypothalamic origin may occur as an isolated disorder, and hypothalamic obesity may occur without hypogonadism. A disturbance of affect frequently accompanies the hypothalamic form of obesity, particularly when it occurs in the adult. This is characterized by unprovoked rages, overt aggression, and antisocial behavior. The precise hypothalamic area involved in man has been documented only infrequently. Lesions of the tuberal and median eminence area of the hypothalamus are usually described (which accounts for the frequent association of obesity, hypogonadism, and diabetes insipidus). Lesions are usually too extensive to provide a useful anatomic correlation.

A case described in some detail by Reeves and Plum[55] has contributed a great deal to an understanding of the precise localization of such lesions in producing this syndrome in man. The patient was a 28-year-old obese woman with a one-year history of excessive eating, polyuria, polydypsia, and amenorrhea (Fig. 6). Neurologic examination was normal; pneumoencephalography showed a filling defect in the anterior third ventricle, but nothing abnormal was found on surgical exploration. Two years later the patient returned with a two-month history of behavioral abnormality characterized by intermittent withdrawal, unprovoked laughing, crying, and at times uncontrolled rages and aggression. On examination, the patient was intermittently confused

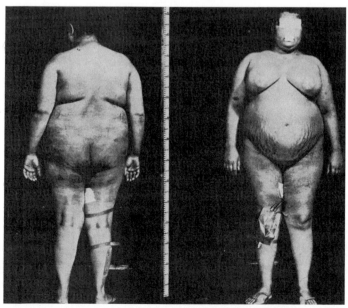

Figure 6. Obesity in a 28-year-old woman with a hypothalamic lesion. Catheter had been inserted for metabolic balance studies. (From Reeves, A. G. and Plum, F.: *Hyperphagia, rage and dementia accompanying a ventromedial hypothalamic neoplasm.* Arch. Neurol. 20:617, 1969, with permission.)

and appeared to have hallucinations. She was even more obese and was extremely un-cooperative and at times physically aggressive. These episodes alternated with periods during which she was cooperative and even apologetic for her behavior. The endocrine studies of the patient were not extensive but indicated borderline-low thyroid and adrenal function. Caloric intake ranged from 8,000 to 10,000 per day and her behavioral outbursts were accentuated by attempts to restrict food intake. The patient died of a pulmonary embolus. Autopsy showed a pale mass that protruded from the basal hypothalamus extending from the posterior optic chiasm to the anterior region of the mammillary bodies. The mass, a hamartoma, was found to have invaded the ventromedial nucleus bilaterally, destroying the median eminence but sparing the lateral hypothalamus (Fig. 7). The lesion extended anteriorly into the anterior hypothalamic-preoptic area.

The clinical-pathologic correlation in this case was remarkable. The symptom complex of excessive appetite, hyperphagia with obesity, diabetes insipidus, amenorrhea, and grossly disordered emotional reactivity was correlated with a lesion destroying the median eminence and the ventromedial hypothalamic nuclei but sparing the lateral zones of the hypothalamus.

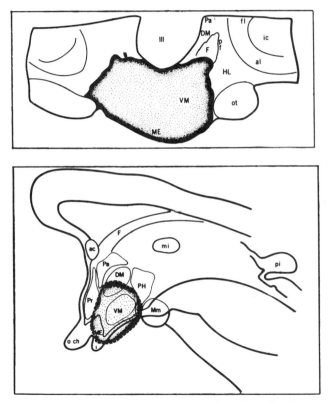

Figure 7. Hypothalamic lesion producing hyperphagia and obesity. The lesion destroyed the ventromedial (VM) nucleus bilaterally and invaded the median eminence (ME). Abbreviations: ac, anterior commissure; al, ansa lenticularis; DM, dorsomedial nuclear region, F, fornix; fl, fasciculus lenticularis; HL, lateral hypothalamus; i, infundibular stalk; ic, internal capsule; mi, massa intermedia; mm, mammillary body; ME, median eminence; o ch, optic chiasm; ot, optic tract; Pa, paraventricular nucleus; ph, pallidohypothalamic tract; pf, perifornical region; PH, posterior hypothalamus; pi, pineal body; Pr, preoptic region; so, supra optic nucleus; t, thalamus; VM, ventromedial nuclear region; zi, zonia incerta; III, third ventricle. (From Reeves, A. G. and Plum, F.: *Hyperphagia, rage and dementia accompanying a ventromedial hypothalamic neoplasm.* Arch. Nurol. 20:621, 1969, with permission.)

259

Most clinical reports of patients with hypothalamic obesity do not show as precise a distribution of lesions as in this case. In most, the lesion is rather ill-defined, and the relationship to obesity not always clear.

Hypothalamic disorders reported to occur in association with obesity have been summarized in a comprehensive review by Bray and Gallagher,[9] which includes eight cases of their own. The most common causes were solid tumors, leukemia, inflammatory disease, external head trauma, and surgical intervention for various tumors or vascular lesions involving the base of the brain. Craniopharyngioma was the most common solid tumor, others included adenoma, angiosarcoma, glioma, cysts, cholesteatoma, hamartoma, ganglioneuroma, epithelioma, meningioma, and chordoma. Inflammatory diseases included sarcoidosis, tuberculosis, arachnoiditis, and encephalitis. In approximately half of these cases endocrine function was abnormal, the most common finding being impaired gonadotropin secretion or diabetes insipidus.

The vastness of the literature on regulation of food intake indicates the complexity of the regulatory process, as well as its importance.[1, 25, 36] Under normal conditions animals, including man, eat appropriately for caloric balance and growth, and in maturity achieve a relatively stable body weight. On a short-term basis, cyclic eating behavior is initiated, then stopped in response to some form of satiety signal. On a long-term basis, mature animals adjust their eating behavior to maintain a constant depot of stored calories in the form of fat. Neural factors are involved in both kinds of homeostatis response, and they are integrated with each other.

Physiologic Sensors of Caloric State

Short-Term Regulation

Extensive ablation studies in the classic era of physiology indicated that afferent stimuli from mouth, throat, and stomach brought about by eating all contribute to the sense of satiety in animals, but these signals are supplemental and not essential for adequate monitoring of food intake.[36, 37] They probably are important in the acquisition and maintenance of conditioned eating responses, i.e., animals will eat "enough" for caloric need and stop eating long before the full metabolic effect of a given meal has been sensed, and bulk distention of the stomach may restrict food intake to some extent. Of greater importance in short-term regulation is probably the hypothalamic system for recognizing blood content of nutrients, particularly glucose. As emphasized by Mayer[41] in his "glucostat" hypothesis, the hypothalamus contains glucose-sensitive neurons, which can monitor either absolute blood glucose, rate of change of blood glucose, or rate of glucose utilization. These glucostat neurons, it is postulated, determine food drive. Experimental findings which support the Mayer hypothesis include the demonstration of neurons in the ventromedial area of the hypothalamus which increase their firing rate in response to increases in blood glucose, and the phenomenon of gold thioglucose-induced obesity. In this experimental model, glucose conjugated with gold, a neurotoxin, is selectively concentrated in the ventromedial nucleus, where it causes both neural destruction and hyperphagia. Gold salts which are not chemical analogues of glucose are not toxic; the effect of the agent is increased by insulin administration which increases gold thioglucose uptake, and the extent of the damage is decreased by diabetes (insulin deficiency), which reduces uptake. Localization of this reaction in the ventromedial nucleus is indicated by the observation that electrolytic destruction of this region (or of adjacent fibers) causes obesity, and electric stimulation of the VMN inhibits eating.

The possibility has been considered that glucoreceptors exist in other regions of the brain, or in the gastrointestinal tract. Russek[57] has proposed that glucose-sensitive hepatocytes can monitor glucose concentrations in the portal vein of the liver. He has recently shown that the transmembrane potentials of the hepatocyte increase after local administration of glucose, and that these detectors signal central regulatory centers via the vagus or the sympathetic nerves. Also, surgical section of the vagi in rats prevents the development of hypothalamic obesity. Not all workers can confirm this claim, however.

Long-Term Regulation

The precision of long-term control of appetite is remarkable. A normal man gains, on the average, 15 pounds in weight between the ages of 20 and 40, representing a daily excess intake of only 16 Calories (equivalent to one teaspoon of sugar). Over this period, he will have ingested a total of approximately 1.5×10^7 Calories, and thus has adjusted intake to need with an accuracy of 0.8 per cent per year, or .001 per cent per meal. Most investigators do not believe that any short-term monitoring system such as receptor afferents from the gastrointestinal tract, or a central glucoreceptor, could possibly provide this extraordinary precision. Moreover, detailed balance studies in man show that most people have rather wide short-term swings in food intake, but on a longer time-scale, intake is quite constant. In experimental animals it is easy to show that forced feeding, which leads to increased fat deposition, is followed by sustained periods of decreased food intake, indicating that the animals adjust to the total fat stores. Even in obesity due to hypothalamic lesions, food intake ceases after a certain weight has been reached. Starvation of such animals followed by free access to food is followed by restitution of the prior (though excess) weight.

On the basis of these observations, Kennedy[36, 37] has proposed that long-term caloric balance is primarily mediated by a "lipostatic" mechanism. In further support of this hypothesis is the experimental finding that rats with hypothalamic hyperphagia and obesity when joined parabiotically to a normal animal cause the normal partner to stop eating and finally to die from cachexia. Moreover, animals whose fat depots have been removed soon gain weight to equalize that of the lost tissue. The mechanism by which fat depots control appetite is unknown; some have postulated that a fat metabolite, such as fatty acids or ketones, is regulatory (modest effects have been demonstrated in ruminants) and others, that fat tissue modifies metabolic degradation of some circulating steroid hormone. Panskepp[50] has proposed the ingenious idea that a fat tissue analogue is present in the hypothalamic appetite-regulating area which reflects the state of peripheral fat tissues.

Neural Organization

Hypothalamus

Hypothalamic mechanisms for regulation of food drive have been well demonstrated. As mentioned previously, lesions of the VMN (or surrounding areas) cause increased eating, while electric stimulation stops feeding.[41, 53] Contrarily, lesions of the lateral hypothalamus (LH) lead to a syndrome of aphagia and adipsia, and stimulation of these regions causes an increase in food intake. Thus, the view has developed of a reciprocal interaction between a lateral food-drive-stimulating region and a VMN satiety mechanism. The VMN includes glucoreceptor elements capable of sensing rising glucose levels. In recent electrophysiologic studies, Oomora and coworkers[49] have shown that about one third of VMN neurons are stimulated by directly applied glucose.

Neuroanatomic studies support the view that there are neural pathways between lateral and medial hypothalamus, and a syndrome identical with that following VMN destruction can be elicited by longitudinal cuts lateral to the VMN.[32] Morgane[43, 44] has shown that the spontaneous electric activity of the lateral hypothalamus is turned off by electric stimulation of the VMN area. Self-stimulation of the lateral hypothalamus (one of the important reward sites) also is inhibited by VMN electric stimulation. LH neurons are inhibited by glucose application. Thus there are distinct types of glucoreceptor neurons, those of the VMN which respond to rising glucose levels, and those of the LH which respond to falling levels. It has been postulated that food drive is tonically maintained by the lateral hypothalamus and is periodically inhibited by VMN influences which reflect glucose level. We think it likely that either of these regions (or both) is controlled by an as yet undefined signal which reflects total body stored calories (Fig. 8)

It is important to recognize that even in LH lesions, control of food intake is not a clearly defined and unique deficit. Such animals also show transient hypodipsia and impaired recognition of external signals of all types. For example, unilateral destruction of the LH region leads to ipsilateral failure to recognize and respond to food placed on the involved side of the animal.

The concept of a VMN "satiety center" and a LH "feeding center" has been challenged repeatedly.[42] VMN-lesioned animals are hyperactive, hyperemotional, and more finicky in food preferences. Since they do not work harder to obtain food it has been argued that motivational systems, not appetite, are affected. LH-lesioned animals are apathetic, hypoactive, and depressed. Morrison and Mayer[45] have suggested that they suffer from an "apraxia of feeding."

Although anatomic connections between the VMN and LH have been demonstrated, it has been proposed that functional connections between these areas important in food intake may be indirect, via the brain stem or limbic system (see Fig. 8). The controversy surrounding this subject has been extensively reviewed by Rabin.[53]

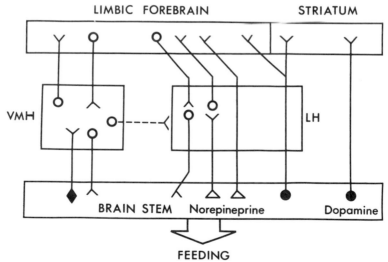

Figure 8. Diagram of the role of the hypothalamus in feeding. Noradrenergic fibers from brain stem project to both lateral hypothalamus (LH) and limbic forebrain. Lesions of these fibers interfere with normal feeding; chemical stimulation via α-receptors stimulates feeding. The ventromedial hypothalamus (VMH) is interconnected with the limbic forebrain and the brain stem. Interactions between a LH "feeding center" and a VMH "satiety center" may thus be indirect via either limbic or brain stem connections. The dotted line between LH and VMH indicates that anatomic connections between these areas do exist. The dopaminergic system to the basal ganglia has been implicated in the motor control of feeding, rather than in the "motivational" aspects.

Peptide Hormones

Direct effects of peptide hormones on appetite regulating areas of the hypothalamus also have been thought to be involved in regulation of feeding. Insulin injections are followed by marked stimulation of food intake in some species. Although it is reasonable to attribute these responses to hypoglycemia, there is also evidence for a direct effect of insulin on the brain, and for the presence of hypothalamic insulin receptors. Glucagon injections are reported to inhibit food intake, an effect possibly related to the induced hyperglycemia. Recently there has been interest in the possible role of gut peptide hormones in the regulation of food intake. It has been proposed by Smith and collaborators[60] that the duodenal hormone pancreazymin-cholecystokinin, which is released in response to feeding serves as a satiety signal. In both rats and monkeys, injections of cholecystokinin (but not other gut hormones) inhibit food intake. Crucial to this claim is whether sufficient amounts of this hormone are released under normal feeding conditions to affect eating behavior. Infusion studies in man suggest that cholecystokinin, when administered in doses equivalent to those that occur naturally after eating, does not suppress appetite. Fed animals are reported to have a circulating peptide or protein "satiety factor" detectable by bioassay.

Neuropharmacologic System

The neural system which regulates food intake includes elements responsive to biogenic amines.[25] In this regard it may parallel the organized biogenic-amine-mediated system involved in determination of affective states and responsible for control of hypophysiotrophic neuron function. Injection of small amounts of norepinephrine into the VMN of food-satiated rats stimulates further food intake; α-blocking noradrenergic agents placed in the same area cause a reduction in food intake.[42] In the lateral hypothalamus, norepinephrine causes a decrease in food intake, an effect blocked by β-receptors. Thus, it has been proposed that the VMN is inhibited by α-receptor activation and the lateral hypothalamus is inhibited by β-receptor activation. Drugs such as amphetamines which inhibit food intake would then be looked on as acting to inhibit lateral hypothalamic function through β-agonist action. Isoproterenol, a β-adrenergic receptor agonist, inhibits food intake in hungry rats; propranolol, a β-blocking drug, increases food consumption. These results support the hypothesis that feeding mechanism may involve both α- and β-adrenergic receptors.

Depletion of central norepinephrine and dopamine by the systemic administration of 6-hydroxydopamine results in a reduction in food intake with a fall in body weight.[42] In contrast, local injections of 6-hydroxydopamine or high-midbrain lesions that interrupt noradrenergic inputs to the hypothalamus result in hyperphagia and obesity. In these studies the histochemical fluorescence of noradrenergic terminals was reduced in the hypothalamic ventromedial nuclei; it was argued that these results indicate an inhibitory role of ascending noradrenergic inputs to the hypothalamus, and suggested that hypothalamic obesity after lesions is due to interruption of this pathway.

Extrahypothalamic Regulation

It would be gross oversimplification to imply that the lateral hypothalamus is the only region of the brain which has an important influence on food intake. The studies of Chi and coworkers[4, 12] have shown that hypothalamic-island procedures that separate the hypothalamus from the rest of the brain, do not necessarily produce aphagia as would be expected if the only region for this drive were located in or restricted to the hypothalamus. Other areas must be capable of initiating this form of behavior. It should not be surprising that such highly integrated activity as seeking, discriminating, and ingesting appropriate quantities of food must involve extensive areas of the limbic brain. Klüver and Bucy[38] described aberrations in discrimination of food following temporal lobe lesions in the monkey, and frontal lobotomy was also sometimes followed by hyperphagia and obesity. Bilateral lesions of the amygdala are reported in several species to produce varying syndromes of adipsia and aphagia, and disorders of perception, recognition, and behavior in respect to food intake have been described in man which have features akin to the Klüver-Bucy syndrome. Extensive neurophysiologic data relating the limbic system to hypothalamic food regulation have been accumulated by Morgane.[44]

Hypothalamic Factors in Human Obesity

While it is generally agreed that obesity may arise from hypothalamic lesions, it is equally likely that in most cases of obesity no significant hypothalamic abnormalities are involved. A number of writers have emphasized the similarities between VMN-lesioned rats and fat humans. As summarized recently by Girvin,[22] both VMN-lesioned rats and fat humans 1) eat more of a good-tasting food, 2) eat less of a bad-tasting food, 3) eat only a slight excess of food during each day, 4) eat fewer meals each day, 5) eat more at each meal, 6) eat more quickly, 7) react more emotionally, 8) are less active, 9) eat more when food is easily accessible, 10) eat less when food is difficult to obtain, and 11) fail to regulate food consumption when the food consumed is preloaded with solids but regulate normally when preloaded with liquids. External controls (tastes, psychic factors, and the social milieu) rather than internal food signals appear to take over regulation of food intake in both obese individuals and VM-lesioned rats. These superficial similarities may be a clue to the pathophysiology of human hyperphagia. Compulsive eating may occur with rather nonspecific brain lesions. Green and Rau[70] have reported a series of 10 such patients, 9 of whom had abnormal EEGs and were successfully treated with anticonvulsants.

Lateral Hypothalamic Lesions: The Lateral Hypothalamic Syndrome in Man

In marked contrast to the VMN syndrome are the effects of lesions in the lateral hypothalamus immediately adjacent to the VMN: these result in aphagia which when severe can lead to cachexia and death.

Anorexia secondary to a hypothalamic lesion is rare. In a case reported by White and Hain,[67] a 62-year-old woman died after progressive emaciation to a final weight of 67 pounds. On postmortem examination, a small discrete cystic lesion in the wall of the third ventricle was noted that had resulted in a decrease in hypothalamic tissue. The primary lesion was in the hypothalamus. More recently, Lewin and coworkers[39] reported the case of a young woman who suffered from severe anorexia nervosa. She was found at autopsy to have an astrocytoma involving the inferior surface of the hypothalamus. A direct correlation between the lateral hypothalamic lesions described in experimental animals and the presence of an anorexia syndrome in man does not appear to have been reported.

Diencephalic Syndrome

A rare disorder of infancy is the diencephalic syndrome caused by a primary neoplasm of the anterior hypothalamic area. No counterpart has been described in experimental animals. The infant, usually a boy, follows a stereotyped course. After normal

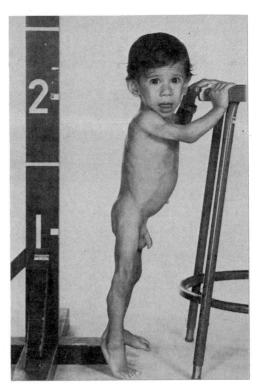

Figure 9. Two-year-old child with diencephalic syndrome due to astrocytoma of anterior hypothalamus. There is loss of subcutaneous fat and growth failure. (Courtesy of H. Guyda.)

birth and early development, the infant starts to lose weight, usually between the third and twelfth months of life, and emaciation becomes progressive despite normal food intake (Fig. 9). In most cases, the infant is described as being unusually cheerful and alert, despite its apparent cachexia. Emaciation is unrelenting and death occurs before the second year. The lesions in these infants have been remarkably consistent, usually being low-grade astrocytomas of the anterior hypothalamus or optic nerve. The pathophysiology of the disturbance is unexplained. It is apparent that this is not an aphagia produced by lateral hypothalamic lesions, as food intake may be increased. Hypothalamic lesions in this age group appear to result consistently in this wasting syndrome rather than the more typical picture of later childhood and adolescence in which similar lesions result in obesity, somnolence, rage, and precocious puberty. The remarkable lack of subcutaneous fat in these cases is so striking as to be of diagnostic assistance on plain roentgenograms of the extremities. Several reports have noted elevated GH levels in cases of diencephalic syndrome due conceivably to loss of the anterior hypothalamic GH-inhibiting pathways. Such lesions might result in uncontrolled secretion of this hormone (see Chapter 7). Further studies will be required to evaluate the role of GH in such cases.

Treatment by surgical removal or irradiation has been effective in some cases (Fig. 10).

DISORDERS OF CONSCIOUSNESS ASSOCIATED WITH HYPOTHALAMIC DISEASE

A disturbance of consciousness attributable to hypothalamic lesions was first described by Gayet in 1875 in a patient with severe somnolence whose autopsy examination disclosed necrotic periventricular lesions of the third ventricle.[66] This was proba-

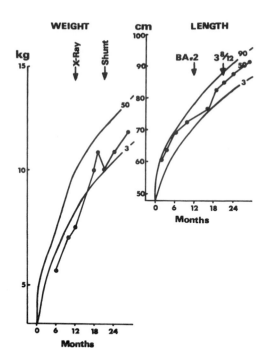

Figure 10. Data on growth failure in child with diencephalic syndrome. Growth failure, which occurred despite elevated GH levels, was corrected by roentgenotherapy. (Courtesy of H. Guyda.)

bly the first description of what was to become known as Wernicke's encephalopathy, the pathology of which was described by him in 1881. This condition commonly is associated with somnolence and confusion in the acute stage. In 1890, Mauthner described several cases of encephalitis in which somnolence was predominent and demonstrated lesions in the basal diencephalon.[66] Probably these cases were early examples of epidemic encephalitis, later described in detail by Von Economo. His descriptions were the first to indicate an association of somnolence with lesions in the posterior hypothalamus. This conclusion has been repeatedly confirmed by both experimental and clinical observations.

Aberrations in the level of consciousness ranging from increased periods of sleeping, from which arousal is easily obtained, to frank coma have been attributed to hypothalamic lesions.[5, 19] This area of investigation, perhaps more than any other aspect of hypothalamic function, has been difficult and poorly documented. The opposite disturbance, insomnia, has rarely been shown to be associated with any specific lesions, with the exception of the reports of Von Economo in which anterior hypothalamic-preoptic lesions were said to be associated with hyperactivity and decreased sleeping periods.

The precise hypothalamic sites that cause a disorder of consciousness have been difficult to obtain from clinicopathologic material. By the time the patient dies, lesions are frequently extensive and the secondary effects of increased intracranial pressure have supervened. Despite this difficulty, one can derive a tentative conclusion with respect to hypothalamic function in the regulation of consciousness which agrees closely with the experimental literature. However, it must be emphasized at the outset that the hypothalamus is neither the sole site of, nor need be implicated at all with lesions that cause a disorder in consciousness.

Regions of the brain, destruction of which result in altered consciousness, range from bilateral cortical lesions to lesions in the caudal pons and possibly the rostral medulla. This subject has been critically reviewed by Plum and Posner.[52] The effect of a given lesion depends to a major degree on the acuteness of onset. A very large lesion in the basal hypothalamus, developing in the course of an expanding tumor, may not be associated with alterations of consciousness, while the abrupt development of a small posterior hypothalamic lesion may produce profound coma. The survival time following an acute lesion also affects the manifestations of that lesion. Remarkable recovery of function following extensive lesions of the upper midbrain and posterior hypothalamus has been reported in patients who have survived for weeks or months after the initial episode. Animal studies closely parallel this finding.

Lesions at a number of diverse sites along the neural axis of the limbic system can produce remarkably similar clinical disorders.[5, 14] Cases from the literature involve lesions of the cingulate gyrus, the hypothalamus, and the midbrain reticular formation, each of which produced a similar clinical abnormality. In the case reported by Neilson and Jacobs,[47] a 46-year-old woman developed a peculiar, abrupt-onset stupor during which she stood immobile with eyes open and a vacant stare, and did not appear to respond to auditory or visual stimuli. She survived several days during which she remained mute and unresponsive, yet frequently appeared to be awake. She was incontinent and made no effort to eat. At autopsy, extensive bilateral lesions were found in the distribution of the anterior cerebral arteries, which had resulted in necrosis of the anterior portions of both cingulate gyri. The corpus callosum was not involved. The authors pointed out the similarities between this case and those of Marchiafava-Bignami disease in which lesions of the corpus callosum occur.

The description of this case is not unlike that of so-called akinetic mutism, a term coined by Cairns in 1941[10] to describe the clinical findings in a 14-year-old girl with a craniopharyngioma extending deeply into the tuberal region of the hypothalamus. The patient had a history of progressive somnolence from which she could not be aroused. At the time of admission, although appearing awake, the patient showed no response to questions and appeared to be in a trance. Her eyes moved to follow an object and she would fixate upon the examiner as if about to speak but nothing was forthcoming. She was mute and showed virtually no spontaneous movement (hence the term akinetic mutism). In addition, she showed minimal responses to painful stimuli with absence of any observable signs of emotional expression. She was able to swallow food and liquid when it was placed in her mouth but made no signs of desiring either. She was incontinent of both feces and urine.

The remarkable feature of this case was that following operative drainage of the tumor under local anesthesia, the patient immediately began to respond and to speak. She had no recollection of the period of coma. This unusual clinical picture has also been referred to as "coma vigil."[11, 13]

Fulton and Bailey[19] described a similar case in a 28-year-old woman with a lesion in the same region. She had suffered for many years from amenorrhea, polyuria, and polydipsia. About five years before death, episodes of drowsiness began to occur, during which the patient would suddenly drop asleep in the midst of an animated conversation or in the middle of routine duties. She could always be aroused from such episodes and they appeared to be normal periods of sleeping rather than seizures. Prior to death, extreme somnolence occurred, progressing to coma. At autopsy, a sarcoma of the tuberal region was found. There was no associated hydrocephalus and the pituitary appeared normal. It is apparent that in such cases the anatomic localization of the defect is not precise. Nor is it always possible to exclude pressure effects on the posterior hypothalamic region or upper midbrain.

A lesion in the posterior-basal hypothalamus was considered to be the cause of somnolence and hypothermia in the case of glioblastoma reported by Davison and Demuth.[14] The tumor in this instance involved the medial posterior hypothalamus and extended from the posterior region of the infundibulum through the mammillary region, but did not extend into the midbrain.

Lesions of the upper mesencephalic reticular formation initially produce profound coma and are usually irreversible.[59, 63] Occasionally, with prolonged survival, recovery to a stage similar to akinetic mutism may occur.[63] It is important to make a distinction with respect to apparent coma secondary to lesions in the pons. Such lesions which interrupt corticospinal, corticobulbar, and corticopontine fibers, can result in total paralysis with preservation of eye or lid movement. The patient may appear superficially to have akinetic mutism. However, consciousness may be entirely preserved and the EEG may show a normal alpha pattern. Recognition of this fact is of upmost importance in the management of the patient. Plum and Posner[52] described this paralytic form as the "locked-in syndrome."

These cases illustrate that no precise anatomic area controls consciousness. The maintenance of normal sleep-waking sequences appear to depend on brain-stem influences as well as those of certain areas of the limbic system. Disturbances at a number of levels may produce profound disorders of consciousness. Having made this generalization, it is still accurate to say that the areas most likely to result in the greatest disturbance of consciousness are the midbrain reticular formation and the posterior hypothalamus.[59, 63, 64]

Experiments in animals confirm this view. Ranson[54] demonstrated in primates that lateral hypothalamic lesions in the regions adjacent to the mammillary bodies produced a syndrome of akinesia, hypothermia, tameness, lethargy, and temporary aphagia. Acute lesions in the mesencephalic tegmentum caused a more severe disorder of consciousness, but Sprague[63] has shown that with careful nursing care during the first weeks following placement of such lesions, survival can be prolonged and accompanied by remarkable recovery. Two-stage operations also result in much less functional disturbance, even when equivalent amounts of tissue are destroyed.

Studies in the cat have also indicated that the degree and persistence of somnolence produced by hypothalamic lesions are proportional to the extent of involvement of pathways from the ventromedial nucleus and posterior hypothalamus to ventral mesencephalic nuclei. Swett[64] recently described in the cat a distinguishing feature of posterior hypothalamic lesions, depending on whether they are medial or lateral. Medial posterior hypothalamic lesions result in minimal disturbance of consciousness, feeding, or grooming, whereas lateral posterior hypothalamic lesions induce drowsiness, cataplexy, and absence of feeding. It was concluded (as Ranson had early suggested) that lateral pathways in or close to the medial forebrain bundle are of great importance in the maintenance of normal alertness.

MEMORY AND THE HYPOTHALAMUS

For many years it was considered likely that lesions of the mammillary bodies which occur in Wernicke's encephalopathy were responsible for a deficit in memory (Korsakoff's psychosis). The extensive studies of Victor and associates[66] have cast some doubt on this hypothesis. The lesions which they found to be most consistently associated with a memory deficit in patients with Wernicke-Korsakoff disease were located in the medial dorsal nucleus of the thalamus. No other evidence for a hypothalamic role in memory function has been produced in man.

PERIODIC HYPOTHALAMIC DISEASE

Kleine-Levin Syndrome

The Kleine-Levin syndrome is characterized by the appearance, usually in adolescent males, of recurrent episodes of somnolence, hyperphagia, and sexual hyperactivity.[7, 15, 21] Individual attacks appear at intervals of three to six months and may last for one to three weeks. During the attack the patient sleeps for extended periods of time, often 18 to 20 hours daily. Episodes of arousal may be associated with gorging of food, masturbation, and overt sexual advances on the nursing staff. The attack is self-limited and there is commonly amnesia for the episode.

During an attack, there is no demonstrable neurologic abnormality and endocrine studies are usually normal. In one report, diurnal variations in steroids were absent during the attack. No structural lesions have been described although occasionally a patient with an encephalitis-like illness may present a similar pattern. One patient was said to have had a recent toxoplasmosis infection.

In the interval between attacks, the patient demonstrates no abnormalities. In general, the disorder is self-limited and disappears by late adolescence or early adult life.

The term Kleine-Levin syndrome was given to this disorder by MacDonald Critchley in 1942.[21] He described two cases of his own and found another 16 in the early literature, the first reports being separate cases reported by Kleine and by Levin.

In recent years, cases of similar periodic disorders have been observed in girls and in adult patients. Because of the characteristic symptoms, the disorder is thought to reflect deranged hypothalamic function, although proof of this is lacking.

Periodic Syndrome of Wolff

In 1964,[68] Wolff described a case of periodic hyperthermia, vomiting, weight loss, and hypercortisolemia that he attributed to cyclic hypothalamic discharge. The attacks occurred with remarkable regularity every three weeks. Treatment with chlorpromazine was effective in controlling the episodes. The relationship of this case to diencephalic epilepsy is not clear at this time.

Diencephalic Epilepsy

Episodes of autonomic dysfunction characterized by tachycardia, flushing, hypertension, salivation, sweating, and deviations in temperature regulation have been called diencephalic epilepsy.[51, 62] The EEG was abnormal in many of the cases reported and about half of the patients have responded favorably to anticonvulsants. In the majority of cases that have been examined at autopsy, a space-occupying lesion has been found in the region of the third ventricle. Cholesteatoma, colloid cyst of the third ventricle, and gliomas have been reported. Paroxysmal attacks of autonomic activation appear, therefore, to be caused by direct pressure effects of obvious anatomic lesions on the hypothalamus. Although rare, when suspected, such cases require complete investigation in an attempt to establish the cause.

MISCELLANEOUS HYPOTHALAMIC SYNDROMES

The association of obesity, hypogonadism and mental retardation has been described in several disorders that are thought to be due to hypothalamic dysfunction.

Prader-Willi Syndrome

A disorder characterized by mental retardation, short stature, hypogonadism (and cryptorchidism), obesity, and neonatal hypotonia was described by Prader, Labhart, and Willi in 1956 and 1963.[69] Over 100 cases that fulfill these criteria have now been reported. The condition occurs sporadically and it is not certain that the syndrome is a single nosologic entity. In fact, the group of symptoms and signs are not dissimilar to so-called Fröhlich's syndrome (adiposogenital syndrome) which is no longer considered to be a specific disorder and which is generally associated with organic brain disease. The disorder is recognized at birth by severe hypotonia and inactivity. The infant is motionless, sleepy, difficult to arouse, and areflexic. Temperature regulation may be abnormal. Tube-feeding is frequently required for several weeks.

Feeding difficulties are replaced by hyperphagia between age 6 months to 2 years. The child eats continuously and seems to lack normal satiety mechanisms. Gross obesity may result. Diabetes mellitus is frequently associated.

The constellation of abnormalities in these patients suggests hypothalamic dysfunction. However, clinical investigations fail to reveal lesions and autopsied cases have not shown any definite abnormalities. Endocrinologic studies have rarely been performed in the postpubertal age group. In the report of Hamilton and coworkers,[27] three patients between the ages of 19 and 23 were studied. Each had evidence of hypogonadotropic hypogonadism and one patient responded to clomiphene with a rise in testosterone that persisted after discontinuation of the drug. TSH, ACTH, and GH responses were normal. It is likely that the disorder is the result of an undefined organic lesion of the hypothalamus that interferes with normal regulation of gonadotropins. The possibility exists that perinatal insult due to an as yet unspecified cause may result in the rather selective hypothalamic abnormality. It is not clear from the literature whether the sense of smell is normal in these patients or whether some may represent a variant of Kallmann's syndrome.

Laurence-Moon-Biedl Syndrome

A hereditary condition characterized by hypogonadism, obesity, retinitis pigmentosa, mental deficiency, and polydactyly has been called the Laurence-Moon-Biedl syndrome. Diabetes mellitus is rare, but diabetes insipidus is common. Other manifestations reported in certain families include nerve deafness and hyperlipemia. Chromosome studies are normal.

Autopsy studies have generally demonstrated normal pituitary architecture and it is assumed that the hypogonadism is secondary to hypothalamic dysfunction. Hypothalamic lesions have not been described. The endocrine manifestations of the syndrome are variable; affected members of a family may show normal gonadal function and pregnancy has been reported to occur.

SUMMARY

Hypothalamic disturbances in man are rare. When they occur they show remarkably close agreement with descriptions found in experimental lesions of the hypothalamus. It is possible to tentatively localize certain disorders of function to hypothalamic regions. Preoptic lesions are associated with autonomic disturbances such as cardiac arrhythmia, bladder incontinence, and pulmonary edema. Hyperthermia is common with acute lesions of the anterior hypothalamic-preoptic region. Lesions of the anterior hypothalamus may produce disturbances in food intake, and in infancy can result in cachexia despite normal food intake. Lesions in the lateral regions of the anterior hypothalamus are associated with loss of thirst drive or with alterations in food intake.

Lesions of the ventromedial hypothalamic area in man produce hyperphagia, obesity, and abnormal emotional states. Lesions in this region that extend into the median eminence also commonly produce endocrine disorders including diabetes insipidus, hypogonadism, and abnormalities of secretion of ACTH, GH, and prolactin. Mid-lateral-hypothalamic lesions have been infrequently documented in man but may cause anorexia and weight loss. Caudal hypothalamic lesions result in disorders in consciousness, somnolence, hypokinesia, and hypothermia or poikilothermia.

REFERENCES

1. ANAND, B. K. AND BROBECK, J. R.: *Hypothalmic control of food intake in rats and cats.* Yale J. Biol. Med. 24:123, 1951.

2. ANDERSSON, B.: *The central control of water and salt balance. In* Mogenson, G. J. and Calaresu, F. R. (eds.): *Neural Integration of Physiological Mechanisms and Behaviour.* University of Toronto Press, Toronto, 1975, p. 213.

3. ARONSOHN, E. AND SACHS, J.: *Die Beziehungen des Gehirns zur Komperwarme und zum Fieber; Experimentelle untersuch Engen.* Arch. Ges. Physiol. 37:232, 1885.

4. BANDLER, R. J., CHI, C. C. AND FLYNN, J. P.: *Biting attack elicited by stimulation of the ventral midbrain tegmentum of cats.* Science 177:364, 1972.

5. BARRETT, R., MERRIT, H. H. AND WOLF, A.: *Depression of consciousness as a result of cerebral lesions. In Sleep and altered states of consciousness.* Res. Pub. Assoc. Res. Nerv. Ment. Dis. 45:241, 1967.

6. BAUER, H. G.: *Endocrine and other clinical manifestations of hypothalamic disease: A survey of 60 cases with autopsies.* J. Clin. Endocrinol. 14:13, 1954.

7. BILLIARD, M., GUILLEMINAULT, C. AND DEMENT, W. C.: *A menstruation-linked periodic hypersomnia. Kleine-Levin syndrome or new clinical entity?* Neurology 25:436, 1975.

8. BLIGH, J.: *Neuronal models of hypothalamic temperature regulation. In* Lederis, K. and Cooper, K. E. (eds.): *Recent Studies of Hypothalamic Function,* S. Karger, Basel, 1973, p. 315.

9. BRAY, G. A. AND GALLAGHER, T. F., JR.: *Manifestations of hypothalamic obesity in man: A comprehensive investigation of eight patients and a review of the literature.* Medicine 54:301, 1975.

10. CAIRNS, H., ET AL.: *Akinetic mutism with an epidermoid cyst of the third ventricle (with a report on the associated disturbance of brain potentials).* Brain 64:273–90, 1941.

11. CAIRNS, H.: *Disturbances of consciousness with lesions of brain-stem and diencephalon.* (Victor Horsley Memorial Lecture) Brain 75:109, 1952.

12. CHI, C. C. AND FLYNN, J. P.: *Neural pathways associated with hypothalamically elicited attack behavior in cats.* Science 171:703, 1971.

13. CRAVIOTO, H., SILBERMAN, J. AND FEIGIN, I.: *A clinical and pathologic study of akinetic mutism.* Neurology 10:10, 1960.

14. DAVISON, C. AND DEMUTH, E. L.: *Disturbances in sleep mechanism: Clinicopathological study; lesions at diencephalic level (hypothalamus).* Arch. Neurol. Psychiat. 55:111, 1946.

15. DUFFY, J. P. AND DAVISON, K.: *A female case of the Kleine-Levin syndrome.* Br. J. Psychiat. 114:77, 1968.

16. FELDBERG, W. AND MYERS, R. D.: *Effects on temperature of amines injected into the cerebral ventricles. A new concept of temperature regulation.* J. Physiol. (Lond.) 173:226, 1964.

17. FOX, R. H., ET AL.: *Spontaneous periodic hypothermia: Diencephalic epilepsy.* Br. Med. J. 2:693, 1973.

18. FRÖHLICH, A.: *Ein Fall von Tumor der Hypophysis cerebri ohne Akromegalie.* Wien. Klin. Wschr. 15:882, 1901.

19. FULTON, J. F. AND BAILEY, P.: *Tumors in the region of the third ventricle: Their diagnosis and relation to pathological sleep.* J. Nerv. Ment. Dis. 69:1, 1929.

20. GALE, C. C.: *Neuroendocrine aspects of thermoregulation.* Ann. Rev. Physiol. 35:391, 1973.

21. GILLIGAN, B. S.: *Periodic megaphagia and hypersomnia—an example of the Kleine-Levin syndrome in an adolescent girl.* Proc. Aust. Assoc. Neurol. 9:67, 1973.

22. GIRVIN, J. P.: *Clinical correlates of hypothalamic and limbic system function. In* Mogenson, G. J. and Calaresu, F. R. (eds.): *Neural Integration of Physiological Mechanisms and Behaviour.* University of Toronto Press, Toronto, 1975, p. 412.

23. GOLDSTEIN, M.: *Brain research and violent behavior (a summary and evaluation of the status of biomedical research on brain and aggressive violent behavior).* Arch. Neurol. 30:1, 1974.

24. GOWERS, W. R.: *Epilepsy and Other Chronic Convulsive Diseases: Their Causes, Symptoms and Treatment.* Dover Publications, New York, 1885.

25. GROSSMAN, S. P.: *Direct adrenergic and cholinergic stimulation of hypothalamic mechanisms.* Am. J. Physiol. 202:872, 1962.

26. GUIHARD, J., ET AL.: *Hypothermie spontanee recidivante avec agenesie du corps calleux. Syndrome de shapiro nouvelle observation.* Ann. Pediat. 18:645, 1971.

27. HAMILTON, C. R., SCULLY, R. E. AND KLIMAN, B.: *Hypogonadotropinism in Prader-Willi syndrome. Induction of puberty and spermatogenesis by clomiphene citrate.* Am. J. Med. 52:322, 1972.

28. HARDY, J. D.: *Control of body temperature. In* Mogenson, G. J. and Calaresu, F. R. (eds.): *Neural Integration of Physiological Mechanisms and Behaviour.* University of Toronto Press, Toronto, 1975, p. 294.

29. HENSEL, H.: *Neural processes in thermoregulation.* Physiol. Rev. 53:948, 1973.

30. HESS, W. R.: *The functional organization of the diencephalon. In* Hughes, J. R. (ed.): Grune and Stratton, New York, 1957, p. 275.

31. HILTON, S. M.: *The role of the hypothalamus in the organization of patterns of cardiovascular response. In* Lederis, K. and Cooper, K. E. (eds.): *Recent Studies of Hypothalamic Function.* S. Karger, Basel, 1973, p. 306.

32. HUANG, Y. H. AND MOGENSON, G. J.: *Neural pathways mediating drinking and feeding in rats.* Exp. Neurol. 37:306, 1972.

33. ISENSCHMID, R. AND KREHL, L.: *Uber den Einfluss des Gehirns auf die Warmerregulation.* Arch. Exp. Path. Pharmakol. 70:109, 1912.

34. JOHNSON, R. H. AND PARK, D. M.: *Intermittent hypothermia.* J. Neurol. Neurosurg. Psych. 36:411, 1973.

35. JOHNSON, R. AND SPALDING, J. M.: *Disorders of the Autonomic Nervous System.* F. A. Davis, Philadelphia, 1975.

36. KENNEDY, G. C.: *Some aspects of the relation between appetite and endocrine development in the growing animal. In* Mogenson, G. J. and Calaresu, F. R. (eds.): *Neural Integration of Physiological Mechanisms and Behaviour.* University of Toronto Press, Toronto, 326, 1975.

37. KENNEDY, G. C.: *The regulation of food intake. Discussion.* Adv. Psychosom. Med. 7:91, 1972.

38. KLÜVER, H. AND BUCY, P. C.: *Preliminary analysis of functions of temporal lobes in monkeys.* Arch. Neurol. Psychiat. 42:979, 1939.

39. LEWIN, K., MATTINGLY, D. AND MILLS, R. R.: *Anorexia nervosa associated with hypothalamic tumour.* Br. Med. J. 2:629, 1972.

40. MARTIN, J. B. AND REICHLIN, S.: *Neural regulation of the pituitary-thyroid axis. In* Kenny, A. D. and Anderson, R. R. (eds.): *Proceedings of the Sixth Midwest Thyroid Conference.* University of Columbia Press, Columbia, Mo., 1970, p. 1.

41. MAYER, J.: *Some aspects of the problem of regulation of food intake and obesity.* N. Engl. J. Med. 274:610, 1966.

42. MOGENSON, G. J.: *Changing views of the role of the hypothalamus in the control of ingestive behaviors. In* Lederis, K. and Cooper, K. E. (eds.): *Recent Studies of Hypothalamic Function.* S. Karger, Basel, 1974, p. 268.

43. MORGANE, P. J.: *Anatomical and neurobiochemical bases of the central nervous control of physiological regulations and behaviour. In* Mogenson, G. J. and Calaresu, F. R. (eds.): *Neural Integration of Physiological Mechanisms and Behaviour.* University of Toronto Press, Toronto, 1975, p. 24.

44. MORGANE, P. J.: *The function of the limbic and rhinic forebrain-limbic midbrain systems and reticular formation in the regulation of food and water intake.* Ann. N.Y. Acad. Sci. 157:806, 1969.

45. MORRISON, S. D. AND MAYER, J.: *Adipsia and aphagia in rats after lateral subthalamic lesions.* Am. J. Physiol. 191:248, 1957.

46. MYERS, R. D.: *Ionic concepts of the setpoint for body temperature. In* Lederis, K. and Cooper, K. E. (eds.): *Recent Studies of Hypothalamic Function.* S. Karger, Basel, 1973, p. 371.

47. NIELSEN, J. M. AND JACOBS, L. L.: *Bilateral lesions of the anterior cingulate gyri.* Bull. Los Angeles Neurol. Soc. 16:231, 1951.

48. NOEL, P., ET AL.: *Agenesis of the corpus callosum associated with relapsing hypothermia: A clinico-pathological report.* Brain 96:359, 1973.

49. OOMURA, Y., ET AL.: *Contribution of electrophysiological techniques to the understanding of central control systems. In* Mogenson, G. J. and Calaresu, F. R. (eds.): *Neural Integration of Physiological Mechanisms and Behaviour.* University of Toronto Press, Toronto, 1975, p. 375.

50. PANSKEEP, J.: *On the nature of feeding patterns — primarily in rats. In* Novin, D., Wyrwicka, W. and Boray, G. A. (eds.): *Hunger: Basic Mechanisms and Clinical Implications.* Raven Press, New York, 1976, p. 369.

51. PENFIELD, W.: *Diencephalic autonomic epilepsy.* Arch. Neurol. Psychiat. 22:358, 1929.

52. PLUM, F. AND POSNER, J.: *The Diagnosis of Stupor and Coma,* ed. 2. F. A. Davis, Philadelphia, 1972.

53. RABIN, B. M.: *Ventromedial hypothalamic control of food intake and satiety: A reappraisal.* Brain Res. 43:317, 1972.

54. RANSON, S. W.: *Somnolence caused by hypothalamic lesions in the monkey.* Arch. Neurol. Psychiat. 41: 1, 1939.

55. REEVES, A. G. AND PLUM, F.: *Hyperphagia, rage and dementia accompanying a ventromedial hypothalamic neoplasm.* Arch. Neurol. 20:616, 1969.

56. ROTHBALLER, A. B.: *Some endocrine manifestations of central nervous system disease. An approach to clinical neuroendocrinology.* Bull. N.Y. Acad. Med. 42:257, 1966.

57. RUSSEK, M.: *Current hypotheses in the control of feeding behaviour. In* Mogenson, G. J. and Calaresu, F. R. (eds.): *Neural Integration of Physiological Mechanisms and Behaviour.* University of Toronto Press, Toronto, 1975, p. 128.

58. SHAPIRO, W. R., WILLIAMS, G. H. AND PLUM, F.: *Spontaneous recurrent hypothermia accompanying agenesis of the corpus callosum.* Brain 92:423, 1969.

59. SKULTETY, F. M.: *Clinical and experimental aspects of akinetic mutism. Report of a case.* Arch. Neurol. 19:1, 1968.

60. SMITH, G. P. AND GIBBS, J.: *Cholecystokin and satiety: Theoretic and therapeutic implications. In* Novin, D., Wyrwicka, W. and Boray, G. A. (eds.): *Hunger: Basic Mechanisms and Clinical Implications.* Raven Press, New York, 1976, p. 349.

61. SMITH, O. A., STEPHENSON, R. B. AND RANDALL, D. C.: *Range of control of cardiovascular variables by the hypothalamus. In* Lederis, K. and Cooper, K. E. (eds.): *Recent Studies of Hypothalamic Function.* S. Karger, Basel, 1973, p. 294.

62. SOLOMON, G. E.: *Diencephalic autonomic epilepsy caused by a neoplasm.* J. Pediatr. 83:277, 1973.

63. SPRAGUE, J. M.: *Chronic brainstem lesions. In Sleep and altered states of consciousness.* Res. Pub. Assoc. Res. Nerv. Ment. Dis. 45:157, 1965.

64. SWETT, C. P. AND HOBSON, J. A.: *The effects of posterior hypothalamic lesions on behavioral and electrographic manifestations of sleep and waking in cats.* Arch. Ital. Biol. 106:283, 1968.

65. VEALE, W. L. AND COOPER, K. E.: *Evidence for the involvement of prostaglandins in fever. In* Lederis, K. and Cooper, K. E. (eds.): *Recent Studies of Hypothalamic Function.* S. Karger, Basel, 1973, p. 359.

66. VICTOR, M., ADAMS, R. D. AND COLLINS, G. H.: *Wernicke-Korsakoff Syndrome,* F. A. Davis, Philadelphia, 1971.

67. WHITE, L. E. AND HAIN, R. F.: *Anorexia in association with a destructive lesion of the hypothalamus.* Arch. Pathol. 68:275, 1959.

68. WOLFF, S. M., ET AL.: *A syndrome of periodic hypothalamic discharge.* Am. J. Med. 36:956, 1964.

69. ZELLWEGER, H. AND SCHNEIDER, H. J.: *Syndrome of hypotonia-hypomentia-hypogonadism-obesity (HHHO) or Prader-Willi syndrome.* Am. J. Dis. Child. 115:588, 1968.

70. GREEN, S. AND RAU, R. H.: *Treatment of compulsive eating disturbances with anticonvulsant medication.* Am. J. Psychiatry 131:428, 1974.

BIBLIOGRAPHY

GOLDSTEIN, M.: *Brain research and violent behavior.* Arch. Neurol. 30:1, 1974.

HAYMAKER, W., ANDERSON, E. AND NAUTA, W. J. H.: *The Hypothalamus.* Charles C Thomas, Springfield, 1969.

JOHNSON, R. AND SPALDING, J. M. K.: *The Autonomic Nervous System.* F. A. Davis, Philadelphia, 1975.

LEDERIS, K. AND COOPER, K. E. (EDS.): *Recent Studies of Hypothalamic Function.* S. Karger, Basel, 1973.

MOGENSON, G. J. AND CALARESU, F. R. (EDS.): *Neural Integration of Physiological Mechanisms and Behaviour.* University of Toronto Press, Toronto, 1975.

NOVIN, D., ET AL.: *Hunger: Basic Mechansims and Clinical Implications.* Raven Press, New York, 1976.

PLUM, F. AND POSNER, J. B.: *Diagnosis of Stupor and Coma.* F. A. Davis, Philadelphia, 1974.

VICTOR, M., ADAMS, R. D. AND COLLINS, G. H.: *The Wernicke-Korsakoff Syndrome.* F. A. Davis, Philadelphia, 1971.

CHAPTER 12

Effects of Hormones on the Brain

Hormones can influence brain function in many different ways.[58] Some act by disturbing the constancy of the internal milieu which is necessary for normal functioning of nerve cells. Others act more directly on neurons, to influence, for example, electrolyte flux and electric properties of cell membranes, the functions of synapses, and the rate of biosynthesis and turnover of central biogenic amines. Certain hormones affect the growth and differentiation of nerve cells and synapses; others react with specific receptors in neurons to activate genetically-programmed patterns of behavior and drive. Specific receptors are involved in feedback control of the pituitary. Because of this complexity of effects, most of which have not been worked out in detail for each hormone, it is often difficult to assign a particular function to a specific hormone.[86] From a pathophysiologic point of view it is relatively easy to explain the general loss of higher functions that follows diffuse brain-cell dysfunction. It is far more difficult to understand how disturbance of a relatively limited aspect of neuron function can appear as a change in affect, mood, or perception. The neural networks responsible for drive can be activated by certain hormones, but current knowledge does not explain how altered neuronal function in certain anatomic systems can lead to certain behaviors. Figure 1 shows various mechanisms by which hormones can affect brain function.

It would be reasonable to suppose that the psychiatric symptoms of an endocrine disorder in any patient result from or are associated with several factors, including the underlying personality and vulnerability of the individual, the chronicity of the disorder, the setting in which the illness occurs, and abnormalities in brain function.[102] However, with few exceptions there is little information to support or disprove these contentions. The brain has a relatively circumscribed range of responses to hormonal or metabolic disturbances, and for this reason psychiatric disturbances tend to be relatively nonspecific. For the most part, the neuroendocrinologist must be content to describe and classify the symptom complexes associated with various states of disturbed brain function, and to analyze the biologic effects of the hormone on brain. The integration of these two domains of knowledge is still elusive. Since endocrine manipulations can lead to concomitant changes in both the physiologic and the psychologic state, endocrine-related brain dysfunction becomes an excellent model for the study of larger questions about the relationship between the brain and the mind.

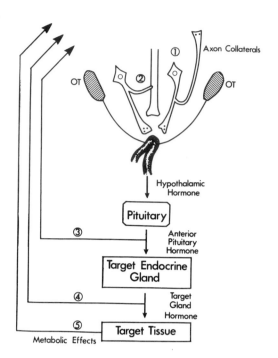

Figure 1. Diagram of mechanisms and routes whereby hormones can affect brain function. Hypophysiotrophic hormones may be released from nerve terminals directly into cerebrospinal fluid (2), or from axon collaterals that terminate on other neurons (1). Pituitary hormones may influence brain function (3), as can target gland hormones (4). Metabolic changes that result from target gland hormones effects may also affect brain (5).

EFFECTS OF HORMONES ON BRAIN DEVELOPMENT AND MATURATION

Endocrine effects on brain development, as the most striking of all hormone-related brain phenomena, are considered first.

Thyroid Function

Thyroid deficiency of onset in utero or early in infancy is termed *cretinism*. The manifestations depend on the time of onset of hypothyroidism in utero and the severity of thyroid hormone deficiency in the infant, and become more recognizable as the infant grows.[12] The diagnosis may be difficult to make at birth. Newly introduced screening methods measuring cord-blood thyroid hormone or TSH indicate an incidence of 1 in 750 newborns.

The most important characteristic of cretinism is mental and growth retardation but this may not become obvious until later in infancy. The first recognizable symptoms include persistent physiologic jaundice of the newborn, poor appetite, failure to thrive, torpid behavior, hypothermia, dry and thickened skin, muscle laxness, umbilical hernia, and a hoarse cry. There is a high correlation between early and adequate thyroid replacement therapy and ultimate IQ attained, but some cretins fail to respond.[66] It is crucial, therefore, that diagnosis and hormone treatment be early, and persistence of treatment also is important.

Thyroid hormone is essential for normal development of the central nervous system.[95, 100] In the brains of cretins, perikarya of neurons in the sensorimotor cortex are decreased in size and closely packed; axons, dendrites, and synapses are hypoplastic. The early postnatal period is critical for brain development in the rat, and in this species, induced thyroid deficiency leads to an analogous abnormal maturation of the cerebral and cerebellar cortex, the principal features of which are decreased size of cell bodies, increased packing density, decreased dendritic development, and decreased myelinization.[25] All of these features are reversed by thyroxine administration. The concentrations of dopamine, norepinephrine, and serotonin are reduced and the development of the rate-limiting enzymes, tyrosine hydroxylase and tryptophan hydroxylase, is also retarded by hypothyroidism and reversed by thyroid hormone administration.

In the cretin, the EEG shows a decreased basic frequency and a flat, uneventful record, features which are normalized by replacement of thyroid hormone.[42]

Hyperthyroidism appears to have little effect on growth and development in the human, even though cell formation and glial development can be increased in the rat by thyroxine administration.[25]

The mechanism of thyroid-hormone action in the developing brain has not been fully elucidated. Thyroid hormone probably acts on nuclear receptors to stimulate differentiation and growth of neurons, as has been reported for a variety of parenchymal tissues.[72]

Gonadal Function

In many species of experimental animals, androgens exert an early organizing effect on brain mechanisms to determine the characteristic male patterns of gonadotropin regulation and sexual behavior after puberty.[7, 30, 31] In the rat, the small amount of androgen secreted by the testis in the first ten days after birth leads to the development of a noncyclic (i.e., male) pattern of gonadotropin regulation; the effect can be blocked by castration, by administration of an antiandrogenic steroid, and with certain neuroleptic drugs such as phenobarbital. In the absence of androgen, the female cyclic-pattern release of gonadotropins develops. Male mounting behavior, a characteristic manifestation of brain sexual dimorphism, is responsive to the same early organizing influences as gonadotropin secretory patterns. Without androgenization a "female" mating response occurs. Periodic running activity, another characteristic of mature female rodents, also is abolished by early androgen administration. Androgenization also may be produced by large doses of estrogen. This may come about because estrogen is converted to androgen. Both the rat and rhesus monkey show sexual dimorphism (morphologic differences between male and female) of brain architecture, including differences in the size of the preoptic-area perikarya (rat) and medial amygdala nuclei (squirrel monkey) (Fig. 2).[11] The relative distribution of synapses on dendritic shafts and spines in the preoptic area of the rat also shows sex differences, with a significantly larger proportion of fibers of nonamygdaloid origin terminating on dendritic spines in the female.[79] As in other sites at which androgens exert effects, the hormone appears to act on a specific nuclear receptor to stimulate growth and differentiation. Antibiotics that block new protein formation also block effects of testosterone on male rat behavior. By analogy with the rhesus monkey, the critical time for brain androgenization in the human is thought to be approximately at the end of the first trimester of pregnancy, but clear-cut human analogues of behavioral androgenization have been difficult to establish with certainty.[32]

Studies in the human have utilized patients inadvertently exposed to androgenic influences in utero.[27, 64, 65, 82] Female pseudohermaphrodites produced by prenatal progesterone treatment (which has an androgenic effect) or secondary to the adrenogenital syndrome (an enzyme defect of the adrenal cortex) are reported to manifest more "tomboy" behavior and have higher intelligence quotients than normal female children. After suitable treatment, unlike the situation in rats, such females can ovulate normally and become pregnant. Similarly, the female rhesus monkey androgenized in utero has also shown normal sex function as an adult. The sex of identification is the sex of rearing, and they are not erotically involved with their own sex. Conversely, the human

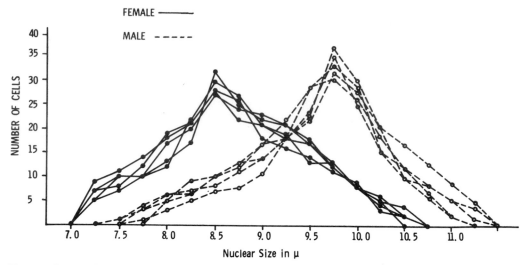

Figure 2. Sexual dimorphism in the nuclear size of amygdalar neurons in the squirrel monkey. Differences in nuclear size may be related to androgenization. Alternately differences may relate to the different hormone environments in male and female monkey. (From Bubenik, G. A. and Brown, G. M.: *Morphologic sex differences in primate brain areas involved in regulation of reproductive activity.* Experientia 29:619, 1973, with permission.)

analogue of the antiandrogen-treated male, the boy with feminizing testis syndrome, appears to be a female and is strongly feminine in behavior. In this condition, there is a defect in androgen receptors in brain and elsewhere, or failure to convert testosterone to an active form in certain target tissues. At present there is no evidence, despite much speculation, that human homosexuality or transsexualism is in any way related to an abnormal androgenization process in utero.[20, 84]

Adrenal Function

Little is known about the effect of adrenal steroids on brain maturation in the human. Cortisol administration in the rat delays development of behavioral responses and causes a delay in CNS maturation, when given in the first seven postnatal days; thereafter, glucocorticoids accelerate maturation. In tissue culture, glucocorticoids cause increased branching of neurons and an increased migration rate of glial cells, as well as induction of the enzyme glycerol phosphate dehydrogenase.

Growth Hormone

Although prenatal administration of growth hormone in the rat leads to increased numbers of cells in the cortex, increased dendrite length, and enhancement of cortically-mediated learning behavior,[25] it is not known whether GH itself influences brain development or psychologic function in man. Dwarfed individuals suffer psychologic distress, especially when entering puberty, but there is no difference between dwarfism caused by GH deficiency and that from other causes. Hypopituitary dwarfs show normal development of IQ but are psychologically immature and hypoactive, with little aggressive drive and a low self-esteem. It is not known whether the emotional problems are secondary to short stature, to GH deficiency, or indeed to deficiency of other pituitary hormones (usually TSH or ACTH). With HGH treatment, there is an initial depression (linked to the low self-esteem), and later helplessness and emotional detachment dominate the clinical picture.[49] The latter symptoms are often related to unrealistic expectations for the treatment program, as well as a lack of sense of identity.

PSYCHOLOGIC DISTURBANCE IN ENDOCRINE DISEASE

Adrenocortical Disease

Cushing's Syndrome

The majority of patients with Cushing's disease show mental changes.[13, 93, 102] A disorder so severe as to be termed psychotic occurs in 5 to 20 per cent of cases. The literature, however, fails to discriminate between the psychic effects of Cushing's syndrome of pituitary (or hypothalamic) versus adrenal origin. This discrimination may be important since ACTH secretion is increased when the disease originates in the pituitary.

Depression is the most common manifestation, and suicide attempts occur in about 10 per cent of cases. Other manifestations include irritability, difficulty in concentration, insomnia, paranoid delusions, and hallucinations. These symptoms often appear very early, before obesity, facial mooning, striae, or muscle wasting is obvious. A wide range of other disturbances occur less commonly: excitement, anxiety, apathy verging on stupor, and delirium manifested by impaired consciousness, disorientation, and loss of recent memory. The acute brain disorder in Cushing's disease is not readily differentiated from that due to various other organic, toxic, or metabolic causes. A schizophrenia-like illness has also been described.

As a result of these varied and often nondescript changes in mood and behavior, many patients with Cushing's disease are treated, inappropriately, for functional psychosis. Dramatic improvements in mental state often occur when the condition is recognized and treated appropriately.

Studies have recently appeared suggesting that mood disturbance is associated with Cushing's syndrome of diencephalic or pituitary origin rather than with Cushing's syndrome due to other causes, e.g., adrenal adenoma or ectopic ACTH-producing neoplasm. The existence of this association suggests that either the affective and neuroendocrine abnormalities have a common basis, or one disturbance produces the other. Based on this reasoning, Carroll has recently hypothesized that a primary diencephalic-limbic disturbance may cause coexistent functional depression and Cushing's syndrome.[14, 15]

In contrast to patients with Cushing's syndrome due to spontaneous endogenous hypercortisolemia, patients treated with pharmacologic doses of glucocorticoids often show euphoria and cheerfulness.[13, 93, 102] These symptoms, observed in three fourths of such patients, are often accompanied by increased appetite and occasionally by increased libido. Although depression is less frequent than in endogenous disease, it may be severe, and a significant number of patients attempt suicide. An acute toxic psychosis with "organic" features also may occur. Some question exists as to whether these effects are dose-related. In certain patients a dose dependency can be demonstrated, so that effective therapeutic dosage with anti-inflammatory steroids may require adjustment to the largest amount that does not produce cerebral manifestations. Other patients may show a psychosis on one occasion and not another, despite a return to the previous dosage of medication. The bulk of evidence indicates that these psychic effects are not related to the patient's premorbid personality. Prior mental disease is not a contraindication to steroid therapy, since such patients do not run a greater-than-normal risk of steroid-induced psychosis. The cause of the high incidence of euphoria and hypomania is not known. In these patients, the entire hypothalamic-pituitary-adrenal axis is suppressed. Direct steroid effects on the sensitive regions of the CNS are the probable cause of the mood alteration.

Psychoendocrinology of Depression

Adrenal hyperfunction occurs commonly in endogenously depressed patients.[13, 15, 89] It is not clear whether the adrenal activation is secondary to the emotional distress or arises as a concomitant manifestation of the depressive disorder. Such patients rarely show clinical evidence of Cushing's disease, but plasma cortisol levels are elevated and fail to show normal diurnal variation. Excess secretion persists during sleep and carefully controlled studies have shown that the adrenal hypersecretion is not due solely to anxiety, nonspecific stress, or the effect of hospital admission. Studies using frequent blood sampling indicate that endogenously depressed patients have episodic bursts of ACTH and cortisol secretion, as occur in normal individuals. However, in contrast to normal subjects, the episodic bursts fail to show a diurnal pattern, so that levels remain high throughout the 24-hour period.[88] Also, depressed patients usually fail to show adequate suppression in response to dexamethasone.[15] These findings point to a possible basic neuroendocrine disorder in severe depression. Recovery from depression is associated with disappearance of the hypersecretion. Other neuroendocrine abnormalities that are described in depression include diminished growth hormone responses to insulin-induced hypoglycemia and to D-amphetamine. Initial reports suggested that GH responses to L-dopa are decreased in depression, but subsequent studies have not confirmed this observation.[87]

A transient antidepressant effect of TRH has been described in some but not all studies.[78] One additional finding suggests that this effect may be significant: depressed patients frequently have diminished TSH responses to exogenous TRH. This finding is so common that it has been suggested as a potentially useful diagnostic test in depression.[26] On the other hand, the prolactin response to TRH has been reported both to be diminished and enhanced in depression. In one study, 8 of 13 patients with depression showed GH release after TRH, an effect not seen in normals. These effects, in general, are reversed after treatment. A significant lowering of plasma LH has also been reported in depressed, menopausal women.

These neuroendocrine abnormalities are found only in endogenously depressed patients. It is tempting to postulate that a common central mechanism is disrupted in such patients, resulting in both endocrine abnormalities and psychiatric symptoms. According to the biogenic amine hypothesis of affective disorders, depressive illness is associated with an absolute or relative deficiency of catecholamines, of serotonin, or of both at some functional site in brain.[1, 53, 89] It is conceivable that an abnormality of biogenic amine function predisposes to both the psychiatric and the endocrine disturbances.

Addison's Disease

Since the original description of adrenocortical deficiency by Addison in 1868, significant change in personality and behavior has been regarded as an almost universal manifestation of this disorder.[13, 93, 102] "Addisonian encephalopathy" in its severe form is recognizable as a typical organic psychosis or delirium, manifested by memory deficit and clouding of consciousness which may progress to stupor and coma. In milder cases, apathy, depression, fatigue, poverty of thought, and lack of initiative are common. The patients are often seclusive, irritable, and negativistic. Patients may be especially sensitive to the euphoriant effect of cortisone.

Evidence of associated brain disturbance is given by the EEG, which shows diffuse, high-amplitude, slow activity. The profound debilitation and weakness may well help to reduce depression. Detailed testing by Henkin and associates revealed that patients with adrenal insufficiency have a lowered threshold of sensitivity to taste, smell, touch, and hearing.[37, 38] Although the detection threshold is lower than normal, judgment and discrimination of sensory input are impaired. The Addisonian patient is notoriously hypersensitive to narcotic agents, particularly barbiturates. These changes in brain function are due principally to glucocorticoid, and not to mineralocorticoid, deficits as evidenced by the fact that administration of salt and deoxycorticosterone acetate (DOCA) does not repair the abnormal EEG, raise sensory thresholds to normal, or rectify the personality disorder. Use of cortisone and other glucocorticoids, on the other hand, completely reverses the behavioral, perceptual, and EEG disturbances.

Mechanism of Corticoid Effects on the Brain

In recent years, the physiologic bases for these neural effects have been better defined, but they are still not fully understood. Electrophysiologic studies have shown that the conduction rate of nerve impulses is not altered by glucocorticoid deficiency, but the latency of transmission at central synapses is prolonged.[16, 100, 103] This is particularly marked in multisynaptic systems such as the reticular activating system, the tonic activity of which is responsible for maintaining alertness and responsivity. High doses of glucocorticoids decrease the latency of synaptic delay. Considerable progress has been made in elucidating the molecular basis of glucocorticoid action on nerve cells. In common with other steroid hormones, the major site of action is on the nucleus. In a manner analogous to that in peripheral tissues, steroid (which is lipid-soluble) readily enters the cell and in the cytosol is linked to a binding protein.[58, 59, 60] The steroid-protein complex (but not the steroid alone) is capable of entering the nucleus and acting at receptor regions on the gene, where it can alter the production of messenger RNA. Both radioautography and uptake studies using tritium-labeled corticosterone demonstrate that corticosteroid binding is greatest in the hippocampus, with most in the large pyramidal neurons of Ammon's horn and less in the small-granule neurons of the dentate gyrus (Fig. 3). Binding is also found in the amygdala, septum, and to some extent the cerebral cortex. In these regions, labeled corticoids localize to specific cytosol binding proteins. In all these sites, corticoids are additionally localized to the cell nucleus. Surprisingly, no major binding has been found in the hypothalamus.

Corticoids stimulate RNA synthesis in neurons and act to regulate important enzymes, notably glycerol phosphate dehydrogenase.[59] Serotonin biosynthesis decreases after adrenalectomy and increases after glucocorticoid administration. Recently, a direct glycolytic action in brain has been shown, and this effect may well be of functional importance. Aldosterone probably regulates Na$^+$ and K$^+$ flux in brain cells as it does in toad bladder and renal tubule. Glucocorticoids have been demonstrated to be neces-

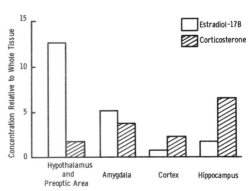

Figure 3. Uptake of 17β-estradiol and corticosterone by rat brain cell nuclei. Patterns of uptake of the two steroids are different in various brain regions.

sary for normal extinction of avoidance behavior. It has also been shown that excess steroids reduce the percentage of time spent in REM sleep.[59] Local effects of the corticoids probably are responsible for certain negative-feedback effects as shown by inhibition of single-neuron unit activity.

Recent studies indicate that ACTH and related peptides affect learning and behavior in rats (see below). The importance of ACTH in the manifestations of Cushing's disease has not been elucidated.

Brain Function in Thyroid Disease

Hypothyroidism

The Myxoedema Commission of 1888, set up by the Clinical Society of London, in examining detailed symptomatology in 109 severely ill patients, found that fully a third had frank and unmistakable psychosis with delusions, dementia, or mania. Asher, who applied A. J. Cronin's term, "myxedema madness," observed 14 cases over a 3-year period in London. The extreme form of hypothyroid encephalopathy is myxedema coma, which frequently is fatal.

Dramatic cases aside, close study of hypothyroid individuals reveals a high proportion with mental disturbance.[101, 102] The slowness and marked latency of response is readily noted and there is deterioration of recent memory and difficulty in concentration. On the Trailmaking Test of Reitan, performance is in the range considered indicative of brain damage. The predominant disorder of affect is a marked depression; sometimes there are paranoid features, while in other cases symptoms are indistinguishable from those of profound melancholia. Psychologic tests indicate mild delirium which, unless searched for, is not readily detectable. A peculiar facetiousness is common, resembling the Witzelsucht of patients with frontal lobe disturbance. The EEG in severe cases shows slowing which is roughly proportional to the depression of metabolic rate.[42, 95] Cerebral blood flow and cerebral oxygen utilization are decreased in proportion to the severity of the clinical manifestations. Seizures may occur in hypothyroid encephalopathy, while they are not increased in thyrotoxicosis.

Further clinical evidence of the brain disturbance in myxedema is abnormal sensitivity to the action of depressant drugs such as morphine and phenothiazines, an effect probably due to reduction in their metabolic degradation, with a resultant elevation in blood levels. Prolonged hypothyroidism can result in a peripheral neuropathy, including spinal and auditory nerves. Selective involvement of the median nerves by connective-tissue compression can result in the carpal-tunnel syndrome. Cerebellar tremor, ataxia, and incoordination also occur. Long-tract signs are observed rarely. Although most patients improve after thyroxine treatment, a proportion do not. Some of these may have a coincidental nonmyxedema psychosis of a usual type, but in the majority of cases the brain deficit may be related to long-standing thyroid deficiency.[42, 95]

Hyperthyroidism

Both cognitive and affective impairment are common in hyperthyroidism.[3, 101, 102] While generalized disruption of intellectual function is seen with both hypothyroidism and hyperthyroidism, the affective disturbance in hyperthyroidism is specifically linked to that condition. Emotional lability, anxiety, "tension," over-reactiveness, poor concentration, restlessness, tremor, sleep disturbance, and frank psychosis are common in thyrotoxicosis. The "nervousness" of the hyperthyroid patient is characterized by motor restlessness and a need to move around, rather than by chronic anxiety. Patients report a loss of "emotional control" and find themselves getting uncontrollably angry out of proportion to the stimulus. A minority of patients, particularly the elderly, become depressed, withdrawn, apathetic, and anorectic. In extremely "toxic" patients, delirium and coma may supervene; indeed, the occurrence of organic delirium in thyrotoxicosis is one of the hallmarks of thyroid storm. Detailed psychologic testing reveals "organic brain damage" in many. As in hypothyroidism, the Trailmaking Test of Reitan shows performance consistent with brain damage as well as impaired performance on the Porteus Maze Test. These features improve following treatment. The organic deficit persists after treatment in a minority of patients, suggesting that severe hyperthyroidism may cause irreversible brain damage.

The role of premorbid personality disturbance in the pathogenesis of Graves' disease is still the subject of debate. Some authors report a high incidence of psychologic abnormality, with a specific type of personality associated with premature assumption of responsibility and a martyr-like suppression of dependency wishes. Others report precipitation by emotional stress, especially with object loss. Still others claim that such abnormalities are due to the disease itself.

Mechanism of Thyroid Hormone Effects on the Brain

In the past, it appeared reasonable to attribute the changes in brain function in hypothyroidism to a lowering of oxygen consumption by neurons. More recently, the role of thyroid hormone in regulating protein metabolism in general has been emphasized. The possibility must be considered, therefore, that the cerebral disturbance in hypothyroidism is due to impaired nucleoprotein and protein synthesis in neurons and synapses. Clear-cut data support this contention for the developing brain, but it has not been demonstrated in mature brains. The function of thyroxine in regulating all aspects of protein turnover and neurotransmitter synthesis in the adult brain has not been defined. Triiodothyronine (T_3) accumulates in the nuclei of certain neurons.[72] Unlike steroid hormones, T_3 goes directly into the nucleus rather than first binding to a specific receptor protein in the cytosol.

The neurophysiologic basis of thyrotoxic encephalopathy has not been established and, in fact, is enigmatic.[100] Surprisingly, cerebral oxygen consumption is not increased in Graves' disease; brain tissue oxygen consumption (measured in laboratory animals), unlike that of liver and skeletal muscle, is unaltered by thyroid administration, and isolated brain mitochondria (unlike those from muscle, kidney, or liver) fail to swell or "uncouple" when exposed to excess thyroxine. These results indicate that hyperthyroid encephalopathy is probably not due to a simple increase in cellular metabolism. Thyroxine appears to produce direct effects on neuronal electric activity. Iontophoretic application produces activation of most neurons. Thyroid hormone increases the sensitivity of neuroreceptors to catecholamine, decreases monoamine oxidase activity, and increases the turnover rate of norepinephrine. These effects may explain in part the enhancement of antidepressant activity of imipramine reported by some workers.

Unlike ACTH, TSH does not appear to regulate its own secretion by feedback effects on the hypothalamus.

Gonadal Steroids and Human Sexual Function

Male Sexual Function

Increased levels of androgenic hormone at puberty are required for normal development of libidinal drive and potency. Once established, acquired androgenic deficiency must be severe before normal male sexual function is seriously impaired, and the onset of impotence and loss of libido lag behind the loss of androgenic function.[20, 40, 83] Boys and girls both have significant increases in circulating androgens at the onset of puberty. In girls, these steroids come mainly from the adrenal gland; in boys the increase in adrenal androgen secretion is paralleled by a much larger increase (about 10 times as great) in the secretion of testosterone by the testes. Although it is frequently stated in the literature that sex drive and potency in normally androgenized men are relatively independent of testosterone level, this is only partially correct; independence is not complete, and there are differences from individual to individual.[70] Men with androgen deficiency who are receiving replacement therapy note a rather close correlation between treatment and psychologic effects, even over a few days. Estrogen therapy in males dramatically inhibits potency and sex drive, presumably due to reduced testosterone secretion. Studies of the effects of castration in male sexual deviants show a decrease in sexual activity, irrespective of the direction of sexual interest, as well as a decrease in aggressiveness (but only if it is sexual). Following castration, sex drive and interest may be maintained despite impotence. The antiandrogens cyproterone or medroxyprogesterone acetate produce a marked reduction of libido and of aggressive acts related to the sex drive, which parallels a drop in circulating androgen.[17, 67] Progesterone derivatives are also reported to lower male sex drive, and female sex drive as well.

Although androgen effects on libido and sex drive are widely known, effects on personality are not limited to sexual behavior. Aggressiveness and the rambunctious behavior of the teenager are well-recognized effects of androgen stimulation. One recent study of aggressive behavior in male prisoners, ages 20 to 35, showed a correlation of high plasma testosterone levels with a history of violent crimes in adolescence, but not with continued aggressiveness.[48] This study and others underline the major impact of testosterone changes during the pubertal period. Among the psychologic side effects of androgen treatment, if the hormone is given in excess, are insomnia and irritability. Testosterone is not an aphrodisiac, as elevation of androgen levels above the normal range does not increase sex drive or potency.[70] Hypogonadal men in addition to diminished libido show marked passivity, poverty of ideation, apathy, hypokinesia, timidity, and a lack of drive and general vigor, and have a higher-than-normal incidence of psychoneurotic symptoms.[40] Patients suffering from Klinefelter's syndrome (who in addition to low testosterone secretion also have a chromosome abnormality) have a subnormal IQ, higher-than-normal incidence of major psychologic disturbance, increased criminality, disorders of sex identification, and transsexualism.

The personality deficits of the hypogonadal man arise in part from difficulties which the physically and sexually inadequate individual experiences in coping with his environment, but an additional important organic component may be androgen deficiency during physical and psychologic development. This conclusion is suggested by the fact that when testosterone treatment is delayed until adulthood the results are variable.[40] Patients may drop out of therapy because they are unable to integrate into their lives the increased sex drive associated with treatment. In others, full development of sex drive may not occur, and many patients show subnormal assertiveness and psychosexual maturity. Several studies indicate that patients treated early with androgen tolerate well the onset of sexual and aggressive impulses.

In men under the age of 50, impotence is almost always due to factors such as neurotic conflict, depression, poor health, fatigue, and fear of erectile failure. Testosterone deficiency is not usually demonstrable in cases of impotence due to psychologic factors, and testosterone treatment does not benefit the patient beyond its use as a placebo. Those few patients with low testosterone levels usually show restoration to the normal range with successful psychotherapy and return of potency. In male rats, access to responsive females can serve as a stimulus to increased testosterone secretion. Anticipation of sexual activity may be a possible stimulus for increased testosterone secretion in the human male. Prolactin hypersecretion has been reported to cause impotence in men (and loss of libido in women). Restitution to normal secretion restores potency. Whether the effect is due to excess prolactin directly or is secondary to gonadotropin-testosterone deficiency has not been determined.

Definitive studies by Kinsey and collaborators demonstrate that male sexual drive and potency reach peak levels in the second decade of life and decline progressively thereafter.[45] This decline is not attributable to androgen deficiency because plasma testosterone levels are maintained relatively constant in almost all men until the sixth decade. The normal decline in male sexual vigor with age probably represents maturation and aging of neural or gonadal structures involved in sexual behavior.[36] The role of modest decline in androgens (within the normal range) over long periods in the course of "normal" decline in potency and vigor of men is unknown. It is folk knowledge that the aging male human not uncommonly seeks to maintain and demonstrate his youthful sexual vigor by seeking out new (and younger) sex partners.

A male climacteric does occur which is much less dramatic than the female counterpart, the menopause.[36] Beginning in the fifth decade, a gradual rise in plasma levels of LH and FSH occurs in most men. This rise indicates reduced feedback signal from the testes. A gradual diminution in sexual competence occurs in later years. The efficacy of androgen treatment of this decreased libido remains to be established. In addition, approximately 15 per cent of older men show evidence of testicular aging by biopsy and by chemical studies of testosterone. A proportion of these men lose libido and manifest autonomic and nervous changes similar to those of the menopause, with restoration of these functions after testosterone administration. This syndrome is not a normal part of the aging process, is uncommon, and may occur at any age. Although some workers dispute the existence of the male climacteric and dismiss the syndrome as being a manifestation of psychoneurosis, it appears reasonable to look for pituitary and testicular deficiency as a cause of loss of libido or potency in men suspected of having the syndrome of the male climacteric, and to judge each case on its merits.

Female Sexual Function

Hormonal regulation of psychosexual function in women is far more complex than in men, involving adrenal androgens as well as cyclic changes in estrogen and progesterone secretion. Most endocrine literature related to hormones and female sexuality concerns the importance of adrenal androgens. Adrenalectomy or hypophysectomy leads to almost complete loss of libido and sex drive, and the reversal of this loss by treatment with testosterone supports the conclusion that androgen and not estrogen is the major determinant of sexual behavior in human females.[83, 91] However, these findings are not necessarily applicable to all women, as the patients studied were for the most part suffering from terminal cancer. Analogous findings are observed in spontaneously occurring pituitary-adrenal disease. High-dosage androgen therapy leads in some cases to enhanced, even pathologic, sex drive. These pathologic changes may be due only to clitoral enlargement and hypersensitivity, or to an additional central component which has not been clearly established.

With respect to estrogens, the situation in the human may differ from that in experimental animals, including both rats and monkeys. In the rat, estrogen alone administered to the adrenalectomized female produces typical lordosis behavior. In the monkey, estrogens administered to females result in their being mounted by males. This appears to be due to two factors which operate together: 1) an increased frequency of the female presenting to the male, and 2) the release of pheromone by the female.[63] The pheromone in the female rhesus monkey which stimulates male sexual activity appears to be a mixture of fatty acids synthesized by bacteria in the vagina as a result of estrogen-induced changes in vaginal pH and secretion. The appearance of this pheromone actually stimulates male courting behavior prior to the appearance of the heightened sexual receptivity of the female, suggesting that the neural response to estrogens in the female has a higher threshold of hormone effect than does the biochemical change in vaginal secretion. Michael and coworkers[61] have recently demonstrated similar fatty acids in the preovulatory phase in 30 per cent of normal women in their sample, which are absent in women on oral contraceptives. It remains to be determined whether attractant pheromones play a role in human sex behavior, but the use of perfumes has a long tradition as a stimulator of sexual arousal. The base of many perfumes is musk or civet, substances which are pheromones in certain animals.

In the human female, sexual function is more independent of hormonal influences than in lower forms. The greater role of the psychic component in female sexuality as compared to the male makes it difficult to evaluate the effects of estrogen and progesterone. Spontaneous or induced menopause produces a marked diminution in the levels of both progesterone and estrogen. Not only are there physical signs of estrogen withdrawal such as vaginal mucosal atrophy, osteoporosis, hot flashes, headache, and backache, but frequently there are depressive symptoms ranging from "blues" to an inability to work and a sense of hopelessness.[47] Coupled with these, there may be a loss of interest in sexual activity. The hot flashes and associated mental symptoms probably are due to estrogen deficiency, as they are also observed with administration of the antiestrogen clomiphene as well as occasionally in hypopituitarism. The regressive changes in the female genitalia induced by estrogen deficiency—thinning and friability of the vulva and vagina and decrease in secretions—may cause dyspareunia. Loss of a sense of well-being also contributes to the loss of sexual feeling. Masters and Johnson[56, 57] claim that continued sexual activity is the single most important factor in maintenance of sexual function in older women, but they also emphasize the importance of adequate replacement therapy to prevent vulvovaginal involution. Most physicians are conservative in their use of endocrine replacement in menopausal women and fail to take into account the affective state, the sexual functioning of the patient, and the presence of unpleasant vasomotor menopausal symptoms. Recent reports linking estrogen therapy to an increased incidence of uterine[54] and possibly breast cancer have made it even more mandatory that the diagnosis of behavioral or affective disorder due to estrogen deficiency be established with certainty, and that the possible disadvantages as well as the benefits of estrogen therapy be carefully considered.

Another estrogen deficiency state is Turner's syndrome, or gonadal dysgenesis. In this syndrome, patients lack one X chromosome and frequently have short stature, webbing of the neck, and deformity of the forearms (cubitus valgus). Individuals with this syndrome are often warm-hearted, friendly, pleasant, and lacking in aggression. They are also reported to have low sex drive. These patients do not have adrenal insufficiency and apparently have normal levels of circulating androgens. The low sex drive, therefore, appears to be due to the low level of estrogen, and is probably related, at least in part, to lack of development of female secondary sex characteristics. Therapy with estrogens restores sex drive. Recent reports linking estrogen treatment with uterine cancer, however, have led to the suggestion that estrogens "should be given at the lowest effective dose for the shortest possible time."[54]

Changes in female sexuality that accompany the normal menstrual cycle are even more complex.[5] These are deeply intertwined with conscious and unconscious conflicts over the significance of the menses themselves. Studies with animals in which sex drive is closely associated with high estrogen levels would lead one to suppose that women should show heightened sexual receptivity at midcycle at a time when gonadal readiness might be expected to coincide with behavioral acceptance. This supposition, based on work in lower animals, appears to hold in part in the human. In a now classic study using a unique longitudinal approach and double-blind methodology, Benedek and

Rubenstein[8] examined mood changes during 152 menstrual cycles in 15 women undergoing psychoanalytic treatment. Vaginal exfoliative cytology was examined and used to divide the cycle into five stages: follicle ripening phase, early ovulation phase, ovulation phase, progesterone (luteal) phase, and premenstrual phase. Although sexual feeling varied throughout the menstrual cycle, and on the average was maximum on the fourteenth day of the cycle, not all women had a peak of sexual interest around the time of ovulation, and some demonstrated increased sexual desire just before and just after the menses. Most women had a decline in sexual feeling during the luteal (postovulatory) phase of the cycle. Hormone changes during these stages of the menstrual cycle have subsequently been well characterized. Estrogen levels rise during the first two stages, peak in the ovulatory phase, remain high in the progesterone phase and drop rapidly in the premenstrual phase. Progesterone level rises only after ovulation and drops together with estrogen in the premenstrual phase.

In a series of married women studied by Udry and Morris,[98] peak frequency of coitus and orgasm was between the fourteenth and sixteenth days of the cycle, with minimum frequency on the fourth day. It is now known that testosterone levels during the menstrual cycle also fluctuate, being significantly higher during the midcycle period than during the follicular or luteal phase. Individuals varied greatly in the timing of the peak.

One of the most consistent findings of change in relation to the menstrual cycle is the "premenstrual tension syndrome." A degree of depression and increased irritability is rather common, and only in the more severe cases does the woman seek medical attention.[94] This syndrome begins as estradiol and progesterone secretion begin to fall rapidly from the postovulatory peak, and is maximum when sex steroid levels are approaching their nadir. The mechanism of this syndrome has not been fully established. Recent studies in patients with premenstrual tension show no difference from normal subjects in the rate or pattern of fall of estrogen and progesterone.[94] It appears that the syndrome is triggered by the fall in these sex steroids in an individual who may be susceptible for, as yet, unknown reasons. A potential etiologic role of prolactin in premenstrual tension has been suggested by preliminary evidence that elevated plasma levels of the hormone may occur in the luteal phase of the cycle in women prone to premenstrual tension. Further evidence for this hypothesis is the observation that some subjects show reduced symptoms after treatment with bromergocryptine, a drug that suppresses prolactin secretion. Much attention has been focused on premenstrual retention of salt and water as an important factor in premenstrual tension. However, many sufferers show no evidence of weight gain, and dehydration measures do not lead to relief except in those cases where fluid retention is obvious. Normally, menstruating women show maximum "negative" affect immediately after, and immediately before, their menses.[94] This is true for both anxiety and hostility. There is a report that 84 per cent of crimes of violence committed by women in Paris occurred during the premenstrual and menstrual phases. About half of the occurrences of industrial sickness, acute psychiatric admissions, and acute medical and surgical admissions coincide with the four premenstrual and four menstrual days.

The normal pattern of anxiety and hostility is observed in women taking sequential contraceptives, but not in those taking combined therapy with estrogens and gestagens (progesterone-like drugs).[19, 29, 39, 43] It appears that gestagens prevent the occurrence of the usual mid-cycle peak of well-being. There is also a slight decrease in menstrual symptomatology. Oral contraceptives of the combined type are said to frequently, but not uniformly, inhibit libido. Up to 10 per cent of women taking oral contraceptives are liable to develop depression symptoms or increased irritability which requires discontinuation of treatment, while a higher percentage (62 per cent in one study) develop lesser symptoms. Risk of depression is higher in those with a history of depressive disorders and in those with premenstrual or menstrual disorders. The relationship of these symptoms to estrogen and gestagen levels is not clear, as a unitary relationship has not been established. Controlled double-blind studies emphasize that placebo effects may play a major role in changing mood and affect.

Influences of Hormones on Headache

Migraine shows a distinct sex difference in adults (but not children), occurring two to three times as often in women as compared with men. Headaches and migraine tend to occur at times of hormonal change: around the time of menstruation, as part of the premenstrual syndrome, at ovulation, at the menarche, or at menopause. During pregnancy, migraine may be more severe during the first three months and improve subsequently, but in some cases pregnancy has no effect.

In some female patients with migraine (probably less than 20 per cent), repeated exacerbation of migraine coincides with the fall in circulating estrogen in the immediate premenstrual phase of the cycle.[33, 94] Headaches in such patients can be produced by administration of long-acting estrogens, the symptoms developing as estrogen levels fall.[96, 97] The management of such patients remains difficult, since continued administration of estrogens is not feasible.[54]

One major side effect of the contraceptive pill is an increased incidence of migraine in susceptible women, particularly with progestogenic pills containing estrogen in low dosage.[22] This combination is the commonest type of oral contraceptive now in use, as it results in a lower incidence of thrombosis. Various mechanisms have been invoked for this migraine susceptibility. Alterations in metabolism of serotonin and noradrenaline (which are implicated in migraine attacks) or effects on vitamin B_6, monoamine oxidase activity, and catechol-O-methyltransferase activity are possible contributory factors.[33]

Mechanism of Sex Steroid Action on the Brain

It is known that progesterone affects the brain directly.[59, 100] This steroid acts on the hypothalamic temperature-regulating area to raise the "set point" for body temperature control. This reaction is the basis for the postovulatory rise in the basal body temperature of normal women. Together with other hormones, it has a synergistic effect on aspects of reproductive function, facilitating sexual behavior and gonadotropin secretion. Some progesterone is essential for the normal induction of the LH surge in rats and guinea pigs. Progesterone depresses the excitability threshold of hypothalamic neurons to reflex stimuli from the genital area and to direct electrical stimulation. The molecular basis of sex steroid action on the brain has received much study, following principles of steroid hormone action developed from experiments on estrogen and progesterone action on reproductive organs. In fact, sexual behavior can be considered to be a sex hormone-dependent secondary sexual characteristic. Two types of progesterone binding have been described, one relatively nonspecific and the other highly specific.[58, 59] Widespread binding of radioactive progesterone in brain tissue has been demonstrated with a gradient of increasing concentrations from anterior hypothalamus through posterior hypothalamus to the region of the cerebral peduncle in the mesencephalon. Corticosterone competes for these binding sites, which appear, therefore, to be glucocorticoid receptor sites. Specific progesterone receptor sites have been found only in the hypothalamus, where they undoubtedly underlie progesterone-induced responses.

Estradiol is localized to specific neurons in the preoptic area, hypothalamus, and amygdaloid region (areas previously shown to be involved in gonadotropin and behavioral regulation) (see Fig. 3).[58, 59] The upper tegmental-posterior mammillary region of

288

the female rhesus monkey is sensitive to estrogen; implants produce an increase in sexual receptivity and, in the male partner an increase in mounting attempts and ejaculations.[63]

Estrogen binds primarily to nuclear receptor sites in neurons, where it may produce effects by an alteration in RNA synthesis.[58, 59, 71] Further evidence for the effect of estrogens on nuclear mechanisms is the demonstration that both the behavioral and negative-feedback effects of estrogens (estrogen-induced estrus, estrogen-induced gonadotropin inhibition) are blocked by treatment with actinomycin D, which inhibits RNA transcription. Estrogen administration also increases monoamine oxidase and alters the turnover of ^{3}H-norepinephrine. An alternative (or complementary) mechanism of estrogen action on brain has recently been proposed by Davies and coworkers.[21] They have shown that estradiol is converted to catechol-estradiol by brain enzyme systems. They postulate that the catechol estrogen and the catecholamines (both of which have a dihydroxy substituted benzene ring) may compete for common substrates and binding sites.

Testosterone, in contrast to estrogen, does not appear to be specifically bound to a receptor protein in the brain and, unlike certain peripheral target tissues, the CNS does not convert testosterone to dihydrotestosterone. Radioautographic studies demonstrate uptake of testosterone in areas of estrogen uptake, and there is evidence that testosterone is aromatized to estrogen in the brain; perhaps testosterone effects on the brain may require this conversion.[85]

Effects of LHRH on the Brain

Recent studies in the rat suggest that LHRH is involved in regulation of sexual activity. Administration of LHRH to the female rat produces an increase in lordosis behavior, even in hypophysectomized recipients; evidently this action is not mediated through pituitary gonadotropins but is a direct one.[69, 76] This effect remains to be demonstrated in other mammals, including man. The administration of LHRH directly into the preoptic area has the same effect, suggesting that there is an LHRH-sensitive "center" for sex drive in the anterior hypothalamus. An anatomic basis for this suggestion comes from immunohistochemical study, which shows in both rats and mice the existence of a LHRH-peptidergic pathway arising in the area of the organum vasculosum (localized in the lamina terminalis at the anterior tip of the third ventricle) and extending posteriorly into the median eminence of the hypothalamus[104] LHRH is found in two distinct regions within the hypothalamus—80 per cent in the median eminence and 20 per cent in the preoptic-region in the area of the organum vasculosum.[10] This latter localization also corresponds to the anterior hypothalamic regions thought to be the site of the ovulatory surge mechanism of LHRH release. Analogous effects have not been demonstrated in other animals or in the human, but are under active study.

Endocrine Changes in Homosexuality and Transsexualism

It has been suggested repeatedly that there may be disturbances of sex steroid secretion in homosexuals.[84] It has been reported (primarily by the Masters' group) that the more "feminine" groups of male homosexuals have testosterone levels significantly lower than normal, and the more "masculine" groups of lesbians have testosterone levels higher than normal for women and a high incidence of menstrual irregularities.[46] Several other groups have failed to confirm these findings.[84] Furthermore, no convincing data link sex-hormone levels with preferences for sex object. Levels appear to be related to general sex drive rather than specific sex orientation.

In the transsexual patient, gonad function is also appropriate to genotype. The endocrinologist may be called on to prescribe appropriate treatment to reverse secondary sexual characteristics, and to advise patients and others as to the management and advisability of the sex-reversal process. This complex and rapidly developing area is discussed in detail by Money and collaborators.[34]

Brain Function in Pituitary Disease

Hypothyroidism, adrenocortical failure, or hypogonadism may give rise to mental disturbance. Consequently, pituitary disease, which produces secondary changes in all three of these functions, is almost invariably accompanied by personality disorder. In one review of 78 cases of hypopituitarism, only six patients were free of psychologic disturbances. Many hypopituitary patients are extremely dependent and psychologic invalids. Early symptoms include fatigability, impotence, and loss of libido, together with loss of body hair and intolerance to cold. Later, apathy, depression, drowsiness, loss of initiative and drive, and mental torpor are the most common manifestations. As pointed out by Michael and Gibbons, "apathy, indifference and inactivity may become so profound that patients rarely leave their living quarters, they lie in bed for much of the day and they neglect even their personal hygiene."[62] Flexor spasm, upper motor neuron signs, and severe contractures may occur. Chronic diffuse brain disturbance with disorientation and loss of memory is common, with delirium and stupor ending in hypopituitary coma in the extreme form.

Adrenal cortex deficiency is the major factor contributing to the mental disturbance of patients with hypopituitarism, as exemplified by the confused or stuporous patient who may rapidly become alert and mentally clear following intravenous therapy with hydrocortisone. Thyroxine, though important, is usually less crucial. For individuals of both sexes, return of libido requires replacement doses of androgenic hormones. In women, an increased sense of well-being often follows estrogen administration.

It is noteworthy that even after all of these replacements have been supplied, certain patients with panhypopituitarism still show residual symptoms such as apathy, lack of drive, and chronic fatigue. The basis for this residual deficiency is unknown; it may be related to deficiency of growth hormone or prolactin, but data to prove this point are lacking. It is also possible that long-standing pituitary insufficiency leads to irreversible brain damage. Although there is a report that growth hormone increases libido, little else is known about its psychologic effects. Acromegalics are said to show lack of initiative and spontaneity and a change in mood. Possible behavioral effects of prolactin are also unknown. Since prolactin affects a wide range of behaviors in lower forms, including the induction of maternal behavior and migratory drive, it is not unreasonable to suppose that there are behavioral effects in the human, and that eventually these will be established.

EFFECTS OF PEPTIDE HORMONES ON THE BRAIN

Recently, a number of important manifestations of peptide hormone action on the brain have been recognized.

Pituitary Peptide Hormones

Certain of the pituitary peptide hormones appear capable of regulating their own secretion through operation of a short-loop feedback control probably at the hypothalamic rather than at the pituitary level (see Fig. 1). Thus, prolactin implants in the hypothalamus inhibit prolactin release, growth hormone implants inhibit GH release, LH implants inhibit LH release, and ACTH implants inhibit ACTH release. An apparent exception to this phenomenon is TSH, implants of which do not inhibit TSH secretion (in most but not all studies).

The reflex release of FSH during copulation in the rabbit appears to be responsible for the sleeplike EEG state of postcoital female rabbits, and FSH is reported to alter catecholamine metabolism in the hypothalamus. Prolactin affects maternal behavior in lower animals; its effects in the human are unknown. Many women who nurse their children describe this experience and the period of nursing as one of special tranquility, but it is not known whether this is a response to the mother-baby psychologic interaction or to the persistent high levels of prolactin in the nursing mother.

Changes in learned behavior and the EEG have been reported to follow injections of α- and β-MSH and of ACTH both in animals and in humans. De Wied and his colleagues have shown in rats that ACTH injections delay the loss of avoidance response in conditioning experiments.[23, 24, 50] This effect can be produced by the amino acid residues 4 to 10 of ACTH, called ACTH 4–10, which unlike ACTH itself, has no effects on the adrenal gland. Moreover, MSH, which contains the identical 4 to 10 amino acid residues, has been shown by Kastin and his colleagues[44] to facilitate learning by improving the ability to pay attention. ACTH 4–10 is reported to produce EEG effects in human subjects indicative of enhanced alertness. ACTH and MSH also increase the excitability of peripheral nerve cells. ADH, like ACTH 4–10, also delays the loss of avoidance responses, but this effect is clearly more prolonged. Animals with hereditary diabetes insipidus characterized by ADH deficiency lose learned avoidance behavior very rapidly unless given ADH.[6] Furthermore, intraventricular administration of ADH antiserum prevents retention of avoidance behavior in normal rats.

Hypophysiotropic Hormones

As described previously (Chapter 9), the secretion of TSH is regulated by the hypothalamic hormone TRH. The wide distribution of TRH outside the brain, and certain behavioral effects, suggest a larger role of TRH as a neurotransmitter or other modulator of brain function. TRH has recently been found to be distributed in all parts of the mammalian brain; 80 per cent of the total TRH of rat brain is found outside the hypothalamus.[81] The widespread distribution of TRH in brain leads to consideration of the possibility that TRH may have effects as a modifier of neuron activity. TRH shortens the sleeping time after pentobarbital and alters the normal temperature response to pentobarbital in mice.[9] Although evidence has been sought, there is no indication to date that TRH influences central catecholamine or indoleamine mechanisms. TRH has been reported to be highly active in the pargyline-dopa mouse activation test which is used extensively to screen drugs for possible antidepressant activity.[9, 52] Administration of the peptide has been reported to cause an elevation of mood, both in patients with unipolar depression and in normal control subjects. Unlike effects of other antidepressant agents, TRH produces a prompt, brief effect. More recent reports from several investigators, however, indicate that the TRH antidepressant effect is not uniformly reproducible.[26] Further investigation will be necessary to clarify this issue.

Direct microiontophoretic application of TRH has a predominantly depressant effect on spontaneous firing of single neurons in hypothalamus, cerebral cortex, cerebellum, and spinal cord. The effect is rapid in onset and low electrophoretic currents are effective, seriously raising the possibility that this is a physiologic effect, and suggesting that such peptides function as neurotransmitters.[55]

The sexual-activity-initiating effect of LHRH has been mentioned above. The tripeptide, Pro-Leu-Gly-NH$_2$ (PLG) was isolated from bovine hypothalamic tissue and is active in some assays in inhibiting MSH release. It also has been reported to have behavioral effects in experimental animals and to be effective in alleviating parkinsonian symptoms in man.[72] The physiologic status of this peptide remains uncertain, since it has no effect on α- or β-MSH secretion in man. However, it has been shown to potentiate the effects of L-dopa in both intact and hypophysectomized rats. It also antagonizes tremor induced by oxotremorine and harmine and can reverse the effects of certain sedative drugs. A recent report suggests that the peptide may have dopaminergic agonist effects. Somatostatin is reported to have a suppressing effect on spontaneous motor activity in the rat and has been observed to have a calming effect in the monkey.[9, 52] Since this substance is found in all areas of the brain, it may have other roles in addition to the function of inhibiting the release of growth hormone from the pituitary. Martin and coworkers[55] have proposed that the various peptidergic systems of the hypothalamus exert effects on other parts of the brain, including the cerebral cortex, through an ascending peptidergic neuronal system analogous to the biogenic amine systems serotonin, dopamine and norepinephrine, which have their origin in the midbrain. Evidence for this concept is still scanty. Lesions of the hypophysiotrophic area of the hypothalamus do not apparently influence cortical content of either TRH or somatostatin.

Angiotensin

Angiotensin II has very potent behavioral effects that suggest a major regulatory role (see also Chapter 4) for this substance in drinking.[2, 28] When given systemically to man or animals or by intraventricular injection to animals, this drug stimulates drinking and the release of ADH. Both the subfornical organ and the preoptic region appear to contain specific receptors for angiotensin II.[92] Lesions of the subfornical organ markedly reduce the drinking response to angiotensin II, and direct application of angiotensin II in the preoptic region induces drinking and influences the rate of firing of single neurons. The effects of injecting hypertonic salt solution into the third ventricle are potentiated by angiotensin II; this hormone may enhance the uptake of salt by osmoreceptors, as it enhances the uptake of salt by vascular structures elsewhere. The human in shock develops severe thirst which may be related to the increased circulating levels of angiotensin II. Anephric humans have blunted thirst responses. The thirst following hypovolemia may thus be a behavioral response to altered renal function.

Substance P

Substance P, an 11-amino-acid peptide, is widely distributed in the nervous system; with high concentrations in the hypothalamus, sensory systems, and substantia nigra.[28.] Substance P has an excitatory effect on central neurons and is postulated to have postsynaptic effects, providing evidence that the peptide may function as a neurotransmitter. The peptide is of particular importance in relay of sensory inputs in the central nervous system.

Sleep and Activity-Producing Peptides

Reports of sleep-promoting factors in blood and cerebrospinal fluid of sleeping experimental animals have appeared at intervals since the early claim of Legendre and Pieron in 1910. A long hiatus ensued, during which interest in this question lagged, but two laboratories, those of Monnier and of Pappenheimer, resumed work in the mid-1960's.[74] Both groups have shown that substances with the properties of peptides can be isolated from either the cerebral blood of rabbits or the third ventricle of sleep-deprived goats, and that injection of these substances into the ventricle of rats or rabbits can cause sleep. The material appears to have a molecular weight of 350 to 700, but a final structure has not been given. It has been proposed that the sleep peptide is part of the mechanism that normally regulates the activity cycle.

During the isolation of the sleep-producing peptide, Pappenheimer and collaborators have isolated a somewhat larger peptide-like substance that has the unexpected property of causing intense motor hyperactivity.[74] The identity and physiologic function of these substances remain to be elucidated.

Learning Peptides

The neurobiologic basis of learning has received much study. One aspect of this work has involved the relationship of peptide hormones to the learning process. This line of approach, initiated by Ungar and his collaborators, has led to the demonstration that a characteristic peptide appears in the brain of rats following a training experience.[99] The first to be isolated and identified is a pentadecapeptide to which the name scotophobin was given. This substance was isolated from the brains of dark-avoidance trained rats. Injection of this substance induces dark-avoidance in untrained rats. The structural formula is Ser-Asp-Asn-Asn-Gln-Gln-Gly-Lys-Ser-Ala-Gln-Gln-Gly-Gly-Tyr NH_2. This substance has never been identified in untrained rat brain, but gradually appears during, and increases to the sixth day of, dark avoidance training; thereafter it decreases. Two thirds of the substance is found in cortex, one fourth in brain stem and cerebellum, and the rest distributed throughout subcortical areas. A second peptide, ameletin, with the tentative structure Pglu-Ala-Gly-Tyr-Ser-Lys, was isolated from the brain of rats habituated to a sound stimulus. In naive recipient animals, it reduces the startle response to the sound stimulus. A number of other peptides with apparent roles related to color discrimination, step-down avoidance, and maze learning are under active investigation. These exciting observations have not as yet been generally confirmed.

Endogenous Opiate-Receptor Peptides

It has been recognized for many years by pharmacologists that drugs act on cells by binding to specific receptors. Development of modern techniques has made it possible to measure the concentrations of morphine receptors in various target tissues including brain and intestine.[105, 107] Within the brain, there are marked regional differences, for the most part believed to be related to the distribution of pain pathways. For example, the medial thalamus is particularly rich in morphine receptors as compared with the lateral thalamus. Although not in the classic nociceptive pathway, the anterior amygdala has the richest concentration of opiate receptors, a regional distribution postulated to be related to the effects of morphine in producing euphoria and behavioral change.

Although the morphine receptor has been studied mainly in relationship to drug effects, several workers have considered the possibility that the morphine receptor might also react with an endogenous substance postulated to play a role in physiologic modulation of the pain stimulus. On the basis of this hypothesis a number of workers have attempted to isolate substances from the brain and from the pituitary gland capable of competing with morphine for receptors in various test systems. This search, initiated by Goldstein and collaborators,[105] led to a systematic search for such substances. In 1975 Hughes and collaborators[41] reported that two peptides isolated from whole brain were active in an opiate-receptor assay. These peptides were named methionine enkephalin and leucine enkephalin. Subsequently, another group of endogenous opiate-like peptides were isolated from hypothalamic extracts by Guillemin and coworkers.[35] The name endorphin (*endo*genous + mor*phine*) was given to these substances which include a 16-amino-acid peptide (α-endorphin), a 31-amino-acid peptide (β-endorphin) and a 17-

amino-acid peptide (γ-endorphin). Hughes recognized that the enkephalin sequences corresponded exactly to peptide sequences in the pituitary hormone β-lipotropin, a linear peptide containing 91 amino acid residues isolated from sheep glands by Choh Hao Li who announced its structure in 1964.[105] The endorphins also correspond to specific sequences in β-liptropin, and Hughes' pentapeptides form part of the endorphin molecule. The endorphins and methionine enkephalin vary considerably in their potency as morphine-like substances in assays of pain threshold and addiction. Many now believe that the major precursor compound is β-endorphin and that the other active compounds are breakdown products.

Although enkephalins and endorphins were first isolated from brain extracts and probably arise in situ, it is also recognized that these compounds can be formed from β-lipotropin by brain enzymes, a finding that suggests a possible role of the pituitary in regulation of brain function. Other sequences of β-lipotropin have previously been recognized to have effects on behavior, neuronal electrical activity, and morphine tolerance. These include β-MSH and a fragment of ACTH (4–10). These homologies and sequences are shown in Fig. 4. Guillemin has pointed out that β-lipotropin, previously a hormone without a function, is the mother compound of a large number of psychoactive peptides. There may be other, as yet unidentified, peptides found in blood and brain extracts that influence behavior or pain threshhold.

Acquisition of new knowledge in the field of endogenous opiate peptides has been explosive because of the important implications for understanding of pain, addiction, behavior, mental disorder, and other brain functions. By means of specific antisera, β-enkephalin has been demonstrated in nerve endings in various parts of the brain corresponding to the site of endogenous opiate receptors. It seems reasonable to conclude that one or more of these substances is, in fact, an authentic neurotransmitter in pain-modifying pathways.

The finding of an endogenous compound that relieved pain initially encouraged

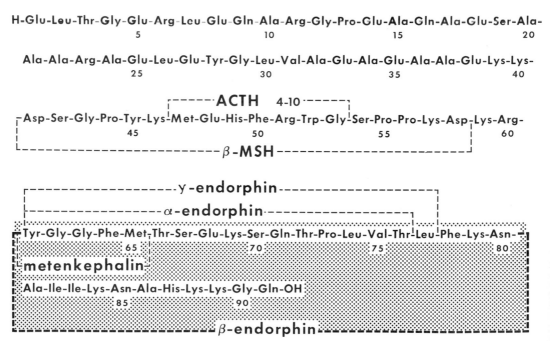

Figure 4. Homologies in structure of sheep β-lipotropin with the ACTH fragment (4–10), β-MSH (41–58), methionine enkephalin (61–65), α-endorphin (61–76), γ-endorphin (61–77), and β-endorphin (61–91).

investigators to believe that the problem of addiction might be solved. This does not appear to be the case because the endorphins are addictive and their effects are blocked by opiate antagonists, such as naloxone. The administration of morphine to experimental animals appears to increase the brain content of enkephalin.

> These observations have led to a powerful new hypothesis of the mechanism of addiction. As outlined by Marx, ". . . investigators hypothesize that the exogenous opiate morphine inhibits, by a feedback mechanism, the firing of neurons that would normally release enkephalins as neurotransmitters. If the peptides are not released they should accumulate in the nerve terminals and their concentrations should increase. This abnormal state, in which there is only exogenous opiate present in the synapses to react with the target neurons, would correspond to tolerance, according to Snyder and Simantov. On abrupt cessation of opiate administration or when naloxone is injected into the animals, the receptors would be temporarily deprived of both enkephalin and morphine. Withdrawal symptoms would result until the enkephalin neurons began firing and releasing the peptides at a normal rate."[106]

Endogenous morphine peptides may also be important in certain psychiatric diseases. Investigators have found that the injection of β-endorphin into the third ventricle of the rat brings about a state of muscular rigidity resembling catatonic schizophrenia.[107] Highly preliminary observations suggest that there may be an increased concentration of endophins in spinal fluid of patients with schizophrenia, and that the administration of naloxone may improve the condition of schizophrenic patients by decreasing their hallucinations and improving the clarity of their thought processes.[107]

The mechanism of action of peptides on brain in general has not been elucidated. They probably act through the cyclic AMP mechanism via specific hormone receptors on the cell membrane (as TRH, LHRH, and somatostatin do in the pituitary), since the brain is rich in adenyl cyclase and cyclic AMP, and striking alterations in function and behavior can be induced by intracerebral injections of cyclic AMP derivatives. Many of these peptide-induced changes in brain function have been recognized only recently. Other peptides, both hormonal and nonhormonal, as yet unrecognized, may profoundly affect mind and behavior.

BRAIN DYSFUNCTION SECONDARY TO HORMONALLY MEDIATED CHANGES IN THE INTERNAL MILIEU

Virtually all of the important plasma constituents whose constancy is normally guarded by homeostatic mechanisms (including those dependent upon hormone action) influence brain function. The major controlled variables are the concentrations in blood of glucose, CO_2, O_2, H^+, Ca^{++}, Na^+, K^+ and osmotically active particles. Gross disturbance of any of these variables can produce metabolic disorder in the brain, with diffuse impairment of higher functions ranging from mild disturbance in consciousness, memory, and judgment through confusion, disorientation, stupor, coma, and death. A variety of symptoms resembling neurasthenia, neurosis, and functional psychosis also can be seen in these syndromes. A detailed account of organic brain disorders is given by Plum.[77] In this section only disturbances in calcium and glucose will be dealt with.

Abnormalities in Plasma Calcium

Hypercalcemia

High blood calcium levels can result from hyperparathyroidism, from vitamin D intoxication, and from carcinomas causing either massive destruction of bone, or a parathyroid-hormone-like syndrome.[80] One of the most dramatic endocrine causes of acute hypercalcemia is infarction of a parathyroid adenoma, which leads to an outpouring of parathyroid hormone.[80] In addition to the relatively unspecific signs of encephalopathy, hypercalcemic patients manifest a variety of poorly-defined neurotic symptoms, fatigue, headache, and organic psychosis. Seizures are exceedingly rare. In an extensive study of the psychiatric aspects of hyperparathyroidism, Peterson[95] evaluated 54 patients. As summarized by Smith and collaborators:

> Personality changes noted in the majority of these patients began with an affective disturbance characterized by lack of initiative and spontaneity, and by depression. This depression was sometimes combined with moroseness, irrascibility or explosiveness. Suicidal tendencies were occasionally noted, although none of the patients had to be hospitalized because of this. Generalized fatigue was a common complaint. Memory impairment, with reduced ability to concentrate, was less common. All these changes developed slowly, sometimes over several years. Acute organic psychosis generally appeared as disorientation, delirium, confusion, paranoid ideas and hallucinations. Severe acute organic psychosis often began abruptly and necessitated rapid surgical correction of hyperparathyroidism. Peterson carefully correlated the degree of psychiatric disturbance with the level of serum calcium. As the level of serum calcium rose, the severity of mental changes increased. This was true whether hypercalcemia was caused by hyperparathyroidism or other causes. When eucalcemia was attained, as by hemodialysis, mental abnormalities disappeared, despite persisting hyperparathyroidism. The serum calcium per se was the determining factor.[93]

Cope,[18] a surgeon with vast experience in the surgical treatment of hyperparathyroidism, emphasized the importance of neurologic and psychiatric symptoms as clues in the evaluation and diagnosis of hyperparathyroidism. The clinical picture of paranoid schizophrenia has been seen in hyperparathyroidism, and its relationship to the illness proven by complete cure after surgery. In Peterson's series,[95] serum calcium levels of 12 to 16 mg./100 ml. were associated with neurasthenic changes, and acute psychosis at values above 16 mg./100 ml.[75] Calcium levels of 16 to 19 mg./100 ml. were associated with alterations in consciousness; somnolence or coma occurred with values over 19 mg./100 ml.

Although many kinds of psychologic disturbance can be seen in patients with hypercalcemia, and blood calcium levels should be measured in all patients with psychiatric problems, it must be emphasized that a modest elevation in blood calcium level is not necessarily the cause of psychiatric illness in a given patient. The true incidence of significant mental impairment is not known. The recent finding of numerous patients with mild hypercalcemia following the application of the multiphasic screening methods has shown that most are asymptomatic. As a practical matter, the likelihood that one is dealing with asymptomatic mild hypercalcemia in a neurotic individual must be borne in mind in differential diagnosis and in the formulation of therapy. Differential diagnosis and treatment of hypercalcemia is dealt with in the literature of internal medicine and endocrinology. Acute management includes hydration and the use of diuretics such as furosemide and high-dosage corticoids. Chronic management includes parathyroidectomy (when the diagnosis of hyperparathyroidism has been established), and administration of phosphates.

Hypocalcemia

Calcium ion is specifically related to neuronal membrane function and synaptic transmission. Low calcium levels such as are seen in *hypoparathyroidism* can lead to a variety of patterns of brain dysfunction. Smith and collaborators provide an excellent summary of these changes:

More than half of the patients with primary idiopathic hypoparathyroidism were noted to have psychological symptoms, in a review of 178 patients. There were no age or socioeconomic differences in the incidence of the disease. The most frequently observed problem was intellectual impairment which was noted in 50 patients. None of these individuals improved spontaneously. However, with treatment of the underlying problem, 23 improved substantially or regained normal intellect. In this group of 178 patients, 43 had an organic brain syndrome (emotional disorder with impaired intellect). Some of these presented with symptoms similar to delirium tremens. In this group, 1 patient improved without treatment; 19 improved or were cured by elevating the serum calcium.

Neurosis and psychosis comprised the third most commonly observed group of symptoms. Functional psychoses were diagnosed in 9 patients. Three died and 2 improved spontaneously. Two patients improved with treatment, and the outcome of the other 2 is unknown. This syndrome can resemble schizophrenia, and some of these patients have been termed *schizoid 1*.

The group termed *neurotic* was composed of 20 patients. In 3 of these, a disturbed emotional state was directly related to the tetanic attacks. Many of the characteristic symptoms of the neuroses were seen—obsessions, phobias, tics, etc. These problems were usually cured when the patient was treated for hypoparathyroidism.[93]

A high incidence of encephalopathy, behavioral disturbance, seizures, tics, and athetoid movements are observed in patients with *pseudohypoparathyroidism,* a disease in which hypocalcemia is due to tissue unresponsiveness to parathyroid hormone.

Vitamin D deficiency due to malabsorption, renal failure, or resistance also may cause hypocalcemia. It should be recalled that diphenytoin can induce vitamin D deficiency in states of marginal function, a caution to be kept in mind in chronic treatment of epilepsy.

The high frequency of neurologic and psychiatric findings in hypocalcemic, as well as hypercalcemic, patients mandates measurement of blood calcium levels in all individuals with psychologic disturbance.

The relation between brain disturbance and gross hypocalcemia is readily apparent. Less certain is the relation between symptoms of neurosis and minimal hypocalcemia. This form of disease is seen with surprising frequency in patients that have been subjected to subtotal thyroidectomy. A few patients have been described who demonstrated impaired parathyroid hormone secretory reserves, and minimal lowering of plasma calcium levels. The frequency of neurosis symptoms is high in such subjects. However, treatment with calcium and vitamin D did not restore normal functioning in the majority of patients, probably because there was no connection between minimal Ca^{++} deficiency and the psychologic status.

Disorders of Carbohydrate Metabolism

Hypoglycemia

In the normal state, the CNS utilizes only glucose as a source of energy, but after prolonged fasting, adaptation of brain enzymes takes place so that normal brain function can take place with only about 30 per cent of the normal glucose uptake, the remaining energy requirement coming from the oxidation of keto acids (β-hydroxybutyrate and acetoacetate).[90] It is not clear that brain adaptation to chronic insulin-induced hypoglycemia is the same as that to chronic starvation. Blood sugar levels between 30 and 40 mg./100 ml. and below frequently cause mild delirium; lower levels are associated with progressive impairment of cerebral function and deep coma results from values below 10 mg./100 ml. The coma that supervenes can be irreversible if hypoglycemia persists, and moderate degrees of neuronal injury follow substantial degrees of hypoglycemia.

The symptomatology of hypoglycemia depends to some extent on the rapidity with which the blood sugar level is lowered. The rate of fall of plasma glucose levels (sensed by central glucoreceptors), rather than absolute levels, determines whether autonomic symptoms due to hypersecretion of catecholamines occur. Thus, a fall from values of 250 to 70 (a glucose concentration still in the "normal range") can result in marked symptoms of "hypoglycemia" which resemble those of anxiety. If the blood sugar level is lowered slowly, or chronically, various types of metabolic encephalopathy and psychologic disturbances can occur. Chronic hypoglycemia can result in syndromes indistinguishable from schizophrenia, depression, and dementia, in the absence of such overt symptoms or signs of epinephrine excess as tachycardia, sweating, anxiety, and pallor.

Reactive (postabsorptive) hypoglycemias are the commonest type of hypoglycemia. Approximately 2 to 3 hours after food intake, there is a dip in blood glucose level followed by a sharp rebound. Symptoms resemble those of anxiety, due primarily to hyperepinephrinemia which is produced by the hypoglycemia. Loss of consciousness and convulsions are rare. Reactive hypoglycemia is seen after subtotal gastrectomy, in early onset diabetes mellitus, and following ingestion of galactose, fructose, or amino acids in sensitive individuals.

Hypoglycemia during the fasting state may be due either to overutilization or to underproduction of glucose. Overutilization of glucose is seen with insulin-secreting tumors, mainly functioning beta-cell tumors of the pancreas, with thyrotoxicosis, massive connective tissue sarcomas, and with growth hormone deficiency, the latter occurring almost exclusively in children. Glucose underproduction may occur with glycogen storage disease, extensive liver damage and with adrenocortical or glucagon insufficiency. In addition, overdosage of insulin or of sulfonylureas may produce hypoglycemia. Initial effects are due to cortical depression with headaches, faintness, confusion, restlessness, clouded consciousness, hunger, irritability, and visual disturbances. Other symptoms, related to epinephrine release, are anxiety, tremor, perspiration, tachycardia, pallor, and tingling of the fingers or around the mouth. With more severe hypoglycemia, or a more rapid onset, progressive changes include loss of environmental contact, myoclonic twitchings, clonic spasms, and increased sensitivity to stimulation. Still further CNS depression leads to tonic spasms, torsion spasms, independent movement of the eyes, and the appearance of long-tract signs. Death may occur. Treatment with glucose alleviates the symptoms, in reverse order, but prolonged or repeated severe hypoglycemia may not be compatible with complete recovery. Unfortunately, the lay public has discovered hypoglycemia as a convenient diagnosis to explain chronic fatigue and depression and other psychoneurotic symptoms, and in recent years an extraordinarily large number of patients are seen whose chief complaint is hypoglycemia.

Crucial to the diagnosis of true hypoglycemia is the demonstration that 1) symptoms are correlated with either a rapid fall in blood sugar level, or with a low absolute value (less than 50 mg./100 ml.), and 2) they respond to treatment with glucose. Many people, when tired or bored, get a "pick-up" from a carbohydrate-rich snack, and this is particularly true of those on weight-reducing diets. This is not evidence of hypoglycemia and is more likely a normal response. Complete analysis of the diagnostic approach to hypoglycemia is dealt with in the endocrine and metabolic literature. It is important to emphasize here that a minimum work-up includes a 5-hour glucose tolerance test after appropriate preparation (300 g. carbohydrate intake daily for 3 days or more). The only test which completely excludes the diagnosis of fasting hypoglycemia is a three-day fast under observation in a hospital setting. Few, if any, patients with pancreatic insulin-producing tumors will fail to show diagnostically low levels of glucose (less than 40 mg./100 ml.) and symptoms by this time. In cases where so-called hypoglycemic symptoms are causing significant disturbance in brain function, this test is mandatory.

Hyperglycemia

High blood sugar levels appear in untreated or poorly treated diabetics, and occasionally in extremely stressed individuals. Values above 1,000 mg./100 ml. are seen almost exclusively in patients with associated renal insufficiency. High blood glucose levels in this range cause cerebral disease through a *hyperosmolarity mechanism,* since gross encephalopathy can be observed even in the absence of ketosis or ketonemia. When severe, *hyperosmolarity coma* is fatal in a high proportion of cases. Even when treated successfully, patients who have experienced a period of hyperosmolar coma may continue to show impairment of higher functions indefinitely, indicating that irreversible neuronal damage has taken place. Autopsy in such cases shows loss of nerve cells. A similar hyperosmolarity state is seen in severe water deficiency, as in untreated diabetes insipidus.

REFERENCES

1. AKISKAL, S. AND McKINNEY, W. T., Jr.: *Overview of recent research in depression.* Arch. Gen. Psychiat. 32:285, 1975.

2. ANDERSSON, B.: *Thirst and brain control of water balance.* Am. Sci. 59:408, 1971.

3. ARTUNKAL, S. AND TOGROL, B.: *Psychological studies in hyperthyroidism. In* Cameron, M. P. and O'Connor, M. (eds.): *Brain-Thyroid Relationships.* Ciba Foundation Study Group No. 18. Churchill, London, 1964, p. 125.

4. BARBEAU, A. AND KASTIN, A. J.: *Double-blind evaluation of oral L-prolyl-L leucylglycine amide in Parkinson's disease.* Can. Med. Assoc. J. 114:120, 1976.

5. BARDWICK, J. M.: *Psychological correlates of the menstrual cycle and oral contraceptive medication. In* Sachar, E. J. (ed.): *Hormones, Behavior and Psychopathology.* Raven Press, New York, 1976, p. 95.

6. BARKER, J. L.: *Peptide regulation of neuronal excitability.* Physiol. Rev. 56:435, 1976.

7. BARRACLOUGH, C. A.: *Modifications in reproductive function after exposure to hormones during the prenatal and early postnatal period. In* Martini, L. and Ganong, W. F. (eds.): *Neuroendocrinology,* vol. 2. Academic Press, New York, 1967, p. 62.

8. BENEDEK, T. AND RUBENSTEIN, B. B.: *The Sexual Cycle in Women, Psychosomatic Medicine Monographs,* vol. 3, nos. 1 and 2. National Research Council, Washington, D. C., 1942.

9. BREESE, G. R., ET AL.: *Interactions of thyrotropin-releasing hormone with centrally acting drugs. In* Prange, A. J., Jr. (ed.): *The Thyroid Axis, Drugs and Behavior.* Raven Press, New York, 1974, p. 115.

10. BROWNSTEIN, M. J., ET AL.: *Distribution of hypothalamic hormones and neurotransmitters within the diencephalon. In* Martini, L., and Ganong, W. F. (eds.): *Frontiers in Neuroendocrinology,* vol. 4. Raven Press, New York, 1976, p. 1.

11. BUBENIK, G. A. AND BROWN, G. M.: *Morphologic sex differences in primate brain areas involved in regulation of reproductive activity.* Experientia 29:619, 1973.

12. CAMERON, M. P. AND O'CONNOR, M. (EDS.): *Brain-Thyroid Relationships.* Ciba Foundation Study Group No. 18. Churchill, London, 1964.

13. CARPENTER, W. T., JR., STRAUSS, J. S. AND BUNNEY, W. E., JR.: *The psychobiology of cortisol metabolism: Clinical and theoretical implications. In* Shader, R. I. (ed.): *Psychiatric Complications of New Drugs.* Raven Press, New York, 1972, p. 49.

14. CARROLL, B. J.: *Psychoendocrine relationships in affective disorders. In* Hill, O. W. (ed.): *Modern Trends in Psychosomatic Medicine.* Butterworth, London, in press.

15. CARROLL, B. J. AND MENDELS, J.: *Neuroendocrine regulation in affective disorders. In* Sachar, E. J. (ed.): *Hormones, Behavior and Psychopathology.* Raven Press, New York, 1976, p. 193.

16. CHAMBERS, W. F., FREEDMAN, S. L. AND SAWYER, C. H.: *The effects of adrenal steroids on evoked reticular responses.* Exp. Neurol. 8:458, 1963.

17. COOPER, A. J., ET AL.: *Antiandrogen (cyproterone acetate) therapy in deviant hypersexuality.* Br. J. Psychiat. 120:58, 1972.

18. COPE, O.: *Hyperparathyroidism: Diagnosis and management.* Am. J. Surg. 99:394, 1960.

19. CULLBERG, J.: *Mood changes and menstrual symptoms with different gestagen/estrogen combinations.* Acta Psychiatr. Scand. [Suppl.] 236:1, 1972.

20. DAVIDSON, J. M.: *Hormones and sexual behavior in the male.* Hosp. Prac. 10:126, 1975.

21. DAVIES, I. J., ET AL.: *The affinity of catechol estrogens for estrogen receptors in the pituitary and the anterior hypothalamus of the rat.* Endocrinology 97:554, 1975.

22. DESROSIERS, J. J.: *Headaches related to contraceptive therapy and their control.* Headache 14:105, 1974.

23. DE WIED, D.: *Pituitary control of avoidance behavior. In* Martini, L. and Fraschini, F. (eds.): *The Hypothalamus.* Academic Press, New York, 1970, p. 641.

24. DE WIED, D., ET AL.: *Hormonal influences on motivational, learning and memory processes. In* Sachar, E. J. (ed.): *Hormones, Behavior and Psychopathology.* Raven Press, New York, 1976, p. 1.

25. EAYRS, J. T.: *Developmental relationships between brain and thyroid. In* Michael, R. P. (ed.): *Endocrinology and Human Behaviour.* Oxford University Press, London, 1968, p. 239.

26. EHRENSING, R. H., ET AL.: *Affective state and thyrotropin and prolactin responses after repeated injections of TRH in depressed patients.* Am. J. Psychiat. 131:714, 1974.

27. EHRHARDT, A. A.: *Prenatal hormonal exposure and psychosexual differentiation. In* Sachar, E. J. (ed.): *Topics in Psychoendocrinology.* Grune & Stratton, New York, 1975, p. 67.

28. FITZSIMONS, J. T.: *The hormonal control of water and sodium intake. In* Martini, L. and Ganong, W. F. (eds.): *Frontiers in Neuroendocrinology,* vol. 2. Oxford University Press, New York, 1971, p. 103.

29. GLICK, I. D. AND BENNETT, S. E.: *Psychiatric effects of progesterone and oral contraceptives. In* Shader, R. I. (ed.): *Psychiatric Complications of Medical Drugs.* Raven Press, New York, 1972, p. 295.

30. GORSKI, R. A. AND WHALEN, R. E. (EDS.): *Brain and Behavior.* In *Proceedings of the Third Conference of the Brain and Gonadal Function.* University of California Press, Berkeley and Los Angeles, 1966.

31. GORSKI, R. A.: *Gonadal hormones and the perinatal development of neuroendocrine function. In* Martini, L. and Ganong, W. F. (eds.): *Frontiers in Neuroendocrinology.* Oxford University Press, New York, 1971, p. 237.

32. GOY, R. W. AND RESKO, J. A.: *Gonadal hormones and behaviour of normal and pseudo-hermaphroditic non-human female primates.* Recent Prog. Horm. Res. 28:707, 1972.

33. GRANT, E. C. G.: *The influence of hormones on headache and mood in women.* Hemicrania 6:2, 1975.

34. GREEN, R. AND MONEY, J. (EDS.): *Transsexualism and Sex Reassignment.* Johns Hopkins University Press, Baltimore, 1969.

35. GUILLEMIN, R., LING, N. AND BURGUS, R.: *Endorphines, peptides d'origine hypothalamique et neurohypophysaire a activite morphinomimetique: Isolation et structure moleculaire d'α-endorphine.* C. R. Acad. Sci. (Paris) 282:1, 1976.

36. HELLER, C. G. AND MYERS, G. B.: *The male climacteric: its symptomatology, diagnosis and treatment.* J.A.M.A. 126:472, 1944.

37. HENKIN, R. I.: *The neuroendocrine control of perception. In* Hamburg, D. (ed.): *Perception and Its Disorders,* vol. 48, Williams & Wilkins, Baltimore, 1970, p. 54.

38. HENKIN, R. I., ET AL.: *Studies in auditory thresholds in normal man and in patients with adrenal cortical insufficiency: The role of adrenal cortical steroids.* J. Clin. Invest. 46:429, 1967.

39. HERZBERG, B., ET AL.: *Oral contraceptives, depression and libido.* Br. Med. J. 3:1, 1971.

40. HUFFER, V. AND SCOTT, W. H.: *Psychological studies of adult male patients with sexual infantilism before and after androgen therapy.* Ann. Intern. Med. 61:255, 1964.

41. HUGHES, J., ET AL.: *Identification of two related pentapeptides from the brain with potent opiate agonist activity.* Nature 258:577, 1975.

42. INGBAR, S. H. AND WOEBER, K. A.: *The thyroid gland. In* Williams, R. H. (ed.): *Textbook of Endocrinology.* W. B. Saunders, Philadelphia, 1974, p. 95.

43. KANE, F. J.: *Psychiatric reactions to oral contraceptives.* Am. J. Obstet. Gyncecol. 102:1053, 1968.

44. KASTIN, A. J., ET AL.: *Psycho-physiologic correlates of MSH activity in man.* Physiol. Behav. 7:893, 1971.

45. KINSEY, A. C. AND POMEROY, W. B.: *Sexual Behavior in the Human Male.* W. B. Saunders, Philadelphia, 1948.

46. KOLODNY, R. C., ET AL.: *Plasma testosterone and semen analysis in male homosexuals.* N. Engl. J. Med. 285:1170, 1971.

47. KOPERA, H.: *Estrogens and psychic functions.* In VanKeep, P. A. and Lauritzen, C. (eds.): *Frontiers of Hormone Research, vol. 2, Aging and Estrogens.* S. Karger, Basel, 1973.

48. KREUS, L. E. AND ROSE, R. M.: *Assessment of aggressive behavior and plasma testosterone in a young criminal population.* Psychosom. Med. 34:321, 1972.

49. KUSALIC, M. AND FORTIN, C.: *Growth hormone treatment in hypopituitary dwarfs.* Can. Psychiatr. Assoc. J. 20:325, 1975.

50. LANDE, S. AND WITTER, A.: *Pituitary peptides—An octapeptide that stimulates conditioned avoidance acquisition in hypophysectomized rats.* J. Biol. Chem. 246:2058, 1971.

51. LEVINE, S. AND MULLINS, R. F., JR.: *Hormonal influences on brain organization in infant rats.* Science 152:1585, 966.

52. LIPTON, M. A., ET AL.: *Behavioral effects of hypothalamic polypeptide hormones in animals and man.* In Sachar, E. J. (ed.): *Hormones, Behavior and Psychopathology.* Raven Press, New York, 1976, p. 15.

53. MAAS, J. W.: *Biogenic amines and depression.* Arch. Gen. Psychiatry 32:1357, 1975.

54. MACK, T. M., ET AL.: *Estrogens and endometrial cancer in a retirement community.* N. Engl. J. Med. 294:1262, 1976.

55. MARTIN, J. B., RENAUD, L. P. AND BRAZEAU, P.: *Hypothalamic peptides: New evidence for peptidergic pathways in the C.N.S.* Lancet 2:393, 1975.

56. MASTERS, W. H. AND JOHNSON, V. E.: *Human Sexual Inadequacy.* Little, Brown and Co., Boston, 1970.

57. MASTERS, W. H. AND JOHNSON, V. E.: *Human Sexual Response.* Little, Brown and Co., Boston, 1966.

58. MCEWEN, B. S.: *The brain as a target organ of endocrine hormones.* Hosp. Prac. 10:95, 1975.

59. MCEWEN, B. S. AND PFAFF, D. W.: *Chemical and physiological approaches to neuroendocrine mechanisms: Attempts at integration.* In Ganong, W. F. and Martini, L. (eds.): *Frontiers in Neuroendocrinology 1973.* Oxford University Press, New York, 1973, p. 267.

60. MCEWEN, B. S., ET AL.: *Steroid hormone interaction with specific brain regions.* In Bowman, R. E. and Datta, S. P. (eds.): *Biochemistry of Brain and Behavior.* Plenum Press, New York, 1970, p. 123.

61. MICHAEL, R. P., BONSALL, R. W. AND KUTNER, M.: *Volatile fatty acids, "copulins", in human vaginal secretions.* Psychoneuroendocrinology 1:153, 1975.

62. MICHAEL, R. P. AND GIBBONS, J. L.: *Interrelationships between the endocrine system and neuropsychiatry.* Int. Rev. Neurobiol. 5:243, 1963.

63. MICHAEL, R. P., ET AL.: *Neuroendocrine factors in the control of primate behavior.* Recent Prog. Horm. Res. 28:665, 1972.

64. MONEY, J.: *Effects of prenatal androgenization and deandrogenization on behavior in human beings.* In Ganong, W. F. and Martini, L. (eds.): *Frontiers in Neuroendocrinology 1973.* Oxford University Press, New York, 1973, p. 249.

65. MONEY, J. AND EHRHARDT, A. A.: *Gender dimorphic behavior and fetal sex hormones.* Recent Prog. Horm. Res. 28:735, 1972.

66. MONEY, J. AND LEWIS, V.: *Longitudinal study of intelligence quotient in treated congenital hypothyroidism.* In Cameron, M. P. and O'Connor, M. (eds.): *Thyroid Relationships.* Ciba Foundation Study Group No. 18. Churchill, London, 1964, p. 75.

67. MONEY, J., ET AL.: *Combined antiandrogenic and counseling program for treatment of 46, XY and 47, XYY sex offenders.* In Sachar, E. J. (ed.): *Hormones, Behavior and Psychopathology.* Raven Press, New York, 1976, p. 105.

68. MOOS, R. H., ET AL.: *Fluctuations in symptoms and moods during the menstrual cycle.* J. Psychosom. Res. 13:37, 1969.

69. MOSS, R. L. AND MCCANN, S. M.: *Induction of mating behavior in rats by luteinizing hormone-releasing factor.* Science 181:177, 1973.

70. NORRIS, R. V. AND LLOYD, C. W.: *Psychosexual effects of hormone therapy.* Medical Aspects of Human Sexuality 3:33, 1973.

71. O'MALLEY, B. W. AND MEANS, A. R.: *Female steroid hormones and target cell nuclei.* Science 183: 610, 1974.

72. OPPENHEIMER, J. H., SCHWARTZ, H. L. AND SURKS, M. I.: *Tissue differences in the concentration of triiodothyronine nuclear binding sites in the rat: liver, kidney, pituitary, heart, brain, spleen and testis.* Endocrinology 95:897, 1974.

73. PAIGE, K. E.: *Effects of oral contraceptives on affective fluctuations associated with the menstrual cycle.* Psychosom. Med. 33:515, 1971.

74. PAPPENHEIMER, V. F., KARNOVSKY, M. L. AND KOSKI, G.: *Peptides in cerebrospinal fluid and their*

relation to sleep and activity. *In* Plum, F. (ed.): *Brain Dysfunction in Metabolic Disorders,* vol. 53. Raven Press, New York, 1974, p. 201.

75. PETERSON, P.: *Psychiatric disorders in primary hyperparathyroidism.* J. Clin. Endocrinol. 28:1491, 1968.

76. PFAFF, D. W.: *Luteinizing hormone-releasing factor potentiates lordosis behavior in hypophysecto-mized ovariectomized female rats.* Science 182:1148, 1973.

77. PLUM, F. (ED.): *Brain Dysfunction in Metabolic Disorders,* vol. 53. Raven Press, New York, 1974.

78. PRANGE, A. J., ET AL.: *Peptides and the central nervous system. In* Iversen, L. L., Iversen, S. D. and Snyder, S. H. (eds.): *Handbook of Psychopharmacology.* Plenum Press, New York, in press, 1976.

79. RAISMAN, G. AND FIELD, P. M.: *Sexual dimorphism in the preoptic area of the rat.* Science 173:731, 1971.

80. RASMUSSEN, H.: *Parathyroid hormone, calcitonin and the calciferols. In* Williams, R. (ed.): *Textbook of Endocrinology.* W. B. Saunders, Philadelphia, 1974, p. 660.

81. REICHLIN, S., ET AL.: *Regulation of the secretion of thyrotropin-releasing hormone (TRH) and luteiniz-ing hormone-releasing hormone (LRH). In* Seeman, P. and Brown, G. M. (eds.): *Neurology and Neu-roscience Research 1974.* Neuroscience Institute, University of Toronto, 1974, p. 48.

82. REINISCH, J. M.: *Effects of prenatal hormone exposure on physical and psychological development in humans and animals: With a note on the state of the field. In* Sachar, E. J. (ed.): *Hormones, Behavior and Psychopathology.* Raven Press, New York, 1976, p. 69.

83. ROSE, R. M.: *The psychological effects of androgens and estrogens—A review. In* Shader, R. I. (ed.): *Psychiatric Complications of Medical Drugs.* Raven Press, New York, 1972, p. 251.

84. ROSE, R. M.: *Testosterone, aggression and homosexuality: A review of the literature and its implica-tions for research. In* Sachar, E. J. (ed.): *Topics in Psychoendocrinology,* Grune & Stratton, New York, 1975, p. 83.

85. RYAN, K. J., ET AL.: *Estrogen formation in the brain.* Am. J. Obstet. Gynecol. 114:454, 1972.

86. SACHAR, E. J.: *Psychiatric disturbances associated with endocrine disorders. In* Reiser, M. (ed.): *Amer-ican Handbook of Psychiatry,* vol. IV. Basic Books, New York, 1975, p. 299.

87. SACHAR, E. J.: *Neuroendocrine abnormalities in depressive illness. In* Sachar, E. J. (ed.): *Topics in Psychoendocrinology.* Grune & Stratton, New York, 1975, p. 135.

88. SACHAR, E. J., HELLMAN, L. AND ROFFWARG, H. P.: *Disrupted 24-hour patterns of cortisol secretion in psychotic depression.* Arch. Gen. Psychiatry 28:19, 1975.

89. SACHAR, E. J. AND COPPEN, A. J.: *Biological aspects of affective psychoses. In* Guall, G. E. (ed.): *Biol-ogy of Brain Dysfunction,* vol. 3. Plenum Press, New York, 1975, p. 215.

90. SACHS, W.: *Disorders of glucose metabolism in brain dysfunction. In* Guall, G. E. (ed.): *Biology of Brain Dysfunction,* vol. 1. Plenum Press, New York, 1973, p. 143.

91. SALMON, U. J. AND GEIST, S. H.: *Effect of androgens upon libido in women.* J. Clin. Endocrinol. 3:235, 1943.

92. SIMPSON, J. B. AND ROUTTENBERG, A.: *Subfornical organ: Site of drinking elicitation by angiotensin-II.* Science 173:1172, 1973.

93. SMITH, C. K., ET AL.: *Psychiatric disturbance in endocrinologic disease.* Psychosom. Med. 34:69, 1972.

94. SMITH, S. L.: *Mood and the menstrual cycle. In* Sachar, E. J. (ed.): *Topics in Psychoendocrinology.* Grune & Stratton, New York, 1975, p. 19.

95. SOKOLOFF, L. AND KENNEDY, C.: *The action of thyroid hormones and their influence on brain develop-ment and function. In* Guall, G. E. (ed.): *Biology of Brain Dysfunction,* vol. 2. Plenum Press, New York, 1973, p. 295.

96. SOMERVILLE, B. W.: *Estrogen-withdrawal migraine: 1. Duration of exposure required and attempted prophylaxis by premenstrual estrogen administration.* Neurology 25:239, 1975.

97. SOMERVILLE, B. W.: *Estrogen-withdrawal migraine: II. Attempted prophylaxis by continuous estradiol administration.* Neurology 25:245, 1975.

98. UDRY, J. R. AND MORRIS, N. M.: *Distribution of coitus in the menstrual cycle.* Nature 220:593, 1968.

99. UNGAR, G.: *Peptides and behavior.* Int. Rev. Neurobiol. 17:37, 1975.

100. VERNIKOS-DANELLIS, J.: *Effects of hormones on the central nervous system. In* Levine, S. (ed.): *Hor-mones and Behavior.* Academic Press, New York, 1972, p. 11.

101. WHYBROW, P. AND FERRELL, R.: *Thyroid state and human behavior: Contributions from a clinical perspective. In* Prange, A. J., Jr. (ed.): *The Thyroid Axis, Drugs and Behavior.* Raven Press, New York, 1974, p. 5.

102. WHYBROW, P. C. AND HURWITZ, T.: *Psychological disturbances associated with endocrine disease and hormone therapy. In* Sachar, E. J. (ed.): *Hormones, Behavior and Psychopathology.* Raven Press, New York, 1976, p. 125.

103. WOODBURY, D. M. AND VERNADAKIS, A.: *Influence of hormones on brain activity. In* Martini, L. and Ganong, W. F. (eds.): *Neuroendocrinology,* vol. 2. Academic Press, New York, 1967, p. 335.

104. ZIMMERMAN, E. A.: *Localization of hypothalamic hormones by immunocytochemical techniques. In* Martini, L. and Ganong, W. F. (eds.): *Frontiers in Neuroendocrinology,* vol. 4. Raven Press, New York, 1976, p. 25.

105. GOLDSTEIN, A.: *Opioid peptides (endorphins) in pituitary and brain.* Science 193:1081, 1976.

106. MARX, J. L.: *Neurobiology: Researchers high on endogenous opiates.* Science 193:1227, 1976.

107. SNYDER, S. H. AND MATTHYSSE, S.: *Opiate receptor mechanisms.* Neurosci. Res. Prog. Bull. 13:1, 1975.

BIBLIOGRAPHY

BROWN, G. M.: *Psychiatric and neurologic aspects of endocrine disease.* Hosp. Prac. 10:71, 1975.

FORD, D. H. (ED.): *Influence of Hormones on the Nervous System.* S. Karger, Basel, 1971.

LEVINE, S. (ED.): *Hormones and Behavior.* Academic Press, New York, 1972.

LISSAK, K. (ED.): *Hormones and Brain Function.* Plenum Press, New York, 1973.

MICHAEL, R. P. (ED.): *Endocrinology and Human Behavior.* Oxford University Press, New York, 1968.

MICHAEL, R. P. AND GIBBONS, J. L.: *Interrelationships between the endocrine system and neuropsychiatry.* Int. Rev. Neurobiol. 5:243, 1963.

PLUM, F. (ED.): *Brain Dysfunction in Metabolic Disorders,* vol. 53. Raven Press, New York, 1974.

REICHLIN, S.: *Neuroendocrinology. In* Williams, R. (ed.): *Textbook of Endocrinology.* W. B. Saunders, Philadelphia, 1974, p. 774.

RELKIN, R.: *Effect of endocrines on central nervous system.* N.Y. State J. Med. 69:2133, 1969.

SACHAR, E. J.: *Psychiatric disturbances associated with endocrine disorders. In* Reiser, M. (ed.): *American Handbook of Psychiatry,* vol. 4. Basic Books, New York, 1975, p. 299.

SACHAR, E. J.: *Psychiatric disturbances in endocrine disease: Some issues for research. In* Plum, F. (ed.): *Brain Dysfunction in Metabolic Disorders,* vol. 53. Raven Press, New York, 1974, p. 239.

SMITH, C. K., ET AL.: *Psychiatric disturbance in endocrinologic disease.* Psychosom. Med. 34:69, 1972.

WHYBROW, P. C. AND HURWITZ, T.: *Psychological disturbances associated with endocrine disease and hormone therapy. In* Sachar, E. J. (ed.): *Hormones, Behavior and Psychopathology.* Raven Press, New York, 1976, p. 102.

CHAPTER 13

Clinical Approach to Diagnosis of Hypothalamic-Pituitary Disease: Neurologic and Roentgenographic Aspects

In the evaluation of patients with suspected disturbance of the hypothalamus or pituitary, it is necessary to assess: 1) the local effects of compression, distortion, or destruction of neural structures, 2) the extent of hormonal disturbance, and 3) alterations in nonendocrine visceral and behavioral functions.[3] As in all clinical medicine, the major clues to the nature of the disorder come from a complete history, general physical examination, and neurologic examination including evaluation of mental status. It is particularly important to interview knowledgeable members of the patient's family or friends, because behavioral disturbance (including sexual dysfunction) is common in both pituitary and hypothalamic diseases and the patient may not be aware of these abnormalities or willing to discuss them. General physical examination is also important because a number of neuroendocrine diseases are manifestations of systemic disorders such as granuloma, diabetes, or malignancy. In this chapter, special aspects of the neurologic examination and of neuroradiologic approaches are reviewed. Hormonal evaluation methods will be discussed in Chapter 14.

SPECIAL ASPECTS OF MEDICAL HISTORY

Headache

Headache due to pituitary tumor is usually bitemporal or bifrontal and may be felt as a deep pain behind the eyes. Headache is thought to result from pressure effects on an intact diaphragma sellae; evidence in support of this is the finding that in some patients the headaches become less severe when the tumor grows into the suprasellar region. Pituitary tumors may be asymmetric and the headaches associated with pressure on the diaphragm may be unilateral. Direct pressure on the optic chiasm or tract may cause visual hallucinatory effects associated with "whiteness," "visual glow," "spots," or "a film of water." Formed images, so-called "peduncular hallucinosis," may occur when large tumors press on the brain stem. Nausea and vomiting, when present, should cause suspicion of increased intracranial pressure. These warning symptoms should not be confused with the pattern of aura, scotomata, pulsating headache, and nausea of classic migraine, which does not occur except by coincidence in pituitary-tumor patients. It should be recalled that migraine may be activated or accentuated by hormone therapy in a hypopituitary patient, or by administration of oral contraceptives to susceptible individuals. A colloid cyst of the third ventricle may cause repeated sudden-onset attacks of bitemporal headaches, which are often positional and associated with drop attacks. Papilledema is frequently present with symptomatic colloid cysts, but in the absence of increased intracranial pressure is not usually seen in hypothalamic or pituitary disease.

Libido

Disturbances of libido frequently occur in patients with tumor of the pituitary. Suppression of libido usually results from gonadal deficiency secondary to pituitary or hypothalamic disease. Elevation of prolactin is frequently associated with decreased sexual activity and with impotence (in men). Whether this is due to the associated gonad-hormone deficiency or to direct effects of prolactin on the brain is unknown, but treatment with bromergocryptine, a drug that lowers plasma prolactin, in some cases restores libido to normal.

Hypersexuality also has been reported in association with hypothalamic lesions. Males with precocious puberty may show precocious sexual interest and drive, but this is much less common than might be anticipated. Increased sexuality with aggressive sex drive has also been seen in the Kleine-Levin syndrome, thought to be an episodic hypothalamic disorder (see Chapter 11).

Sleep

Alterations in sleep which may occur with pituitary or hypothalamic disease (see Chapter 11) include hypersomnia, inability to sleep, and reversal of day-night rhythms. Somnolence is a common presenting complaint in hypothalamic tumors. Headaches or diabetes insipidus also may interfere with sleep.

SPECIAL DIAGNOSTIC METHODS

Vision and Visual-Field Evaluation

The boundaries of the sella turcica are contiguous with a number of neural structures whose functions must be assessed in suspected disorders of the hypothalamus and pituitary. Because the ventral hypothalamus and pituitary are so close to the optic nerves, optic chiasm, and optic tracts, careful testing of visual acuity and visual fields is an essential part of the clinical evaluation. Serial measurements help to follow progress of the clinical disturbance and of the effects of therapy. The state of visual function is also often crucial in determining the type and urgency of the therapy to be used. Lateral extension of pituitary tumors may compromise the function of the third, fourth, or sixth cranial nerves within the cavernous sinus, resulting in diplopia (Fig. 1). The ophthalmic division of the fifth cranial nerve also may be affected in the cavernous sinus, to diminish the corneal reflex or decrease facial sensation on the same side. Lateral involvement of the cranial nerves is much less frequent than is involvement of the visual system.

Initial assessment of visual fields by confrontation is relatively reliable provided certain precautions are followed. The use of finger movements is *not* adequate. A small, round object such as the head of a pin, measuring 2 to 3 mm. in diameter, is a satisfactory test object. The periphery of the visual fields can be compared with that of the examiner; a red object provides a more sensitive index of loss of vision within a portion of a field than does a white object. The size of the blind spot can be assessed by confrontation. It should be remembered in confrontation testing that the object must be placed equidistant between the examiner and the patient. Visual acuity can be assessed by the use of a Jaegher reading card or a miniaturized Snellen chart held at a prescribed dis-

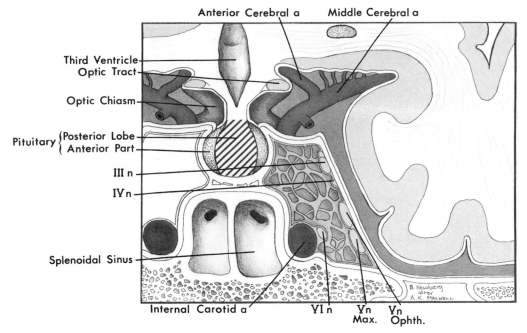

Figure 1. Diagramatic representation of the anatomic relations of the pituitary fossa and cavernous sinus. The lateral wall of the sella turcica is formed by the cavernous sinus. The sinus contains the carotid artery, two branches of the fifth cranial nerve (ophthalmic and maxillary), the III nerve (oculomotor), IV nerve (trochlear), and VI nerve (abducens). The optic chiasm and optic tract are located superior and lateral, respectively, to the pituitary. (Drawing by B. Newberg, modified from A. K. Maxwell in *Gray's Anatomy*, ed. 35. W. B. Saunders, Philadelphia, 1973.)

tance of 14 inches. In patients with glasses, visual acuity should be tested both with and without glasses.

Accurate assessment of visual fields, particularly in early cases of compression, requires evaluation by tangent screen and perimetry. The tangent screen permits identification of focal visual defects (scotomata) within the field of vision near the point of fixation. Perimetry is used to assess the peripheral fields of vision; with use of variable sizes and colors it is possible to construct an accurate contour of visual acuity at various angular distances from the central point of fixation (Fig. 2).

The particular pattern of visual symptoms produced by tumors of the hypothalamus and pituitary in an individual case depends on anatomic features such as the position of the chiasm in relation to the pituitary fossa, the configuration of the diaphragma sellae, and the size and rate of growth of the tumor.[13] The decussating fibers in the optic chiasm are arranged in well-defined laminae. Nasal retina fibers, which constitute approximately 50 to 60 per cent of the total retina fibers from one eye, cross over to join the temporal fibers of the opposite eye to form the optic tract. These fibers subserve vision in the temporal field. The ventral fibers, which subserve the upper temporal fields, are located in the anterior, inferior part of the chiasm; they form a short loop that extends into the optic nerve of the opposite side before passing backward to form the optic tract. The dorsal fibers, which subserve the lower temporal field, loop into the ipsilateral optic tract before crossing in the posterosuperior chiasm to form a portion of the contralateral optic tract. Fibers from the macular region of the retina occupy the posterior part of the chiasm.

The visual disturbance produced by a lesion in the parasellar region depends on the

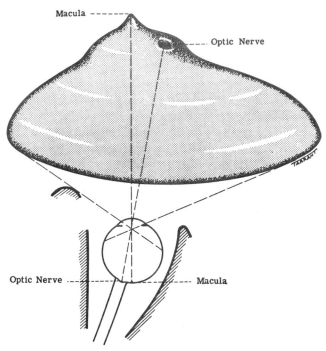

Figure 2. Diagram of island of vision subserved by one eye. The macular area is represented as the apex of the cone-shaped field of vision. The optic nerve head forms the blind spot. (From Holmes Sellors, P. J.: *Visual abnormalities in pituitary tumors. In* Jenkins, R. (ed.): *Pituitary Tumours.* Butterworth, London, 1973, with permission.)

part of the chiasm compressed. Midline pressure on the optic chiasm from below first affects the fibers subserving vision in the upper temporal field, leading to a characteristic bitemporal hemianopia (Fig. 3). However, because of the complex pattern of fiber crossover, visual defects are commonly asymmetric. With further chiasm compression, visual loss in the temporal field progresses circularly from the upper temporal to the lower temporal region. Complete bitemporal hemianopsia occurs with transection of the chiasm. Visual acuity is normal in bitemporal hemianopsia unless there is also involvement of the uncrossed fibers from the macular region of the same eye. Commonly, visual-field loss is greater in one eye, due to a predominantly lateral involvement of the chiasm as the tumor mass extends upward asymmetrically.

Lesions impinging on the posterior chiasm may result in bitemporal hemianopic scotomas due to macular-fiber involvement (Fig. 4). Visual acuity remains normal in such cases unless the adjacent optic nerve is also affected, resulting in disturbance of nasal macular fibers. Recent studies have emphasized that vascular impairment secondary to compression is the most important mechanism of the visual disturbance.

Chiasm lesions occasionally produce a central unilateral scotoma that may be confused with papillitis or retrobulbar neuritis. Papilledema rarely occurs and develops only when the tumor extends into the third ventricle and causes obstructive hydrocephalus and increased intracranial pressure. A large tumor that compresses one optic nerve and also causes increased intracranial pressure may result in pallor of the ipsilateral optic nerve associated with papilledema in the opposite eye (Foster-Kennedy syndrome).

The location of the chiasm in relation to the sella may be important in some cases in determining the extent of visual symptoms. In the majority of cases (approximately 75

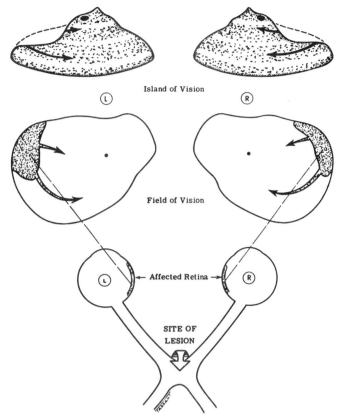

Island of Vision

Field of Vision

Affected Retina

SITE OF
LESION

Figure 3. Diagram of classic bitemporal hemianopia produced by a lesion impinging on the anterior optic chiasm. The field deficit is first evident in the superior temporal field and progresses inward and downward as indicated by the arrows. (From Holmes Sellors, P. J.: *Visual abnormalities in pituitary tumors. In* Jenkins, R. (ed.): *Pituitary Tumours.* Butterworth, London, 1973, with permission.)

per cent), the chiasm lies directly over the dorsum sella; in 15 to 20 per cent the chiasm lies more anteriorly over the tuberculum sellae (prefixed chiasm), and in a small number (less than 5 per cent) it is situated behind the dorsum sellae (postfixed).[4] The position of the chiasm also is important in the transfrontal surgical approach to the sellar region, as a prefixed chiasm limits visualization of the sellar region. The pituitary stalk is always posterior to the chiasm.

Loss of visual acuity accompanied by optic disk pallor, particularly in the temporal zone, is common in chiasm lesions. The pallor is due to decreased vascularity of the optic nerve head.

Tumors arising above the stalk lead initially to loss of acuity in the outer, lower quadrants of the visual field. Either suprasellar or infrasellar lesions may cause a combination of total blindness in one eye and an opposite temporal hemianopia.

In a series of 1,000 cases of pituitary adenomas reported by Hollenhorst and Younge[12] from the Mayo Clinic, 421 presented with visual complaints (Table 1). This was by far the commonest symptom associated with pituitary tumor. Diplopia was rare (seven cases) and other CNS signs and symptoms (seizures, dizziness, confusion, subarachnoid hemorrhage) occurred in 24. Diabetes insipidus was a symptom in 10 cases and CSF rhinorrhea in five. Headache and complaints referrable to acromegaly were less frequent than visual complaints.

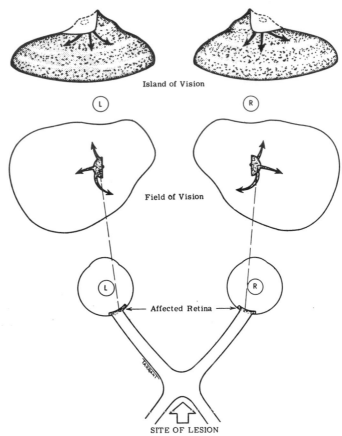

Figure 4. Diagram of visual field disorder produced by a lesion impinging on the posterior chiasm. Bitemporal hemianopic scotomas occur which progress laterally to further compromise the temporal fields. This disturbance is more common in the presence of a "prefixed" chiasm. (From Holmes Sellors, P. J.: *Visual abnormalities in pituitary tumors. In* Jenkins, R. (ed.): *Pituitary Tumours.* Butterworth, London, 1973, with permission.)

In this large series of cases, visual-field findings varied. Bitemporal hemianopsia was found in 300 cases of which half had acromegaly (Table 2). A superior bitemporal defect was present in an additional 101 cases; blindness in one eye with a temporal defect in the other occurred in 81 and a combined central and temporal hemianopic scotomas in 56. A homonymous hemianopia occurred in 42 patients (Fig. 5). Central scotomas, which are usually attributed to papillitis or retrobulbar neuritis, occurred in only eight patients. Of the total group, 70.1 per cent had defects in the visual fields. In this series, 228 patients were acromegalic.

Optic pallor correlated closely with loss of visual acuity and was present in 18 per cent of the total series. Papilledema occurred in only three patients, each of whom had large tumors invading the third or a lateral ventricle. Fifteen patients had significant hemorrhage into the tumor; these patients presented with severe headaches, acute visual loss, severe weakness, or endocrine symptoms (amenorrhea, acromegaly).

Symptoms of chiasm compression can occur with lesions located outside the pituitary fossa. Meningiomas of the tuberculum sellae or sphenoid wing, and suprasellar craniopharyngiomas may duplicate precisely the symptoms and signs of visual disturbance associated with an intrasellar pituitary adenoma. Classic symptoms of chiasm

310

Table 1. Presenting Complaints in 1,000 Cases of Pituitary Adenoma

Complaint		Cases
Visual disturbances		421
Headache		137
Acromegaly		136
Related to hypopituitarism		95
Amenorrhea		48
Diplopia		7
Others		156
Pain unrelated to tumor	44	
Cushing's syndrome	29	
CNS signs or symptoms*	24	
Diagnosis and treatment elsewhere	19	
Tumor found on routine physical	10	
Diabetes insipidus	10	
ENT	6	
CSF rhinorrhea	5	
Enlarged sella (noted elsewhere)	5	
Multiple adenomatosis	4	
Total		1000

*Syncope 5, seizures 5, dizziness 9, confusion 4, subarachnoid hemmorrhage 1.
(Adapted from Hollenhorst, R. W. and Younge, B. R.: *Ocular manifestations produced by adenomas of the pituitary gland: Analysis of 1000 cases. In:* Kohler P. O. and Ross, G. T. (eds.): *Diagnosis and Treatment of Pituitary Tumors.* Exerpta Medica, Amsterdam, 1973, p. 53.)

compression have also been described in the empty-sella syndrome in the absence of direct pressure from a tumor.[14] In such cases, chiasm damage occurs by herniation of the optic chiasm into the pituitary fossa; repeated pulsations of CSF or of adjacent arteries of the circle of Willis are believed to account for the progressive damage.

One of the hazards of transfrontal hypophysectomy is the possibility of damage to

Table 2. Defects in Visual Fields in 1,000 Cases of Pituitary Adenoma

Defect	Acromegaly	No Acromegaly	Total
None	144	155	299
Bitemporal hemianopia	28	272	300
Superior bitemporal defect	31	70	101
Blind (1 eye), temporal defect (other eye)	3	78	81
Central or temporal scotoma (1 eye), superior temporal scotoma (other eye)	3	53	56
Homonymous hemianopia	3	39	42
Central or temporal scotoma (both eyes)	4	23	27
Superior temporal defect (1 eye)	4	29	33
Temporal scotoma (1 eye)	1	11	12
Central scotoma (1 eye)	0	8	8
Inferior temporal defect (1 eye)	0	4	4
Arcuate scotoma (1 eye)	0	4	4
Inferior temporal defect (both eyes)	3	0	3
Arcuate scotoma (1 eye), temporal defect (other eye)	0	3	3
Miscellaneous	4	23	27
Total	228	772	1000

(Adapted from Hollenhorst, E. W. and Younge, B. R.: *Ocular manifestations produced by adenomas of the pituitary gland: Analysis of 1000 cases. In* Kohler, P. O. and Ross, G. T. (eds.): *Diagnosis and Treatment of Pituitary Tumors.* Exerpta Medica, Amsterdam, 1973, p. 53.)

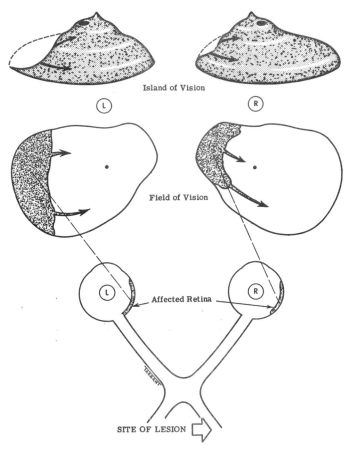

Figure 5. Diagram of homonymous hemianopia caused by a lateral lesion impinging on the optic tract posterior to the chiasm. The hemianopia begins laterally and progresses toward the central area of vision. (From Holmes Sellors, P. J.: *Visual abnormalities in pituitary tumors. In* Jenkins, R. (ed.): *Pituitary Tumours.* Butterworth, London, 1973, with permission.)

the optic nerves or chiasm at the time of surgical exploration. In general, these effects are due to interruption of the vascular supply to the chiasm, which is provided not by a single artery but by an arterial plexus derived from branches of the anterior cerebral, anterior communicating, internal carotid, hypophysial, and posterior communicating arteries.[1] The optic nerves are relatively resistant to radiation and rarely does loss of visual function occur as a complication of radiation to the pituitary or hypothalamic area.

Oculomotor Function

Ocular palsy occurs in 10 to 15 per cent of patients with large pituitary tumors.[5, 12] The third cranial nerve is most commonly involved, resulting in lid ptosis and weakness of adduction of the affected eye.[7] Pupillary involvement is unusual, the clinical presentation thus resembling that in third-nerve lesion of diabetes mellitus. The sixth cranial nerve is the second most frequently involved.

Smell

Assessment of olfaction is important because lesions in the region of the tuberculum sellae may compress the olfactory bulbs to cause unilateral or bilateral anosmia. Meningiomas in particular affect olfaction. Head trauma commonly disrupts the olfactory nerves at the level of the cribriform plate. Patients with congenital hypogonadism often have hyposmia or anosmia (Kallmann's syndrome).

Smell can be tested with a variety of common materials. Soap or tobacco can provide an initial screening. Each nostril should be tested separately, the patient being asked to close his eyes and to sniff two or three times, trying to identify the substance. If initial testing suggests a deficit, more careful testing is required using stronger scents such as oil of wintergreen, cloves, or strawberry extract. Irritative compounds such as ammonia and alcohol are to be avoided because they may stimulate receptors of the fifth cranial nerve to give a false-positive test. Henkin[11] has described more precise methods for testing olfaction; these are important in quantitation of abnormalities of smell such as occur in patients with thyroid or adrenal dysfunction.

Pineal Tumors

Tumors of the pineal or other structures in the posterior region of the third ventricle can result in distinctive clinical manifestations. Pressure on the posterior commissure and superior colliculi causes paralysis of conjugate upward gaze (Parinaud's syndrome), which may be associated with pupillary asymmetry and, rarely, with nystagmus retractorius, a condition in which the eyes move rhythmically inward and outward. Pupillary abnormalities with epithalmic lesions result from interruption of pretectal and posterior commissure connections to the oculomotor-nerve nucleus. These pathways subserve the light reflex (pupillary vasostriction). Argyll Robertson pupils (nonreactive to light but reactive to accommodation) may be present. Defects in downward gaze are rare and are associated with lesions of the midbrain tegmentum below the aqueduct, superior and medial to the red nucleus.

Compression of the aqueduct of Sylvius results in obstructive hydrocephalus, headaches, vomiting, and papilledema. Pressure on the upper brain stem in advanced cases can result in cerebellar ataxia, pyramidal-tract signs (weakness, spasticity, and extensor plantar responses) and coma.

Other Neurologic Manifestations

Lateral extension of pituitary tumors into the medial part of the temporal lobe may result in seizures, often with gustatory or olfactory auras. Lateral extension into the internal capsule may result in hemiplegia. Hypothalamic lesions may cause disorders of temperature regulation, emotionality, thirst, appetite, or level of consciousness (for detailed discussion see Chapters 4 and 11).

RADIOLOGIC ASSESSMENT

Radiologic assessment of the skull is important in all patients with suspected hypothalamic-pituitary disorders, unexplained visual disturbance, optic atrophy, or diplopia.[16, 17] Anteroposterior and lateral views of the skull should be screened for evidence of calcification, increased intracranial pressure, and focal erosions in the region of the sella turcica. Views of the optic canal are important if glioma of the optic nerve is considered. Complete examination of the sella turcica, particularly in suspected microadenomata of the pituitary, requires tomography even if the initial skull roentgenograms appear normal.

Sella Turcica

The normal sella turcica, as seen on lateral projection, consists of the posterior part of the planum sphenoidale, the tuberculum sellae, the anterior clinoid processes, the floor, and the dorsum sellae; the latter includes the posterior clinoid processes and the adjacent part of the sphenoid and occipital bone that form the clivus (Fig. 6)[5]

Size

There are three normal variations in the shape of the sella; oval, round, and flat. A small sella turcica has no particular significance, although long-standing pituitary insufficiency may occasionally result in a small fossa. Enlargement of the sella is an important finding and requires careful delineation of the cause.[16] The anteroposterior diameter of the sella, determined by measuring the maximum distance from the anterior concavity of the sella to the anterior rim of the dorsum sellae, varies from 5 to 16 mm. with an average of 10.5 mm. The depth of the pituitary fossa is measured as the greatest distance from the floor to a perpendicular line drawn between the tuberculum sellae and the top of the dorsum sellae. The upper limit is usually stated as 13 mm. The width of the sella is determined in films taken in an anteroposterior projection by calculating the distance across the floor of the sella, which can be seen as a thin, horizontal plate of bone approximately 1 cm. below the anterior clinoid processes. The normal width varies from 10 to 15 mm. Mahmoud,[15] in a series of 100 normal sellae, calculated the area of the sella by planimetry as visualized on lateral projection. The range was 22 to 130 mm.[2] In 45 of 49 patients with pituitary tumors, the area was 130 to 823 mm.[2]; four patients had sellae measurements slightly below 130 mm.[2]

The volume of the sella can be calculated using a formula derived by Di Chiro and Nelson.[9, 10] Anteroposterior, depth, and width measurements are multiplied, and then divided by two. The volume of the sella was considered to be abnormal when it exceeded 1092 mm.[3]; the mean volume was 594 mm.[3] In practice there is considerable variation and one cannot always decide with certainty whether a particular sella is enlarged or not.[2] In general, changes in contour or asymmetry, demineralization, and local erosions or resorption are more reliable indicators of intrasellar disease.

Calcification

Calcification of sellar or extrasellar contents may occur normally, particularly in an elderly subject. A curved arch of calcification evident in the center of the sella on lateral view is often due to calcification in the internal carotid artery (Fig. 7). A line of calcification extending posterolaterally from the dorsum sella is a normal finding, the consequence of calcification in the petroclinoid ligaments (Fig. 8). Occasionally, one may see bridging of the anterior and posterior clinoid processes by a linear line of calcification along the intraclinoid ligaments. Craniopharyngiomas (60 to 70 per cent) and meningiomas (30 per cent) are commonly calcified; pituitary adenomas, almost never (less than 5 per cent).

Causes of Enlargement

The sella may be enlarged secondary to increased pituitary size, increased intracranial pressure, defective diaphragm (empty sella), or erosion caused by extracellular struc-

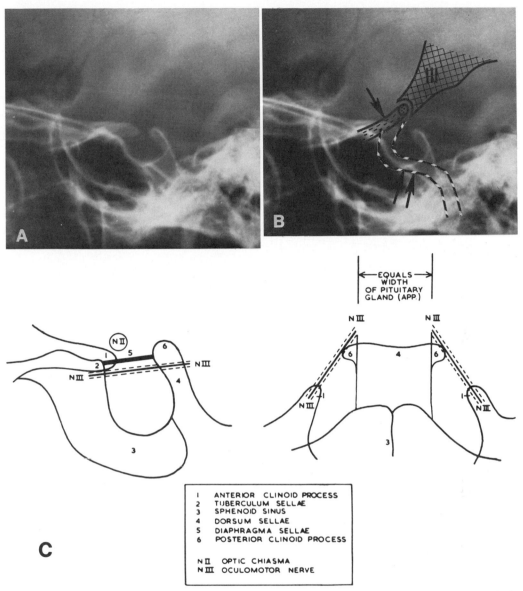

Figure 6. *A,* Radiologic view of the normal sella in lateral projection. *B,* Lateral view of the sella turcica indicating carotid artery *(double arrows),* optic nerve *(single arrow),* and anterior third ventricle *(III). C,* Diagram of relations of the pituitary gland and radiologic landmarks of the sella turcica. (From Bloch, H. J. and Joplin, G. F.: *Some aspects of the radiological anatomy of the pituitary gland and its relationship to surrounding structures.* Br. J. Radiol. 32:531, 1959, with permission.)

tures.[16, 17] Long-standing hypothyroidism also can cause enlargement of the pituitary fossa due to secondary pituitary enlargement. Common intrasellar lesions are pituitary adenomas, craniopharyngiomas, and pituitary cysts. Rarely, tumors of the nasopharynx extend superiorly into the sella. Parasellar lesions may mimic intrasellar tumors and therefore must be considered in the differential diagnosis. Aneurysms of the internal carotid artery arising in the cavernous sinus or at the origin of the anterior cerebral artery may cause lateral erosion and enlargement of the sella turcica.[6, 7] Radiologic find-

315

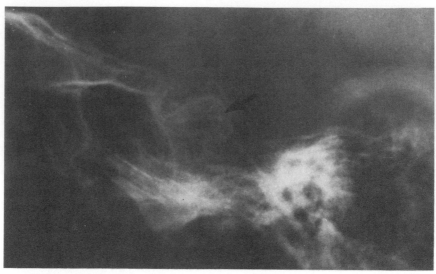

Figure 7. Calcification of an intracavernous portion of the internal carotid artery *(arrow)*. The artery is tortuous and displaced upwards.

ings in this condition may resemble in every respect an enlarging asymmetric pituitary tumor and can be distinguished only by carotid angiography.

Increased intracranial pressure, particularly when accompanied by dilatation of the third ventricle, may rarely lead to sellar enlargement. Such enlargement more commonly occurs without increased intracranial pressure; it results from extension of the subarachnoid space through a defective diaphragma sellae (empty-sella syndrome). It is believed that continued pulsations within the subarachnoid space transmit hydraulic forces which remodel the bone and eventually enlarge the sella. Although the pituitary

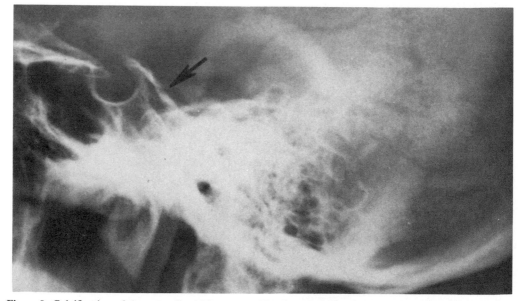

Figure 8. Calcification of the petroclinoid ligaments. The linear calcification is evident posterior to the sella turcica.

Table 3. Common Tumors of the Sellar Region

Intrasellar tumors	*Anterior suprasellar tumors*
Adenomas	Meningiomas
Craniopharyngiomas	Optic gliomas
Meningioma	*Posterior suprasellar tumors*
Pituitary cyst	Adenoma
Glioma	Meningioma
Suprasellar tumors	Craniopharyngioma
Adenomas	Chordomas
Craniopharyngioma	Epidermoid cysts
Ependymoma	*Intraventricular tumors*
Hamartoma—infundiboloma	Colloid cyst
Glioma	Arachnoid cyst
Teratoma—germinoma, ectopic pinealoma	Papilloma
Meningioma	Astrocytoma
Arachnoid cysts	Craniopharyngioma

is compressed into a rim of tissue around the wall of the sella, function usually remains surprisingly normal (see Chapter 15). By conventional roentgenography, one cannot distinguish an enlarged sella turcica due to an intrasellar lesion from an empty-sella syndrome. This differentiation can only be made definitively with pneumoencephalography. During pneumonencephalography, it is essential to position the head so that air can enter the cavity in the pituitary fossa through the diaphragma sellae. The usefulness of computed axial tomography (CAT scan) is under study. In many cases, the CAT scan is diagnostic, but we have seen several cases in which the CAT scan failed to detect the empty sella. Empty sella in association with benign intracranial hypertension has been reported. Rarely, intrasellar extension of a suprasellar or tuberculum sellae meningioma may give the appearance of an enlarged pituitary fossa. Common tumors of the sellar and parasellar region are summarized in Table 3.

Intrasellar tumors typically produce an asymmetric ballooning of the sella, with undercutting of the clinoid processes either anteriorly or posteriorly (Fig. 9).[15, 18] Mi-

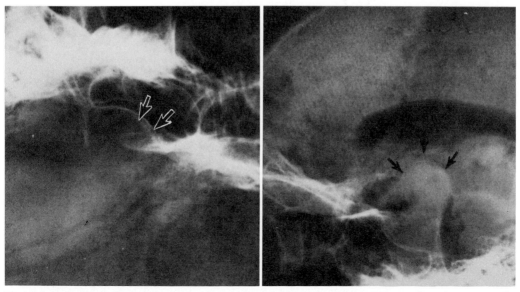

Figure 9. *Left,* Asymmetric enlargement of the sella turcica produced by a GH-secreting adenoma. *Right,* Pneumoencephalogram shows suprasellar extent of tumor *(arrows).*

croadenomas may cause asymmetric focal erosion of the floor of the sella, which may be evident only on lateral or anteroposterior tomography. With experience gained from transsphenoidal surgery, it is now evident that microadenomas as small as 3 to 5 mm. in diameter can cause erosion of the floor. This sign is of particular importance in the diagnosis of prolactin-secreting microadenomata.

Radiologic Signs of Increased Intracranial Pressure

The earliest detectable radiologic sign of increased intracranial pressure is erosion of the anterior aspect of the dorsum sellae; the cortical bone on the inside of the fossa becomes thin and indistinct. This is followed by atrophy of the superior margins of the posterior clinoid processes. Long-standing increases in intracranial pressure result in complete loss of the tips of the posterior clinoids. By this time, changes are also usually evident in the floor of the fossa, with thinning of the cortical bone; this is followed by enlargement of the pituitary fossa. Eventually, changes can occur also in the anterior clinoid processes.

Brain Scan

The radioisotope brain scan has only limited value in the assessment of suprasellar or hypothalamic lesions.[8] Poor contrast results from uptake of isotope by the temporal muscles on lateral view, and by the proximity of the sella to other bones at the base of the skull. The brain scan is not generally useful in detection of small suprasellar extensions of pituitary adenomas; only tumors extending well above the sella can be detected reliably. Radioactive 99m technetium is the isotope most commonly used, at the recommended dose of approximately 8 to 10 mCi. The half-life of the isotope is 6 hours; as a result, the total dose of body radioactivity is very small (less than 0.13 rad per 10 mCi IV dose). The radioisotope brain scan provides a simple, safe, noninvasive preliminary screening test. Suprasellar chromophobe adenomas (Fig. 10), craniopharyngiomas, meningiomas, and teratomas can often be visualized on brain scan. The scan is of little use for detection of aneurysms of the internal carotid or circle of Willis. The brain scan is commonly positive with tumors in the pineal region.

LUMBAR PUNCTURE

Evaluation of the cerebrospinal fluid is important for exclusion of granulomas or meningeal infection in cases of diabetes insipidus, or where a subarachnoid hemorrhage

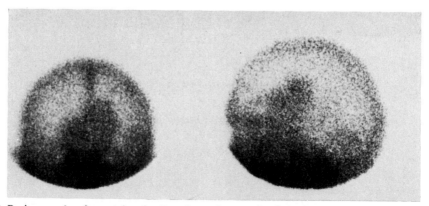

Figure 10. Brain scan showing uptake of radioactive technetium in a large suprasellar chromophobe adenoma.

318

must be excluded. In diabetes insipidus, elevated protein or increased cells in the CSF may provide clues to the diagnosis of sarcoidosis, histiocytosis, or malignancy. The CSF sugar is usually reduced in CNS sarcoidosis and in meningeal carcinomatosis. In patients with suspected pituitary apoplexy, the examination of the CSF may be necessary to differentiate subarachnoid hemorrhage, as signs and symptoms of the two conditions may be confused. In subarachnoid hemorrhage, the CSF is usually grossly bloody with a xanthrochromic supernatant, whereas in pituitary apoplexy, red cells may be present, but rarely in sufficient numbers to give evidence of gross bleeding.

It has been suggested that measurement of anterior pituitary hormones in spinal fluid may detect suprasellar extension of pituitary tumors. ACTH and growth hormone have been reported with suprasellar extension. This is not now a standard procedure, but is under investigation in several centers.

Lumbar puncture should never be performed when increased intracranial pressure is suspected or when papilledema is present. It is also unwise to perform lumbar puncture if obstructive hydrocephalus may be present. In such cases the patient should be investigated first with CAT scan, echoencephalography, or carotid angiography and, where indicated, by ventriculography.

ECHOENCEPHALOGRAPHY

The echoencephalogram is a useful noninvasive technique for detection of ventricular dilatation or midline shift of the ventricular system. It cannot be used reliably to outline a mass, although techniques for this type of investigation are being improved rapidly.

COMPUTED AXIAL TOMOGRAPHY (CAT SCAN)

The CAT scan, in some cases, can demonstrate an empty sella, and visualizes suprasellar extension if the lesion is more than 1 cm. above the sella turcica. It accurately displays cerebroventricular dilatation. Hypothalamic and other tumor masses are well visualized. Cystic craniopharyngiomas located above the sella usually can be visualized also.

ELECTROENCEPHALOGRAPHY

Information gained from EEG evaluation in patients with basilar lesions of the hypothalamus or midbrain is of limited value. In cases of akinetic mutism or of the "locked-in" syndrome, the EEG may be important because it can demonstrate normal alpha activity and indicate that the patient may not be unconscious.

Patients with "diencephalic epilepsy" may have normal EEGs. The pathophysiology of this disorder is not known.

PNEUMOENCEPHALOGRAPHY AND VENTRICULOGRAPHY

Pneumoencephalography is performed by introduction of air into the lumbar subarachnoid space via a lumbar-puncture needle. The test is important to demonstrate suprasellar extension of the pituitary tumor, to exclude an empty sella (Fig. 11) as a cause of enlargement of the pituitary fossa, and to determine displacement of the third and fourth ventricles due to lesions of the hypothalamus or pineal. Pneumoencephalography is contraindicated when papilledema is present.

Ventriculography, a neurosurgical procedure, is performed when there is hydrocephalus or evidence of increased intracranial pressure. Pneumography is generally required

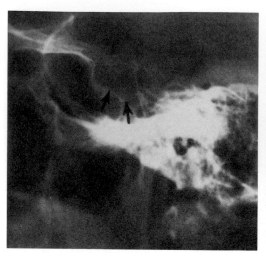 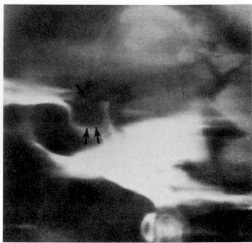

Figure 11. *Left,* Empty-sella in a patient with enlarged pituitary fossa. Arrows indicate double floor of sella. *Right,* Air is evident within the sella turcica on pneumoencephalogram and the pituitary gland is compressed to the wall of the fossa.

before a surgical approach to the pituitary is undertaken, whether by a transfrontal or transsphenoidal approach.[3, 8] Pneumography not only permits accurate visualization of the tumor but may also provide important information concerning the anatomic relationships of structures in the suprasellar region. In the case of transsphenoidal microsurgery, pneumoencephalography is necessary in most cases to provide a clear delineation of the extent of suprasellar tumor, and to detect an empty sella. Transsphenoidal surgery in the latter case may lead to a persistent CSF fistula.

CEREBRAL ANGIOGRAPHY

Cerebral angiography of the internal carotid artery and its branches and of the vertebrobasilar system is done either by direct puncture of the vessels or by selective catheterization by the femoral-aortic route. Angiography carries a 2 to 5 per cent risk of morbidity associated with transient or permanent neurologic deficit or vascular occlusion. This hazard is substantially increased in elderly patients, in severe atherosclerosis, in diabetes, and in hypertension. Although increasing use of CAT scans has greatly reduced the need for angiography, its use is still advocated to exclude a parasellar or suprasellar aneurysm as a cause of radiographic changes in the sella or parasellar region; to outline cerebral vessels, in particular the internal carotid and its branches that form the anterior circle of Willis in cases where surgery is envisioned; and to demonstrate lateral displacement of the carotid within the cavernous sinus, since this region cannot be adequately visualized by the CAT scan.[1, 3] Because of the risk of hemorrhage from an unsuspected aneurysm, angiography is considered by most neurosurgeons to be mandatory when direct surgical intervention is planned, whether by the transfrontal or transsphenoidal route.

CAVERNOUS SINUS VENOGRAPHY

Radiologic visualization of the cavernous sinus is possible by cannulation of a superficial facial vein and retrograde injection through the venous plexus of the posterior orbit. This technique, although not widely used, is useful in proving lateral extension of pituitary tumors. It is commonly performed where stereotactic thermal or proton-beam ablation of the pituitary gland is planned.

REFERENCES

1. BAKER, H. L., JR.: *The angiographic delineation of sellar and parasellar masses.* Radiology 104:67, 1972.

2. BATZDORF, U. AND STERN, W. E.: *Clinical manifestations of pituitary adenomas: A pilot study using computer analysis. In* Kohler, P. O. and Ross, G. T. (eds.): *Diagnosis and Treatment of Pituitary Tumors.* Excerpta Medica, Amsterdam, 1973, p. 17.

3. BENTSON, J. R.: *Relative merits of pneumographic and angiographic procedures in the management of pituitary tumors. In* Kohler, P. O. and Ross, G. T. (eds.): *Diagnosis and Treatment of Pituitary Tumors.* Excerpta Medica, Amsterdam, 1973, p. 83.

4. BERGLAND, R. M., ET AL.: *Anatomical variations in the pituitary gland and adjacent structures in 225 human autopsy cases.* J. Neurosurg. 28:93, 1968.

5. BLOCH, H. J. AND JOPLIN, G. F.: *Some aspects of the radiological anatomy of the pituitary gland and its relationship to surrounding structures.* Br. J. Radiol. 32:527, 1959.

6. BULL, J. W. D. AND SCHUNK, H.: *The significance of displacement of the cavernous portion of the internal carotid artery.* Br. J. Radiol. 35:801, 1962.

7. COGAN, D. G.: *Neurology of the Visual System.* Charles C Thomas, Springfield, 1966.

8. DECK, M. D. F.: *Radiographic and radioisotopic techniques in diagnosis of pituitary tumors. In* Kohler, P. O. and Ross, G. T. (eds.): *Diagnosis and Treatment of Pituitary Tumors.* Excerpta Medica, Amsterdam, 1973, p. 71.

9. DI CHIRO, G.: *The width (third dimension) of the sella turcica.* Am. J. Roentgenol. 84:26, 1960.

10. DI CHIRO, G. AND NELSON, K. B.: *The volume of the sella turcica.* Am. J. Roentgenol. 87:989, 1962.

11. HENKIN, R. J.: *The neuroendocrine control of perception. In* Hamburg, D. (ed.): *Perception and Its Disorders,* vol. 48. Williams & Wilkins, Baltimore, 1970, p. 54.

12. HOLLENHORST, R. W. AND YOUNGE, B. R.: *Ocular manifestations produced by adenomas of the pituitary gland: Analysis of 1000 cases. In* Kohler, P. O. and Ross, G. T. (eds.): *Diagnosis and Treatment of Pituitary Tumors.* Excerpta Medica, Amsterdam, 1973, p. 53.

13. HOLMES SELLORS, P. J.: *Visual abnormalities in pituitary tumors. In* Jenkins, J. S. (ed.): *Pituitary Tumors.* Butterworth, Boston, 1972, p. 106.

14. KAUFMAN, B., ET AL.: *Radiographic features of intrasellar masses and progressive, asymmetrical nontumorous enlargements of the sella turcica, the "empty" sella. In* Kohler, P. O. and Ross, G. T. (eds.): *Diagnosis and Treatment of Pituitary Tumors.* Excerpta Medica, Amsterdam, 1973, p. 100.

15. MAHOMOUD, M. S.: *The sella in health and disease: Value of the radiographic study of the sella turcica in morbid anatomical and topographic diagnosis of intracranial tumors.* Br. J. Radiol. Suppl. 8:1, 1958.

16. MCLACHLAN, M. S. F., ET AL.: *Estimation of pituitary gland dimensions from radiographs of the sella turcica; a post-mortem study.* Br. J. Radiol. 41:323, 1968.

17. MCLACHLAN, M. S. F., ET AL.: *Applied anatomy of the pituitary gland and fossa; a radiological and histopathological study based on 50 necropsies.* Br. J. Radiol. 41:782, 1968.

18. ROSS, R. J. AND GREITZ, T. V. B.: *Changes of the sella turcica in chromophobe adenomas and eosinophilic adenomas.* Radiology 86:892, 1966.

CHAPTER 14

Clinical Approach to Diagnosis of Hypothalamic-Pituitary Disease: Endocrinologic Aspects

Knowledge of the physiologic control of pituitary secretion has led to the development of newer, more specific tests of pituitary secretory reserve; the introduction of three of the hypothalamic hypophysiotrophic hormones (TRH, LHRH, and somatostatin) into clinical medicine has made it possible to assess directly the functional capacity of the pituitary gland. These developments have depended on the use of radioimmunoassay which has made it possible to assess the secretion of each of the known hormones of the pituitary by direct measurement in plasma. These advances have both increased the accuracy of diagnosis and made it more complex.

RADIOIMMUNOASSAY

This technique has so revolutionized the diagnostic resources of the clinical neuroendocrinologist that it merits brief outline of the principles involved.[22, 24, 31] Before 1960, it was difficult or impossible to determine the concentration of most protein hormones in blood, except in cases of marked elevation. Also, it was not clearly understood that the secretions of the pituitary, as a general rule, varied from time to time during the day, and that in most instances secretion was episodic or pulsatile. The bioassays then in use were laborious, required large volumes of plasma (and hence could not detect short-term alterations), and were not adequately specific. Radioimmunoassay (RIA) was developed by a number of workers among whom Berson and Yalow, Ekins, Greenwood and Hunter, Talmadge and Skom, Daughaday, and Utiger gave early impetus to the field.[3, 11, 16, 24] First applied to the assay of insulin by Berson and Yalow, the method was soon adapted to measurement of GH,[12] LH, TSH, and other peptides.[8] By means of haptene-coupling methods, small-molecular-weight hormones such as the thyroid hormones T_3 and T_4, and the steroid hormones cortisol, estradiol, progesterone, testosterone, aldosterone and ADH have been rendered antigenic so that specific antibodies can be developed.[2, 4, 5-7, 26, 27, 32] More recently, immunoassays for the hypothalamic hormones TRH, LHRH, and somatostatin have been introduced into clinical investigation.[1, 13] The RIA technique has led to methods for measurement of drugs such as digoxin, morphine, and marijuana derivatives, and a number of enzymes. A list of substances that can be measured by RIA is presented in Table 1.

The underlying principles of RIA are not complex (Fig. 1). The basis of the assay procedure is the competition for binding between specific antibody on the one hand with isotopically labeled antigen (Ag*) and unlabeled antigen (Ag) on the other. In the presence of large amounts of unlabeled ("cold") Ag, the amount of Ag* bound to anti-

Table 1. Substances That Can Be Measured by Radioimmunoassay

Protein and Polypeptide Hormones	Pharmacologically-Active Substances
Anterior pituitary hormones	*Drugs*
GH	Cardiac glycosides
FSH	Morphine
	LSD
	Canabis
	Anticonvulsants
ACTH	*Miscellaneous*
α-MSH	Prostaglandins
β-MSH	Vitamins
Hypothalamic hormones	
TRH	*Hematologic Substances*
LHRH	Fibrinogen
Somatostatin	Plasminogen
Posterior pituitary hormones	Antihemophilic factor
Vasopressin	Vitamin B_{12}
Oxytocin	Folic acid
Neurophysin	Australia antigen
Other peptide hormones	Erythropoietin
Glucagon	
Insulin	*Viruses*
Pro insulin	
Parathormone	*Cyclic Nucleotides*
Gastrin	3′,5′-cyclic AMP
Secretin	3′,5′-cyclic GMP
Human placental lactogen	
Human chorionic gonadotropin	*Enzymes*
Renin	Dopamine β-hydroxylase
Angiotensin	Creatinine phosphokinase
Calcitonin	
Bradykinin	*Tumor-Associated Antigens*
	Carcinoembryonic antigen
Nonpeptide Hormones	α-feto protein
Thyroxinc	
Triiodothyronine	
Testosterone	
Progesterone	
Aldosterone	
Cortisol	
Dihydrotestosterone	
Estrone	
Estradiol	
Melatonin	

body is reduced or abolished by displacement. In the absence of cold Ag, most of the labeled compound will be bound by the antibody. Standard displacement curves are derived using known concentrations of the Ag (usually a hormone) (Fig. 2). The amount of displacement produced by an unknown concentration of hormone can then be measured, and its equivilance in hormonal units determined. For practical reasons, a number of technical aspects of the assay must be considered. The concentration of Ag* and antibody are carefully adjusted to give optimum binding, within the range of the expected hormone levels. Sometimes the assay must be repeated because values fall outside the displacement curve. The antibodies must be specific, and the Ag* virtually pure. Interfering substances in the samples being examined must be excluded.

Although RIA has provided a powerful tool for measurement of substances that exist in low concentrations in plasma, the methods require considerable care for routine use and present several problems that need to be recognized and understood.

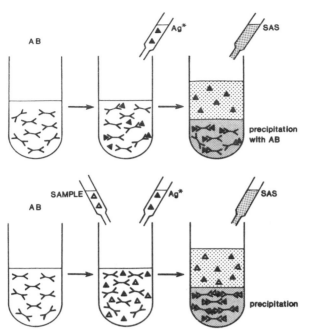

Figure 1. Diagram of principles of radioimmunoassay. Upper part shows addition of Ag* to antibody (AB) and precipitation of the labeled hormone with saturated ammonium sulfate (SAS). In lower part, addition of unknown sample results in competition with Ag* for AB. The reduction in Ag* bound to AB results in fewer counts in precipitate.

It must be emphasized that RIA measures immunologic and not biologic activity. This is particularly important with respect to polypeptide and protein hormones. Repeated injections of a hormone during the immunization procedure can result in formation of multiple antibodies that may combine with any of several immunologically active sites on the hormone molecule. It is increasingly recognized that full biologic activity may reside in only a small portion of the polypeptide. Since fragments of the hormone may also circulate, the immunologic components measured by RIA may have little or no biologic activity and may not accurately reflect the actual biologic activity of the substance.

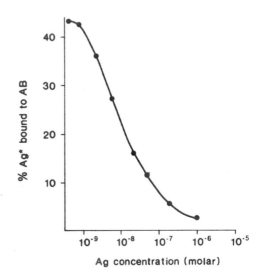

Figure 2. Standard displacement curve used in radioimmunoassay. Increased concentrations of unlabeled antigen (abcissa) result in decreased binding of labeled antigen (Ag*) to antibody. The curve is approximately linear when plotted against log dose of antigen.

325

RIA determinations, while permitting measurement of substances in the picomole range, still suffer from some technical problems. Even well-established assays can produce rather disturbing day-to-day variations in results. It is therefore important that appropriate controls be used to establish the extent of such interassay and intra-assay variation.

Nonspecific interference with the RIA by materials in serum or plasma may give rise to special problems. Interference by anticoagulants, the presence of normal serum proteins, and various inhibitors of the antibody-antigen reaction found in the blood may result in difficulties in measurement of a given substance. In many instances, a hormone or other substance is easily determined in tissue extracts, but reliable determination in blood may be troublesome and difficult. This has been particularly true, for example, in the radioimmunoassay for ACTH, and for the hypothalamic hormones TRH, LHRH, and somatostatin.

Blood Samples for Hormone Assays

The pituitary hormones GH, prolactin, TSH, LH, and FSH are usually assayed in serum (clotted blood). The assay for ACTH requires special care and handling of blood collections because it binds to glass surfaces. Analysis of steroid hormones (cortisol, estrogen, progesterone, and testosterone) is usually performed on heparinized samples. In general, all samples should be taken in the fasting state.

The tubes should be carefully labeled with the patient's name and sample time. Most hormones are stable in whole blood for several hours at 0° to 4° C, but longer delays in separation of serum or plasma should be avoided. Serum or plasma may be stored frozen at −20° C for many months.

TESTING OF SPECIFIC HORMONE SECRETION

One need not carry out all possible endocrine evaluation tests, and clinics differ in the emphasis placed on one or another of these. A distinction also should be made between tests needed for precise diagnosis and the determination of therapy, and those that are primarily investigative. The tests commonly used for diagnosis on our services are summarized in Table 2. A form for recording results of pituitary evaluation as developed by Jackson and Canalis is shown in Fig. 3.

Growth Hormone

Normal basal serum levels of GH (in the early morning, at rest) rarely exceed 5 ng./ml. and are usually less than 2 ng./ml., even in the normal subject. Spontaneous bursts of GH release may occur at any time and can result in values as high as 20 to 30 ng./ml. The emotional stress of venipuncture also can raise GH levels in normal persons. Plasma levels of GH are elevated (over 10 ng./ml.) in infants during the first few weeks of life, with values as high as 30 to 50 ng./ml. During the early part of nocturnal sleep, especially in adolescents, GH values may rise to 20–50 ng./ml.

It is important to determine the status of GH secretion in cases with suspected pituitary deficiency and in cases with suspected GH excess. The strategies of differential diagnosis of these two conditions differ. To determine GH insufficiency, it is necessary to provoke stimulation, and in the case of hypersecretion, to determine whether physiologic stimuli can suppress the elevated GH levels.[23] Because random values in normal persons may fall into the "hypopituitary" or the "acromegalic" range, it is necessary to carry out standard provocation tests.

Growth Hormone Secretory Reserve Tests

It is often most convenient, especially in children seen as outpatients, to carry out provocative screening tests. The easiest of these is the exercise test, consisting of 15

Table 2. Recommended Routine Studies for Evaluation of Endocrine Disturbances in Hypothalamic-Pituitary Disease

Acromegaly or Gigantism

1. Plasma GH levels at rest in fasting state on three occasions.
2. Three-hour glucose tolerance test with GH and glucose samples taken at 0, 15, 30, 60, and 120 minutes.
3. Evaluation of other pituitary hormones.
   a. ACTH-adrenal function
      1. Diurnal cortisol rhythm (8 A.M., 4 P.M.).
      2. ACTH reserve (either insulin tolerance or oral metyrapone test).
   b. Pituitary-thyroid
      1. Plasma TSH, thyroxine (T_4) and triiodothyronine (T_3).
   c. Prolactin
      1. Random serum sample at rest in fasting state.
   d. Gonadotropin
      1. Plasma testosterone or estradiol.
      2. LH and FSH.
      3. If above are abnormal, LHRH test (if available).
   e. ADH
      1. If urine volume less than 2,000 ml./day and urine gravity of 1.012 or more in overnight specimen, no further tests are indicated.

Galactorrhea or Hyperprolactinemia

1. Prolactin
   a. Three random samples at rest in fasting state.
   b. If prolactin values over 100 ng./ml., L-dopa administration, 500 mg. p.o. Plasma samples removed for prolactin determination at 0, 30, 60, and 120 minutes. Bromergocryptine 1.0 or 2.5 mg. p.o. Plasma samples at 0, 60, and 120 minutes. TRH test, 400 μg. IV.
2. Growth hormone
   a. One random sample at rest in fasting state.
   b. GH secretory reserve (either usually hypoglycemia or L-dopa, see below).
3. ACTH-adrenal
   a. Diurnal cortisol rhythm.
   b. ACTH reserve.
4. Pituitary-thyroid
   a. Plasma TSH, T_4, and T_3.
5. Gonadotrophins
   a. Plasma testosterone or estradiol.
   b. LH and FSH.
   c. LHRH Test.
6. ADH
   a. If urine volume less than 2,000 ml./day, or first A.M. urine specimen with specific gravity 1.012 or more, no further test indicated.

Panhypopituitarism

1. Growth hormone
   a. Insulin tolerance test (0.05 U./kg. b.w.). Blood sugar must be reduced to 40 mg./100 ml. or 50% of initial blood sugar or less. Blood samples taken for GH and glucose at 0, 20, 40, and 60 minutes. Test terminated with IV glucose, 10 gm.
   Test contraindicated in older individuals, those with heart disease or long-standing hypothyroidism. Patient must be observed to avoid serious problems. If IV insulin test is not feasible, recommend L-dopa test.
   b. L-dopa test, 500 mg. p.o. Blood samples taken for GH assay at 0, 15, 30, and 60 minutes.
2. Prolactin
   a. A.M. sample in resting state.
   b. TRH, 500 μg. IV. Blood samples taken at 0, 15, 30, 60, and 90 minutes. Samples at 0 and 30 minutes are usually sufficient.
3. ACTH-adrenal
   a. Diurnal cortisol rhythm.
   b. ACTH reserve test either IV insulin or metyrapone.
4. Pituitary-thyroid
   a. Plasma TSH, T_4, and T_3.
   b. TRH test, 500 μg. IV. Blood samples at 0, 15, 30, 60, and 90 minutes. A sample at 0 and 30 minutes is usually sufficient, but in differentiating hypothalamic and pituitary abnormality may require more samples.
5. Gonadotrophins
   a. Plasma testosterone or estradiol.
   b. Serum LH and FSH.
   c. LHRH test, 100 μg, IV or SC. Samples drawn for LH (FSH is optional) at 0, 15, 30, and 60 minutes.

PITUITARY WORKUP SHEET

NEW ENGLAND MEDICAL CENTER HOSPITAL

Name _____ NEMCH# _____

Age _____ Sex _____ Diagnosis _____ Drugs _____

HGH and Prolactin

Time	ITT Gluc	Cort-isol	GH	Prol	L Dopa GH	L Dopa Prol	Thorazine GH	Thorazine Prol	H₂0 Load Prol	H₂0 Load Osm.
0										
15										
30										
60										
90										
120										
180										
240										

****

TRH Test **T4I** **T3 Resin** **LRH Test** **Other**

Time	TSH	T3	Prol	GH	LH	FSH	GH
0							
15							
30							
60							
90							
120							
150							

****

GTT **Cortisol Cortrosyn Test** **DR**

Time	Gluc	GH	Ins	Glucag
0				
30				
60				
90				
120				
180				
240				
300				

0	30	60	PM	AM

Figure 3. Form for recording results in hypothalamic-pituitary tests (based on record used at New England Medical Center, courtesy of I. M. D. Jackson and E. Canalis).

minutes of rapid stair-climbing or the Bovril test (an oral amino acid mixture). Blood is taken at the completion of the exercise or 15 to 30 minutes after taking the Bovril. An increase in GH of 5 ng./ml. or more constitutes a normal secretory reserve and unless the index of suspicion of GH deficiency is very high, most endocrinologists do not proceed further. About 25 per cent of normal persons (including children) do not respond to these stimuli and require further testing. Hypogonadism (whether primary, acquired, or associated with the normal preadolescent state) impairs the GH response to these and other provocative stimuli. The pituitary can be sensitized by the administration of an estrogen for one to three days. A standard method is administration of conjugated estrogens 2.5 mg. p.o., or diethylstilbestrol 1.0 mg. p.o., daily for one to three days. It is important to emphasize that failure of GH to respond is not evidence of deficiency unless associated hypogonadism has been rectified. In the hospital setting, or in cases that fail to respond to appropriate "screening" tests, more formal tests are required. The chief tests are the insulin hypoglycemia test, the L-dopa test, and a few workers use the apomorphine test.

INSULIN HYPOGLYCEMIA TEST

Substance	Crystalline zinc insulin administered intravenously.
Dose	0.1 U./kg. (normal patient); 0.05 U./kg. (suspected hypopituitary patient).
Principle	Insulin given IV causes hypoglycemia which is monitored by CNS glucoreceptors. Stimulation of GH release occurs in 30 to 60 minutes provided significant hypoglycemia (usually less than 50 per cent of pretest levels) is induced.
Method	The patient should be fasted and on bed rest after midnight. Any symptoms or signs of hypoglycemia should be recorded. Blood samples for glucose, GH and cortisol are taken at 0, 30, 60, 90, and 120 minutes.
Possible adverse effects	Symptomatic hypoglycemia is necessary for adequate stimulation of GH secretion, but in the event of marked CNS signs or symptoms, glucose should be given intravenously. Care should be taken with suspected hypopituitary patients who may have insufficiency of both GH and adrenal functions and who may show exaggerated responses to hypoglycemia. Elderly subjects and those in whom heart disease is suspected should not be given insulin.
Interpretation	A majority of normal subjects who show a fall in plasma glucose to less than 40 mg./100 ml. will respond with a rise in GH above 10 ng./ml. In many laboratories, an increase of 6 ng./ml. is considered normal. In one recent study,[10] the mean GH response in 20 normal subjects was 28.7 ng./ml. Only two of the 20 subjects failed to respond. Failure of GH to respond to adequate hypoglycemia cannot be taken as absolute proof of GH insufficiency as 10 to 15 per cent of normal subjects may not respond in a given test.

The insulin hypoglycemia test can also be used to assess ACTH-adrenal reserve. A majority of normal subjects (90%) show a rise in plasma cortisol of $10-20$ μg./100 ml. after adequate hypoglycemia.

The insulin hypoglycemia test is generally considered to be the most useful test of pituitary GH reserve, and has the advantage that it tests ACTH and prolactin secretory reserve as well. It may be abnormal with lesions of the hypothalamus, pituitary stalk, or pituitary gland.

L-DOPA TEST

Substance	L-dopa is a precursor of dopamine and norepinephrine and readily crosses the blood-brain barrier.

Dose	0.5 g. by mouth at beginning of test.
Principle	L-dopa, by conversion to the catecholamines, causes GH release, probably by an effect at a hypothalamic level to stimulate GRH release. L-dopa causes depression of prolactin secretion, due either to stimulation of release of PIF, or to direct action at the pituitary level.
Method	The patient should be fasted and on bed rest after midnight. Blood samples are taken at 0, 30, 60, and 90 minutes for GH and PRL.
Possible adverse effects	Nausea or vomiting occurs in 10 to 15 per cent of patients 45 to 60 minutes after oral L-dopa. The GH response does not depend on this stress effect, however.
Interpretation	Approximately 80 per cent of normal subjects have a GH response greater than 6 ng./ml. The mean maximal response in the recent study cited above was 28.2 ng./ml. The GH response is often defective in lesions of the hypothalamus or pituitary. This test is widely used in combination with insulin hypoglycemia to determine GH reserve. It is safer than insulin in older patients.

Apomorphine Test

Substance	Apomorphine, a derivative of morphine, has no narcotic effect and is given in a dose that rarely causes nausea or vomiting.
Dose	Apomorphine hydrochloride 0.75 mg.s.c.
Principle	Apomorphine, a highly specific dopamine agonist, causes GH release by action on the hypothalamus, and PRL inhibition by direct effects on hypothalamic or pituitary sites.
Method	The patient should be fasted and on bed rest after midnight. Blood samples are taken at 0, 30, 45, 60, and 90 minutes for GH and PRL.
Possible adverse effects	Nausea or vomiting occurs in 10 to 15 per cent of subjects.
Interpretation	We have found the apomorphine test to be very reliable in assessing GH reserve (Fig. 4). The peak response occurs at 45 to 60 minutes and is greater in men than in women. In a consecutive series of more than 30 men, we have not found a single false negative. In women, however, 10 to 15 per cent fail to show a response greater than 6 ng./ml. In our experience, apomorphine has proven to be more reliable and effective than L-dopa for assessing GH reserve. Apomorphine also causes prolactin suppression in patients with prolactin-secreting tumors.

Other Tests

Arginine by intravenous infusion is a reliable stimulus for GH.[9] The usefulness of this test is restricted by the fact that solutions of arginine appropriate for testing are not widely available in hospital pharmacies. Arginine also causes prolactin release in some normal subjects and may be useful for simultaneous testing of both hormones. The mechanism of arginine-induced GH or PRL release is unknown. The procedure is the least unpleasant stress test of GH secretion. Glucagon, administered intramuscularly or intravenously, also is effective in stimulating GH release.

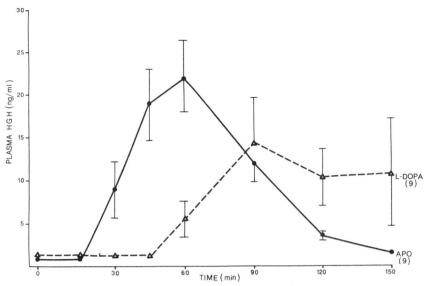

Figure 4. Plasma GH responses to apomorphine (solid line) and L-dopa (dotted line) in nine normal males. The peak response to subcutaneous apomorphine occurs at 45 to 60 minutes, the response to oral L-dopa somewhat later.

Growth Hormone Suppression Test

In patients with acromegaly or gigantism, random GH levels are usually consistently above 10 ng./ml. Many patients have extremely high values, reaching several hundred ng./ml. These high values in acromegaly are not suppressible below 10 ng./ml. by glucose administration, although there may be a slight decrease in plasma levels in approximately half of the cases.

GLUCOSE GROWTH HORMONE SUPPRESSION TEST

Substance	Oral glucose, as used in the glucose tolerance test, is used.
Dose	75 to 100 g. glucose p.o.
Principle	Glucose, acting via the hypothalamus, suppresses GH release. Acromegalics usually fail to suppress GH after glucose or may show a paradoxic response.
Method	The patient should be fasted and on bed rest after midnight. Oral glucose is administered and blood samples for GH and glucose are taken at 0, 30, 60, 90, 120, and 180 minutes.
Possible adverse effects	None, although an occasional subject is nauseated due to gastric irritation.
Interpretation	Normal subjects almost invariably show suppression in GH to less than 5 ng./ml. by 90 to 180 minutes. Patients with acromegaly, starvation, anorexia nervosa, and certain other conditions may fail to suppress, or show a paradoxical rise.

Patients with acromegaly also show, in about one third of cases, a moderate to marked increase in plasma GH following the intravenous injection of a standard dose of TRH (see below). Normals do not show this kind of response; a proportion of patients with depression or renal failure, however, are said to show a GH response to the tripeptide.

Prolactin Secretion

Determination of plasma prolactin levels has become a valuable part of the workup for hypothalamic and pituitary disease, even in patients without galactorrhea. Normally, prolactin levels in men are 1 to 20 ng./ml., in nonpregnant women 1 to 25 ng./ml. In the majority of normal subjects, serum prolactin levels are less than 10 ng./ml. In a large series reported by Frantz,[34] men had a mean serum prolactin level of 4.7 and women 8.0 ng./ml. Normal children have values in the same range, but neonatal infants (during the first four weeks) have elevated levels (as high as 50 to 150 ng./ml.). In normal subjects, prolactin levels are slightly elevated during the early morning hours 3 to 7 A.M. Most patients with galactorrhea have elevated serum prolactin levels. On the other hand, galactorrhea is observed in only 1 of 6 patients with hyperprolactinemia. In patients with chromophobe adenomas, 30 to 50 per cent have elevated prolactin levels, indicating that the tumor is hypersecretory. Lesions of the hypothalamus may also cause an elevation. In such cases, even minimal amounts of residual pituitary may be capable of maintaining normal levels of prolactin, due presumably to loss of PIF activity. Stimulatory tests for prolactin release are not useful in distinguishing pituitary from hypothalamic causes of hyperprolactinemia.

Prolactin Deficiency

Prolactin deficiency is usually seen as part of severe panhypopituitarism due to pituitary disease, and only rarely as an isolated manifestation of pituitary insufficiency. Failure of prolactin response to TRH administration (see below for technique) usually indicates intrinsic pituitary failure. The chlorpromazine procedure is useful in assessing pituitary prolactin reserve.

CHLORPROMAZINE TEST

Substance	Chlorpromazine.
Dose	25 mg. intramuscularly.
Principle	Chlorpromazine antagonizes the dopaminergic system, causing secretion of prolactin by removing tonic inhibition normally exerted by endogenous dopamine, through suppression of PIF, or by direct effects on the pituitary.
Method	The patient should be fasted and on bed rest after midnight. Samples are taken at 0, 1, 2, and 3 hours.
Possible adverse effects	Minimal, but include drowsiness, hypotension, and mild parkinsonian effects.
Interpretation	Early reports suggested that the response to chlorpromazine may distinguish between hypothalamic and pituitary lesions, the response being absent with hypothalamic lesions. This differentiation is not always valid, since there is growing evidence that dopamine receptors exist on pituitary prolactin-secreting cells and that chlorpromazine and L-dopa may act directly at the pituitary level.

Prolactin Hypersecretion

Suppression and stimulation tests have had relatively little value in differentiating tumor from other causes of increased plasma prolactin. In all cases, a careful roentgenographic evaluation should be made for tumor. The higher the plasma prolactin levels, the more likely is the diagnosis of tumor. Almost all patients with values over 200 ng./ml. and most with values over 100 ng./ml. have tumors, but there are some exceptions. Most patients with tumors show normal suppression of prolactin levels after administration of L-dopa, apomorphine, and bromergocryptine, as do patients with "functional" pituitary disease. However, failure to inhibit with these agents is highly suggestive of tumor since other cases uniformly are inhibited. Acute suppression tests with L-dopa and apomorphine are carried out as described above. Bromergocryptine also can be used to assess PRL suppression. The drug is administered in a dose of 2 mg. p.o. and plasma prolactin levels are followed at one-hour intervals for six hours. Water loading was also proposed recently as a test of suppressibility of "functional" prolactin hypersecretion, but a number of workers now report that this reaction is not uniform, either in normal persons or in "functional" galactorrhea; suppression may occasionally be seen in patients with tumor. This is our own experience. The LHRH test (see below) may be of some value. If patients with amenorrhea and galactorrhea fail to respond to LHRH injection, it is likely that tumor is present and has destroyed much of the pituitary. Most patients with galactorrhea-amenorrhea, however, respond to LHRH even if they have prolactin-secreting pituitary adenomas.

ACTH Secretion

Direct measurements of plasma ACTH are not as readily available as other tests of anterior pituitary secretion, and generally are used in differentiating causes of Cushing's syndrome. The techniques of diagnosis of states of adrenal cortical hyperfunction are outlined in Chapter 8. The levels of sensitivity of assays for ACTH are generally not adequate for the diagnosis of ACTH deficiency. Instead, indirect techniques based on plasma cortisol measurements and urinary cortisol and cortisol metabolites are widely used. Since adrenal function is only an indirect measure of ACTH secretion, one needs to show that the adrenal cortex can respond normally by determining effects of ACTH injection.

Diurnal Variation in Cortisol

Measurement of plasma cortisol levels in the morning and evening is important in the assessment of normal diurnal variation and gives clues to the possibility of hypersecretion or of adrenal failure. Normal levels at 8 A.M. range from 10 to 25 μg./100 ml. There is normally a fall to below 10 μg./100 ml. in random values measured from 3 to 6 P.M. Adrenal failure is suggested by plasma cortisol levels persistently below 8 μg./100 ml. in the morning. Episodic secretion of cortisol may mask a normal diurnal variation, depending on whether samples are taken at peak or at trough of a secretory burst. Hospitalized patients under stress may lose diurnal variations. If diurnal variation has not been established on first sampling, repeat sampling on the following day will usually be definitive. High-normal values in both the morning and evening may indicate Cushing's disease; 24-hour urinary cortisol determinations will confirm this.

ACTH Test

This test is usually carried out by giving synthetic ACTH 1-24, 25 μg. IV over a period of 4 to 8 hours. The material is dissolved in 500 ml. of normal saline containing 5 per

333

cent glucose. Plasma cortisol is determined before and at the end of the infusion. Urine 17-hydroxysteroids are measured for 24 hours before and after the infusion. Plasma steroid levels should increase to the normal range (15 to 25 μg./100 ml.) after the stimulation, and urine excretion should increase by at least 100 per cent. For convenience, and as a screening test for Addison's disease, many endocrinologists administer ACTH gel IM and measure plasma cortisol as well as urinary corticoids before and four hours later. It is important to note that prolonged ACTH deficiency may lead to decreased or absent adrenal sensitivity to ACTH. This is also true after prolonged administration of corticosteroid, and for this reason, the initial injection of ACTH may not increase corticosteroid secretion appreciably and it may be necessary to stimulate daily for three days to restore normal sensitivity. Day-by-day responses will be found to increase progressively.

Pituitary ACTH Reserve

METYRAPONE TEST. Pituitary ACTH reserve is usually tested by administering metyrapone, which inhibits 11-β-hydroxylase, the enzyme that catalyzes the final step in the biosynthesis of cortisol. A decrease in cortisol secretion after administration of metyrapone reduces negative-feedback effects on ACTH, resulting in a compensatory rise in ACTH secretion which stimulates increased steroid biosynthesis. The increased secretion of total 17-hydroxycorticosteroids indicates an adequate ACTH reserve. The significance of an impaired metyrapone test has been debated, since either hypothalamic or pituitary disease can cause abnormal responses. We believe that normal response to decreased plasma cortisol levels (the basis of the metyrapone test) requires a certain number of functioning ACTH cells in the pituitary, and a certain amount of CRF secretion. Loss of either of these components of ACTH regulation may result in failure of the response, and for this reason, the test does not discriminate adequately between hypothalamic and pituitary abnormalities.

The standard test is performed by administering metyrapone in a total of six doses of 10 mg./kg. each, administered every four hours. Many workers use as a standard dose 750 mg. every four hours for six doses. Pituitary, hypothalamic, or adrenal failure can cause impaired responses. In Cushing's disease, the response is supranormal. A normal response consists of a twofold or greater increase in urinary 17-hydroxycorticosteroids on the day of administration or the day following, compared with preadministration values.

STRESS-INDUCED ACTH RESPONSES. The administration of insulin, pyrogens, and ADH have all been used to stimulate ACTH secretion. The most readily available clinical test, the insulin hypoglycemia test, can be combined with the GH stimulation test as described above.

All stress tests are at best unpleasant, and at worst dangerous. Both hypoglycemia and ADH can induce coronary insufficiency, and are contra-indicated in older patients or those with known heart disease. Neither pyrogen administration nor ADH evokes stimulatory responses in 100 per cent of normal persons, and for this reason, failure to respond is not an absolute indicator of hypothalamic-pituitary failure. In practise, it is sometimes useful to evaluate ACTH, GH, and prolactin secretory reserve by measuring plasma hormone levels after the patient has completed a stressful diagnostic procedure such as pneumoencephalography. A patient with suspected ACTH deficiency should never be exposed to severe stress without adequate pretreatment with corticoids. This applies particularly to angiography, pneumoencephlography, and surgical procedures.

An abnormal stress test does not differentiate adequately between hypothalamic and pituitary causes of insufficiency.

TSH Secretion

The clinician almost never has to deal with problems of TSH hypersecretion due to primary pituitary disease, there being at most a handful of cases in the world literature with hyperthyroidism due to primary pituitary disease (see Chapter 9). On the other hand, hypothyroidism is relatively common and the differential diagnosis between primary thyroid failure (primary hypothyroidism), TSH deficiency due to intrinsic pituitary disease (secondary hypothyroidism), and TSH deficiency due to hypothalamic TRH deficiency (tertiary hypothyroidism) often must be made. Intrinsic thyroid disease is the most common and hypothalamic disease the least common of the three. Aside from clinical features which may suggest the diagnosis of intrinsic thyroid disease such as goiter, evidence of thyroiditis, and prior thyroidectomy or radioiodine treatment, more than 90 per cent of patients with intrinsic thyroid insufficiency have elevated levels of plasma immunoassayable TSH (normal level is 1 to 8 μU./ml.). Clinical and laboratory evidence of hypothyroidism (plasma T_4 levels less than 5 μg./100 ml., plasma T_3 levels less than 80 ng./ml., in association with normal plasma thyroid hormone-binding proteins), if present in association with low or normal TSH levels, is highly suggestive of TSH failure. Usually, patients with pituitary or hypothalamic disorders that cause hypothyroidism have low TSH levels, and the differential diagnosis is made between these two entities by overall consideration of the clinical picture, and by use of the TRH stimulation test (see below).

As noted in Chapter 9 and above, clinical tests of pituitary-thyroid function have generally conformed to the widely accepted theory of control of the pituitary thyroid axis: TSH levels are high in primary thyroid disease and low in pituitary or hypothalamic disease. The TRH test is of greatest value in diagnosis of hypothyroidism, is useful in a minority of cases with primary thyroid failure who do not have elevated plasma TSH levels, and helps to differentiate between pituitary and hypothalamic hypothyroidism.

TRH Test

Substance	TRH is a synthetic tripeptide.
Dose	The usual test dose is 100 to 400 μg. IV. TRH has been released in Canada in 400 μg. dosage.
Principle	TRH acts directly on pituitary cells, probably via cyclic AMP, to cause release of both TSH and prolactin.
Method	TRH is administered IV over a 30-second period after an initial baseline blood sample has been taken. Subsequent samples are taken at 15, 30, 60, and 90 min. For simplicity and economy, samples taken prior to injection and at 15 and 30 minutes are usually sufficient. If the test is being done to distinguish between pituitary and hypothalamic disease, several authors have suggested that the full five-sample procedure be carried out, because "hypothalamic" hypothyroid cases are more likely to have a delayed peak response. However, patients with pituitary disease occasionally show this same response.
	Because some patients show slight hypertension (less than 20 per cent) or occasionally hypotension, patients should be kept prone for 15 minutes after injection.
Possible adverse effects	Symptoms in about 50 per cent of subjects include flushing, sweating, palpitations, nausea, sensation of urinary urgency, mild hypertension, or mild hypotension. No serious complications have been

reported. Probably a somewhat slower administration (2 to 3 minutes instead of a single bolus injection) is equally effective without causing side effects, but tests done this way have not been standardized.

Interpretation   A TSH response to TRH greater than 2 μU./ml. occurs in over 95 per cent of normal persons, the average being 20 to 30 μU./ml. The lower responses are seen primarily in men over age 40. Ninety-eight per cent of hyperthyroid patients fail to show a response to TRH. Therefore, a normal response almost completely excludes the diagnosis of thyrotoxicosis. In hypothyroidism, about 70 per cent of patients have a response greater than the normal, and also prolonged. However, the overlap between normal and hypothyroid patients makes this test valuable only in the group of hyper-responders.

In the differential diagnosis of secondary and tertiary thyroid failure, complete absence of pituitary TSH response to TRH is strong evidence of intrinsic pituitary disease. However, an appreciable number (approximately 20 per cent) of cases of intrinsic pituitary disease show TSH secretory responses in the low-normal range, and in this group, hypothalamic failure cannot now be distinguished from pituitary failure. Most patients with proven hypothalamic disorder show TSH responses within the normal range; a few are hyper-responsive. Thus in this group of patients, complete absence of the TSH response is indicative of pituitary disease, but a modest response does not, of itself, distinguish between pituitary and hypothalamic disease, although it favors the latter. The clinician must take into account the entire clinical presentation, including evidence of the site of lesion. Unlike the situation with LHRH (see below), prolonged TRH deficiency does not appear to lead to a secondary loss in pituitary responsiveness to TRH.

The TRH test is also of value in stimulating prolactin release. Most patients with prolactin-secreting tumors respond to TRH. Nonfunctional pituitary adenomas, due to compromise of lactotropes by compression, may cause diminished responsiveness of prolactin to TRH. In 60 to 80 per cent of acromegaly cases, TRH causes GH release, unlike the normal situation where TRH has no effect on GH secretion.

In the last two or three years, several investigators have called attention to the paradoxic finding that a few patients with hypothryoidism due to pituitary or hypothalamic disease have high-normal plasma TSH levels. Two possible explanations for this effect have been offered, neither of which has been proved. It has been suggested that a biologically inactive but immunologically similar TSH molecule is secreted in these cases, or alternatively that prolonged TSH deficiency has led to impaired thyroid function, which in turn has evoked a compensatory increase in TSH secretion. Neither explaination seems particularly likely. These cases also may be caused by a combination of intrinsic thyroid disease and pituitary failure, neither of which alone would have been capable of causing clinical disease. This peculiar syndrome should be borne in mind in the evaluation of hypothyroidism with normal levels of TSH.

Patients with long-standing primary hypothyroidism may develop enlargement of the pituitary fossa together with marked TSH hypersecretion. Until careful hormonal studies have been carried out, including assay of plasma TSH levels, the clinician's first impression may be that these are cases of primary pituitary tumor with secondary thyroid failure.

Gonadotropic Hormone Secretion

Primary hypersecretion of gonadotropic hormones by the pituitary is an extremely rare clinical entity. The pattern of gonadotropic and gonadal hormone secretion in precocious puberty resembles that of normal adults. On the other hand, hypogonadism is an extremely common feature of hypothalamic and pituitary disease, and is observed as a functional disturbance in "hypothalamic amenorrhea" and anorexia nervosa (see Chapter 5). The diagnosis of gonadal failure can usually be made on clinical grounds by failure to develop normal secondary sex characteristics in adolescents, and by loss of established sexual function in adults. Women first lose the ovulatory pattern of LH release, which gives rise to amenorrhea, or show irregular, scanty periods (oligomenorrhea) due to breakthrough bleeding. Later, basal FSH and LH secretion is reduced, and variable degrees of estrogen deficiency ensue ranging from partial to complete. Estrogen deficiency causes amenorrhea, atrophy of the breasts, uterus, and genitalia, decrease in body hair growth, and premature osteoporosis. In men, loss of potency is probably the earliest manifestation of testosterone deficiency, followed by loss of libido, decrease in growth of facial and body hair, decrease in muscle strength and mass, and general loss of vigor.

The determination of plasma gonadal steroids (testosterone in men, 17-β-estradiol in women) confirms the diagnosis of gonadal deficiency. Normal testosterone values in men are 3 to 9 μg./ml. Estradiol in normal women ranges from 20 to 60 pg./ml. in the follicular phase, 330 to 700 pg./ml. during midcycle, and 100 to 200 pg./ml. in the luteal phase. Primary gonadal failure can be distinguished from hypothalamic-pituitary disease by measurement of plasma gonadotropins. If gonadotropins are elevated, the disease lies in the gonad; if low or in the normal range in the face of testosterone or estrogen deficiency, this inappropriately low level indicates gonadotropin deficiency, permitting the diagnosis of hypogonadotropic hypogonadism. Normal values for FSH and LH in men are 5 to 25 mIU./ml. and 6 to 30 mIU./ml., respectively. Normal values for LH in women are 5 to 30 mIU./ml. in the follicular phase, 40 to 200 mIU./ml. midcycle and 5 to 40 mIU./ml. in the luteal phase. Normal values for FSH in women range from 5 to 40 mIU./ml. during various phases of the cycle.

LH and FSH are secreted episodically, with a periodicity of about 1 to 1.5 hours; the fluctuations are particularly great in hypogonadal individuals who may show, at times, values within the normal range. For this reason, it may be necessary to collect repeated samples at intervals of 15 to 30 minutes. A valid method is to collect three separate samples at 15-minute intervals and to pool them for immunoassay.

Urine gonadotropic hormones traditionally have been measured by bioassay, but this procedure has been outmoded by modern diagnostic methods for plasma measurement. The urine methods are both expensive and inaccurate.

Hypogonadotropic Hypogonadism

The finding of hypogonadotropic hypopgonadism requires further testing to determine whether the disease is hypothalamic or pituitary in origin, and whether it is due to structural abnormalities, or is "functional."

DELAYED PUBERTY. Puberty normally occurs between the ages of 10 and 15 in the female and between the ages of 11 and 16 in the male. The time of onset of puberty has decreased in the Western world by about two years in the last century. If growth is otherwise normal and the plasma GH reserve is normal, isolated gonadotropic hormone deficiency must be considered as the cause of delayed puberty. Family history of delayed puberty, presence of chromosomal abnormalities (Turner's syndrome in the female, Klinefelter's syndrome in the male), and the finding of hyposmia or anosmia give clues to the diagnosis. If none of these is present, the differential diagnosis lies between "constitutional" delayed puberty and organic disease. We have seen at least two patients with hypothalamic primary amenorrhea, in which prolactin hypersecretion caused the delayed puberty. If all other pituitary functions are normal and there are no localizing neurologic findings, including normal visual fields and skull roentgenograms, then more aggressive diagnostic procedures such as pneuoencephalography are not usually recommended. Tests of gonadotropic secretory reserve (clomiphene, LHRH, see below) do not help to differentiate delayed puberty from organic hypothalamic-pituitary disease, because clomiphene cannot stimulate LH release unless hypothalamic mechanisms for LH control have matured, and LHRH is only marginally effective in prepubertal children. In prepubertal children, FSH responses to LHRH are relatively greater than are LH responses. This may prove to be of value in differential diagnosis. We recommend careful follow-up in such cases, with special emphasis on hypothalamic-pituitary function. Puberty may commence as late as age 18 in females and 20 in males, although this is rare. The recommendation of prolonged observation does not imply that no treatment is indicated. Because of the severe psychologic effects of hypogonadism, and the crucial requirement of sex hormones for normal brain development (including psychosocial maturation), in most cases it is advisable to commence substitution therapy in either sex by age 15. In boys treatment with HCG or with testosterone may stimulate the development of testes function. In girls, cyclic estrogen-progesterone therapy is indicated. Periodically, the therapy should be discontinued to permit the evaluation of pituitary-gonad function. In boys, testes growth during the course of testosterone therapy usually means that normal gonadotropic function has returned, and that replacement therapy need not be continued.

HYPOGONADOTROPIC HYPOGONADISM IN THE ADULT. *Male:* Persistently low gonadotropic hormone levels in the presence of otherwise normal pituitary function suggests isolated gonadotropic deficiency. Other evidence of hypothalamic or pituitary disease should be sought to help make this differential diagnosis. If all other functions are normal (including GH and ACTH secretory reserves), and the visual fields and routine skull roentgenograms are normal, then more intensive neurodiagnostic procedures usually do not help, and the patient is followed carefully over a period of years. Progressive hypothalamic or pituitary disease may subsequently appear in patients with isolated gonadotropin failure. Clomiphene has been used to stimulate LH release in such patients (see below), but the response is usually minimal and the drug does not help to differentiate pituitary and hypothalamic causes. LHRH has been used to distinguish hypothalamic from pituitary etiologies of hypogonadotropism (see below). If the patient shows a normal response to LHRH, endogenous LHRH deficiency probably is present, due to a lesion of either the hypothalamus or the pituitary stalk. On the other hand, failure to release LH in response to a single dose of LHRH does not necessarily indicate that pituitary function is primarily disordered. Long-standing LHRH deficiency can prevent pituitary response to exogenous LHRH. Similarly, prepubertal children or those with constitutionally delayed puberty show minimal or no response to LHRH. The responsivity of the pituitary to LHRH can be restored in such cases by prolonged treatment with the hormone. Recent studies indicate that the best treatment routine is 500 μg. LHRH administered three times daily s.c. Smaller doses (100 μg. b.i.d.) may suffice to restore pituitary responsiveness. The LHRH test has not been completely validated in differentiating between pituitary and hypothalamic disease. It is likely that a residuum of functioning pituitary cells can be stimulated by a regimen of LHRH administration, and several cases have now been reported in males in which this has been the case.

Female: In the evaluation of anovulatory amenorrhea, it is essential to determine that the uterus and vagina are normal and responsive to sex steroids. In practise, persistent amenorrhea (defined as absence of menses for at least three months in a nonpregnant woman) is initially evaluated by administering a progesterone compound such as progesterone acetate 100 to 150 mg. i.m., or medroxyprogesterone 10 mg. daily for five days. Menstruation within two to seven days after commencing therapy indicates that the uterus has been previously stimulated by estrogen and that the uterus and vagina are probably normal. Because progesterone and its derivatives may be harmful to the developing fetus, the test should only be done after laboratory test show that the patient is not pregnant. If bleeding fails to occur, the patient should be treated for one or two months with an estrogen (1.25 or 2.5 mg. daily for 24 days) plus medroxyprogesterone 10 mg. daily on days 20 to 24 of each cycle. If menstruation ensues, uterine-response capacity is intact; if it does not, the disorder is in the uterus. If nonmenstrual bleeding occurs, then further testing of hypothalamic, pituitary, and ovarian function is required. Ovarian failure can be excluded as a cause of amenorrhea by measurement of plasma gonadotropins. If they are low, attention is drawn to disorder of hypothalamic-pituitary function. Skull roentgenograms and evaluation of other endocrine functions are indicated.

Clomiphene. Approximately 60 to 80 per cent of women with "functional amenorrhea" respond to the administration of clomiphene, which acts as an "antiestrogen" at estrogen receptor sites in hypothalamus and pituitary to bring about a functional estrogen-deficiency state. The block of negative-feedback effects of estrogen triggers gonadotropin release. The criterion of response to clomiphene is a normal menstrual period approximately 12 days after administration of the drug, or evidence of ovulation as reflected in change in body temperature. A positive response is assumed to mean that hypothalamic function was abnormal. Clomiphene effects can be demonstrated also by measurement of plasma LH 12 to 16 days after the first day of administration of clomiphene. Plasma LH levels should be in the ovulatory range.

The usual starting dose of clomiphene is 50 mg. daily for five days followed by no therapy for 25 days. If two consecutive months of therapy are ineffective, the dose is increased to 100 mg. daily for five days for a further two months. Some recommend doses as high as 150 or 200 mg. daily if lower doses are ineffective. In addition to establishing a diagnosis of "functional amenorrhea" clomiphene therapy commonly leads to ovulation in women who want to become pregnant. It is believed that some patients with intrinsic pituitary disease also may respond to clomiphene. The efficacy of treatment is greater in women with relatively normal basal estrogen levels, but some relatively estrogen-deficient women also may release LH in response to the drug. If the clomiphene test is abnormal and other aspects of pituitary function are intact, the LHRH provocative test (see below) may provide further clues to the site of the abnormality.

Differential diagnosis of causes of amenorrhea includes disease of the ovary such as the polycystic ovary syndrome, virilizing disorders of the ovarian medullary tissue such as hyperthecosis and thecoma, and adrenal disorders such as the adrenogenital syndrome (which may be due to enzymatic defects in the adrenal cortex) or tumor of endocrine tissue (adenoma or carcinoma). Cushing's disease is also a cause of amenorrhea. Usually disorders of this general type are accompanied by clinical evidence of virilization or hirsutism which may include excessive hair growth on face and body, acne, increased muscle mass, and in severe cases, clitoral enlargment. Differentiation of primary gonadotropin failure from disorders due to excessive production of androgenic hormones is therefore usually made on clinical grounds, but in questionable cases, workup should include a study of urinary and plasma adrenal and ovarian steroids. Details of this approach are found in textbooks of clinical or gynecologic endocrinology.

LHRH Test

Substance	LHRH, a synthetic decapeptide.
Dose	100 μg. IV or SC.

339

Principle	LHRH directly stimulates the pituitary to release LH and FSH, probably acting via cyclic AMP.
Method	With the patient at rest during the test, blood samples are taken at 0, 30, 45, 60, and 90 minutes after administration. Plasma determinations of LH are usually sufficient for diagnostic purposes, but FSH also should be measured if possible.
Interpretation	An increase in plasma LH of 10 to 20 mIU./ml. is considered normal. FSH usually shows a lesser response and the peak is delayed. In some patients with hyperprolactinemia, the FSH response is exaggerated, and in prepubertal children FSH response is greater than LH response. A response within the normal range indicates that the pituitary is intrinsically normal, and it may be inferred that the cause of the amenorrhea is endogenous LHRH deficiency. However, failure to respond does not always indicate that the pituitary is abnormal. As in male patients with hypogonadotropic hypogonadism, longstanding LHRH deficiency can cause secondary unresponsiveness to exogenous LHRH, and normal responsivity can be restored by prolonged stimulation. Proper criteria for the longer-term diagnostic stimulation of LH and FSH have not been developed. An example of this problem is anorexia nervosa, in which a single injection of LHRH is often ineffective in stimulating the pituitary until the patient has regained some body weight.

Combined Test of Pituitary Function

Several groups of workers have advocated the use of a combined test of pituitary functional reserve that can be carried out in a few hours at one sitting and thereby can eliminate costly, prolonged hospitalization. It has been shown in the triple-stimulation test that the response to one stimulus does not interfere with the responses to the others. Although it is recommended that all six pituitary hormones be determined at each interval, as a general rule reasonably useful data will be obtained if only 0-, 30-, and 60-minute samples are taken. When prolactin abnormalities are suspected, insulin and TRH should be given separately.

TRIPLE STIMULATION TEST

Substances	The simultaneous administration of insulin, TRH, and LHRH provides rapid assessment of all six pituitary hormones. TRH together with crystalline zinc insulin is given IV and LHRH is given SC or IV.
Dose	Insulin 0.1 U./kg. IV (normal patient); 0.05 U./kg. IV (suspected hypopituitary patient); TRH 100 to 400 μg. IV and LHRH 100 μg. SC.
Principle	Insulin, by causing hypoglycemia, stimulates GH, ACTH, and prolactin. TRH directly stimulates the pituitary to release both TSH and PRL. LHRH directly stimulates the pituitary to release both LH and FSH.
Method	The patient should be fasted and on strict bed rest after midnight. Blood samples are taken at 0, 30, 45, 60, 90, and 120 minutes.
Interpretation	The triple test has been useful in screening for possible pituitary insufficiency, since all hormones can be assessed.

340

USE OF RELEASING HORMONES

Both TRH and LHRH have been used extensively in the investigation of hypothalamic-pituitary disorder in man. On the basis of knowledge of the physiology of anterior pituitary regulation, it would be expected that use of the releasing hormones would permit a clear distinction between hypothalamic and pituitary failure. However, experience with these substances indicates that this expectation is generally but not totally fulfilled in the case of TRH, and is only partially fulfilled in the case of LHRH.

TSH Responses to TRH

The minimal effective intravenous dose of TRH in normal man is 15 μg. and doses between 100 and 500 μg. give effects that are indistinguishable from one another. There appears to be a dose-response relationship for patients when considered as a group, but there is substantial intrapatient variation in sensitivity. Normal TSH responses are summarized in Table 3 which presents values from a few representative studies. Men tend to have lower responses than do women in the reproductive age (presumably due to estrogen sensitization of the pituitary), and men over the age of 40 have rather meager responses, so that increments of 2 μU./ml., a relatively modest response and one that is barely in the range of most immunoassays, may be seen in normals of this age group.

Criteria for abnormality must therefore be adjusted for age and sex. Although the dose of 500 μg. given intravenously as a bolus over 30 seconds has been widely used for testing in the United States and Canada, it is likely that a smaller dose, given over a somewhat longer time, would be equally effective and would have the advantage of producing fewer side effects. Proper clinical trials in large numbers of patients have not been carried out using this more conservative regimen, and for this reason diagnostic standards do not exist for doses lower than 200 μg. The effects of estrogen priming have not been standardized for clinical testing.

TRH Test

In at least two major types of pituitary-hypothalamic disease, TRH testing has proved to be of definitive value. The first group consists of children with *idiopathic hy-*

Table 3. Normal TSH Responses to TRH

Sex	Dose (μg IV)	Response ($\mu U./ml.$)	Investigator
Women	500	>6	Snyder et al.[29]
Men			
age <30	500	>6	Snyder et al.[29]
age 40–79	500	>2	
Men and women	500	Mean 15 (8.5–27.0)*	Fleischer et al.[13]
Men and women	25 to 200	>5.9	Sakoda et al.[27]
Men	200	3.5 to 15.6	Ormston et al.[25]
Women	200	6.5 to 20.5	Ormston et al.[25]
Men	200	3.5 to 15.0	Faglia et al.[12]
Women	200	6.0 to 30.0	Faglia et al.[12]
Men	200 (60-min. infusion)	mean 10.4 (6.8–23.3)*	Lundberg and Wide[20]
Women	200 (60-min. infusion)	mean 15.7 (10.8–23.7)*	Lundberg and Wide[20]
Children (1-10/12 to 14-3/12	500	23.3 ± 3.3 SEM	Kaplan et al.[18]

*Range of responses.

popituitarism, whether hypothyroid or not, all of whom have responses to TRH in the normal range for their age (Table 4). Moreover, in this group, the response to TRH is frequently prolonged with peak values occurring as late as 60 minutes. The second group of patients in whom TRH testing is definitive are those with hypothyroidism due to *Sheehan's syndrome* in which responses are almost always low or absent.

A hypothalamic versus pituitary etiology for hypothyroidism with TSH deficiency can be distinguished by the TRH test in most patients; those that fail to respond to TRH have intrinsic pituitary disease and those with normal responses to TRH have hypothalamic failure. However, some patients do not fall into this simple classification and a proper decision can be made in some cases only on the basis of results of other pituitary tests and after radiologic evaluation of the hypothalamic-pituitary region (Table 5). This differential diagnosis is more difficult to make in men over the age of 40 because the normal response may be as low as 2 mU./ml., a value sometimes achieved after stimulation in patients with pituitary lesions. In Snyder's large series of patients with pituitary lesions giving rise to hypothyroidism, an abnormal response was observed in 24 of 26 cases.[29] However, a normal response does not exclude pituitary disease. In the series of Faglia and coworkers,[12] several patients with pituitary disease and secondary hypothyroidism had responses to TRH within the normal range. In a series of 76 hypothyroid patients with pituitary disease of all types collected by Abbott Laboratories[14] not classified by sex, 60 per cent had TSH responses that were less than 2 μU./ml, and an additional 23 per cent had responses less than 6 μU./ml. In this series, 17 per cent fell within the normal range of responses.

The identification of patients with hypothalamic failure as a cause of hypothyroidism *(hypothalamic hypothyroidism, tertiary hypothyroidism)* may also be difficult at times. The true incidence of this condition as assessed by review of cases reported in the literature may be hard to ascertain because diagnostic criteria used often include demonstration of normal TRH responsiveness. However, normal or delayed responses to TRH do not prove that the defect lies in the hypothalamus. In the series reported by Snyder and coworkers[29] responses of this type occurred in nine patients with hypothyroidism secondary to documented intrasellar tumor. That this was not due to pressure on the stalk of the hypothalamus was shown by the finding that these patients did not have elevated prolactin levels.

An important aspect of TRH testing of patients with hypothalamic-pituitary disease is that responsiveness may be abnormal even in patients who are not clinically hypothyroid. For example, in Snyder's series, 9 of 13 women had impaired responses while only five were hypothyroid. In men, 5 of 11 without hypothyroidism had impaired responses. Therefore the TRH test can be used in some patients to demonstrate hypo-

Table 4. TRH Responses in Pituitary-Hypothalamic Disease in Children

	Mean Peak TSH *(μU./ml.)*	*Peak Prolactin* *(ng./ml.)*
Normal Children (Age 1-10/12 to 14-3/12)	23.3 ± 3.3 (SEM)	25.9 ± 1.8 (SEM)
Isolated GH Deficiency (Age 5 to 25)	20.7 ± 2.8	30.7 ± 4.1
Multiple Hypopituitarism (Age 5-1/2 to 24-10/12)	27.7 ± 4.4	25.9 ± 1.8

(Adapted from Kaplan, S. L., et al.: *Thyrotropin-releasing factor (TRF) effect on secretion of human pituitary prolactin and thyrotropin in children and in idiopathic hypopituitary dwarfism: Further evidence for hypophysiotropic hormone deficiencies.* Endocrinol. Metab. 35:825, 1972.)

Table 5. TRH Responses in Pituitary-Hypothalamic Disease in Adults

Diagnosis	No. of Cases	Response	Author
Acromegaly	16 Euthyroid	43% Impaired	Snyder et al.[29]
	10 Hypothyroid	7 Normal	Faglia et al.[12]
		0 Absent	
		2 Impaired	
		1 Exaggerated	
Nonfunctioning pituitary tumor with hypothyroidism	12	7 Absent or impaired	Snyder et al.[29]
	8	2 Absent, 2 impaired	Faglia et al.[12]
	6	6 Absent	Fleischer et al.[13]
Hypothalamic disease	4 Hypothyroid	2 Normal	Snyder et al.[30]
	2 Euthyroid	1 Impaired	Snyder et al.[30]
Craniopharyngioma	3 Hypothyroid (includes above)	2 Reduced	Snyder et al.[30]

thalamic-pituitary disease even in the absence of demonstrable TSH insufficiency.

In patients with acromegaly, evaluation of TSH responsiveness to TRH is complicated by the fact that growth hormone excess appears to interfere with TRH effects on TSH responses. Impairment of the TSH response cannot be taken therefore to be unequivocal evidence of destruction of thyrotropic cell mass. In the combined series of Snyder[29] and Faglia[12] and their collaborators, of 16 euthyroid acromegalics, 43 per cent had responses below normal.

TRH testing has proved of great value in the diagnosis of *thyrotoxicosis*. Even minimal degrees of hyperthyroidism are sufficient to block responses to TRH. Perhaps 98 per cent or more of hyperthyroid patients have impaired or absent TRH responses, thus making this test the single most reliable index of the hyperthyroid state. In primary hypothyroidism (that due to intrinsic thyroid failure), approximately 80 per cent of cases have increased responsiveness which is of diagnostic value. However, the finding of low T_4 (or T_3) and elevation of plasma TSH levels is usually sufficient to make the diagnosis without a TRH stimulation test.

PROLACTIN SECRETORY RESERVE. In addition to causing discharge of TSH, TRH evokes the release of prolactin. The prolactin-secreting function of the pituitary is the most resistant of all secretions to local damage, presumably due to the fact that these cells function well in the absence of hypothalamic hormonal inputs. For this reason, patients with pituitary insufficiency may respond to TRH. On the other hand, failure to discharge prolactin after TRH injection is definitive evidence of severe intrinsic pituitary disease. Prolactin secretory reserve is frequently evaluated in patients with hyperprolactinemia in an attempt to differentiate between hypothalamic or functional disease on the one hand, and pituitary adenomas on the other. Unfortunately, most patients with tumors respond to a standard dose of TRH, and for this reason the test is not a valuable aid in differential diagnosis. The majority of cases with adenoma show an excessive response of plasma prolactin, whereas the response to chlorpromazine is disproportionately small (see Chapter 6).

LHRH Test

LHRH has been administered for diagnostic and physiologic test purposes in doses ranging from 25 to 100 μg. intravenously, subcutaneously, or by continuous infusion for up to 24 hours. There appears to be no advantage of one route over the other, but most workers now prefer to administer 100 μg. intravenously or subcutaneously. No side effects have been observed with this dose. LH secretion begins within two minutes, and reaches a peak by 20 to 40 minutes in most cases. FSH secretion usually does not begin until 10 to 20 minutes and reaches a peak at a later time (Table 6). In most patients, the LH secretory response to LHRH is much greater than the FSH response. For this reason, except in special cases (see below), it is generally sufficient to measure LH levels only. Failure of a normal person to show an LH response to 100 μg. of LHRH is rare. The authors have not seen a single instance of this in over 200 tests, and we are not aware that this has been reported by other workers. On the other hand, it is not uncommon to find almost no change in plasma FSH after injection of LHRH.

Normal ranges of response are recorded in Table 7, based on several large series. In men over age 60, responses are slightly less than in younger subjects. If compared on a weight basis, infants also appear to have somewhat lower LH responses to LHRH than do adult men. It is of interest that children, unlike adults, have greater FSH responses to LHRH than LH responses. It is believed that this difference is due to the state of development of the germ cells in ovary and testis. The germ cells produce the hormone "inhibin," which acts on the pituitary to selectively inhibit FSH secretion, both spontaneously and in response to LHRH. Inhibin is not secreted by the prepuberal gonad.

Responses to LHRH in sexually mature women depend on the stage of the menstrual cycle. The increase in LH is least during the follicular phase of the cycle, higher during the luteal phase, and greatest during the ovulatory surge. FSH responsiveness does not share these marked changes at different stages of the menstrual cycle. As noted in Chapter 5, cyclic changes in sensitivity in women are due to steroid effects, and possibly also to changes in endogenous LHRH secretion. In considering criteria for abnormality of response in hypogonadal states, it is usual to take as the lower limit of normal the response in women during the follicular phase, when responsivity is least.

The LHRH test has been mainly applied to the diagnosis of hypogonadotropic hypogonadism since either hypothalamic failure or pituitary failure can bring about a decrease in LH or FSH secretion. The most complete study of LHRH in diagnostic testing is that of Mortimer and colleagues,[21] who utilized 100 μg. intravenously as the test dose and measured responses at 20 and 60 minutes in 155 patients with hypogonadism (Table 8). Their findings indicate that in 31 patients with hypogonadism due to nonfunctioning pituitary tumors (presumably chromophobe adenomas), 11 had normal LH responses, 19 were impaired, and only one had an absent LH response. Impaired FSH responses occurred in only three cases. Thus, pituitary destruction sufficient to cause hypogonadism commonly does not destroy enough gonadotropic cells to block responses to presumably supramaximal amounts of LHRH.

Table 6. Range of LH and FSH Responses to 100 μg. Intravenous Bolus of LHRH in Normal Adults

Time (min.)	Male (n = 39)		Female (n = 7)*	
	LH (mU./ml.)	FSH (mU./ml.)	LH (mU./ml.)	FSH (mU./ml.)
0	3.2 – 8.6	1.4 – 7.8	3.2 – 5.6	3.8 – 8.3
20	8.4 – 34.0	1.6 – 10.5	9.0 – 22.0	4.3 – 10.0
60	5.8 – 34.0	1.2 – 11.0	6.0 – 18.4	6.0 – 12.0

*The females were in the follicular phase of the menstrual cycle.
(Adapted from Mortimer, C. H. et al.: *Luteinizing hormone and follicle-stimulating hormone-releasing hormone test in patients with hypothalamic-pituitary-gonadal dysfunction.* Br. Med. J. 4:73, 1973.)

Table 7. Normal Responses to LHRH

	Mean Max. Δ LH (mIU. ± S.D.)	Mean Max. Δ FSH (mIU. ± S.D.)	Investigator
Men			
50 µg. IV			Snyder et al.[30]
Age 21–30	37.7 ± 9.6	2.0 ± 0.3	
250 µg. IV			Snyder et al.[30]
Age 20–39	53.7 ± 31.7	3.0 ± 2.8	
Age 40–49	54.3 ± 29.0	2.9 ± 2.3	
Age 60–79	37.9 ± 18.5	1.1 ± 2.7	
100 µg. IV			Lemarchand-Beraud[19]
Age 18–40	32.2 ± 6.2	3.0 ± 1.4	
Age >65	22.6 ± 3.8	3.2 ± 0.8	
25 µg. IV			Pimstone et al.[26]
Infants 8–35 months	10.28 ± 2.01 (3.75–19.8)*	18.47 ± 6.43 (9.25–67.50)*	
Women			
100 µg. IV			Lemarchand-Beraud et al.[19]
Follicular phase	17.5 ± 2.7	3.1 ± 0.6	
Around LH peak	162.0 ± 49.0	7.6 ± 2.6	
Luteal phase	49.6 ± 8.2	2.5 ± 0.4	

*Range of responses.

LHRH testing in patients with known hypothalamic disease may also give ambiguous responses. In the Mortimer series,[21] patients with isolated gonadotropin deficiency, believed by most workers to be due to hypothalamic disease, had impaired or absent responses in 11 of 15 cases. In craniopharyngiomas, thought to have destroyed the hypothalamus or stalk region or both (and not the pituitary), more than half of the cases had impaired or absent responses to LHRH. FSH responses generally, but not always, followed LH changes. These observations, made by a number of other workers as well, indicate that long-standing hypothalamic disease that has led to LHRH failure causes a loss of sensitivity of the pituitary to LHRH. This is true whether the insufficiency arises from organic disease of the hypothalamus or to the "functional disturbance" seen in anorexia nervosa or psychogenic amenorrhea. In patients with anorexia nervosa, responsivity to LHRH returns with clinical recovery.

The loss of sensitivity to LHRH is restored by giving repeated injections of LHRH. Responses, initially absent, may thus be restored to normal. Since this may occur in some patients with intrinsic pituitary disease (as well as in patients with hypothalamic disease), it is likely that LHRH can stimulate the function (or hyperplasia) of remnant gonadotropic cells. Even though gonadotropic failure is one of the earliest manifestations of hypothalamic or pituitary disease in many patients, LHRH responsiveness is retained even when ACTH, TSH, or GH deficiency is present.

The foregoing discussion indicates that the LHRH test alone given as a single bolus injection is of limited value in differentiating between hypothalamic and pituitary disease. On the other hand, in states of primary gonadal insufficiency, LHRH-induced LH and FSH responses are usually exaggerated, suggesting that the hyperfunctional state in some way is a hyper-responsive state. This is also true in postmenopausal women.

In prepubertal children, responses to LHRH are absent or minimal. This may be due to the low gonadal hormone levels or, more likely, to the fact that endogenous LHRH is not being secreted. It is probable that endogenous LHRH, released as puberty unfolds, accounts for pubertal development of the pituitary and of its sensitization.

It can be anticipated that the LHRH test will be refined for diagnostic purposes by

345

Table 8. Serum LH and FSH Responses to LHRH in 155 Patients with Hypothalamic-Pituitary-Gonadal Dysfunction

Condition	Total	LH				FSH			
		Normal	Absent	Impaired	Exaggerated	Normal	Absent	Impaired	Exaggerated
Hypothalamic disease									
Isolated gonadotrophin deficiency	15	4	3	8		9	3	3	
Craniopharyngioma	10	4	5	1		2	5	3	
Isolated TRH deficiency	1			1		1			
Tumors	2		1	1		1		1	
Pituitary disease									
Nonfunctioning pituitary tumors	31	11	1	19		28		3	
Acromegaly	27	6		21		11		16	
Cushing's disease	3	1		1	1	2		1	
Sheehan's syndrome	2			2		2			
Idiopathic hypopituitarism	6	1	4	1		4	2		
Amenorrhea syndromes									
Delayed puberty—primary amenorrhea	4	1		2	1	2		2	
Anorexia nervosa	13	6		2	5	8		2	3
Secondary amenorrhea and galactorrhea	15	7			8	14			1
Polycystic ovary syndrome	3	2			1	2		1	
Turner's syndrome	2				2				2
Male syndromes									
Delayed puberty	3	3				2		1	
Precocious puberty	1	1				1			
Testicular feminization	1				1				1
Primary gonadal failure	7	2			5	1		1	6
Anorexia nervosa	1			1				1	
Galactorrhea	3	2	1			2		1	
Gynecomastia	2	2				2			
Miscellaneous									
Internal hydrocephaly	2	1	1			2			
Werner's syndrome	1				1				1
Total	155	54 (35%)	16 (10%)	60 (39%)	25 (16%)	95 (61%)	10 (7%)	36 (23%)	14 (9%)

(Adapted from Mortimer, C. H., et al.: *Luteinizing hormone and follicle stimulating hormone-releasing hormone test in patients with hypothalamic-pituitary-gonadal dysfunction.* Br. Med. J. 4:73, 1973.)

means of various steroid priming regimens and by the use of more precisely determined doses, but data of this sort have not yet been accumulated in sufficient amount.

REFERENCES

1. BASSIRI, R. M. AND UTIGER, R. D.: *The preparation and specificity of antibody to thyrotropin releasing hormone.* Endocrinology 90:722, 1972.

2. BEARDWELL, C. G.: *Radioimmunoassay of arginine vasopressin in human plasma.* J. Clin. Endocrinol. 33:254, 1971.

3. BERSON, S. A. AND YALOW, R. S.: *General principles of radioimmunoassay.* Clin. Chim. Acta 22:51, 1968.

4. BERSON, S. A. AND YALOW, R. S.: *Radioimmunoassay for ACTH in plasma.* J. Clin. Invest. 47:2725, 1968.

5. BOYD, G. W., LANDON, J. AND PEART, W. S.: *Radioimmunoassay for determining plasma levels of Angiotensin II in man.* Lancet 2:1002, 1967.

6. CHOPRA, I. J., HO, R. S. AND LAM, R.: *An improved radioimmunoassay of triiodothyronine in serum: its application to clinical and physiological studies.* J. Lab. Clin. Med. 80:729, 1972.

7. COHEN, E. L., ET AL.: *Accurate and rapid measurement of plasma renin activity by radioimmunoassay.* J. Lab. Clin. Med. 77:1025, 1971.

8. COYOTUPA, J., PARLOW, A. F. AND ABRAHAM, G. E.: *Simultaneous radioimmunoassay of plasma for testosterone and dihydrotestosterone.* Anal. Lett. 5:229, 1972.

9. DEFTOS, L. J., ET AL.: *Immunoassay for human calcitonin. II. Clinical studies.* Metabolism 20:1129, 1971.

10. EDDY, R. L., ET AL.: *Human growth hormone release. Comparison of provocative test procedures.* Am. J. Med. 56:179, 1974.

11. EKINS, R. P.: *Basic principles and theory in radioimmunoassay and saturation analysis.* Br. Med. Bull. 30:3, 1974.

12. FAGLIA, G., ET AL.: *Plasma thyrotropin response to thyrotropin-releasing hormone in patients with pituitary and hypothalamic disorders.* J. Clin. Endocrinol. Metab. 37:595, 1973.

13. FLEISCHER, N., ET AL.: *Synthetic thyrotropin releasing factor as a test of pituitary thyrotropin reserve.* J. Clin. Endrocrinol. Metab. 34:617, 1972.

14. GANTT, M.: Personal communication.

15. GLICK, S. M, ET AL.: *Immunoassay of human growth hormone in plasma.* Nature (London) 199:784, 1963.

16. JAFFE, B. M. AND BEHRMAN, H. (EDS.): *Methods of Hormone Radioimmunoassay.* Academic Press, New York, 1974.

17. JEFFCOATE, S. L., ET AL.: *Radioimmunoassay of luteinizing hormone releasing factor.* J. Endocrinol. 57: 189, 1973.

18. KAPLAN, S. L., ET AL.: *Thyrotropin-releasing factor (TRF) effect on secretion of human pituitary prolactin and thyrotropin in children and in idiopathic hypopituitary dwarfism: further evidence for hypophysiotropic hormone deficiencies.* Endocrinol. Metab. 35:825, 1972.

19. LEMARCHAND-BERAUD, T., ET AL.: *Influence of different physiological conditions on the gonadotropins and thyrotropin response to LH-RH and TRH. In* Luft, R. and Yalow, R. S. (eds.): *Radioimmunoassay: Methodology and Applications in Physiology and in Clinical Studies, Hormone and Metabolic Research,* Supplement Series, vol. 5. Georg Thieme, Stuttgart, 1974, p. 170.

20. LUNDBERG, P. O. AND WIDE, L.: *The response to TRH, LH-RH, metyrapone and vasopressin in patients with hypothalamus-pituitary disorders.* Europ. J. Clin. Invest. 3:49, 1973.

21. MORTIMER, C. H., ET AL.: *The luteinizing hormone and follicle stimulating hormore-releasing hormone test in patients with hypothalamic-pituitary-gonadal dysfunction.* Br. Med. J. 4:73, 1973.

22. NABARRO, J. D. N. (ED.): *Radioimmunoassay and saturation analysis.* Brit. Med. Bull. 30:1, 1974.

23. NELSON, J. C., KOLLAR, D. J. AND LEWIS, J. E.: *Growth hormone secretion in pituitary disease.* Arch. Int. Med. 133:459, 1974.

24. ODELL, W. D. AND DAUGHADAY, W. H. (EDS.): *Principles of Competitive Protein-Binding Assays.* Lippincott, Philadelphia, 1971.

25. ORMSTON, B. J., ET AL.: *Thyrotropin-releasing hormone as a thyroid-function test.* Lancet 1:10, 1971.

26. PIMSTONE, B. L., BECKER, D. J. AND KRONHEIM, S.: *FSH and LH response to LH releasing hormone in*

normal and malnourished infants. In Luft, R. and Yalow, R. S. (eds.): *Radioimmunoassay: Methodology and Applications in Physiology and in Clinical Studies, Hormone and Metabolic Research.* Supplement Series, vol. 5, Georg Thieme, Stuttgart, 1974, p. 179.

27. SAKODA, M., ET AL.: *Effect of synthetic thyrotropin-releasing factor (TRF) on pituitary TSH secretion in men.* Endocrinol. Jpn. 17:541, 1970.

28. STEINER, A. L., KIPNIS, D. M. AND UTIGER, R.: *Radioimmunoassay for the measurement of adenosine 3',5'-cyclic phosphate.* Proc. Natl. Acad. Sci. U.S.A. 64:367, 1969.

29. SNYDER, P. J., ET AL.: *Diagnostic value of thyrotrophin-releasing hormone in pituitary and hypothalamic diseases; assessment of thyrotrophin and prolactin secretion in 100 patients.* Ann. Int. Med. 81:751, 1974.

30. SYNDER, P. J., REITANO, J. F. AND UTIGER, R. D.: *Serum LH and FSH responses to synthetic gonadotropin-releasing hormone in normal men.* J. Clin. Endocrinol. Metab. 41:938, 1975.

31. SPECTOR, S.: Radioimunoassay. *Ann. Rev. Pharmacol.* 13:359, 1973.

32. UNDERWOOD, R. H. AND WILLIAMS, G. H.: *The simultaneous measurement of aldosterone, cortisol and corticosterone in human peripheral plasma by displacement analysis.* J. Lab. Clin. Med. 79:848, 1972.

33. WU, C. H. AND LUNDY, L. E.: *Radioimmunoassay of plasma estrogens.* Steroids 18:91, 1971.

34. FRANTZ, A. G.: Personal communication.

BIBLIOGRAPHY

BERSON, S. A. AND YALOW, R. S.: *General principles of radioimmunoassay.* Clin. Chim. Acta 22:51, 1968.

EKINS, R. P.: *Basic principles and theory in radioimmunoassay and saturation analysis.* Br. Med. Bull. 30:3, 1974.

JAFFE, B. M. AND BEHRMAN, H. (EDS.): *Methods of Hormone Radioimmunoassay.* Academic Press, New York, 1974.

NABARRO, J. D. N. (ED.): *Radioimmunoassay and saturation analysis.* Brit. Med. Bull. 30:1, 1974.

ODELL, W. D. AND DAUGHADAY, W. H. (EDS.): *Principles of Competitive Protein-Binding Assays.* Lippincott, Philadelphia, 1971.

CHAPTER 15

Treatment of Hypothalamic-Pituitary Disease

PITUITARY ADENOMAS

Pituitary adenomas account for approximately 5 to 10 per cent of all symptomatic intracranial tumors. Autopsy studies show that 10 to 20 per cent of pituitary glands contain small discrete adenomas, half of which are asymptomatic,[2, 6] More than 75 per cent of pituitary adenomas in adults are classified as chromophobes on the basis of classic histologic stains and light microscopy. More recently, studies by electron microscopy have shown that the cells of most, if not all, chromophobe adenomas contain secretory granules. After the development of prolactin radioimmunoassays, it became apparent that up to 30 to 50 per cent of such tumors secrete prolactin, with similar incidences in men and women. That many of these tumors were originally thought to be nonfunctional can be attributed to the fact that hyperprolactinemia may not produce recognizable symptoms, particularly in men. Pituitary adenomas are rare in childhood and when they occur, are most often associated with GH secretory excess, i.e., gigantism.

Eosinophile adenomas account for approximately 10 to 15 per cent of pituitary tumors.[6] They are usually associated with excessive secretion of GH or prolactin, and occasionally, of both. Basophile adenomas of the pituitary are associated with excess ACTH and, more rarely, with excess TSH secretion; these tumors are usually small and do not commonly produce significant enlargement of the sella turcica. Skull roentgenograms of patients with Cushing's disease may show decreased bone density due to cortisol-induced osteoporosis. Enlargement of the pituitary may occur after adrenalectomy for Cushing's disease (Nelson's syndrome). Such enlargement is due to hyperplasia and hypertrophy of ACTH-secreting cells which may result in enlargement of the pituitary fossa, headaches, and local extension. Basophile tumors of this type, the most invasive of the pituitary adenomas, may become inoperable. Rarely, pituitary tumors may secrete two hormones. Cases of tumors that secreted both prolactin and GH, ACTH and GH, ACTH and prolactin, and GH and TSH have been reported.

Nonfunctioning Adenomas

In addition to the frequent finding of small, asymptomatic microadenomas at autopsy, in other cases evident enlargement and erosion of the pituitary fossa have been noted without symptoms of pituitary disease during life.[18] On the other hand, most patients in whom the diagnosis of chromophobe adenoma has been made on the basis of an enlarged sella or local compression signs, will show continued tumor growth requiring treatment. In the series reported by Sheline,[33] 16 cases were followed for four to twenty years without treatment (because the patient had refused it, or because the doctor believed that the disease was not progressive). Of tumors in these 16 patients, only two showed neither clinical nor roentgenographic evidence of growth. The other 14 showed changes as early as six months and as late as 15 years from the time of initial diagnosis, and all required treatment. Among the manifestations of tumor growth were increasing sella size, shrinking of visual fields,[14] and headaches. For this reason, careful differential diagnosis and treatment of asymptomatic pituitary enlargement is recommended. In the case of functioning tumors, such as eosinophile, basophile, and prolactin-secreting adenomas, treatment is indicated for the reduction of the abnormal secretion as well as for prevention or amelioration of local compression manifestations. Due to the relatively frequent occurrence of "empty sella," differential diagnosis should be made before treatment with roentgenotherapy.

Surgery

The earliest treatment used for adenomas was surgical. As early as 1906 Horsley approached the pituitary by way of the middle cranial fossa, and Schloffer in 1907 operated by the extracranial, transsphenoidal route.[31] According to MacCarty and col-

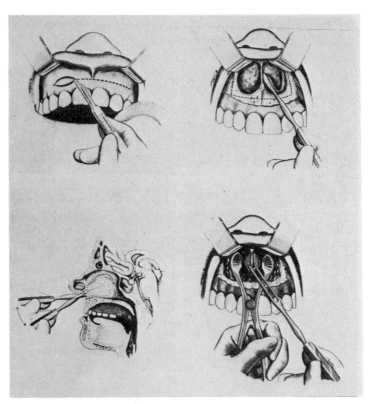

Figure 1. Surgical approach to transsphenoidal hypophysectomy. Incision is made in mucosa of upper jaw and the maxillary and sphenoid sinuses are opened to approach the anterior, inferior margin of the pituitary fossa (From Hardy, J.: *Transsphenoidal surgery of hypersecreting pituitary tumors. In* Kohler, P. O. and Ross, G. T. (eds.): *Diagnosis and Treatment of Pituitary Tumors.* American Elsevier, New York, 1973, with permission.)

leagues,[25] the first successful endonasal, transsphenoidal approach was that of Hirsch, who in 1910 removed two tumors. Cushing initially favored the extracranial approach, but later developed the transfrontal procedure which became the most widely used technique. More recently, the development of microsurgical methods,[12, 13] the availability of antibiotics, and improved roentgenologic techniques[3, 5, 30] have repopularized the transsphenoidal approach which is now gaining increasing acceptance for most types of pituitary tumor.

The classic transfrontal, intracranial approach to the pituitary is still indicated in several circumstances, which include the presence of significant optic-chiasm or optic-nerve compression, compression of the hypothalamus, visual disturbance in the empty-sella syndrome (due to herniation of the optic chiasm into the pituitary fossa), and suprasellar extension when the intracranial portion is separated from the intrasellar portion by a narrow neck.[7, 17, 22, 25] Pituitary apoplexy and invasive adenomas may be treated by the transfrontal or transsphenoidal approach. The transfrontal approach is not without substantial risk, although some surgeons have reported series with almost no mortality. In the pre-cortisone era, Cushing had a mortality rate of 2.4 per cent in his last 205 operations. Bronson Ray reported no deaths in a series of 80 patients treated with benefit of cortisone.[25] At the Mayo Clinic, an overall operative mortality of 6.8 per cent was recorded which in the steroid era was reduced to only 3 per cent.[25] With massive extrasellar extension, mortality is greater. Wound infection occurs in 3 to 4 per cent of cases, and postoperative convulsive disorders occur in 3 to 4 per cent of cases operated via the transfrontal route. Unilateral or bilateral loss of the sense of smell is frequent after the transfrontal approach, and there is some threat to vision, since the blood supply to the optic chiasma is readily damaged by even minor manipulation in this area.

Transsphenoidal microsurgery has gained increased prominence through the work of Guiot[12] and Hardy.[13] The subnasal, midline rhinoseptal transsphenoidal approach is now mainly used. The sphenoid sinus is exposed by dissection of the cartilaginous nasal septum and the sphenoid sinus entered (Figs 1 and 2). The anterior wall of the pituitary fossa is removed under direct observation with a dissecting microscope and the tumor excised by a combination of blunt dissection and aspiration. Adenomas do not have a clearly defined capsule. An effort is made to separate tumor from normal pituitary so as to preserve normal function. Guiot recommends the transsphenoidal approach in five situations: 1) elderly patients, 2) patients almost blind because of long-standing optic chiasmal compression, 3) pituitary apoplexy, 4) invasive adenomas, and 5) downward

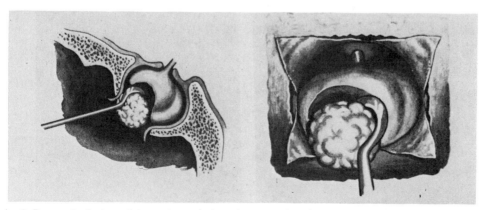

Figure 2. Removal of microadenoma from pituitary by transsphenoidal approach (from Hardy,: *Transsphenoidal surgery of hypersecreting pituitary tumors. In* Kohler, P. O. and Ross, G. T. (eds.): *Diagnosis and Treatment of Pituitary Tumors.* American Elsevier, New York, 1973, with permission.)

351

tumor extension. Hardy[13] emphasizes both endocrinologic and compressive indications for transsphenoidal microsurgery. These include functioning pituitary adenomas of all kinds. Hardy recommends transsphenoidal removal of some large suprasellar extensions and even some craniopharyngiomas. He believes that removal from below permits many suprasellar tumors to drop down into the sella where they may be removed. Complications of the transsphenoidal approach include CSF rhinorrhea (9 of 475 in Guiot's series), meningitis (3 of 475) and sudden worsening of vision. This last condition may be due to blood clots or herniation of the optic nerves into the fossa. In the case of functioning adenomas, residual hypersecretory tissue may be left behind (see below).

Radiation Therapy

Roentgenotherapy (conventional or supervoltage) is widely used in the treatment of chromophobe adenomas, either alone or in addition to surgical therapy.[11, 21]

The series of Sheline[33] is representative of radiation treatment of chromophobe adenomas, and utilized bilateral opposed fields using 1 MeV. or higher-energy photon beams with total doses to the pituitary of 4,000 to 5,000 rads over a period of five to six weeks with five fractions per week. Lower doses appear to be less effective. No evidence of further tumor growth, with maintenance of any improvement in symptoms or signs, was taken as evidence of control. As a practical matter, visual-field deterioration was used as the chief indicator of tumor growth. A total of 133 patients with chromophobe adenomas were included in this study. Twenty received radiation alone, 36 had surgical decompression, and 77 had a combination of surgery and radiation therapy. Immediate improvement during the first one to two years was similar in all three groups, but recurrence was much more frequent in the surgically treated group who did not receive radiation therapy. The addition of surgery to radiation was no better than radiation alone at either five or ten years after treatment. Because the recurrence rate after surgery alone is much greater, Sheline, and most others, recommends radiation therapy of *all* surgically treated chromophobe adenomas. No complications were definitely attributed to radiation treatment. Kjellberg[38] does not routinely recommend irradiation after surgical removal of a chromophobe adenoma. Instead, he places a radiopaque marker above the pituitary at the time of resection, and observes this marker by serial x-ray studies over time. Only if the marker shows signs of tumor growth does he then advocate radiation therapy.

In the management of hyperfunctioning adenomas, betatron therapy[23] has been widely used in addition to conventional radiotherapy, and, in two centers in the United States, proton-beam irradiation.[10, 19] Other ablative approaches include stereotaxic transsphenoidal cryohypophysectomy,[28] stereotaxic transsphenoidal thermal coagulation, and direct implantation of radioactive substances such as yttrium or gold.[8, 9] Pituitary ablation has also been carried out in the palliative treatment of carcinoma of the breast and prostate, and in diabetic retinopathy.[9, 28, 31]

Hyperfunctioning Adenomas

The objective of treatment of GH-, prolactin-, and ACTH-secreting adenomas includes a reduction in secretion rate as well as management of the local space-occupying manifestations.

Acromegaly

Management of acromegaly must take into consideration a number of factors: presence of local damage, severity of diabetes and other manifestations caused by growth-hormone hypersecretion, age, general health, and the importance of preserving residual pituitary function. Ideal therapy of acromegaly requires that morbidity and mortality be less than that of the untreated disease, that GH levels be reduced to less than 5 ng./ml. without induction of hypopituitarism, that extrasellar-pressure effects are prevented or cured, and that the reduction in GH levels be rapid when the clinical situation so demands. No single mode of treatment presently available fully meets these requirements.

Therapeutic benefit is demonstrated objectively by a decline in the elevated levels of GH, and by the regression of characteristic acromegalic signs and symptoms (Fig. 3). When GH levels are reduced, most acromegalic patients show improved carbohydrate tolerance, although the abnormality may not clear completely, and the increased sweating decreases or disappears. Surprisingly, the soft-tissue overgrowth, so common a feature of acromegaly, may show remarkable regression. The hands and feet decrease in volume, nasal prominence decreases, and the skin becomes much less coarse. These changes, which can occur over a few days or weeks after hypophysectomy, are accompanied by marked excretion of nitrogenous products in the urine. Back pain and other skeletal complaints also may improve dramatically, and blood pressure often falls into the normal range. It is, of course, essential to determine the effects of treatment on other pituitary tropic functions, such as thyroid and adrenal regulation, and give appropriate hormone replacement therapy.

Most neurosurgeons believe that acromegalic patients with significant suprasellar extension, giving rise to either hypothalamic or optic chiasmal compression, require surgical hypophysectomy via the transfrontal approach. The question of whether such patients should ever be operated by the transsphenoidal route remains unsettled at this time. The results obtained by Hardy[13] have been encouraging but the number of patients thus treated remains small. Others do not advocate transsphenoidal surgery for patients with severe visual disturbance. In general, the current practice in most North American centers is to decompress by the transfrontal approach all tumors that extend into the suprasellar area.

In the absence of neurologic involvement the choice in acromegaly is among a) no treatment, b) irradiation, c) surgery, d) drugs.

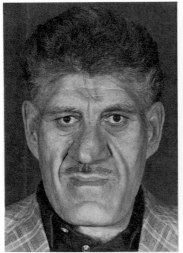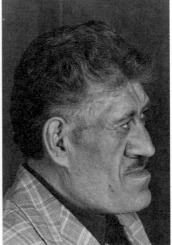

Figure 3. 56-year-old man with acromegaly. Serum GH levels were 220 ng./ml. Skull roentgenogram showed a large pituitary erosion extending deep into the sphenoid sinus. Visual fields were normal.

No Treatment

The older literature commonly referred to "burned-out" acromegaly. The development of radioimmunoassays for GH has largely put this notion to rest; virtually all cases of untreated acromegaly have elevated GH levels.[11] Acromegaly is a progressive disease and a decision not to treat must take into consideration the fact that morbidity and mortality in acromegaly are twice that expected in the general population. The progression of the disease and its complications do not correlate with levels of radioimmunoassayable GH in plasma; a definition of "mild" acromegaly is, therefore, difficult to find. Most patients should be treated unless age, general health, or psycho-social factors supervene.

Radiation Therapy

Conventional high-voltage or betatron radiation of the pituitary has long been the standard form of radiation therapy for acromegaly, but the value of this form of treatment is still a subject of controversy. Conventional therapy is defined by Sheline as being "megavoltage radiation given in a single fractionated course of about 5 treatments per week to a total dose of approximately 5,000 rads in 5 to 6 weeks."[33] By clinical criteria (and before immunoassay was developed) it was believed that 50 to 75 per cent of treated patients had a remission of their disease, but early studies utilizing radioimmunoassay indicated that most patients (75 per cent) did not have a decrease in GH levels below 7.5 ng./ml. As experience has accumulated, a number of workers have pointed out that a large proportion of patients show adequate benefit after conventional treatment but this response takes a long time to develop fully. For example, in the series of Sheline,[33] 13 of 17 patients studied between 2 and 24 years after therapy had complete return to normal GH levels. Similar findings by Gorden and Roth[11] indicate that in patients followed for three to six years after treatment with 4,000 to 4,500 rads, almost 75 per cent had GH levels under 10 ng./ml. and almost 50 per cent had GH concentrations of 5 ng./ml. or less. Conventional radiation has the further advantages of being available in most communities, being applicable to patients with irregularly shaped tumors with lateral or inferior extension, having a very low incidence of complications such as visual disturbance, and rarely causing pituitary insufficiency.

The main disadvantage of conventional radiation is the long delay in ablating GH hypersecretion, no effect usually being seen before six months. In cases of severe diabetes, skeletal manifestations, and cardiac disease, this long lag may not be tolerable. Other disadvantages are that a significant proportion of patients are not brought under control (as many as 25 per cent at five years), the treatment requires daily visits to the hospital for five to six weeks and thus may not be feasible for many patients, and epilation is extremely common.

The most widely used alternative form of radiation therapy in the United States and Canada is the proton beam. This technique, pioneered by Lawrence and coworkers[23, 24, 39] in the Donner Laboratory, California, and by Kjellberg and Kliman at the Massachusetts General Hospital in Boston,[19] depends on the availability of cyclotron-generated protons delivered to the pituitary region under carefully controlled conditions. Because the energy release of protons is highly localized (as compared with electrons or x-rays) it is possible to deliver as much as 12,000 to 15,000 rads to the pituitary without damaging skin or skull. The intensity of this form of energy necessitates extremely careful control to avoid damage to optic nerves, cranial nerves, temporal lobe, and hypothalamus. The method is appropriate only in patients whose lesions are confined to the pituitary fossa, are regular in outline, and are unaccompanied by local signs of hypothalamic or optic-chiasm compression. The procedure also requires preliminary pneumoencephalography and cavernous sinograms to outline the tumor adequately. At least 53 per cent of cases so treated show a fall of GH to the normal range, and in most of the others some degree of reduction in GH occurs. Proton-beam radiation has the following advantages: it produces maximum effects within two years (in contrast to three years or longer with conventional therapy), requires only a two- or four-day hospitalization instead of a six-week course of daily treatments, and is usually unaccompanied by epilation. The incidence of side effects, however, is somewhat greater after proton-beam radiation than after conventional radiation. In the compliation of Kjellberg and Kliman[19] of their second 100 cases (in which most of the technical problems of radiation, dosimetry, and localization had been resolved), the following complications were observed: temporary disturbance in extraocular movements, 12 per cent; visual impairment, 2 per cent; partial hypopituitarism, 3 per cent; total hypopituitarism, 6 per cent; transient diabetes insipidus, 3 per cent; seizures, 2 per cent. Other complications, observed in a small number of cases, were minor temporal-lobe disturbance (episodes of sensory or olfactory aura) requiring anticonvulsants, and disturbed mentation.

Proton-beam radiation has the disadvantages of requiring high-level technology available only in two centers in the United States, being applicable only when the tumor is confined to the sella, and not being fully effective in an appreciable number of cases.

Because of the high incidence of optic-nerve and cranial-nerve damage and brain necrosis in patients treated with more than 5,000 rads by conventional methods or 15,000 rads by proton beam, it is widely recommended that patients not be given a second course of radiation therapy if they have already received one full course. Also the incidence of sarcoma of the pituitary is increased in patients given more than one course of treatment.

Another radiation method which has been used in an attempt to destroy the pituitary (both adenomas and the normal gland, in metastatic cancer of the breast or diabetes mellitus) is the implantation of particles of radioactive yttrium (^{90}Y) or of radioactive gold (^{198}Au) by means of a transsphenoidal stereotaxic approach.[9] ^{90}Y is a hard beta emitter, and ^{198}Au a moderate gamma emitter; both have been shown to be capable of destroying pituitary tissue. A number of studies were reported using these techniques in the late 1950s and early 1960s, but they have been given up in most centers because of the relatively high frequency of complications. In the series of 12 patients reported by Fraser and coworkers[9] using ^{90}Y, two patients developed meningitis, two incurred a permanent rhinorrhea, and two had field defects. In Rand's series,[31] 12 to 15 per cent of patients had delayed radionecrosis of the floor of the sella with subsequent cerebrospinal rhinorrhea and meningitis. Radioactive gold causes fewer complications and effectively destroys normal pituitary tissue, but is less effective in treatment of tumors, particularly acromegaly. In the 1961 series of Joplin[17] (before the immunoassay era), insulin resistance improved in 7 of 11, and 9 of 10 patients had regression of headache, but only 1 of 15 had a decrease in hand volume.

These specialized radiation methods have mainly been abandoned in favor of surgical ablation including cryohypophysectomy, diathermic hypophysectomy, and transsphenoidal microsurgery.

Transsphenoidal Cryohypophysectomy and Thermal Hypophysectomy

Several groups of neurosurgeons have used intense cold to destroy the pituitary gland, using an extracranial transsphenoidal stereotaxic approach with a cryoprobe cooled with liquid nitrogen. The probe is placed in a paracentral position on each side of the midline of the pituitary and the tip cooled for increasingly long periods of time. In order to avoid damage to surrounding nerve tissue, the patient is obliged to remain awake and cooperative. In Rand's 1973 series,[32] 19 of 27 acromegalic patients showed cure of the disease as demonstrated by serum GH levels below 4 ng./ml.; in seven, values ranged between 5 and 10 ng.; and one had a GH level of 12 ng./ml. These 27 successfully treated cases were from a larger group of 32 cases. Meningitis and rhinorrhea developed in one case. This procedure cannot be used in patients with significant suprasellar growth. In another series, 76 per cent of cases had GH values of 10 ng./ml. or less after treatment, but in those with preoperative values over 40 ng./ml., only 50 per cent were cured. Cryosurgery does not have a great advantage over conventional radiation therapy for acromegaly, except that the response is rapid, and in some hands, a somewhat higher remission rate is obtained. Only a few surgical centers are equipped for this procedure. On the other hand, cryosurgery is a reasonable alternative to transsphenoidal hypophysectomy for removal of normal pituitaries.

Thermal ablation by radiofrequency-heated electrodes has been pioneered by Zervas.[37] In this procedure, the transnasal transsphenoidal approach is used and the electrode inserted on each side of the midline. A specially designed electrode permits the heating of up to 1 cm. of tissue on each side of the midline, and a series of 18 to 30 overlapping lesions are made with an electrode temperature of 80° C for 30 to 60 seconds. Immediate clinical remission was observed in 16 of 18 patients reported by Zervas, and levels of GH less than 10 ng./ml. were noted in 15 cases. The response required six to twelve weeks. The complications of the procedure included one case of partial oculomotor nerve palsy and one case of intrasellar hemorrhage requiring decompression. No meningitis or rhinorrhea developed, and in only one case (the first patient treated) has there been a relapse, after follow-ups of six months to six years. All patients became hypopituitary and diabetes insipidus appeared transiently in two. This method has been used mainly in one hospital center, and has the disadvantage of producing the highest incidence of panhypopituitarism of any modality of treatment other than transfrontal hypophysectomy.

MICROSURGERY

This technique, first used by Cushing, was later abandoned in favor of the transfrontal approach but was re-established by Guiot[12] in 1958 in France. Subsequently, Hardy,[13] in Montreal, developed a number of technical improvements and extended the indications for use of the modified approach to the treatment of other tumors, including craniopharyngioma, chordoma, and occasionally ectopic pinealoma or teratoma. The results of transsphenoidal treatment in acromegaly have been encouraging but the series reported remain small in number. Hardy has reported a reduction in GH to normal levels in 63 of 79 operations since 1962.[40] The morbidity was minimal; patients routinely were up and about on the day after surgery and discharged from hospital within seven to fourteen days. There was no death in his series. Endocrine replacement was required in less than 15 to 20 per cent of cases; recurrence was rare in patients who had not received prior radiation and who had normal postoperative GH levels. In a series of 100 cases of acromegaly reported by Williams and coworkers[36] in London, the initial treatment of 68 was surgical (nine underwent transfrontal hypophysectomy and 59 transsphenoidal hypophysectomy). The remainder were not treated because of age, concurrent illness, apparent mildness of the condition, or refusal of treatment. There was no death due to treatment in the 59 patients operated by the transsphenoidal route; one patient died at home six weeks later of a pulmonary embolus, one developed CSF rhinorrhea that stopped spontaneously after two weeks, and three suffered acute frontal sinusitis that responded to antibiotics. The results of this series are shown in Figure 4. A satisfactory response to operation, defined as a fall in plasma GH to less than 5

TRANSPHENOIDAL SURGERY FOR ACROMEGALY

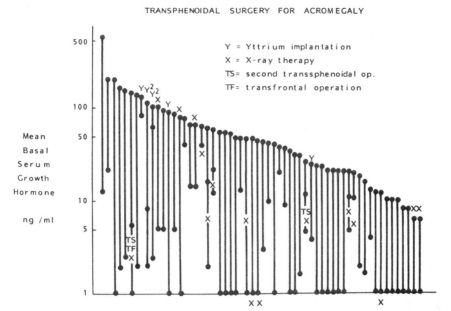

Figure 4. Decline in serum growth-hormone levels in 59 cases treated with transsphenoidal hypophysectomy. (From Williams, R. A., et al.: *The treatment of acromegaly with special reference to trans-sphenoidal hypophysectomy.* Quart. J. Med. 44:85, 1975, with permission.)

ng./ml. was achieved in 39 of 59 patients (66 per cent). Seven patients required subsequent treatment consisting of either roentgenotherapy (five patients) or implantation of radioactive yttrium (two patients).

Atkinson and associates[1] have reported a series of 17 patients in which serum GH decreased to less than 5 ng./ml. in seven of nine previously untreated cases. They emphasized, as did Hardy, that prior radiation or radioactive implants make the microsurgery more difficult and reduce the chance of "cure." In this series, one patient died of meningitis and another patient became blind after orbital fracture. The authors emphasize that the transsphenoidal approach requires great surgical care and that new surgical teams must be properly trained in the technique.[29] They emphasize that some suprasellar tumors can be removed via the transsphenoidal route because evacuation of the sella turcica often allows the suprasellar portion of the tumor to collapse back into the fossa.

Relief of headache and sweating, two prominent complaints in acromegaly, is frequently noted immediately after the operation. Symptoms of carpal-tunnel compression often clear during the first postoperative week, and a reduction in soft-tissue thickening is evident within a month. The resolution of signs and symptoms correlates closely to GH levels (i.e., reduction to less than 5 ng./ml.). In the Williams series,[36] carbohydrate tolerance improved significantly in all patients when GH was reduced to normal levels. The majority of patients operated on via the transsphenoidal approach recover without deficit of other anterior pituitary hormones. We believe that this is related primarily to the fact that hypothalamic-pituitary connections are preserved, and that even small amounts of residual pituitary tissue can return to normal function under normal hypothalamic drive.

As transsphenoidal microsurgery has advanced technically, we have increasingly recommended this form of surgical approach in patients with small tumors and no major

357

suprasellar extension, in young patients in whom preservation of gonadotropin function is important, and in patients in whom rapid decrease in GH levels is necessary.

PHARMACOLOGIC TREATMENT

ESTROGENS. The earliest pharmacologic treatment for acromegaly was estrogen therapy, which produces in some cases a decrease in the severity of the metabolic disturbance. The basis of this treatment has recently been shown to be a suppression in the formation of somatomedin, the intermediary of GH action on the skeleton. Estrogen therapy does not depress the secretion of GH, and, in fact, may increase GH secretion, due presumably to direct stimulation of somatotrope cell function. In experimental animals, estrogen administration sensitizes the pituitary to GH releasing-factor and, after prolonged administration, may induce mammotrophic-somatotrophic pituitary tumors. The use of estrogen therapy in treatment of acromegaly fell into disrepute following the observation that a large proportion of patients so treated developed pituitary apoplexy. The possibility that estrogens may stimulate the tumor directly, and the modest benefits of the treatment have led clinicians away from estrogen therapy, but an adequate trial using modern techniques for evaluation, particularly in cases resistant to other forms of therapy, should be carried out. Gordon and Roth[11] have reported favorable results in a few cases.

PROGESTERONE. A number of workers have studied the effects of progesterone derivatives on GH secretion. In particular, medroxyprogesterone acetate (MPA) has been shown in some cases to reduce GH levels. In the early report of Lawrence and Kirsteins,[24] 10 of 12 patients had a decline in plasma GH levels after six days of treatment, together with a blunting of the GH response to arginine. In later studies of Malarkey and Daughaday[26] and of Jackson and Ormston,[16] less than 50 per cent of cases had a lowering of GH levels, and in most cases, the GH concentration failed to fall to the normal range. MPA, like estrogen therapy, has been discarded as primary therapy. A trial of combined estrogen and progesterone has not, as far as we know, been reported.

CHLORPROMAZINE. In 1971, Kolodny and coworkers[20] reported that treatment of one patient with chlorpromazine led to a reduction in plasma GH levels from 18 to 4 ng./ml. Unfortunately, other workers have failed to confirm this finding. There has been no systematic study of single and combined neuroleptic agents designed to inhibit all three of the biogenic amines thought to be involved in physiologic GH regulation of GH secretion, i.e., dopaminergic, serotonergic and catecholaminergic factors. The identification of paradoxic suppression of GH in acromegaly by dopaminergic agents has, however, led to trials with other pharmacologic agents.

BROMERGOCRYPTINE. Bromergocryptine is the first drug to be shown to have significant and meaningful effects in reducing GH secretion. This drug initially gained notice by virtue of its potent and sustained (up to eight hours) suppression of prolactin in patients with galactorrhea (see below). Several recent investigations have provided unequivocal evidence that up to 60 to 80 per cent of acromegalics show suppression in response to bromergocryptine; improvement in clinical symptoms in some cases is dramatic.[34] We are currently using this agent in patients in whom surgical or radiation treatment has failed to produce a definitive cure.

SOMATOSTATIN. The use of somatostatin in acromegaly is under investigation. Infusions of the peptide are effective in depressing GH, but the action is brief. Rebound secretion occurs within 15 to 30 minutes after infusion and the levels of GH reached are often higher than those present prior to infusion. A protamine-zinc suspension of somatostatin is reported to increase the duration of effect up to six hours. Long-acting analogues of somatostatin are being sought.

OVERVIEW OF THERAPEUTIC APPROACHES

In patients with suprasellar extension (judged by visual-field examination and pneumoencephalogram) transfrontal craniotomy is indicated unless an experienced neurosurgeon believes that the tumor can be removed by transsphenoidal hypophysectomy. In patients with tumor restricted to the pituitary fossa with little or no invasion of surrounding structures, the choice depends on the intensity of disease and the availability of skilled neurosurgeons and specialized radiation facilities. If the degree of GH hypersecretion is modest (less than 40 ng./ml.), one may consider conventional radiotherapy, proton-beam therapy, transsphenoidal hypophysectomy, thermal hypophysectomy, and cryohypophysectomy; all will yield approximately the same cure rate. The first is the most available and has the smallest number of complications, but takes the longest time to be effective. Of the other forms of therapy, the proton beam carries the lowest complication risk and has a relatively short lag time of effectiveness, but can be carried out in only a few centers. If therapy is urgent, transsphenoidal hypophysectomy is probably the best approach, but cryohypophysectomy and thermal hypophysectomy should be considered if the facility is available.

If the tumor has invaded the sphenoid sinus, with or without suprasellar invasion, transsphenoidal hypophysectomy is indicated unless other features of the case contraindicate this course.

If hypersecretion of GH persists after transsphenoidal hypophysectomy, reoperation is indicated. This procedure will increase the likelihood of panhypopituitarism (since the surgeon will be less scrupulous in removing questionable tissue), and of CSF rhinorrhea. If GH levels are still elevated, some form of radiation therapy is indicated. Since the effects of surgical hypophysectomy by any route are readily followed by measuring GH levels (unlike the situation with chromophobe adenomas), roentgenotherapy is not routine after hypophysectomy. If relapse occurs after transsphenoidal hypophysectomy, it usually happens within a few months.

The most distressing therapeutic problem in acromegaly, seen in an uncomfortably large proportion of cases (about 15 per cent), is persistent hypersecretion following surgery and radiation therapy. Such patients have either locally invasive eosinophilic tumors (a few of which have the histologic character of carcinomas) in the sphenoid sinus, the cavernous sinus, or even the temporal lobe, or have intrasellar tumors so large and extensive that ablation is impossible. Repeated courses of radiation carry the risk of inducing brain necrosis or sarcoma.

At this time, bromergocryptine will probably prove to be the best mode of treatment. Other alternatives, all less satisfactory, include MPA and estrogen administration. Somatostatin analogues may prove to be valuable in this situation. It must be admitted that some patients with acromegaly continue to show progressive damage from persistent GH hypersecretion unresponsive to current modes of treatment.

Prolactin-Secreting Tumors

The management of patients with hyperprolactinemia and prolactin-secreting pituitary tumors has evolved rapidly since the advent of the prolactin radioimmunoassay in 1971. In males, the primary symptoms and signs that bring a prolactin-secreting adenoma to the attention of the physician are the local tumor effects or loss of other pituitary functions.[35] Galactorrhea is relatively rare. In women, on the other hand, galactorrhea is common and amenorrhea is usually present. These changes are the presenting manifestations more commonly than local signs, such as headache and compromise of other pituitary functions. It should be re-emphasized that in both men and women loss of gonadotropic functions does not necessarily mean that either hypothalamus or pituitary is directly damaged since prolactin suppresses gonadotropic secretion by effects at the hypothalamic level.

As with acromegalic and chromophobe tumors (see above), management depends on the anatomic extent of the tumor as well as possible functional consequences. In males, management of small prolactin-secreting tumors (without suprasellar or local invasive features) is by either bromergocryptine administration, transsphenoidal hypophysectomy, conventional radiation therapy, or proton-beam radiation. In many cases, it may be advisable to follow the patient closely with repeated roentgenographic studies and measurement of prolactin levels, and to withhold treatment. If there is evidence of further tumor growth, conventional radiation can be considered since this form of treatment is the one most widely available. Transsphenoidal removal, as in the female, can produce a cure at least in so far as available follow-up studies indicate.

The management of female patients who present with the amenorrhea-galactorrhea syndrome has evolved rapidly in the past few years. This is due to: 1) the increasing proof that many such patients have small prolactin-secreting pituitary tumors, 2) the development of transsphenoidal microsurgical techniques that permit selective removal of the microadenoma, and 3) the increasing availability of bromergocryptine.

The initial assessment of such patients should include measurement of serum prolactin, careful roentgenographic studies of the sella turcica (including tomograms of the pituitary fossa obtained in both an anterior-posterior and lateral projection), and documentation of gonadotropin, estrogen, and progesterone secretion.[27] The great majority of such patients have low estrogen levels, low-normal values of serum LH and FSH, and a normal response to exogenous LHRH. Failure to respond to LHRH suggests that the tumor has destroyed most of the normal pituitary.

Serum prolactin levels in excess of 150 ng./ml. almost invariably indicate a tumor. Recent experience suggests that levels over 100 ng./ml. also usually indicate the presence of a tumor as opposed to a functional disturbance of inhibitory hypothalamic control. On the other hand, levels below 100 ng./ml. do not exclude the possibility of a tumor; we have investigated and operated on several patients with levels of 50 to 100 ng./ml. who have been found to have discrete tumors and who have been cured by the operation. Experience in several centers has now shown that prolactin stimulation by chlorpromazine or TRH, or inhibition by L-dopa or bromergocryptine is of limited value in distinguishing a hypothalamic versus pituitary etiology of hyperprolactinemia.

In most series, 5 to 10 per cent of prolactin-secreting tumors also secrete GH. Most of these cases present with acromegaly and are incidentally discovered on testing to have elevated PRL levels.

Tomographic examination of the sella turcica is now recognized to be of major importance in the detection of small microadenomas.[13, 27] A small asymmetric erosion of the floor of the sella is often not visible on plain skull films. Adenomas 3 to 5 mm. in diameter may produce radiologic changes that are detectable by tomography. On the other hand, the finding of an asymmetric sella is not diagnostic of a tumor. Congenital asymmetry of the sella without demonstrable functional pituitary tumor is occasionally found. Some of these cases may represent the nonfunctional pituitary adenomas that are found in 10 to 20 per cent of routine autopsies. Hardy[13] has emphasized that microadenomas can be localized to different regions of the gland, depending on the hormone that they secrete (Fig. 5).

A major problem at this time is how to manage a patient with elevated prolactin levels (greater than 100 ng./ml.) in whom tomography fails to demonstrate abnormality. In collaboration with Dr. Jules Hardy, Notre Dame Hospital, Montreal, we have had one such patient treated by transsphenoidal surgery, with removal of a microadenoma, re-

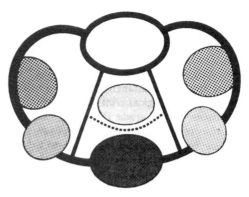

Figure 5. Diagramatic representation of regional distribution of pituitary microadenomas. Growth-hormone and prolactin tumors are usually in the lateral wing of the gland. TSH and ACTH tumors are midline (From Hardy, J.: *Transsphenoidal surgery of hypersecreting pituitary tumors.* In Kohler, P. O. and Ross, G. T. (eds.): *Diagnosis and Treatment of Pituitary Tumors.* American Elsevier, New York, 1973, with permission.)

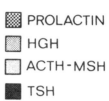

▨ PROLACTIN
▧ HGH
☐ ACTH-MSH
■ TSH

turn of fertility, pregnancy, and complete preservation of other pituitary trophic function.

After transsphenoidal hypophysectomy, there is rarely any need for postoperative replacement with cortisol or thyroxine. Diabetes insipidus may occur transiently for one to two weeks after removal of large tumors, but is almost never observed with microadenomas. The morbidity and mortality of the transsphenoidal technique in expert hands are very low. The placement of a muscle graft into the sella has greatly reduced the incidence of CSF rhinorrhea and meningitis. Follow-up of operated patients has been gratifying; prolactin levels frequently return to normal by the end of the operation and normal menses commonly reappear two to four months later.

Bromergocryptine Therapy

Administration of bromergocryptine in a dose of 2.5 to 7.5 mg. daily in divided doses exerts a rapid and sustained suppressive effect on prolactin secretion, both in functional hyperprolactinemia (due to hypothalamic disturbance) and in most prolactin-secreting pituitary tumors.[35] A single dose of bromergocryptine (1 or 2.5 mg. p.o.) reduces prolactin levels within one to two hours and the effect persists for six to eight hours. Administration of 2.5 mg. three times per day produces virtually total suppression of prolactin secretion throughout the 24-hour period. Over 90 per cent of female patients receiving this treatment show a return of ovulatory menstrual cycles within six weeks to two months after initiation of treatment. Side effects of the drug have been minimal; initially postural hypotension and nausea and vomiting are troublesome in some patients, as is true of L-dopa, but these are not usually sustained for more than a few days to a week. Maximum daily doses used have reached 15 to 20 mg., but we have rarely found it necessary to give more than 10 mg.

A Canadian multicenter trial of the efficacy of bromergocryptine in treatment of amenorrhea-galactorrhea has been summarized recently.[35] Of a series of 77 cases, 40 were functional (cause undetermined), 21 had microadenomas, eight had macroadenomas (greater than 10 mm. in diameter), and eight were postsurgical. Serum prolactin was elevated (above 30 ng./ml.) in 59 cases; there was no correlation between degree of galactorrhea and serum prolactin level. Prolactin levels were higher in patients with tumors, but in 10 cases of microadenoma values were under 100 ng./ml. Bromergocryptine caused suppression of prolactin in every case, regardless of etiology (Fig. 6). Fifty-seven patients had return of ovulatory cycles within six months of the initiation of bromergocryptine therapy; in 46 of the cases, the first ovulation occurred within two months of the start of treatment. Side effects were minimal in most patients, consisting of nausea or vomiting (eight cases), dizziness or postural hypotension (two cases), weight gain (one case), tender breasts (three cases), and anorexia (one case). Five patients discontinued the medication, usually after two to three weeks, because of side effects. At this writing, 22 patients have become pregnant, of whom five aborted (not greater than usual incidence), 12 have been delivered of healthy newborns, and five have not yet given birth.

By 1976, 94 pregnancies after bromergocryptine treatment had been reported throughout the world, and the outcome of pregnancy was known in 47 cases. There were three cases of malformation: one of kidney aplasia, one of pulmonary artery atresia, and one of inguinal hernia. There were seven spontaneous abortions.

It is not necessary to continue treatment during pregnancy; we recommend that the drug be stopped as soon as pregnancy is confirmed. Normal pregnancy is maintained despite a rapid return to very high prolactin levels after discontinuation of the drug. This has resulted, however, in a recently recognized complication of pregnancy in such patients. Of 22 patients, four developed marked enlargement of the sella turcica during pregnancies following bromergocryptine therapy. Roentgenograms before pregnancy showed only equivocal enlargement of the sella turcica. This observation draws attention to the fact that estrogen secretion during pregnancy, which is known to stimulate prolactin secretion (and increase the number of lactotropes), can endanger the patient. Sudden, rapid enlargement of the gland, as noted years ago by Cushing, can lead to visual disturbance that may go undetected. Very close observation of visual fields is indicated. It should be recalled that hypophysectomy after the third month of pregnancy does not necessarily cause abortion.

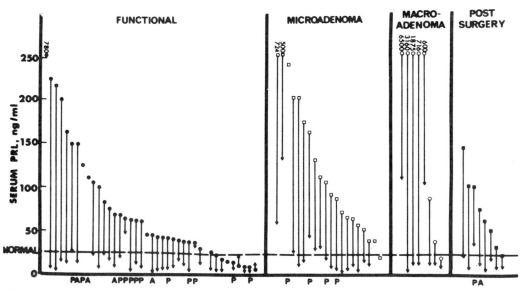

Figure 6. Serum prolactin levels before and after treatment with bromergocryptine. Arrows indicate fall in prolactin after treatment. (Courtesy of H. G. Friesen and G. Tolis.)

In the United States, investigators using bromergocryptine for treatment of galactor-rhea-amenorrhea have been informed by the Food and Drug Administration that the drug should not be used in patients with tumors, that patients should use birth control techniques to avoid pregnancy while on the drug, and that the drug should not be continued if the patient becomes pregnant. One of the major questions is the role of brom-ergocryptine in inducing ovulation, and indirectly, pregnancy. If a woman has a tumor and wishes to become pregnant, microsurgery seems the best approach.

There is evidence that bromergocryptine can reduce the size of a pituitary tumor in nonpregnant women, but this effect has not been completely proven. In one of our recent cases, a large pituitary tumor associated with severe headaches and serum prolactin levels of 1600 ng./ml. responded rapidly to bromergocryptine; prolactin levels fell to less than 5 ng./ml., the headaches abated, menses returned, and libido was re-established. Others have reported an improvement of visual fields in both prolactin-secreting tumors and acromegaly after administration of the drug. It appears that this drug will become one of the important agents for the management of both amenorrhea-galactor-rhea and acromegaly.

One of the disappointments with bromergocryptine is the observation that galactor-rhea almost invariably returns after discontinuation of treatment. This suggests that the drug acts to suppress abnormal secretion but has no long-term effects on the underlying pathophysiologic disturbance. We have been increasingly impressed that many of these patients go on to develop tumors that are best treated by transsphenoidal removal.

SURGERY

The question of when to operate on patients with prolactin-secreting microadenomas has become an important one. Despite increasing use of the transsphenoidal technique throughout the world, most neurosurgeons still hesitate to operate on patients with small pituitary tumors. Hardy[13] has accumulated the largest series of such patients. In more than 100 operated cases with elevated prolactin levels, a pituitary tumor has been found and removed in all but two patients. Four of these patients were operated on successfully despite absence of sellar erosion on roentgenograms.

RADIATION THERAPY

Radiation therapy may also be considered in the treatment of prolactin-secreting adenomas. There are few accumulated data on the effects of conventional radiation. We have observed one patient who showed a decline of plasma prolactin levels from 350 ng./ml. to 75 ng./ml. following a dose of approximately 7,000 rads by proton-beam radiation, but the patient still has not menstruated normally despite the fact that her pituitary responded to LHRH. Since most chromophobe adenomas (studied in the pre-prolactin immunoassay era) showed regression after conventional radiation, it is reasonable to suggest that this might be a highly useful form of therapy, and would carry a low complication rate.

We are not aware of any series of patients with roentgenographically negative functional amenorrhea who have been treated with conventional radiation. Most physicians do not regard galactorrhea and amenorrhea as serious enough to warrant radiation to the pituitary; the use of bromergocryptine, however, may make it possible for such women to become pregnant.

ACTH-Secreting Tumors

The management of Cushing's disease due to ACTH-secreting tumors has been discussed previously in Chapter 8.

Case Reports

Case 1: Acromegaly with Cure after Transsphenoidal Hypophysectomy[15]

D.R., a 28-year-old woman, was admitted to the hospital because of suspected acromegaly.

Three years before admission, she developed progressive bilateral numbness and tingling in the hands due to a carpal tunnel syndrome.

The patient had noticed occasional throbbing bitemporal headaches, coarsening of the hair, enlargement of the face and jaw, deepening of the voice, increase in shoe and glove size, and increase in body hair and sweating. She had noted scant nipple discharge on two occasions. She was nulligravida, her menstrual periods were normal, and she had no other endocrine complaints. There was no family history of neuroendocrine disease.

Her temperature was 37° C and vital signs were normal.

Physical examination revealed coarse scalp and body hair, a protuberant nose and slight prognathism; the mandibular teeth were separated and the tongue was enlarged. Proptosis was present and the eyelids were puffy. The hands and feet were enlarged and broadened. The fundi and visual fields were normal. Neurologic examination revealed decreased touch and pinprick sensation in the median-nerve distribution of both hands.

Results of hematologic studies and urinalysis were normal. Serum electrolytes, Ca and PO_4, and tests of liver and kidney function were all normal. Fasting blood glucose was 80 and the two hour postprandial value 82 mg./100 ml. The spinal fluid was normal. The ECG, EEG, and brain scan were normal. Skull roentgenograms, including sellar tomograms demonstrated asymmetric erosion of the sella turcica, greater on the left, with extension of a soft tissue mass into the sphenoid sinus (Fig. 7). A bilateral carotid angiogram showed slight elevation of the horizontal portion of the right anterior cerebral artery; a pneumoencephalogram demonstrated a suprasellar extension of approximately 5 mm. (Fig. 8). The EMG demonstrated mild slowing of sensory and motor conduction across both wrists, consistent with the diagnosis of carpal tunnel syndrome.

Endocrinologic evaluation revealed the following: T_4 6.1 μg./100 ml.; plasma cortisol at 8 A.M. 110 and at 4 P.M. 35 ng./ml.; serum TSH 7.5 μU./ml; serum LH 7.3 and FSH 7.2 mIU./ml. Basal serum GH was persistently elevated, ranging from 14.0 to 33.0 ng./ml. An oral glucose tolerance test had no effect on the GH levels, while insulin hypoglycemia resulted in a slight GH rise. The administration of L-dopa and apomorphine caused a fall in GH (Fig. 9). TRH administration caused a marked rise in GH (Fig. 10) and a significant prolactin response. The LH and FSH responses to LHRH were normal.

The patient underwent transsphenoidal removal of the pituitary adenoma by Dr. Gilles Ber-

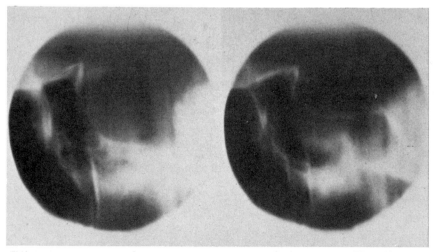

Figure 7. Tomograms of sella turcica in lateral projection. *Left,* A large erosion of the sella. *Right,* A near-normal configuration. This case illustrates the asymmetric lateral position of most GH-secreting adenomas.

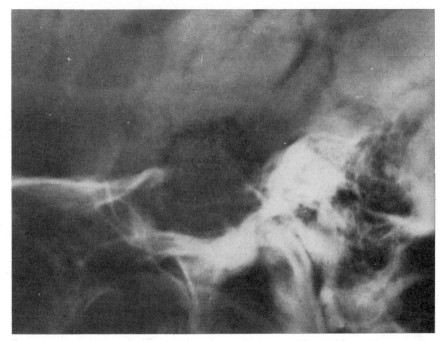

Figure 8. Pneumoencephalogram showing bulging of tumor into suprasellar position.

trand at the Montreal Neurological Hospital. The tumor extended into the anterior wall of the sella, mainly on the left side. The remainder of the gland appeared normal. The patient quickly recovered from surgery and was discharged home on the fifth postoperative day. The only postoperative medication was cortisone acetate 12.5 mg. orally, three times a day, which was tapered and discontinued over three weeks.

Two months postoperatively the patient was feeling well, her carpal tunnel symptoms were

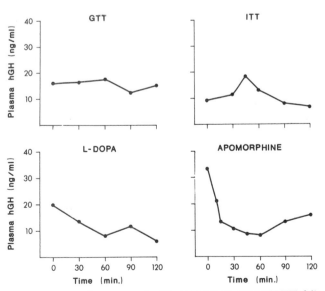

Figure 9. Growth-hormone responses in acromegaly. Glucose tolerance test (GTT) fails to suppress GH and response to insulin (ITT) is minimal. Both L-dopa and apomorphine induce "paradoxic" fall in GH.

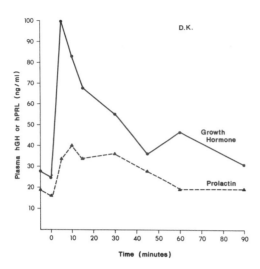

Figure 10. Serum GH and prolactin response to TRH in acromegaly.

gone, and the soft tissue edema of the face had disappeared. Menstrual cycles were regular and the patient had no symptoms of ADH deficiency or excess. Provocative tests of GH secretion were repeated.

Several baseline GH levels were normal (less than 5 ng./ml.). The administration of L-dopa and apomorphine resulted in a GH rise. TRH had no effect on GH but again caused a normal prolactin response. Insulin hypoglycemia resulted in an elevation in plasma cortisol to twice basal levels at 60 minutes and an increment in GH of 30 ng./ml. at 120 minutes. Plasma cortisol at this time was 104 ng./ml. at 8 A.M. and 48 ng./ml. at 4 P.M. The T_4 was 7.1 µg./100 ml. and the rest of the laboratory tests remained normal. Thirty-six months postoperatively, the patient is well with no evidence of active acromegaly; baseline GH remains normal.

Discussion

This patient demonstrated paradoxic GH responses but showed complete reversion to normal GH responsiveness following pituitary adenomectomy. The responses to L-dopa and apomorphine postoperatively were normal. Insulin hypoglycemia, which caused little effect preoperatively, resulted in a clearly normal GH response postoperatively.

The complete postoperative reversion to normal GH responsiveness suggests that the primary disorder was in the pituitary gland. There are several possible explanations for paradoxic GH responses and their reversion to normal. The pituitary somatotropes comprising the tumor may have possessed altered receptors. resulting in aberrant GH responses; the pituitary tumor may have physically compressed the adjacent hypothalamus, causing paradoxic inhibition of GH-releasing factor secretion; or the short-loop negative-feedback system may have been reset by the elevated circulating GH levels. This could result in paradoxic inhibition of GH release on stimulation of hypothalamic mechanisms by dopaminergic agonists.

In support of an altered pituitary receptor mechanism is the finding of GH release after administration of TRH and LHRH. After removal of the tumor, the GH response to TRH was normal. In our case, the postoperative reversion to normal GH responsiveness after TRH also implicates the pituitary as the site of the primary abnormality. The observation of TRH-induced GH release in acromegaly may thus be best explained by altered somatotrope receptors, possibly due to dedifferentiation of the tumor cells.

An unanswered paradox in acromegaly is the failure of elevated serum GH levels to suppress GH responses to provocative stimuli. Further characterization of normal feedback control, whether by GH itself (short-loop feedback) or secondary to somatomedin, will be required before the question can be resolved.

This case report demonstrates that certain cases of acromegaly are probably due to pituitary dysfunction alone. Although the patient may conceivably have a recurrence, we believe, based on our experience, that she is cured. Acromegaly may prove to be due to several causes; some

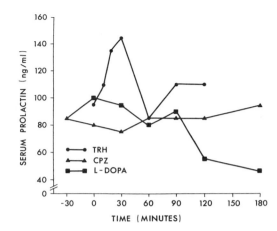

Figure 11. Serum prolactin responses to TRH, chlorpromazine (CPZ), and L-dopa in patient with amenorrhea-galactorrhea syndrome. TRH results in prolactin rise, CPZ has no effect, and L-dopa causes suppression.

may arise from pituitary tumors, other from excessive hypothalamic secretion of GRF (or deficiency of somatostatin).[4]

Case 2: Postpartum Amenorrhea-Galactorrhea Syndrome with Pituitary Tumor

C.M., a 25-year-old woman, was admitted for investigation of galactorrhea-amenorrhea. She had a normal menarche at age 12. Five years before admission, she took oral contraceptives for eight months. Ten months after discontinuing the medication she became pregnant and delivered a normal male. She did not breast-feed the baby but developed persistent postpartum galactorrhea-amenorrhea. Clomiphene therapy was unsuccessful.

Physical examination was normal except for galactorrhea. Neurologic examinations and visual fields by perimetry were normal.

The serum T_4 was 4.8 μg./100 ml., prolactin 95 ng./ml., LH 0.9 and FSH 12.5 mIU./ml. Infusion of 400 μg. of TRH caused a rise in PRL from 95 to 145 ng./ml. at 30 minutes (Fig. 11); intramuscular injection of 50 mg. of chlorpromazine caused a slight prolactin rise from 85 to 95 ng./ml. at 180 minutes. L-dopa (500 mg. orally) caused a fall in serum prolactin from 100 to 46 ng./ml. at 180 minutes. The subcutaneous administration of 100 μg. of LHRH resulted in a normal LH response and an exaggerated FSH response (Fig. 12). Skull roentgenograms showed slight sellar asymmetry but no clear evidence of pituitary tumor.

Treatment with bromergocriptine was begun at a dose of 1 mg. t.i.d. and increased to 2.5 mg. b.i.d. after one month. The breast fullness disappeared and menses resumed within four weeks;

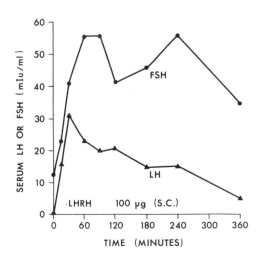

Figure 12. Serum FSH and LH responses to LHRH in amenorrhea-galactorrhea syndrome.

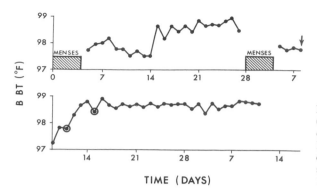

Figure 13. Daily basal body temperatures (BBT) in patient during treatment of amenorrhea-galactorrhea with CB-154. A rise in BBT occurs on day 14 of first cycle. Medication was stopped on 9th day *(arrow)* of second cycle. Intercourse occurred on days 12 and 15 with pregnancy resulting.

basal body temperatures revealed ovulatory cycles (Fig. 13). Serum prolactin was <3 ng./ml. After two normal ovulatory menstrual cycles, the patient wished to become pregnant, but was reluctant to do so while taking medication. Accordingly, bromergocryptine 2.5 mg. b.i.d. was given for the first seven days of her next cycle and then discontinued. Conception occurred on day 11 or day 15; body temperatures revealed that ovulation had probably occurred on day 11 (see Fig. 13). Pregnancy was uneventful and a healthy male infant was delivered at term.

Postpartum, the galactorrhea-amenorrhea recurred although the patient did not breast-feed. Serum prolactin was 94 ng./ml. Tomograms of the sella turcica demonstrated a marked change with a right-sided expanding intrasellar lesion and erosion of the floor of the sella (Fig. 14).

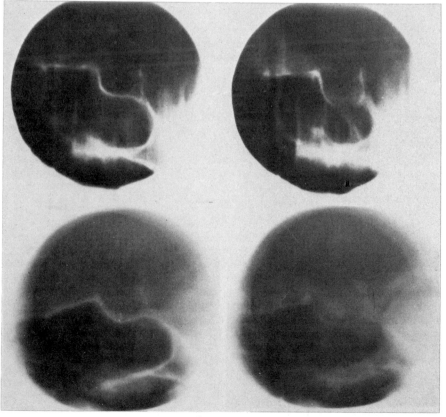

Figure 14. Tomograms of sella turcica (lateral view) before *(upper figures)* and after *(lower figures)* pregnancy. There is marked enlargement of the right side of the sella.

The patient was referred to Dr. Jules Hardy, Notre Dame Hospital, Montreal, who removed a 5.5 mm. microadenoma from the right lateral wing of the pituitary gland. Postoperatively, the galactorrhea regressed over an eight-week period, with return of breast size to normal and establishment of regular menstrual cycles. Serum prolactin is 17 ng./ml. She has remained normal for three years and is not on replacement medication.

Discussion

This patient presented at first as a Chiari-Frommel syndrome (postpartum galactorrhea) without definite evidence of a tumor. After successful treatment with bromergocryptine, she became pregnant. The effect of pregnancy on the tumor was dramatic, emphasizing that great care must be taken with patients who become pregnant. We recommend careful follow-up with repeated visual-field testing to detect the development of optic nerve compression.

Case 3: Amenorrhea-Galactorrhea with Microadenoma and Normal Skull Roentgenograms

D.T., a 27-year-old woman, presented with an 18-month history of amenorrhea and galactorrhea. Menarche was at age 11 and menses were normal until age 18, when irregular cycles began. She was treated for three years with oral contraceptives. Amenorrhea and galactorrhea developed after discontinuation of medication at age 26.

Physical examination was normal except for profuse bilateral galactorrhea. Neurologic and visual-field examinations were normal. Serum prolactin was 54 ng./ml. (normal: 1 to 25 ng./ml.) and skull roentgenograms including tomograms were normal. Treatment with thyroxine and L-dopa were unsuccessful; serum prolactin rose to 195 ng./ml.

The patient was referred to Dr. Jules Hardy, Notre Dame Hospital, Montreal, who explored the sella by the transsphenoidal route. A 6-mm. violaceous microadenoma was selectively removed from the left lateral wing of the pituitary gland. The patient recovered quickly from surgery and was discharged from the hospital on no replacement therapy.

Galactorrhea stopped immediately after surgery and menses resumed normally one month later. An intravenous injection of TRH (500 μg.) showed a normal TSH and prolactin response. Basal prolactin was 8 ng./ml. Plasma cortisol, T_4 and urinary estrogens were normal.

The patient became pregnant 12 months after operation and delivered a healthy male infant. Postpartum the galactorrhea-amenorrhea recurred transiently, but normal periods resumed several months later. Serum prolactin was 27 ng./ml.

Discussion

This patient was operated on because serum prolactin was high despite a normal series of sellar tomograms. Removal of the tumor restored menses and fertility.

PITUITARY INSUFFICIENCY

Chronic Replacement

ACTH Deficiency

In the evaluation of patients with pituitary insufficiency, the identification of ACTH deficiency is of paramount importance; the consequent adrenal insufficiency can be life-threatening, particularly in stress. Most patients are well controlled on 25 mg. of cortisone or the equivalent (20 mg. hydrocortisone or 5 mg. prednisone) per day, given in two, equal, divided doses. Some patients feel perfectly well on a single daily dose. A few patients require a larger dose for regular maintenance, e.g., 37.5 mg. of cortisone per day (30 mg. hydrocortisone or 7.5 mg. prednisone given as 5 mg. in the morning and 2.5 mg. at night). We noted that many hypopituitary patients given the higher dose of cortisone or prednisone as a standard dose develop mild signs of steroid overdosage.

The benefit from the use of hydrocortisone or cortisone is no greater than from predni-sone; the much lower cost of the latter and the longer duration of action (due to slower degradation), in fact, make prednisone superior. Because ACTH deficiency does not lead to complete mineralocorticoid (aldosterone) deficiency, hypopituitary patients, un-like addisonian patients, rarely require supplemental treatment with synthetic mineralo-corticoids such as desoxycorticosterone acetate (DOCA) or fludrocortisone acetate. During stress, patients must increase the dosage two- or threefold, and they must also be instructed to contact a physician if they are unable to take medications by mouth. It is imperative to instruct and repeatedly remind the patient of the necessity for close medical supervision, particularly if under stress. It is also imperative that the patients carry identification (wallet card, necklace, or bracelet) indicating that they are "corti-sone dependent." If medical attention will not be available in an emergency, as for ex-ample when traveling in an undeveloped country or in a wilderness area, we insist that our patients be accompanied by a companion and carry a vial or two of a soluble prepa-ration of steroid. Monitoring the adequacy of adrenal steroid replacement includes eval-uation of appetite, weight, sense of well being, and measurements of plasma sodium concentration and appropriate postural blood pressure changes. There is no completely objective measure of adequacy of corticoid replacement independent of careful and ex-perienced clinical judgment.

Thyroid Deficiency

Most TSH-deficient patients are well treated with 100 to 200 μg. per day of synthetic L-thyroxine given as a single dose. Monitoring the adequacy of replacement involves clinical evaluation, but measurements of plasma T_4 and T_3 are a good guide to therapy since they accurately reflect circulating hormone; values should fall within the usual normal range. Because of the danger of precipitating angina, coronary insufficiency, and arrhythmia in patients with long-standing pituitary disease, thyroid hormone replace-ment is usually initiated stepwise: in an older person, 25 μg. T_4 for two weeks, 50 μg. for the next two weeks, and then 100 μg. per day for two weeks. Additional incre-ments of 50 μg. per day are then given at two-week intervals until full replacement is achieved.

Gonadotropin Deficiency

Unless the patient wants to have children, gonadotropin deficiency is well managed with gonadal steroid replacement therapy. In the adult male, most workers recommend testosterone dosage equivalent to 12 to 15 mg. per day, given IM in a long-acting prepa-ration every two or three weeks. This form of treatment is the least expensive. Thus, testosterone enanthate or propionate can be given in a dose of 200 to 300 mg. every two or three weeks. The patient is usually instructed in self-administration. Testosterone can also be administered by mouth in the form of fluoxymesterone tablets, the only commercially available derivative of testosterone that is absorbed readily by the gut. Absorption of this form is somewhat irregular, and all orally taken testosterone prepa-rations have the potential to cause cholangitis with the appearance of obstructive jaun-dice. Parenteral preparations are free of this problem. The criteria for adequate replace-ment include maintenance of beard growth, libido, and potency. Excess dosage may result in edema formation, gynecomastia, disturbing sexual drive, nightmares, and acne. Because hypogonadal men do not express genetically determined baldness, normal re-placement doses may bring about baldness in those who are susceptible, which in a sense can be regarded as a side effect of therapy. It is important to inform the patient of this possibility. Long-standing gonadal insufficiency may require many months of therapy before adequate sexual drive and performance can be restored. The longer the deficiency has been present, the longer it takes to achieve the desired response, and if the patients have been untreated for many years, particularly in the teens and early twenties, full restoration of normal male development may never occur. This lack of sex drive may lead to the peculiar situation in which the patient is not motivated to maintain adequate sex hormone replacement therapy. Another point of practical importance is that a surprisingly large number of individuals may have been hypogonadal for many years prior to its recognition and have therefore adopted a life style appropriate to hypogonadism. This can include the choice of marital partner or of vocation. Replacement therapy may create difficulties in such patients, since it may threaten a harmonious marriage or cause sex drive which cannot be fulfilled. The physician must exercise broad judgment in his institution of gonad replacement therapy.

In women, adequate sex hormone replacement therapy is given with one of several estrogenic preparations (ethinyl estradiol 10 to 15 μg. per day, conjugated estrogens 0.65 to 2.5 mg. per day). Diethylstilbestrol, the least costly of the estrogens, has been declared by the FDA to have carcinogenic potential and is no longer used for replacement treatment. Therapy is given for 25 days of each month, and a menstrual period induced by the administration, on days 21 to 25 inclusive, of an orally-effective progestin such as medroxyprogesterone 5 to 10 mg. per day. Other acceptable regimens include one of the birth control pills in daily doses not to exceed the equivalent of 25 μg. per day of estradiol; doses in the range of 10 μg. per day are probably adequate. Recent evidence indicates that the administration of estrogenic hormones increases the frequency of endometrial carcinoma approximately fivefold. For this reason we now insist that patients given hormone replacement take regular progestin treatment to induce menses (because of the finding that progesterone reverses endometrial hyperplasia) and have gynecologic evaluations at yearly intervals. The smallest dose that is effective is the one that should be used. In young women, the advantage of taking estrogen replacement includes the maintenance of secondary sex characteristics, reduced risk of cardiac disease, sense of well being, breast size, vaginal and vulvar tissue turgor, and bone integrity. Whether these advantages persist after the mid-forties is still a matter of controversy. The physician and the patient together should discuss the pros and cons of therapy and decide, in the individual case, how replacement therapy will be managed. We advise sex-hormone replacement in young hypopituitary women who may have greater need and desire for restoration and maintenance of normal physiologic function. Cervical exfoliative cytology ("Pap test") and breast examinations should be evaluated at six-month intervals in women on estrogen replacement therapy.

Estrogenic hormones alone do not usually restore normal libido to the panhypopituitary woman. The addition of small amounts of an androgenic hormone is required to make up for the loss of adrenal androgen secretion. This can be accomplished by the administration of a long-acting testosterone preparation such as testosterone enanthate or testosterone proprionate in oil, 50 mg. every 4 to 6 weeks. Fluoxymesterone 5 to 10 ng. p.o. also can be given one or two days a week. Excessive dosage is indicated by the development of hirsutism. Clinicians usually fail to ask their women hypopituitary patients about abnormalities in libido, and many patients are unaware that anything can be done about their loss of sex drive. This can be of extreme importance in maintenance of a happy family life.

Infertility

It is now possible to restore fertility in more than half of gonadotropin-deficient men and women by means of substitution therapy.

WOMEN. In women with functional amenorrhea, ovulation commonly follows the

371

administration of clomiphene citrate. If successive trials of clomiphene fail to induce ovulation, the patient is a candidate for combined treatment with a FSH-like preparation followed by an ovulation dose of an LH preparation. A FSH-rich preparation, menotropins, is now available commercially and when administered over a two-week period can stimulate the normal growth of the follicle. Menotropins are extracted from the urine of menopausal women; the preparation is moderately expensive, has the potential for producing multiple births, and must be administered by a physician experienced in this method. Ovulation is brought about by the injection of human chorionic gonadotropin, with a success rate of about 60 to 70 per cent. The cost of a one-month course of treatment for hormone alone is at present approximately $300.00 to $600.00. Before contemplating a course of menotropins-HCG, patients require the usual infertility evaluation, which includes study of the husband's semen.

MEN. To ripen the sperm requires chronic therapy with menotropins for 70 or more days and with HCG for about 20 days. Such treatment is approximately 30 per cent successful in inducing maturation of live sperm. Recently, the demonstration that chronic treatment with LHRH can induce normal spermatogenesis in most hypogonadotropic men, even those with intrinsic pituitary disease, suggests a better approach; LHRH, a synthetic peptide, can be produced at a lower cost than the gonadotropin preparations, and appears to stimulate testis growth and function more physiologically. This material is still being used as a research tool. Unfortunately, it requires the systemic administration of hormone at least twice daily for as long as three months. Orally effective derivatives have been developed on an experimental basis. Androgen replacement is not needed during therapy with LHRH.

Fertile men who are to undergo ablative surgery in the pituitary-hypothalamic area should consider the advisability of placing their sperm in a sperm bank, even if they are not married and do not contemplate having children. Sperm can be kept viable for seven years or more in such banks, at this time.

ADH Deficiency

The treatment of diabetes insipidus has been discussed previously in Chapter 4.

Growth Hormone or Prolactin Deficiency

The use of growth-hormone replacement is limited to the pediatric age group, and is seldom of value if bone age is in excess of 14 years. Endocrine texts should be consulted for an approach to management of GH deficiency. There is no clear evidence that GH is needed for normal functioning in adults. This is also true for prolactin. The effect of prolactin on any aspect of physical or psychologic functioning of the hypopituitary patient is unknown, since no primate prolactin has been available for clinical investigation.

Treatment of Acute Severe Hypopituitarism

Particularly in stressed individuals, it may be necessary to give treatment on an emergency or semiemergency basis. ACTH deficiency is best treated with a glucocorticoid preparation. Treatment can be initiated with intravenous injection of a soluble solution of cortisol or hydrocortisone in doses of 100 to 300 mg. per day, which are from 3 to 10 times the normal replacement doses. Cortisone can be given as an intramuscular injection in a similar dose. In this form, it is absorbed somewhat more slowly, but also somewhat less dependably. Oral absorption is equal to or better than absorption following IM injection, and for this reason the latter route should not be used as the sole method in a critically sick patient. Patients with long-standing hypopituitarism given usual or large replacement doses of corticoids may abruptly develop euphoria, or even acute psychotic reactions; for this reason, it is generally better to avoid large doses unless the clinical situation is urgent.

In the treatment of pituitary coma or precoma, both corticoid and thyroid-hormone replacement is urgently indicated. However, excessively rapid thyroid-hormone replacement can result (in susceptible patients) in the precipitation of coronary insufficiency, myocardial infarction, angina, or arrhythmias. The clinician must often steer the difficult course between life-threatening myxedema coma and potential cardiac disturbance. Given a patient with severe TSH-thyroid deficiency requiring urgent treatment, most clinicians now administer the usual normal daily requirement of thyroid hormone for two or three days by mouth, if possible, or otherwise by vein (50 μg. per day of T_3, or 150 μg. per day of T_4). The dose is decreased after three to four days of treatment to 50 to 100 μg. of thyroxine per day, and a week to ten days later, after the urgent situation is past, therapy is increased in the usual way (see above).

REFERENCES

1. ATKINSON, R. L., ET AL.: *Acromegaly. Treatment by trans-sphenoidal microsurgery.* J.A.M.A. 233: 1279, 1975.

2. BATZDORF, U. AND STERN, W. E.: *Clinical manifestations of pituitary adenomas: A pilot study using computer analysis. In* Kohler, P. O. and Ross, G. T. (eds.): *Diagnosis and Treatment of Pituitary Tumors.* American Elsevier, New York, 1973, p. 17.

3. BENTSON, J. R.: *Relative merits of pneumographic and angiographic procedures in the management of pituitary tumors. In* Kohler, P. O. and Ross, G. T. (eds.): *Diagnosis and Treatment of Pituitary Tumors.* American Elsevier, New York, 1973, p. 86.

4. DAUGHADAY, W. H., ET AL.: *The role of the hypothalamus in the pathogenesis of pituitary tumors. In* Kohler, P. O. and Ross, G. T. (eds.): *Diagnosis and Treatment of Pituitary Tumors.* American Elsevier, New York, 1973, p. 26.

5. DECK, M. D. F.: *Radiographic and radioisotopic techniques in diagnosis of pituitary tumors. In* Kohler, P. O. and Ross, G. T. (eds.): *Diagnosis and Treatment of Pituitary Tumors.* American Elsevier, New York, 1973, p. 71.

6. EARLE, K. M. AND DILLAR, S. H., JR.: *Pathology of adenomas of the pituitary gland. In* Kohler, P. O. and Ross, G. T. (eds.): *Diagnosis and Treatment of Pituitary Tumors.* American Elsevier, New York, 1973, p. 3.

7. FAGER, C. A., ET AL.: *Indications for and results of surgical treatment of pituitary tumors by the intracranial approach. In* Kohler, P. O. and Ross, G. T. (eds.): *Diagnosis and Treatment of Pituitary Tumors.* American Elsevier, New York, 1973, p. 146.

8. FRASER, R., ET AL.: *The assessment of the endocrine effects and the effectiveness of ablative pituitary treatment by* ^{90}Y *and* ^{198}Au *implantation. In* Kohler, P. O. and Ross, G. T. (eds.): *Diagnosis and Treatment of Pituitary Tumors.* American Elsevier, New York, 1973, p. 35.

9. FRASER, R., ET AL.: *Needle implantation of yttrium seeds for pituitary ablation in cases of secondary carcinoma.* Lancet 1:382, 1959.

10. GARCIA, J. F., ET AL.: *Treatment of pituitary tumors with heavy particles. In* Kohler, P. O. and Ross, G. T. (eds.): *Diagnosis and Treatment of Pituitary Tumors.* American Elsevier, New York, 1973, p. 253.

11. GORDEN, P. AND ROTH, J.: *The treatment of acromegaly by conventional pituitary irradiation. In* Kohler, P. O. and Ross, G. T. (eds.): *Diagnosis and Treatment of Pituitary Tumors.* American Elsevier, New York, 1973, p. 230.

12. GUIOT, G.: *Transsphenoidal approach in surgical treatment of pituitary adenomas: General principles and indications in non-functioning adenomas. In* Kohler, P. O. and Ross, G. T. (eds.): *Diagnosis and Treatment of Pituitary Tumors.* American Elsevier, New York, 1973, p. 159.

13. HARDY, J.: *Transsphenoidal surgery of hypersecreting pituitary tumors. In* Kohler, P. O. and Ross, G. T. (eds.): *Diagnosis and Treatment of Pituitary Tumors.* American Elsevier, New York, 1973, p. 179.

14. HOLLENHORST, R. W. AND YOUNGE, B. R.: *Ocular manifestations produced by adenomas of the pituitary gland: Analysis of 1000 cases. In* Kohler, P. O. and Ross, G. T. (eds.): *Diagnosis and Treatment of Pituitary Tumors.* American Elsevier, New York, 1973, p. 53.

15. HOYTE, K. M. AND MARTIN, J. B.: *Recovery from paradoxical growth hormone responses in acromegaly after transsphenoidal selective adenomectomy.* J. Clin. Endocrinol. Metab. 41:656, 1975.

16. JACKSON, I. M. D. AND ORMSTON, B. J.: *Lack of beneficial response of serum GH in acromegalic patients treated with medroxy progesterone acetate (MPA).* J. Clin. Endocrinol. Metab. 35:413, 1972.

17. JOPLIN, G. F., ET AL.: *Partial pituitary ablation.* The Lancet. 2:1277, 1961.

18. KAUFMAN, B., ET AL.: *Radiographic features of intrasellar masses and progressive asymmetrical nontumorous enlargements of the sella turcica, the "empty" sella. In* Kohler, P. O. and Ross, G. T. (eds.): *Diagnosis and Treatment of Pituitary Tumors.* American Elsevier, New York, 1973, p. 100.

19. KJELLBERG, R. N. AND KLIMAN, B.: *A system for therapy of pituitary tumors. In* Kohler, P. O. and Ross, G. T.: *Diagnosis and Treatment of Pituitary Tumors.* American Elsevier, New York, 1973, p. 234.

20. KOLODNY, H. D., ET AL.: *Acromegaly treated with chlorpromazine.* N. Engl. J. Med. 284:819, 1971.

21. KRAMER, S.: *Indications for, and results of, treatment of pituitary tumors by external radiation. In* Kohler, P. O. and Ross, G. T. (eds.): *Diagnosis and Treatment of Pituitary Tumors.* American Elsevier, New York, 1973, p. 217.

22. KRUEGER, E. G. AND UNGER, S. M.: *Extrasellar extension of pituitary adenomas: Clinical and neuroradiological considerations.* American J. Roentgenol. Radium Ther. Nucl. Med. 98:616, 1966.

23. LAWRENCE, A. M. AND HAGEN, T. C.: *Alternatives to ablative therapy for pituitary tumors. In* Kohler, P. O. and Ross, G. T. (eds.): *Diagnosis and Treatment of Pituitary Tumors.* American Elsevier, New York, 1973, p. 297.

24. LAWRENCE, A. M. AND KIRSTEINS, L.: *Progestins in the medical management of active acromegaly.* J. Clin. Endocrinol. Metab. 30:646, 1970.

25. MacCARTY, C. S., ET AL.: *Indications for and results of surgical treatment of pituitary tumors by the transfrontal approach. In* Kohler, P. O. and Ross, G. T. (eds.): *Diagnosis and Treatment of Pituitary Tumors.* American Elsevier, New York, 1973, p. 139.

26. MALARKEY, W. B. AND DAUGHADAY, W. H.: *Variable response of plasma GH in acromegalic patients treated with medroxy progesterone acetate.* J. Clin. Endocrinol. Metab. 33:424, 1971.

27. NEWTON, T. H. AND WEINSTEIN, M.: *The sella turcica in Nelson's syndrome.* Radiology 118(2):363, 1976.

28. NORRELL, H. A., ET AL.: *A clinicopathologic analysis of cryohypophysectomy in patients with advanced cancer.* Cancer 25(5):1050, 1970.

29. PENN, W. H. AND RHOTON, A. L.: *Microsurgical anatomy of the sellar region.* J. Neurosurg. 43:288, 1975.

30. POWELL, D. F., BAKER, H. L., JR. AND LAWS, E. R., JR.: *The primary angiographic findings in pituitary adenomas.* Radiology 110:589, 1974.

31. RAND, R. W.: *Hypophysectomy in endocrine disorders.* Clin. Neurosurg. 17:226, 1970.

32. RAND, R. W., ET AL.: *Stereotaxic cryohypophysectomy: Ten year experience with pituitary tumors. In* Kohler, P. O. and Ross, G. T. (eds.): *Diagnosis and Treatment of Pituitary Tumors.* American Elsevier, New York, 1973, p. 277.

33. SHELINE, G. E.: *Treatment of chromophobe adenomas of the pituitary gland and acromegaly. In* Kohler, P. O. and Ross, G. T. (eds.): *Diagnosis and Treatment of Pituitary Tumors.* American Elsevier, New York, 1973, p. 201.

34. THORNER, M. O., ET AL.: *Bromocriptine treatment of acromegaly.* Br. Med. J. 1:299, 1975.

35. TOLIS, G. AND FRIESEN, H. G.: *A clinical study of the use of bromergocryptine: The Canadian experience.* Clin. Endocrinol., in press.

36. WILLIAMS, R. A., ET AL.: *The treatment of acromegaly with special reference to trans-sphenoidal hypophysectomy.* Quart. J. Med. 64:79, 1975.

37. ZERVAS, N. T., ET AL.: *Experimental induction healing hypophysectomy.* Confin. Neurol. 35:129, 1973.

38. KJELLBERG: Personal communication.

39. LAWRENCE, J. H., ET AL.: *Heavy particle therapy in acromegaly and Cushing's disease.* J.A.M.A. 235:2307, 1976.

40. HARDY, J.: Personal communication.

CHAPTER 16

Special Problems
in Hypothalamic-Pituitary Disease

The clinical manifestations of hypothalamic-pituitary disease can usually be predicted on the basis of anatomic and physiologic principles. On the other hand, the natural history of an individual case depends on the etiology of the underlying disease. This is also true in considering diagnostic and therapeutic approaches. In this chapter, a number of specific causes of hypothalamic-pituitary dysfunction and their pathogenesis are discussed.

NONPITUITARY TUMORS OF THE THIRD-VENTRICLE REGION

The midline region around the third ventricle is a common site of involvement by a variety of tumors, particularly those arising from cell rests or developmental abnormalities (Table 1).[11, 28] The effects of such tumors depend on the location of the tumor, its rate of growth, and the occasional production of hormones by tumor cells. Tumors in the region of the anteromedial basal hypothalamus or inferior part of the third ventricle produce disorders of neuroendocrine regulation and of visual and olfactory functions. Tumors of the anterior-superior portion of the third ventricle may give rise to hydrocephalus by obstructing the foramina of Monro. Dementia may occur as a result of interruption of connections between the dorsomedial thalamic nucleus and the frontal lobe. Papilledema, loss of vision, headaches, and vomiting may supervene. Mass le-

Table 1. Nonpituitary Tumors of the Third Ventricular Region

I. Cell-rest tumors	III. Glial tumors
1. Rathke's-cleft cyst	1. Astrocytoma
2. Craniopharyngioma	2. Oligodendroglioma
3. Epidermoid, cholesteotoma	3. Ependymoma
4. Colloid cyst	4. Pituicytoma, infundibuloma
5. Arachnoid cyst	5. Microgliomatosis
6. Hamartoma, infundibuloma	IV. Choriod plexus papilloma
7. Chordoma	V. Meningioma
8. Lipoma	VI. Angioma, angioblastoma
II. Germ-cell tumors	VII. Infections
1. Pinealoma	1. Tuberculoma
2. Ectopic pinealoma	2. Cystocercosis
3. Germinoma	3. Echinococcal cyst
4. Dermoid	
5. Teratoma	

375

sions in the epithalamic or pineal region of the third ventricle cause Parinaud's syndrome (paralysis of conjugate vertical gaze), pupillary abnormalities, nystagmus, and brain-stem signs. Obstruction of the aqueduct of Sylvius results in increased intracranial pressure. Posteroinferior involvement commonly causes hydrocephalus, ocular palsies, cerebellar ataxia, and pyramidal-tract signs.

Craniopharyngioma and Pituitary Cysts

Rathke's-Cleft Cysts

Cysts of Rathke's pouch occur in vestigial remnants of the craniopharyngeal anlage that gives rise to the anterior pituitary, the intermediate lobe, and the pars tuberalis.[10, 65] In the third or fourth week of gestation, the roof of the stomodeum folds intracranially to form Rathke's pouch. The pouch elongates into the craniopharyngeal duct, and by the seventh week, the cranial portion of the duct obliterates, leaving a small pouch in the pituitary.[69] Remnants of the pituitary portion of the pouch form the vestigial intermediate lobe. The pouch is usually obliterated by infoldings of epithelial tissues, but small portions of lumen may be recognized microscopically, and the residual cavity, called Rathke's cleft, is lined with ciliated, cuboidal or columnar epithelium and secretes mucin. According to some studies, 13 to 22 per cent of randomly examined pituitary glands contain small microscopic clefts.

Only rarely are pituitary cysts symptomatic. Compression of surrounding pituitary tissue may result in partial or complete hypopituitarism. Extension above the pituitary fossa, with compromise of vision, has been reported.

Craniopharyngioma

The second most common pituitary tumor (after adenoma) is the craniopharyngioma.[53, 55, 69] The craniopharyngioma differs histologically from Rathke's cleft in that it contains stratified squamous epithelium and lacks cuboidal or columnar cells. The histologic pattern frequently resembles that of the primitive enamel of the tooth bud, and accordingly, the terms adamantinoma or ameloblastoma are used. The tumor is thus believed to arise from epithelial cell rests carried with Rathke's pouch into the pituitary fossa or region of the pars tuberalis. The tumors are commonly well-encapsulated, and may be either cystic or solid. Cysts are often multiloculated and contain dark brown, oily fluid in which can be found debris and cholesterol crystals. They may be as large as 8 to 10 cm. in diameter. About two thirds arise above the sella turcica, and in 70 per cent of cases a portion of the tumor is calcified, forming a linear, granular or amorphous mass that can be seen in lateral roentgenograms of the skull. The most common site is suprasellar, but in 75 per cent of cases there is evidence of radiologic abnormality within the sella turcica. Craniopharyngiomas do not synthesize or secrete a hormonal product.

CLINICAL MANIFESTATIONS. Although craniopharyngioma is primarily a condition of the first two decades of life, symptoms may emerge as late as the seventh or eighth decade. In one series, 24 of 68 patients were over 50 years of age and nine were over 70. In children, the common presenting manifestations are headache, vomiting, visual loss, growth failure, and diabetes insipidus. Obstruction of the cerebral aqueduct or foramina of Monro can result in increased intracranial pressure and papilledema. Sixth-nerve palsies may occur. In the adolescent, diabetes insipidus and hypogonadism are frequent. In adult patients, diabetes insipidus, visual-field defects, and dementia are most common. Craniopharyngiomas occasionally arise within the third ventricle and may mimic a colloid or arachnoid cyst.[68]

In the series of 57 childhood cases reported by Matson and Crigler,[55] intracranial calcification was present in 56, retarded bone growth in 38, abnormal sella turcica in 34, and hydrocephalus in 24. Involvement of the visual fields is common; in a series reported by Love and Marshall,[53] progressive loss of vision was the most common presenting symptom. Since the tumor is often above optic chiasm, early visual involvement may first affect the inferior temporal fields. Asymmetric visual involvement is frequent with decreased visual acuity in one eye and a temporal hemianopia in the other. In some cases, because of the posterior position of the tumor, there may be involvement of one optic tract producing a contralateral homonymous hemianopia. Anosmia may occur with anterior extension of the tumor. Examination of CSF usually shows a modest elevation of protein, normal sugar, and no cells. Craniopharyngiomas may present as a neurologic emergency, with sudden development of ophthalmoplegia, severe headache, meningeal signs, coma, and seizures. Examination of CSF shows abnormalities suggesting that a cystic cavity has ruptured into the subarachnoid space.

The differential diagnosis of craniopharyngioma includes pituitary adenoma, ectopic pinealoma, teratoma, or germinoma in the pediatric age group, and meningioma in older patients. The diagnosis should be kept in mind whenever a combination of neurologic and endocrine dysfunction occurs. Diabetes insipidus rarely occurs with pituitary adenoma, but is common with craniopharyngioma and with granulomatous, inflammatory, or infiltrative lesions at the base of the brain.

TREATMENT. The treatment of craniopharyngioma, usually surgical, is difficult at best. The choice of radical versus partial removal of the cyst is still debated. In the pediatric series reported by Matson and Crigler,[55] 57 of 74 children underwent radical excision. Remarkably, in the 40 that had not been previously operated on, there were no deaths. Of the total series, 40 cases were judged by long-term follow-up to represent a good result. Recurrences were rare. In adults, such radical removal is more difficult and accompanied by much higher mortality, up to 30 to 40 per cent in some series. Recently, there has been increasing evidence that radiation may help arrest growth of the remaining tumor. Consequently, excision may not always be advisable; aspiration of the cyst and postoperative radiation may provide better management. Each case must, however, be considered individually.

Epidermoid Tumors (Cholesteatomas)

Epidermoid tumors are benign and arise from epithelial cell rests. According to Russell and Rubenstein,[69] epidermoid tumors cannot be clearly differentiated from craniopharyngiomas, since both commonly contain histologic features of squamous epithelium and contain cholesterol crystals. The relationship of craniopharyngioma and epidermoid cyst to Rathke's pouch and its derivatives has never been firmly established. Multiple sectioning of craniopharyngioma tissue almost invariably results in some sections that resemble in every respect the classic picture of the epidermoid cyst. It would thus appear that separation of the two tumor types is artificial.

Hamartomas, Infundibulomas, and Pituicytomas

Hamartomas are defined by Blackwood and coworkers[11] as "congenital malformation with a potentiality for growth which does not exceed that of the normal tissue in which they are situated." In most instances, such tumors represent ectopias, or abnormal localization of neural tissue in the brain. Hamartomas may arise spontaneously and singly or they may occur in multiple sites in combination with hereditary disorders such as tuberous sclerosis, Lindau's syndrome, von Recklinghausen's neurofibromatosis, and perhaps Sturge-Weber disease.

Hamartomas occur rather commonly in the tuberal region of the hypothalamus, both as isolated tumors as reported in the case of Reeves and Plum (see page 258), and in combination with the syndromes described above. They do not usually produce hormones, with the exception of LHRH, thought in some cases to induce precocious puberty (see Chapter 5). Other space-occupying lesions identically placed are rarely associated with precocious puberty.

The other symptoms that arise are due to local pressure which disturbs endocrine and autonomic functions of the hypothalamus. Tuberous sclerosis has been reported to cause growth failure, hypogonadism, or precocious puberty. Neurofibromatosis may result in diabetes insipidus and anterior pituitary deficiency. A curious, unexplained clinical observation is the association of neurofibromatosis with excessive somatic growth and of cerebral gigantism (see page 173). These patients do not secrete GH excessively, and the mechanism of the growth acceleration is unknown.

The term infundibuloma was originally applied to tumors of the infundibular region that were thought to arise from pituicytes. The true histologic nature of these tumors is in some doubt and Russel and Rubenstein[69] argue that they are likely astrocytomas. Tumors may arise in the neurohypophysis itself and have been called pituicytomas. They are exceedingly rare.

Arachnoid Cysts

Fluid-filled cysts arising from arachnoid membrane may occur in the suprasellar subarachnoid space and in the third ventricle.[70, 71] The latter are believed to develop from entrapments of arachnoid that occur during development.

Arachnoid cysts occur predominantly in childhood and may give rise to rather specific neurologic signs. Russman and coworkers[71] reviewed the neurologic and endocrinologic abnormalities in four cases reported in the literature and included three of their own. The cysts, most commonly intraventricular, resulted in macrocephaly (hydrocephalus) and head and trunk tremor. The head tremor was characterized in most cases by a rhythmic bobbing. The ventricle was dilated. Endocrinologic abnormalities included precocious puberty, diabetes insipidus, obesity, hypothyroidism, and adrenal insufficiency. Arachnoid cysts of the suprasellar area may give rise to visual-field defects and blindness. It is important to recognize this syndrome in children, because the cysts are benign and can be removed surgically with a good prognosis.

Chordomas

A chordoma is a tumor of the notochord, the embryologic anlage of the neural tube. Both sacral and head regions may be involved. Within the cranium, the tumor arises most commonly along the clivus of the sphenoid bone posterior to the sella turcica. Anterior extensions of the tumor into the suprasellar region do occur and can cause optic-tract or chiasm compression. Endocrinologic disturbances may occur if the hypothalamus or pituitary stalk is invaded.

Lipomas

Lipomas arising within the cranial cavity are believed to represent maldevelopment.[69] They are reported with an incidence of about 0.1 per cent in routine autopsies. Intracranial lipomas are usually in or close to the midsagittal plane and are most common over the corpus callosum. They may also occur in the infundibular region and, when large, may cause local symptoms. They occasionally are located inside the ventricular system and can lead to hydrocephalus. Histologically, the tumors may contain muscle and foci of calcification.

Glial Tumors

Malignant astrocytomas (glioblastomas) may arise in the hypothalamus or may infiltrate from adjacent structures. Infiltration of the columns of the fornix is relatively common with lesions of the cerebral hemisphere. In the hypothalamus proper, astrocytomas are the most common form of glial tumor; ependymomas rarely occur above the tentorium of the cerebellum. Astrocytomas can fungate into the third-ventricle space and cause obstruction, mimicking the signs and symptoms of a colloid cyst.

Colloid Cyst

The colloid cyst, a benign tumor, usually arises *in* the roof of the third ventricle,[44][51] although rarely, the cyst may occur *above* the diencephalic roof of the third ventricle, between the leaves of the septum pellucidum.[18] The origin of these tumors is debated; for many years they were thought to arise from the paraphysis. More likely, they represent embryonic vesicular infolding of choroid and neuroepithelial tissue. It has been suggested on this basis that the colloid cyst be termed a neuroepithelial cyst. Microscopically, the cyst is characterized by a single layer of cuboidal or columnar epithelium surrounding a gelatinous center.

The classic clinical presentation of the colloid cyst is a paroxysmal headache of rapid onset with vomiting, blindness, and drop attacks with or without loss of consciousness. The patients are usually adolescents or young adults. Bifrontal, intense headache is the most common symptom. Sometimes relief can be obtained by lying flat. Positional aspects are often emphasized, with the headache or drop attack occuring in a particular position, presumably due to obstruction of the CSF pathway at the foramen of Monro or the aqueduct of Sylvius. If obstruction is not relieved, coma and death may ensue.

This typical presentation does not always occur, however; in the reviews of 78 cases of colloid cyst by Kelly[44] and Little and MacCarty,[51] it is emphasized that other symptoms may be found and that vomiting and papilledema need not be present. In the series of Little and MacCarty,[51] 8 of 38 cases presented with progressive dementia and gait disturbance, without papilledema—findings reminiscent of "normal-pressure" hydrocephalus. Sudden deterioration and death occur in about 10 per cent of all cases and the cyst may only be found at autopsy.

In patients with drop attacks, consciousness is commonly not lost; the patient reports headache, a sudden weakness of the legs, and collapse without mental change. Echoencephalography often aids diagnosis, showing dilatation of the anterior third ventricle and of the lateral ventricles. Ventriculography usually is the definitive procedure by which the lesion is diagnosed. In the absence of papilledema, pneumoencephalography may be undertaken, provided the diagnosis is suspected and neurosurgical preparations have been made in case obstruction occurs suddenly. Large colloid cysts may be visualized by computed axial tomography. Endocrine studies in patients with colloid cysts have not been well systematized; no consistent abnormalities have been reported.

The treatment of the colloid cyst is surgical. The tumor is usually approached via the foramen of Monro, through a transcortical incision in the nondominant hemisphere.

Metastatic Tumors

A solitary metastasis to the pituitary gland is occasionally reported at autopsy in cases of carcinoma of the lung or breast. The lesion is usually asymptomatic. Meningeal invasion by metastatic carcinoma or leukemic infiltrates is more frequent and may cause visual symptoms, cranial nerve palsies, diabetes insipidus, hypopituitarism, and obesity. Leukemic involvement is particularly common in children where hyperphagia, personality change, and diabetes insipidus signal the need for intrathecal treatment.

AQUEDUCT STENOSIS

Obstruction of the aqueduct of Sylvius may occur as a hereditary, congenital, post-infectious, or postinflammatory condition. Congenital cases are associated with stricture or forking of the aqueduct, or with formation of a membrane that occludes part or all of the lumen. A partial stricture may not become symptomatic until adulthood. The obstruction to CSF circulation results in hydrocephalus with dilatation of the third and lateral ventricles. Neurologic manifestations are due to increased intracranial pressure and include vomiting, headaches, papilledema, ataxia, spasticity and extensor plantar responses. Enlargement of the head can occur in childhood, leaving signs of increased intracranial pressure which may be evident on skull roentgenograms in the adult.

Few studies have been done to characterize endocrine function in these patients. In early reports it was suggested that panhypopituitarism might occur, and enlargement of the sella turcica has been described. In a recent report of three cases of congenital stenosis of the aqueduct, Fiedler and Krieger[27] conducted detailed endocrine assessments and reviewed the endocrine status of five other cases from the literature. The clinical presentations varied in these cases and endocrine disturbances were mild; hypogonadism and abnormalities in dynamic GH and ACTH secretion were the commonest disorders. Improvement in endocrine status was observed in some cases after surgical placement of a shunt.

VASCULAR LESIONS OF THE HYPOTHALAMIC-PITUITARY REGION

Aneurysms

Aneurysms are uncommon causes of pituitary destruction. Cushing was the first to point out that an aneurysm can simulate an adenoma, although he never encountered such a lesion; but the first case was reported much earlier, by Silas Weir Mitchell in 1888.[20]

In a dramatic account, White[99] records the difficulty in distinguishing between an expanding intrasellar aneurysm and a hypophysial tumor by roentgenographic means. He illustrated his paper with a series of roentgenograms reproduced in a standard textbook to show progressive sellar destruction by a pituitary adenoma. "Unfortunately, the lesions turned out to be an aneurysm and the error in diagnosis caused this patient her life." In this case, a large aneurysm arising from the infraclinoid portion of the right internal carotid artery had compressed the optic nerves, eroded into the pituitary fossa, and destroyed the pituitary by pressure. In White's review of the literature, and collection of unpublished cases, he was able to discuss 36 examples in which "the differential diagnosis between hypophysial tumor and intrasellar aneurysm without routine angiography would have been difficult or impossible." Less than 1.9 per cent of all intracranial aneurysms manifest this abnormality. The average age was 46.5 years, the oldest 67, and the youngest 16. An aneurysm presenting as diabetes insipidus was seen in a 6-month-old boy by Shucart and Wolpert.[86] There seems to be no sex difference in aneurysm distribution. Most aneurysms arise from the internal carotid, and in this group the infraclinoid portion is the most frequent site of origin. Rarely the anterior cerebral, or posterior communicating or basilar arteries are the site of the lesion. Progressive loss of anterior pituitary function and optic nerve compression are the most common manifestations. Cranial nerve compression giving rise to ocular palsies has occurred in less than 15 per cent of the cases. Headaches occur, but not in all cases. Due to the fact that the aneurysm may become thrombosed, even bilateral arteriography may not reveal the presence of abnormality in every case.

Hypothalamic Damage Following Rupture of a Berry Aneurysm

Following the rupture of an anterior communicating aneurysm, insufficiency of pituitary-adrenal function[23] or the syndrome of inappropriate secretion of ADH[41] may appear. In an extensive study of the hypothalamus, Crompton[20] observed three types of hypothalamic lesions in 61 per cent of cases. Anterior and posterior communicating aneurysms were most frequently the cause. The lesions were those of ischemia, varying from minute foci of necrosis to large areas (5 mm. in diameter or more). Small or large hemorrhagic lesions were also observed. Massive hemorrhages occurred in the path of rupture of an aneurysm into the lateral ventricles. "Microhemorrhages usually consisted of subarachnoid blood that was forced up the perivascular sheathes of the perforating arteries, greatly distending the sheathes and then rupturing out into the cerebral parenchyma through the wall of the sheath to form ball hemorrhages along the course of the vessel."[20] The microhemorrhages were often localized in the paraventricular and supraoptic nuclei, which were completely destroyed if the hemorrhage became confluent. Though not discussed by Crompton, it is important that these two nuclei are richly supplied with blood. Extensive endocrine testing has not been carried out in such patients,[61] but in one series, Jenkins and collaborators[38] showed a high frequency of impaired responses to metyrapone, and loss of the usual diurnal cortisol rhythm.

Pituitary Apoplexy

Acute hemorrhage into the pituitary gland was first reported in 1905 by Bleibtrau, and at the time of Rovit and Fein's 1972 review[67] approximately 180 cases had been reported in addition to their own personally observed series of nine cases. Hemorrhage almost always occurs in a previously abnormal gland, most commonly a functioning adenoma.[23, 52, 91] Precipitating causes include anticoagulant therapy, head trauma, radiation therapy, estrogen therapy, and upper respiratory infection. Spontaneous hemorrhage unrelated to any antecedent event occurs most frequently.

Rovit and Fein proposed the following course of events in the pathogenesis of this disorder.

An epithelial tumor, probably a chromophobe adenoma, gradually enlarges, expanding the pituitary fossa and compressing the remnants of functioning contiguous pituitary tissue. As the tumor continues to enlarge, it gains additional room for expansion by stretching the diaphragma sella. Further expansion superiorly may be accomplished if the attenuated diaphragm splits or if the diaphragmatic notch itself is unusually voluminous. Otherwise the neoplasm must squeeze itself through a narrow channel between the firm fibrous peripheral limbs of the diaphragma sella and the hypophysial stalk centrally. It is precisely at this juncture where we believe the chain of events leading to pituitary apoplexy occurs. . . .

Virtually all the afferent blood supply destined for the pars distalis and the tumor itself is contained in a fine complex of vessels lying within and adjacent to the now compressed and distorted hypophysial stalk. Impairment of the infundibular circulation by impaction of tumor at the diaphragmatic notch may accordingly render virtually the entire anterior lobe ischemic, necrotic and hemorrhagic, as well as the tumor, and so produce the clinical and pathological concomitants of the condition known as pituitary apoplexy. The cavernous sinuses are acutely stretched, thus leading to compression of the oculomotor nerves and attenuation of the intracavernous internal carotid and inferior hypophysial arteries. . . . The hypophysial infarction may be so extensive as to disrupt the capsule of the tumor, allowing escape of necrotic tissue and red cells into the chiasmatic cisterns and thence into the general subarachnoid fluid circulation.[67]

Their pathologic account explains the common clinical presentation with sudden onset of severe headache in a patient with pre-existing (though not necessarily recognized) intrasellar tumor. In most patients the headache is initially bifrontal, but when blood escapes into the subarachnoid space, occipital pain and stiff neck occur. Any degree of impairment of mental functioning can occur, including profound stupor and death. Ophthalmoplegia, a common finding, can be either bilateral or unilateral. Papilledema is usually not present. Eyelid edema may result from cavernous sinus compression. Abnormalities in CSF can usually be detected, and resemble the findings in subarachnoid hemorrhage.

Most cases should be considered as neurosurgical emergencies warranting immediate intervention. However, Dawson and coworkers[23] have recently emphasized that a threat to vision is the only pressing indication for craniotomy. A number of cases have been managed by the use of high-dose corticoids alone. The relative benignity of transsphenoidal hypophysectomy, however, which is now being widely developed in many centers, makes it, together with high-dose corticoid therapy, probably the treatment of choice for most patients.

Ischemic Pituitary Necrosis

Ischemic necrosis of the pituitary is a relatively common cause of hypopituitarism. The most frequent pathologic event leading to this disorder is severe hemorrhage in a pregnant woman at the time of delivery.[100] Other less frequent causes are diabetes (in both men and women), and shock due to nonobstetric causes such as trauma, hemorrhage, infection, anesthesia, transfusion reactions, burns, poisoning, anoxia, low atmospheric pressure, heat stroke, and anaphylaxis.[2, 24, 36, 56, 88] Pituitary necrosis, presumably ischemic in origin, has been observed also in patients with increased intracranial pressure,[101] head injury, and sickle cell anemia. Pituitary necrosis is a frequent finding in epidemic hemorrhagic fever, in which cases it probably is due to direct capillary damage by a virus.

Postpartum Pituitary Necrosis

In his complete review of ischemic necrosis, Kovacs[46, 47] noted that the first reported case of postpartum pituitary necrosis was by a Polish pathologist, Glinski, who in 1913 published the case of a 37-year-old woman who suffered severe uterine bleeding due to uterine atony in the course of her delivery. She died nine days later as a result of puerperal sepsis, and at autopsy was found to have extensive necrosis of the pituitary. Glinski postulated that the pituitary infarction was due to thrombosis of the pituitary vascular supply, leading to pituitary insufficiency, which in turn led to uterine atony, hemorrhage, and collapse. Soon thereafter, in 1914, Simmonds[87] reported his classic case of a 46-year-old woman who had suffered from severe puerperal sepsis at the age of 36 and had not menstruated since. Her chief symptoms were weakness and emaciation, and she died in coma. At autopsy, the pituitary gland was found to be shrunken and replaced by a fibrous scar. Simmonds postulated that pituitary destruction had occurred because minute bacterial emboli had lodged in the sinusoids of the pituitary gland.

Modern views of the pathogenesis of postpartum pituitary necrosis date to Sheehan,[77-84] whose extensive writings on the subject have delineated the syndrome in detail, and after whom the disease has been named. He wrote:

> From a histological study of the lesions which develop in the vessels of the human pituitary gland during the first two days after the onset of postpartum necrosis of the anterior lobe, it is concluded that the primary vascular disturbance is a spasm involving the arteries which supply the anterior lobe and the stalk. This arrests the portal blood supply and also the direct arterial blood supply to the lobe, but permits a slight circulation to continue in the stalk. If the spasm is relieved within about an hour the parenchyma suffers only a transient functional damage. If it continues for several hours, all the tissues in the anterior lobe are killed and, when blood finally attempts to flow into the dead vessels, stasis and thrombosis occurs. This thrombosis is a secondary phenomenon and is not the cause of the necrosis. Variations in the extent and the duration of the spasm account for the variations in the size of the necrosis; in about half the cases the lesion involves 97 to 99% of the anterior lobe, but the pars tuberalis and a small amount of the pars interloralis always survive. The arterial spasm is certainly related to a severe general circulatory collapse at the time of delivery, but the reason for its very specific localization to the anterior lobe of the pituitary gland remains obscure.[70]

In his interpretation of the pathogenesis of the disorder, Sheehan was struck by the highly convoluted and muscular-walled vessels of the human primary portal plexus (named the gomitolus by Fumagalli), a structure more complex than the simple loops of most other animals. However, proof that the vessels go into spasm during shock has not been adduced. In the rat and the mouse, moreover, shock leads to dilatation of the portal vessels. In Sheehan's syndrome it is equally possible that decreased blood flow alone may be the principal vascular disturbance, rather than vasospasm.

Vascular insufficiency alone cannot account for the high frequency with which this condition follows pregnancy. The hyperplastic, highly vascular pituitary of the pregnant woman is especially sensitive to ischemic insult. It has been reported that the average sella size in such patients is smaller than normal. The crowding of tissue may contribute to its vulnerability to loss of blood flow. The bulk of new cells are lactotropes arising under stimulation of placental estrogens. It is most likely that Sheehan's syndrome arises when this highly vascular gland, with its high rate of metabolism, is suddenly deprived of blood flow due to shock. The role of local spasm and of circulating vasoconstrictor substances has not been fully evaluated. Rarely, postpartum necrosis may occur in the absence of any evidence of hemorrhage.

The observed frequency of Sheehan's syndrome is to some extent a function of the adequacy of obstetric care. In 1963, Sheehan estimated, on the basis of the occurrence in routine autopsies and on the mean survival (22 years) of his patients, that in Liverpool 55 patients per million had severe hypopituitarism, and a similar number moderate hypopituitarism.[80] The estimated maximum was between 240 and 350 live patients per million. Sheehan stated that if a woman dies in the puerperium, there is a 38 per cent chance that a massive or large pituitary necrosis will be found at autopsy. It is likely that many patients suffer from unrecognized mild pituitary failure following childbirth.

Pituitary Necrosis of Diabetes

Although the histologic findings and course in pituitary necrosis of diabetes resemble those of postpartum pituitary necrosis, there is no convincing explanation for the occurrence of this disorder in the diabetic. Stalk vessels occasionally appear to be sclerotic in diabetics, but in most cases the blood supply is not abnormal. The high prevalence of diabetes in men, moreover, excludes the role of estrogen-stimulated lactotrope hyperplasia as a factor. Infarctions have also been reported in young diabetics under the age of 20.

Clinical Manifestations

Ischemic necrosis causes no local symptoms or signs; rather, the manifestations are due to partial or complete loss of anterior pituitary secretions. Rarely, the onset of hypopituitarism may be abrupt, leading to severe ACTH-adrenal insufficiency, and thus complicating the clinical management of shock. Usually, hypopituitarism appears more gradually. Commonly, milk is not produced, due to prolactin deficiency; normal menses are never resumed, due to gonadotropin deficiency; weakness, loss of body hair, and loss of libido ensue, due to ACTH insufficiency; and varying degrees of hypothyroidism may be noted. Because so many women are given estrogens at the time of delivery to prevent lactation, and birth control pills to prevent subsequent pregnancy, the usual hallmarks of Sheehan's syndrome may be missed for months or years. Hypopituitarism may develop after a few apparently normal periods. Although it is usual for amenorrhea to occur in such cases, there have been reports of patients with normal periods in whom deficiencies of the other pituitary hormones occurred. Pregnancies occur in a few such patients, some only after thyroxine replacement therapy.

In the diabetic, the occurrence of ischemic infarction is announced by the sudden amelioration of the severity of the carbohydrate disturbance, including a marked decrease in insulin requirement. In fact, a sudden decrease in insulin requirement in a diabetic suggests pituitary infarction. This occurrence is the clinical analogue of the "Houssay phenomenon" in the dog: the amelioration of postpancreatectomy diabetes following hypophysectomy. Infarction may beneficially affect the course of the disease. In the classic case of Poulson,[63] pituitary infarction led to a reversal of the changes of diabetic retinopathy. This observation, in fact, was one of the important findings that led to the widespread use of hypophysectomy and stalk section in man for the management of vascular disease in diabetes.

RADIATION-INDUCED HYPOTHALAMIC-PITUITARY DYSFUNCTION

Although the normal pituitary resists radiation damage, a number of patients have developed pituitary insufficiency after radiation of the head for various malignant conditions, including carcinoma of the nasopharynx, carcinoma of the maxillary sinus, intracranial medulloblastoma, glioma, ependymomas, and angiomas.[20, 21, 26, 30] The dose of radiation responsible for this effect is variable.

The most frequent manifestation of pituitary insufficiency is growth failure following radiation in children.[37, 75] Growth hormone secretory reserve is diminished in these cases — 11 of 16, for example, in the series of Shalet and coworkers,[75] studied a year or more after treatment. The importance of GH deficiency in growth failure was demonstrated by showing adequate growth after replacement therapy. Secondary amenorrhea due to gonadotropin failure has also been reported. Growth disturbance occurs so frequently that it should be evaluated routinely in all children receiving roentgenotherapy to the head. In adults, deficiency of all anterior pituitary functions has been demonstrated after head radiation. In several cases studied more recently, the use of the thyrotropic-hormone-releasing-hormone test has shown that pituitary responses are normal; from this it has been inferred that the disorder is caused by a radiation-induced hypothalamic lesion.[48]

The hypothalamus, in common with all other neural tissues, is relatively sensitive to the damaging effects of ionizing radiation, and, as shown by Arnold and collaborators[1] in the monkey, is more sensitive than is the pituitary.[14] Gross necrosis of the hypothalamus and other parts of the brain in man has been produced by repeated courses of radiation to resistant acromegalics (doses recorded by Peck and McGovern[59] were 9,775, 8,150, and 10,126 r). The late clinical manifestations of postradiation necrosis can include the appearance of localizing neurologic signs, papilledema, and dementia. Sarcoma and malignant change in the brain also has been reported following ionizing radiation.[32, 33] Fortunately, the routine use of prophylactic cerebral radiation of children being treated for acute leukemia has not been followed by demonstrable impairment of intelligence. In a study of 34 children by Soni and collaborators[90] treated prospectively with 2,400 rads from ^{60}Co, there was no disturbance in neurologic or psychologic function 18 months later. Eleven other patients studied four years after radiation also were indistinguishable from a control group.

Several authors have given estimates of the maximum dose that can be tolerated by brain tissue. Boden[14] estimated that the largest dose the brain stem can tolerate is 4,500 r in 17 days (250 KV) for small- and medium-sized fields, and 3,500 r in 17 days for large fields over 100 cm³. Arnold and collaborators[1] suggest a dose not to exceed 4,500 r in 30 days for centrally-located tumors. According to Peck and McGovern, "the degree of radionecrosis is proportional to the total size of the dose and time factors in its administration."[59] It becomes more pronounced as the time interval from radiation is lengthened. Lindgren[49] calculated time-dose relationship curves for human brains on the basis of 13 cases adequately described in the literature, plus four of his own drawn from previously-radiated autopsied gliomas. He stated that the minimal dose which produced necrosis on delivery of the rays through medium-sized fields was between 4,500 and 5,000 r in 30 days. Peck and McGovern recommend "a mid-plane tissue dose of 4,000 r through stationary fields in 28 days using 4 × 4 cm. portals at the surface. . . . There is little excuse for repeated courses of therapy."

Peck and collaborators note that "the relative radiosensitivity of the brain varies from one region to another. The cortex and immediate subcortical medullary region are less sensitive than the deep-seated white matter. The sensitivity of the latter also appears to vary from region to region. . . ."[59]

There are two phases to the radiation injury. Initially, there is an acute inflammatory vasculitis, meningitis and choroid plexitis, with leukocytic infiltration.[6, 73] The nuclei of the granular cells of the cerebellum show contraction and pyknosis. These early changes are established within 2 hours of irradiation, increased over 8 to 24 hours, and regress by 4 days. The delayed response, weeks and months later, includes damage to glia, astrocytosis, vascular endothelial proliferation, hyalinization of basement membranes, and necrosis.[34, 93] The neuron damage may be due in part to the ischemic change.

There is no known treatment for radiation-induced brain damage. Only preventive measures can be used, i.e., restricting doses to maximum recommended levels of 4,000 r to central brain structures. Radiation-induced hypothalamic injury should be considered in the differential diagnosis of hypothalamus-pituitary insufficiency in patients who have received head or upper-neck radiation.

HISTIOCYTOSIS X

Histiocytosis X is a granulomatous disease of unknown etiology and highly variable course, characterized by solitary or multiple lesions that can involve virtually any tissue in the body and, although most common in early childhood, can occur at any age.[4, 5, 94] It is important to the clinical neuroendocrinologist in causing lesions of the hypothalamus. The term histiocytosis X includes several clinical varieties of disease, now believed by most pathologists to be different manifestations of a single underlying pathogenetic defect. The most common variety is termed *Hand-Schüller-Christian dis-*

ease, so named because of classic descriptions of cases, the first reported by Hand in 1893. This patient had the so-called classic triad: polyuria, exophthalmos, and skull defects. Much less common is the type termed *Letterer-Siwe disease,* seen in infants in a rapidly progressive form with widespread parenchymal involvement. The term *eosinophilic granuloma* was originally applied to solitary bone lesions. Since the identical cytologic finding can be demonstrated in each of the forms of histiocytosis X, this term has come into common use.

Diabetes insipidus is the most frequent endocrine manifestation of histiocytosis and occurs in somewhat less than half of the cases of the chronic disseminated type (Hand-Schüller-Christian disease).[45, 58] It is often seen in partial form, and can present as the earliest sign of the disease in the absence of any other manifestation. Other endocrine abnormalities, of much less frequency, are impaired growth,[15] hypogonadism, and partial and complete hypopituitarism.[25, 89] The growth failure can be due in part to uncontrolled diabetes insipidus or to GH deficiency. Other, less common, neurologic findings include those due to mass lesions in the basal third ventricle and hypothalamus, indistinguishable from those due to any type of localized hypothalamic disease. The lesion in the basal hypothalamus usually consists of a localized granulomatous lesion, poorly or well circumscribed in nodular form, of histiocytic character with eosinophile elements.[4, 5, 9] The usual cause of diabetes insipidus is nodule involvement of the tuber cinereum and hypothalamus. The nodules may involve the dura also, and distort the adjacent pituitary. Localized tumor-like infiltrations have been observed also in the hypothalamus.[45] It is uncommon for the tumor to replace the pituitary; evidently hypopituitarism in these cases is generally caused by damage to the hypothalamus or stalk.

Diagnosis and Course

The diagnosis of histiocytosis X should be the first consideration in differential diagnosis of diabetes insipidus in infants or young children. In fully established cases, 90 per cent will show skeletal lesions in some part of the body, especially in membranous bone of the skull. Lesions of the hypothalamus rarely give rise to roentgenographic changes in the sella, and cases have been observed showing sellar lesions without hypopituitarism. Exophthalmos, usually unilateral, rarely bilateral, and much less common, is caused by retrobulbar infiltration of granulomatous tissue. Early in the illness, and sometimes even after the illness is well established, diabetes insipidus may be the only neuroendocrine abnormality present, and even pneumoencephalography may fail to demonstrate a mass lesion. Such presentations are difficult to diagnose; the first clue to the nature of the illness may come from biopsy of the intracranial lesion.

The course of histiocytosis X is highly variable. Patients with single skeletal lesions (common in the jaw or mastoid) may be managed with local treatment such as roentgenotherapy or curettage, and have no further manifestations. Others may follow a smoldering course, with new lesions occurring from time to time over many years, and a few who present with parenchymal infiltration may show a rapid and explosive course. Most cases fit the second category, and the prognosis for the disease as a whole is generally good, with a mortality rate of less than 15 per cent for all cases.

Treatment

The variable and indolent nature of the disease has made it difficult to evaluate therapy.[22] There is no evidence that therapy directed at the CNS can reverse damage already inflicted, but it may arrest further progress of disease. In contrast, skeletal lesions can heal completely. Among the modalities that have been used are local excision and curettage of accessible lesions, and roentgenotherapy for well-circumscribed or inaccessible lesions. High-dosage steroid (prednisone) therapy has been useful in treating the systemic manifestations, such as pulmonary involvement, which can be immediately life-threatening. Some patients have been reported to go into remission for 12 to 30 months after this treatment, and others require continued low-dose treatment for active peripheral manifestations such as infiltration of lung and skin.

The most significant advance in the treatment of disseminated histiocytosis has been the introduction of chemotherapy. Vogel and Vogel[94] summarize the results of therapy with alkylating agents, such as nitrogen mustard, cyclophosphamide, and methotrexate, to show an 80 to 90 per cent remission rate. Leukoblastine has been used most frequently, with a remission rate of approximately 80 per cent.

Whether one gives a single course of therapy or an initial course followed by low-dose maintenance therapy, depends upon one's concept of therapy. Experts in cancer chemotherapy tend to try for a cure, by giving high doses and repeated courses in order to decrease tumor cell mass and to destroy resistant cells. Since the nature of histiocytosis X (neoplasm versus infection) has not been established, no dogmatic position can be followed on this question. It is obvious that a proper approach to patients with histiocytosis requires collaboration with experienced chemotherapists and roentgenotherapists.

SARCOIDOSIS OF THE HYPOTHALAMIC-PITUITARY UNIT

Sarcoidosis is a granulomatous illness of unknown etiology that can involve any part of the body. First described by Boeck in 1899 as a skin lesion, the systemic form of the disease was recognized by Schaumann in 1914, and diabetes insipidus due to sarcoid was first described by Tilligren in 1935.[92] The course can be relatively benign and self-limiting, or progressive. Evidence of systemic infection is often completely absent. CNS involvement is relatively uncommon, but by 1948, Colover[19] could report 118 cases, including three of his own. The brain can be involved very early in the course of the illness, so that the common systemic manifestations are inapparent, or can appear late.[3] The pituitary gland is particularly liable to damage by sarcoidosis, as evidenced by the finding that 35 per cent of the reported cases with neurologic findings presented symptoms of diabetes insipidus at some time during the course of their illness.[12, 60, 64] The special vulnerability of the stalk probably reflects its superficial location in relation to a basilar meningitis: an infiltrative basilar meningitis extends upward into the hypothalamus along the perivascular cuffs.[31, 62, 74] Infiltrative nodules may also appear in the hypothalamus and pituitary. All degrees of pituitary insufficiency have been reported, ranging from total panhypopituitarism to partial syndromes.[74, 76, 92] Other evidence of hypothalamic involvement, such as somnolence and hyperphagia, has also been reported.[3] Optic atrophy and bitemporal or homonymous hemianopia may result from local pressure on the visual system. Extension of granulomatous tissue along the base of the brain is common and results in unilateral or bilateral cranial nerve palsies.

Patients with cerebral sarcoidosis usually have abnormal CSF findings: protein concentration is slightly or markedly elevated, a modest pleocytosis is present, and in many patients low CSF sugar is reported. One case studied by Pennell[64] had values as low as 10 mg./100 ml. Thus, the appearance of tuberculosis is mimicked. It is obvious that sarcoidosis should be considered in the differential diagnosis of any patient with localized hypothalamic or pituitary disorder, particularly in young adult Blacks, in whom the disease is most common in North America. The only known treatment of sarcoidosis is the use of corticosteroids in anti-inflammatory doses. One patient has been reported to have had a prolonged remission of diabetes insipidus after such treatment, and remained in remission despite the progress of other systemic manifestations of the disease.

EMPTY-SELLA SYNDROME

The term empty-sella syndrome refers to enlargement of the sella turcica secondary to extension of the subarachnoid space through a partially defective diaphragma sellae.[42, 43] Although the pituitary gland becomes compressed to the rim of the fossa, hypothalamic-pituitary connections are usually preserved and endocrine disturbances, if any, are minimal.[8] Radiologically, the enlarged pituitary fossa cannot be readily distinguished from that due to an expanding intrasellar tumor.[98]

Etiology

The term empty-sella was first applied to this condition by Busch in 1951.[16] Early descriptions emphasized the development of the disorder after operative or x-ray ablation of pituitary tumors. More recently, it has been shown that the condition frequently occurs spontaneously in patients with no history of pituitary disease.[42] The abnormality is commonly first noted on routine skull roentgenograms taken in patients who present with headaches. Such cases are referred to as the *primary* empty-sellae syndrome.

Several theories have been proposed with respect to the etiology of primary empty-sella syndrome.[42, 43] Kaufman has emphasized that the condition develops because of a congenitally defective sella turcica. The condition is more common in females, particularly in the obese, and may occur with associated conditions such as benign intracranial hypertension,[97] pickwickian syndrome,[98] extrasellar tumor, hydrocephalus, and congestive heart failure. However, the majority of cases occur in the absence of these conditions and without evidence of increased intracranial pressure.

Careful autopsy studies, as reported by Busch,[16] have indicated that the diaphragma sellae was partially incomplete in 58 per cent of cases. Of these, only 5.5 per cent were associated with remodelling of the pituitary fossa. As this indicates, the condition is not uncommon, and several cases are seen each year on any major endocrine service.

Clinical Manifestations

Neurologic

In the series of 31 cases reported by Neelon and coworkers,[57] 87 per cent were females and 93 per cent were obese. Headache was the presenting symptom in 71 per cent, and 29 per cent had hypertension. The ages of onset centered in the fifth decade but ranged from the third to the eighth. Nontraumatic CSF rhinorrhea or visual-field disturbances occur rarely. The occurrence of visual-field disturbance is attributed to herniation of the optic chiasm into the sella turcica, with vascular or compressive neuropathy.

Four patients in this series had papilledema due to benign intracranial hypertension. The sella turcica was enlarged by measurement in 26 of the 31 patients but the configuration remained normal in 15. The result was a "symmetrically ballooned sella."

Endocrine

In the patients reported by Neelon and coworkers,[57] the endocrine status was normal in 63 per cent of cases, panhypopituitarism existed in four cases, and acromegaly was diagnosed in four cases. Testing of pituitary-hormone reserve indicated partial hypopituitarism in 11 patients, the most common abnormality being a decreased response of plasma GH to insulin-induced hypoglycemia. Reduced levels of LH were present in five cases but FSH was normal. Diabetes insipidus and disturbance of other hypothalamic functions were extremely rare. Secondary amenorrhea and hyperprolactinemia with galactorrhea have been reported in primary empty-sellae syndrome.[7, 85]

Management

The primary diagnostic problem with empty sella is to distinguish it from an enlarging intrasellar pituitary tumor. This differentiation can be definitively made only with pneumoencephalography (See Chapter 13). Normal pituitary tissue lining the rim of the sella is often visible, but there is no correlation between this observation and the likelihood of pituitary insufficiency. In some cases, the CAT scan can outline the fluid-filled fossa, but this is not usually sufficiently reliable to take the place of pneumoencephalography (PEG). The use of the CAT scan for evaluation of empty sella is currently under investigation.

The rare association of the condition with other causes of increased intracranial pressure should lead to the search for the possibility of benign intracranial hypertension,[97] abnormalities of cardiac or pulmonary function[98] and, rarely, of extrasellar brain tumor. These associations are fortunately uncommon.

A difficult clinical problem is the question of whether headaches are caused by the empty sella. A few case reports have appeared in which surgical repair by muscle grafting of the defective diaphragma sellae has resulted in remission of headache. However, no clear presenting feature of the headache permits separation from the much more common tension or muscle-spasm headache, and it is often very difficult to decide, in a given case, whether the headache is in fact related to the presence of the empty sella.

Occasionally, surgery is required in empty sella (whether primary or secondary) because of visual-field disturbances. In a recent case seen at the Montreal Neurological Hospital, the presence of optic atrophy and visual-field abnormality were shown at surgery to be associated with entrapment of the optic chiasm into the superior portion of the sella turcica by arachnoid-tissue adhesions. The excision of these tissues was followed by complete recovery of visual function.

BENIGN INTRACRANIAL HYPERTENSION

The syndrome of benign intracranial hypertension (pseudotumor cerebri) presents clinically as a combination of headache, papilledema, and raised intracranial pressure in the absence of a space-occupying lesion of the brain or of obstructive hydrocephalus.[13, 39, 40] The CSF pressure is invariably increased but its protein and sugar concentrations are normal, and diagnostic studies including EEG, brain scan, and cerebral angiography are normal. Pneumoencephalography usually shows normal or small cerebral ventricles; in a small number of cases, the ventricles are slightly enlarged. If these criteria are strictly applied, over 95 per cent of cases are self-limiting and follow-up fails to reveal underlying disturbance.

Etiology

A small percentage of cases have been shown to occur in relation to dural venous sinus occlusion, toxic agents, antibiotics, and excessive vitamin A therapy, and a causative relationship with these factors is suggested (Table 2). In the large series reported by Weisberg[95, 96] and by Johnston and Paterson,[39, 40] the majority of cases were idiopathic and occurred most frequently in obese females in the third or fourth decade of life. An association with minor menstrual irregularities, contraceptive medication, or pregnancy has been noted by several investigators but the frequency of these conditions in the general population makes definite correlation impossible.[66] Steroid therapy

Table 2. Differential Diagnosis of Syndrome of Benign Intracranial Hypertension (Papilledema, Headache, and Increased Intracranial Pressure)

I. Endocrine	IV. Circulatory diseases
Steroid administration and withdrawal	Congestive heart failure
Contraceptive medication	Chronic pulmonary hypoventilation
Addison's disease	Mediastinal obstruction
Obesity	Hypertensive encephalopathy
Pregnancy	V. Vascular or infectious diseases
II. Metabolic diseases	Disseminated lupus erythematosus
Uremia	Bacterial endocarditis
Hypocalcemia-hypoparathyroidism	Lateral-sinus thrombosis
Diabetic ketoacidosis	Meningitis or encephalitis
Eclampsia	VI. Hematologic diseases
III. Toxic agents	Iron deficiency anemia
Heavy metal poisoning	Infectious mononucleosis
Hypervitaminosis A	Idiopathic thrombocytopenia purpura
Tetracycline	Polycythemia
Nalidixic acid	VII. Hydrocephalus

with subsequent withdrawal of adrenal corticoids has been one of the more common events believed to play a role in the development of the condition.[13, 17]

The intracranial hypertension is due to an increase in cerebral tissue-fluid content (cerebral edema). Brain edema, as defined by Fishman,[29] is due to an increase in brain water content. Generally speaking, this state may occur secondary to vascular damage (vasogenic edema), to cell injury (cytotoxic edema) or secondary to disruption of normal CSF circulation and reabsorption (interstitial edema). Biopsies of the cerebral cortex in patients with benign intracranial hypertension, as reported by Sahs and Joynt,[72] showed both intracellular and extracellular edema. Mathew and coworkers,[54] using isotope studies have shown that patients with the syndrome have an increase in cerebral blood volume and a decrease in cerebral blood flow. They postulated that such alterations in cerebral blood dynamics could be accounted for by a compensatory dilation of cerebral veins in the face of elevated intracranial pressure. However, their studies showed that reduction of intracranial pressure by removal of CSF through lumbar puncture did not significantly alter the cerebral blood volume. They interpreted these data to indicate that a primary disorder of cerebral vascular regulation occurs in benign intracranial hypertension. Other workers have postulated that the predominant pathophysiologic mechanism is a defect in CSF transfer to veins through the arachnoid villi, leading to interstitial edema.[39, 40] A comparable disturbance can be produced by occlusion of the large cerebral veins and this is a common cause of the syndrome in places where middle ear disease and lateral sinus occlusion occur (otitic hydrocephalus). Such an etiology, however, is rare in North America. In view of the variety of factors associated with the syndrome, probably no single abnormality can account for all instances of the disorder. In the case of adrenal corticoid deficiency or steroid withdrawal, it is likely that the syndrome results from effects of corticoids on the permeability of cerebral capillaries. The relative steroid deficiency may result in alteration of transport of fluid across the blood-brain barrier, resulting in increased brain water.

The frequent occurrence of benign intracranial hypertension in women, and its occurrence after contraceptive use and during pregnancy has resulted in the listing of "endocrinopathy" as an etiologic factor. Estrogens are known to cause relaxation of vascular smooth muscle and to decrease the elasticity within blood vessels, factors that are thought to contribute to venous stasis and phlebothrombosis in the leg veins. There are, however, no data to confirm or deny a specific effect of estrogens on brain vessels.

Treatment

Treatments for benign intracranial hypertension are difficult to assess because the disorder ordinarily is self-limiting. Some clinicians have advocated the use of adrenal steroids, but carefully controlled trials have not been carried out.

The administration of glycerol by mouth, 1.5 g./kg. three times daily, is an effective treatment in some cases and may be safer than adrenal steroids. Acute symptoms are often relieved by removal of CSF (25 to 40 ml.), and some clinicians use this procedure for treatment. In severe cases, temporal decompression may be required, but fortunately this is rarely necessary. Relapse after recovery occurs in less than 10 per cent of cases.

REFERENCES

1. ARNOLD, A., BAILEY, P. AND HARVEY, R. A.: *Intolerance of the primate brainstem and hypothalamus to conventional and high energy radiations.* Neurology (Minneap.) 4:575, 1954.

2. ARRAS, M. J., JR. AND SAUNDERS, A. M.: *Renal cortical necrosis with pituitary infarction in a nonpregnant woman.* Arch. Pathol. 85:262, 1968.

3. ASZKANAZY, C. L.: *Sarcoidosis of the central nervous system.* J. Neuropath. Exp. Neurol. 11:392, 1952.

4. AVERY, M. E., McAFEE, J. G. AND GUILD, H. G.: *The course and prognosis of reticuloendotheliosis (eosinophilic granuloma, Schüller-Christian Disease and Letterer-Siwe Disease).* Am. J. Med. 22:636, 1957.

5. AVIOLI, L. V., LASERSOHN, J. T. AND LOPRESTI, J. M.: *Histiocytosis X (Schüller-Christian disease): A clinicopathological survey, review of ten patients and the results of prednisone therapy.* Medicine (Baltimore) 42:119, 1963.

6. BAILEY, O. T.: *Basic problems in the histopathology of radiation of the central nervous system. In:* Haley, T. J. and Snider, R. S. (eds.): *Response of the Nervous System to Ionizing Radiation.* Academic Press, New York, 1962, p. 783.

7. BAR, R. S., MASSAFERRI, E. L. AND MALARKEY, W. B.: *Primary empty sella, galactorrhea, hyperprolactinemia, and renal tubular acidosis.* Am. J. Med. 59:863, 1975.

8. BERKE, J. P., BUXTON, L. F. AND KOKMEN, E.: *The 'empty' sella.* Neurology 25:1137, 1975.

9. BERNARD, J. D. AND AGUILAR, M. J.: *Localized hypothalamic histiocytosis X.* Arch. Neurol. 20:368, 1969.

10. BERRY, R. G. AND SCHLEZINGER, N. S.: *Rathke-cleft cysts.* Arch. Neurol. 1:648, 1959.

11. BLACKWOOD, W., ET AL.: *Neuropathology.* Williams & Wilkins, Baltimore, 1973.

12. BLEISCH, U. R. AND ROBBINS, S. S.: *Sarcoid-like granuloma of the pituitary gland.* Arch. Int. Med. 89:877, 1952.

13. BODDIE, H. G., BANNA, M. AND BRADLEY, W. G.: *"Benign" intracranial hypertension. A survey of the clinical and radiological features, and long-term prognosis.* Brain 97:313, 1974.

14. BODEN, G.: *Radiation myelitis of the brain-stem.* J. Fac. Radiol. 2:79, 1950.

15. BRAUNSTEIN, G. D. AND KOHLER, P. O.: *Pituitary function in Hand-Schüller-Christian Disease. Evidence for deficient growth-hormone release in patients with short stature.* N. Engl. J. Med. 286:1225, 1972.

16. BUSCH, W.: *Die Morphologie der Sella Turcica und ihre beziehungen zur Hypophyse.* Arch. f. Path. Anat. 320:437, 1951.

17. CARLOW, T. J. AND GLASER, J. S.: *Pseudotumor cerebri syndrome in systemic lupus erythematosus.* J.A.M.A. 228:197, 1974.

18. CIRIC, I. AND ZIVIN, I.: *Neuroepithelia (colloid) cysts of the septum pellucidum.* J. Neurosurg. 43:69, 1975.

19. COLOVER, J.: *Sarcoidosis with involvement of the nervous system.* Brain 71:451, 1948.

20. CROMPTON, M. R.: *Hypothalamic lesions following the rupture of cerebral berry aneurysms.* Brain 86:301, 1963.

21. CROMPTON, M. R. AND LAYTON, D. D.: *Delayed radionecrosis of the brain following therapeutic x-radiation of the pituitary* Brain 84:85, 1961.

391

22. DARGEON, H. W.: *Considerations in the treatment of reticuloendotheliosis. The Janeway Lecture, 1964.* Am. J. Roentgenol. 93:521, 1965.

23. DAWSON, B. H. AND KOTHANDARAM, P.: *Acute massive infarction of pituitary adenomas.* J. Neurosurg. 37:275, 1972.

24. DONIACH, I. AND WALKER, A. H. C.: *Combined anterior pituitary necrosis and bilateral cortical necrosis of kidneys following concealed accidental hemorrhage.* J. Obstet. Gynecol. Br. Emp. 53:140, 1946.

25. EZRIN, C., CHAIKOFF, R. AND HOFFMAN, H.: *Case Report: Panhypopituitarism caused by Hand-Schüller-Christian disease.* Can. Med. Assoc. J. 89:1290, 1963.

26. FADELL, E. J.: *Necrosis of brain and spinal cord following x-ray therapy.* J. Neurosurg. 11:353, 1954.

27. FIEDLER, R. AND KRIEGER, D. T.: *Endocrine disturbances in patients with congenital aqueductal stenosis.* Acta Endocrinol. 80:1, 1975.

28. FINN, J. E. AND MOUNT, L. A.: *Meningiomas of the tuberculum sellae and planum sphenoidale. A review of 83 cases.* Arch. Ophthalmol. 92:23, 1974.

29. FISHMAN, R. A.: *Brain edema.* N. Engl. J. Med. 293:706, 1975.

30. GHATAK, N. R. AND WHITE, B. E.: *Delayed radiation necrosis of the hypothalamus.* Arch. Neurol. 21:425, 1969.

31. GJERSOE, A. AND KJERULF-JENSEN, K.: *Hypothalamic lesion caused by Boeck's sarcoid.* J. Clin. Endocrinol. 10:1602, 1950.

32. GOLDBERG, M. B., SHELINE, G. E. AND MALAMUD, N.: *Malignant intracranial neoplasms following radiation therapy for acromegaly.* Radiology 80:465, 1963.

33. GREENHOUSE, A. H.: *Pituitary sarcoma: a possible consequence of radiation.* J.A.M.A. 190:269, 1964.

34. HAGER, H., HIRSCHBERGER, W. AND BRIET, A.: *Electron microscope observations on the x-radiated central nervous system of the Syrian hamster. In* Halèy, T. J. and Snider, R. S. (eds.): *Response of the Nervous System to Ionizing Radiation.* Academic Press, New York, 1962, p. 783.

35. HAMILTON, C. R., JR., SCULLY, R. E. AND KLIMAN, B.: *Hypogonadotropinism in Prader-Willi Syndrome.* Am. J. Med. 52:322, 1972.

36. HARLIN, R. S. AND GIVENS, J. R.: *Sheehan's syndrome associated with eclampsia and a small sella turcica.* South. Med. J. 61:900, 1968.

37. HARROP, J. S., ET AL.: *Pituitary function after treatment of intracranial tumors in children.* Letter to the Editor. Lancet 2:231, 1975.

38. JENKINS, J. S., ET AL.: *Hypothalamic pituitary-adrenal function after subarachnoid hemorrhage.* Br. Med. J. 2:707, 1969.

39. JOHNSTON, I. AND PATERSON, A.: *Benign intracranial hypertension. I. Diagnosis and prognosis.* Brain 97:289, 1974.

40. JOHNSTON, I. AND PATERSON, A.: *Benign intracranial hypertension. II. CSF pressure and circulation.* Brain 97:301, 1974.

41. JOYNT, R. J., AFIFI, A. AND HARBISON, J.: *Hyponatremia in subarachnoid hemorrhage.* Arch. Neurol. 13:633, 1965.

42. KAUFMAN, B.: *The "empty" sella turcica—a manifestation of the intrasellar subarachnoid space.* Radiology 90:931, 1968.

43. KAUFMAN, B., PEARSON, O. H. AND CHAMBERLIN, W. B.: *Radiographic features of intrasellar masses and progressive, asymmetrical nontumorous enlargements of the sella turcica, the "empty" sella. In* Kohler, P. O. and Ross, G. T. (eds.): *Diagnosis and Treatment of Pituitary Tumors.* Excerpta Medica, Amsterdam, p. 100.

44. KELLY, R.: *Colloid cysts of the third ventricle. Analysis of twenty-nine cases.* Brain 74:23, 1951.

45. KEPES, J. J. AND KEPES, M.: *Predominantly cerebral forms of histiocytosis-X. A reappraisal of "Gagel's hypothalamic granuloma", "Granuloma infiltrans of the hypothalamus" and "Ayala's disease" with a report of four cases.* Acta Neuropathol. (Berl.) 14:77, 1969.

46. KOVACS, K.: *Necrosis of anterior pituitary in humans. I.* Neuroendocrinology 4:170, 1969.

47. KOVACS, K.: *Necrosis of anterior pituitary in humans. II.* Neuroendocrinology 4:201, 1969.

48. LARKINS, R. G. AND MARTIN, F. I. R.: *Hypopituitarism after extracranial irradiation. Evidence for hypothalamic origin.* Br. Med. J. 1:152, 1973.

49. LINDGREN, M.: *On tolerance of brain tissue and sensitivity of brain tumors to irradiation.* Acta Radiol. [Suppl.] 170, 1958.

50. LISSER, H. AND CURTIS, L. E.: *Treatment of posttraumatic Simmonds' disease with methyl testosterone linguets.* J. Clin. Endocrinol. 5:363, 1945.

51. LITTLE, J. R. AND MACCARTY, C. S.: *Colloid cysts of the third ventricle.* J. Neurosurg. 39:230, 1974.

52. LOCKE, S. AND TYLER, H. R.: *Pituitary apoplexy.* Am. J. Med. 30:643, 1961.

53. LOVE, J. G. AND MARSHALL, T. M.: *Craniopharyngiomas (pituitary adamantinomas).* Surg. Gynecol. Obstet. 90:591, 1950.

54. MATHEW, N. T., MEYER, J. S. AND OTT, E. O.: *Increased cerebral blood volume in benign intracranial hypertension.* Neurology 25:646, 1975.

55. MATSON, D. D. AND CRIGLER, JR., J. F.: *Management of craniopharyngioma in childhood.* J. Neurosurg. 30:377, 1969.

56. MURDOCH, R.: *Sheehan's syndrome. Survey of 57 cases since 1950.* Lancet 1:1327, 1962.

57. NEELON, F. A., GROEE, J. A. AND LEBOVITZ, H. E.: *The primary empty sella: Clinical and radiographic characteristics and endocrine function.* Medicine 52:73, 1973.

58. OLIN, P.: *Growth hormone response to insulin induced hypoglycemia in a boy with diabetes insipidus and short stature before and after treatment with vasopressin.* Acta Paediatr. Scand. 59:343, 1970.

59. PECK, F. C. AND MCGOVERN, E. R.: *Radiation necrosis of the brain in acromegaly.* Neurosurgery 25:536, 1966.

60. PENNELL, W. H.: *Boeck's sarcoid with involvement of the central nervous system.* Arch. Neurol. Psych. 66:728, 1951.

61. PITTMAN, J. A., JR., ET AL.: *Hypothalamic hypothyroidism.* N. Engl. J. Med. 285:844, 1971.

62. PLAIR, C. M. AND PERRY, S.: *Hypothalamic-pituitary sarcoidosis.* Arch. Path. 24:527, 1962.

63. POULSEN, J. E.: *Diabetes and anterior pituitary insufficiency. Final course and postmortem study of a diabetic patient with Sheehan's syndrome.* Diabetes 15:73, 1966.

64. PURNELL, D. C., ET AL.: *Postpartum pituitary insufficiency (Sheehan's syndrome): Review of 18 cases.* Mayo Clin. Proc. 39:321, 1964.

65. RINGEL, S. P. AND BAILEY, O. T.: *Rathke's cleft cyst.* J. Neurol. Neurosurg. Psych. 35:693, 1972.

66. ROTHNER, A. D. AND BRUST, J. C. M.: *Pseudotumor cerebri. Report of a familial occurrence.* Arch. Neurol. 30:110, 1974.

67. ROVIT, L. AND FEIN, J. M.: *Pituitary apoplexy: A review and reappraisal.* J. Neurosurg. 37:280, 1972.

68. RUSH, J. L., ET AL.: *Intraventricular craniopharyngioma.* Neurology 25:1094, 1975.

69. RUSSEL, D. S. AND RUBINSTEIN, L. J.: *Pathology of Tumors of the Nervous System.* Williams & Wilkins, Baltimore, 1963.

70. RUSSO, R. H. AND KINDT, G. W.: *A neuroanatomical basis for the bobble-head doll syndrome.* J. Neurosurg. 41:720, 1974.

71. RUSSMAN, B. S., TUCKER, S. H. AND SCHUT, I..; *Slow tremor and macrocephaly: Expanded version of the bobble-head doll syndrome.* J. Pediatrics 87:63, 1975.

72. SAHS, A. L. AND JOYNT, R. J.: *Brain swelling of unknown cause.* Neurology (Minneap.) 6:791, 1956.

73. SCHOLZ, W., SCHLOTE, W. AND HIRSCHBERGER, W.: *Morphologic effects of repeated low dosage and single high dosage application of x-irradiation to the central nervous system. In* Haley, T. J. and Snider, R. S. (eds.): *Response of the Nervous System to Ionizing Radiation.* Academic Press, New York, 1962, p. 783.

74. SELENKNOW, H. A., ET AL.: *Hypopituitarism due to hypothalamic sarcoidosis.* Am. J. Med. Sci. 238:456, 1959.

75. SHALET, S. M., ET AL.: *Pituitary function after treatment of intracranial tumours in children.* Lancet 2:104, 1975.

76. SHEALY, C., N., ET AL.: *Hypothalamic-pituitary sarcoidosis.* Am. J. Med. 30:46, 1961.

77. SHEEHAN, H. L. AND MURDOCH, R.: *Postpartum necrosis of anterior pituitary; Production of subsequent pregnancy.* Lancet 1:818, 1939.

78. SHEEHAN, H. L.: *The frequency of postpartum hypopituitarism.* J. Obstet. Gynecol. Br. Commonw. 72:103, 1965.

79. SHEEHAN, H. L. AND SUMMERS, V. K.: *Syndrome of hypopituitarism.* Quart. J. Med. 18:319, 1949.

80. SHEEHAN, H. L. AND WHITEHEAD, R.: *The neurohypophysis in postpartum hypopituitarism.* J. Pathol. Bacteriol. 85:145, 1963.

81. SHEEHAN, H. L.: *The repair of postpartum necrosis of the anterior lobe of the pituitary gland.* Acta Endocrinol (Kbh) 48:40, 1965.

82. SHEEHAN, H. L.: *Neurohypophysis and hypothalamus. In* Bloodworth, J. M. B., Jr., (ed.): *Endocrine Pathology.* Williams & Wilkins, Baltimore, 1968, p. 12.

83. SHEEHAN, H. L. AND STANFIELD, J. P.: *The pathogenesis of postpartum necrosis of the anterior lobe of the pituitary gland.* Acta Endocrinol. (Kbh) 37:479, 1961.
84. SHEEHAN, H. L. AND MURDOCH, R.: *Postpartum necrosis of anterior pituitary; effect of subsequent pregnancy.* Lancet 2:132, 1938.
85. SHREEFTER, M. J. AND FRIEDLANDER, R. L.: *Primary empty sella syndrome and amenorrhea.* J. Obstet. Gynecol. 46:535, 1975.
86. SHUCART, W. A. AND WOLPERT, S. A.: *An aneurysm in infancy presenting with diabetes insipidus.* J. Neurosurg. 37:368, 1972.
87. SIMMONDS, M.: *Ueber Hypophysisschwund mit Todlichem ausgang.* Deut. Med. Wschr. 40:322, 1914.
88. SMITH, C. W., JR. AND HOWARD, R. P.: *Variations in endocrine gland function in postpartum pituitary necrosis.* J. Clin. Endocrinol. 19:1420, 1959.
89. SMOLIK, E. A., ET AL.: *Histiocytosis X in optic chiasm of an adult with hypopituitarism.* J. Neurosurg. 29:290, 196.
90. SONI, S. S., ET AL.: *Effects of central-nervous-system irradiation on neuropsychologic functioning of children with acute lymphocytic leukemia.* N. Engl. J. Med. 293:113, 1975.
91. TAYLOR, A. L., ET AL.: *Pituitary apoplexy in acromegaly.* J. Clin. Endocr. 28:1784, 1968.
92. TILLGREN, J.: *Diabetes insipidus as a symptom of Schaumann's disease.* Brit. J. Dermat. 47:223, 1935.
93. VOGEL, F. S.: *Effects of high dose gamma radiation on the brain and on individual neurones. In:* Haley, T. J. and Snider, R. S. (eds.): *Response of the Nervous System to Ionizing Radiation.* Academic Press, New York, 1962, p. 240.
94. VOGEL, J. M. AND VOGEL, P.: *Idiopathic histiocytosis: A discussion of eosinophilic granuloma, the Hand-Schüller-Christian syndrome and the Letterer-Siwe syndrome.* Seminars in Hemat. 9:349, 1972.
95. WEISBERG, L. A.: *Benign intracranial hypertension.* Medicine 54:197, 1975.
96. WEISBERG, L. A.: *The syndrome of increased intracranial pressure without localizing signs: A reappraisal.* Neurology 25:85, 1975.
97. WEISBERG, L. A., HOUSEPIAN, E. M. AND SAUR, D. P.: *Empty sella syndrome as complication of benign intracranial hypertension.* J. Neurosurg. 43:177, 1975.
98. WEISBERG, L. A.: *Asymptomatic enlargement of the sella turcica.* Arch. Neurol. 32:483, 1975.
99. WHITE, J. C.: *Aneurysms mistaken for hypophyseal tumors.* J. Clin. Neurosurg. 10:224, 1964.
100. WHITEHEAD, R.: *The hypothalamus in postpartum hypopituitarism.* J. Pathol. Bacteriol. 86:55, 1963.
101. WOLMAN, L.: *Pituitary necrosis in raised intracranial pressure.* J. Pathol. Bacteriol. 72:575, 1956.
102. ZELLWEGER, H. AND SCHNEIDER, H. J.: *Syndrome of hypotonia-hypomentia-hypogonadism-obesity (HHHO) or Prader-Willi Syndrome.* Am. J. Dis. Child. 115:588, 1968.

Index

Serotonin — *Continued*
  storage of, 53
  synthesis of, 52–53, 232
  thyrotropin-releasing hormone secretion and,
    220
Serum levels
  growth hormone, 326
  prolactin, 129–131
    in newborn, 139
  thyrotropin, 201
Sex steroids
  classes of, 95
  gonadotropic hormone regulation and, 103
  homosexuality and, 289
  mechanisms of action of, on brain, 288–289
  prolactin secretion and, 136
  transsexualism and, 289–290
Sexual function
  effects of gonadal steroids on, 283–288
  luteinizing hormone-releasing hormone and,
    289
SFO. See Subfornical organ.
Sheehan's syndrome
  diabetes insipidus and, 81
  TRH test and, 341–342
Short-loop feedback control
  of growth hormone secretion, 168–169
  of prolactin secretion, 135–136
Sleep
  diagnosis of hypothalamic-pituitary disease
    and, 306
  growth hormone secretion and, 153–154, 174
  pituitary-adrenal rhythms and, 183–184
  prolactin secretion and, 137–138
Sleep-producing peptides, 292–293
SME. *See* Stalk-median eminence.
Smell, evaluation of, in diagnosis of hypotha-
    lamic-pituitary disease, 313
Sodium metabolism, neuroendocrine regulation
    of, 77–79
Somatomedins, 148
  growth hormone secretion and, 168–169
Somatostatin, 159
  actions of, 305, 159–160
  clinical use of, 160–162
  identification of, 208
  in treatment of acromegaly, 358
  localization of, 162
  thyrotropin secretion and, 208
Somatotropes, 147
Somnolence, hypothalamic lesions and, 265–268
Spontaneous periodic hypothermia, 256–257
Stalk section
  effects of, 18
  thyrotropin secretion and, 208
Stalk-median eminence, 22
Steroid hormones, 95
  mechanism of action of, on brain, 288–289
  prolactin secretion and, 136
Stimulus
  electric
    of hippocampus, growth hormone secretion
      and, 164

  of hypothalamus, growth hormone secretion
    and, 156–157
  thyrotropin secretion and, 206–207
  suckling, 110
    lactation and, 138
    prolactin secretion and, 135
Stimulus-secretion-coupling mechanism of
    hormonal release, 8
Storage
  dopamine, 49
  norepinephrine, 49
  serotonin, 53
Stress
  adrenocorticotropic hormone secretion and,
    185
  antidiuretic hormone secretion and, 74
  growth hormone secretion and, 152–153
  pituitary-adrenal axis and, 185
  prolactin secretion and, 135–137
  thyrotropin secretion and, 211–212
Stress tests of pituitary adrenocorticotropic
    hormone reserve, 334
Subcommissural organ, 241
Subfornical organ, 242
Substance P, 292
α-Subunit of thyrotropin, 201
β-Subunit of thyrotropin, 201
Suckling stimulus, 110
  lactation and, 138
  prolactin secretion and, 135
Surgery
  adenomas and, 350–352
  prolactin-secreting tumors and, 363
Syndrome(s)
  adiposogenital, 270
  Albright, 121
  amenorrhea-galactorrhea, 112
    case report of, 367–369
    post-pill, 142
  Chiari-Frommel, 139–140
  Cushing's, 190–197, 279–280
  diencephalic, 264–265
  ectopic ACTH, 192
  ectopic humoral, 86
  empty-sella, 388–389
  Frölich's, 270
  Kallmann's, 115, 313
  Kleine-Levin, 268–269
  lateral hypothalamic, 264
  Laurence-Moon-Biedl, 270
  maternal deprivation, 170
  Nelson's, 196
  of inappropriate secretion of antidiuretic
    hormone, 85–88
  of primary hypothyroidism, thyrotropin
    hypersecretion, and pituitary
    enlargement, 223
  Parinaud's, pineal tumors and, 239
  periodic, of Wolff, 269
  Prader-Willi, 269–270
  premenstrual tension, 287
  psychosocial deprivation, 170
  Schwartz-Bartter, 85–88